Evaluation and Treatment of the Neurogenic Bladder

Evaluation and Treatment of the Neurogenic Bladder

Edited by

Jacques Corcos MD
Department of Urology
McGill University
Sir Mortimer B Davis-Jewish General Hospital
Montréal PQ
Canada

Erik Schick MD
Department of Urology
University of Montréal
Maisonneuve-Rosemont Hospital
Montréal PQ
Canada

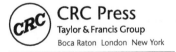

CRC Press
Taylor & Francis Group
Boca Raton London New York

CRC Press is an imprint of the
Taylor & Francis Group, an **informa** business

CRC Press
Taylor & Francis Group
6000 Broken Sound Parkway NW, Suite 300
Boca Raton, FL 33487-2742

First issued in paperback 2019

© 2005 by Taylor and Francis Group, LLC
CRC Press is an imprint of Taylor & Francis Group, an Informa business

No claim to original U.S. Government works

ISBN-13: 978-1-84184-557-9 (hbk)
ISBN-13: 978-0-367-39343-4 (pbk)

A CIP record for this book is available from the British Library.

Visit the Taylor & Francis Web site at
http://www.taylorandfrancis.com

and the CRC Press Web site at
http://www.crcpress.com

Contents

Contributors vii
Preface xi

Part I
Evaluation of neurogenic bladder dysfunction **1**

1. Clinical evaluation: history and physical examination 3
  Gary E Lemack

2. Quality of life assessment in neurogenic bladder 7
  Patrick Marquis

3. The voiding diary 15
  Martine Jolivet-Tremblay and Pierre E Bertrand

4. The pad test 29
  Martine Jolivet-Tremblay and Erik Schick

5. Endoscopic evaluation of neurogenic bladder 35
  Jacques Corcos and Erik Schick

6. Imaging techniques in the evaluation of neurogenic bladder dysfunction 43
  Walter Artibani and Maria A Cerruto

7. Normal urodynamic parameters in children 51
  Steven P Lapointe and Diego Barrieras

8. Evaluation of neurogenic bladder dysfunction: basic urodynamics 57
  Christopher E Kelly and Victor W Nitti

9. Urodynamics in infants and children 67
  Kelm Hjälmås and Ulla Sillén

10. Electrophysiological evaluation: basic principles and clinical applications 83
  Simon Podnar and Clare J Fowler

11. Practical guide to diagnosis and follow-up of patients with neurogenic bladder dysfunction 105
  Erik Schick and Jacques Corcos

Part II
Classification **109**

12. Classification of lower urinary tract dysfunction 111
  Anders Mattiasson

Part III
Treatment **123**

Non-surgical

13. Conservative treatment 125
  Jean-Jacques Wyndaele

14. Systemic and intrathecal pharmacological treatment 137
  Shing-Hwa Lu and Michael B Chancellor

15. Intravesical pharmacological treatment 149
  Carlos Silva and Francisco Cruz

16. Transdermal oxybutynin administration 161
  G Willy Davila

17. Management of autonomic dysreflexia 167
  Waleed Altaweel and Jacques Corcos

Electrical

18. Peripheral electrical stimulation 171
  Magnus Fall and Sivert Lindström

19. Emptying the neurogenic bladder by electrical stimulation 177
  Graham H Creasey

20. Central neuromodulation 189
  Philip EV Van Kerrebroeck

21. Intravesical electrical stimulation
     of the bladder   193
     Helmut G Madersbacher

Surgical

22. Surgery to improve reservoir function   199
     Manfred Stöhrer

23. Surgery to improve bladder outlet function 207
     Gina Defreitas and Philippe Zimmern

24. Urinary diversion   241
     Greg G Bailly and Sender Herschorn

Future developments

25. Tissue engineering applications for patients
     with neurogenic bladder   259
     Anthony Atala

26. Restoration of complete bladder function by
     neurostimulation   267
     Michael Craggs

27. Neuroprotection and repair after spinal
     cord injury   279
     W Dalton Dietrich

Part IV
Synthesis of treatment   **285**

28. Treatment alternatives for different
     types of neurogenic bladder dysfunction
     in adults   287
     Erik Schick and Jacques Corcos

29. Treatment alternatives for different
     types of neurogenic bladder dysfunction
     in children   297
     Roman Jednak and Joao Luiz Pippi Salle

30. The vesicourethral balance   309
     Erik Schick and Jacques Corcos

Part V
Complications   **315**

31. Complications related to neurogenic
     bladder dysfunction – I: infection, lithiasis
     and neoplasia   317
     Andrew Z Buczynski

32. Complications related to neurogenic
     bladder dysfunction – II: reflux and
     renal insufficiency   325
     Imre Romics, Antal Hamvas, and Attila Majoros

     Index   335

Contributors

Waleed Altaweel MD
Resident in Urology
Department of Urology
McGill University
Montreal
Quebec
Canada

Walter Artibani MD
Professor and Chairman
Department of Urology
University of Verona
Verona
Italy

Anthony Atala MD
Associate Professor of Surgery
Director, Center for Genitourinary Tissue Reconstruction
Children's Hospital and Harvard Medical School
Boston MA
USA

Greg G Bailly MD FRCSC
Fellow in Urodynamics and Reconstruction
Sunnybrook and Women's College Health
Sciences Centre
University of Toronto
Ontario
Canada

Diego Barrieras MD FRCSC
Assistant Professor of Urology
Division of Urology
Hôpital Sainte-Justiné-University of Montréal
Montreal, PQ
Canada

Pierre E Bertrand MD FRCSC
Assistant Professor of Urology
University of Montreal
Maisonneuve-Rosemont Hospital
Montreal
Quebec
Canada

Andrew Z Buczynski MD PhD
Urologist and Orthopedic Surgeon
Head, Department of Neurourology
Metropolitan Rehabilitation Center
Konstancin/Warsaw
Poland

Maria A Cerruto MD
Resident in Urology
University of Verona
Verona
Italy

Michael B Chancellor MD
Professor of Urology
Department of Urology
University of Pittsburgh Medical Center
Pittsburgh, PA
USA

Jacques Corcos MD FRCSC
Associate Professor of Urology
Department of Urology
Jewish General Hospital
McGill University
Montreal, Quebec
Canada

Michael Craggs
Professor, Spinal Research Centre
Royal National Orthopaedic Hospital
Stanmore, Middlesex
UK

Graham H Creasey MB ChB FRCSEd
Functional Electrical Stimulation Center
Case Western Reserve University
Cleveland, OH
USA

Francisco Cruz MD PhD
Professor of Urology, Faculty of Medicine of Porto
Vice-Chairman, Department of Urology
Hospital de S. João
Porto
Portugal

G Willy Davila MD
Chairman of the Department of Gynecology
Head of the Section of Urogynecology and
Reconstructive Pelvic Surgery
Cleveland Clinic Florida
Weston, FL
USA

Gina Defreitas MD
Fellow in Female Urology
Division of Urology
University of Texas Southwestern
Medicine School
Dallas, TX
USA

W Dalton Dietrich PhD
The Miami Project to Cure Paralysis
Department of Neurological Surgery
University of Miami School of Medicine
Miami, FL
USA

Magnus Fall MD PhD
Professor, Department of Urology
Institute of Surgical Sciences
Sahlgrenska University Hospital
University of Göteborg
Sweden

Clare J Fowler MBBS MSC FRCP
Reader and Consultant in Neuro-Urology
Department of Uro-Neurology
The National Hospital for Neurology and
Neurosurgery
London
UK

Antal Hamvas MD PhD
Associate Professor
Department of Urology
Semmelweis University
Budapest
Hungary

Sender Herschorn BSC MDCM FRCSC
Professor and Chairman, Division of Urology
University of Toronto
Director of Urodynamics and Attending Urologist
Sunnybrook and Women's College Health
Sciences Centre
Consultant Urologist Toronto Rehabilitation
Institute
Toronto, Ontario
Canada

Kelm Hjälmås MD DMSC
Associate Professor of Pediatric Urology
Department of Pediatric Surgery/Urology
Göteborg University
Göteborg
Sweden

Roman Jednak MD FRCSC
Assistant Professor of Urology
Division of Pediatric Urology
The Montreal Children's Hospital/McGill University
Health Center
Montreal, Quebec
Canada

Martine Jolivet-Tremblay MD FRCSC
Assistant Professor of Urology
University of Montreal
Division of Urology
Maisonneuve-Rosemont Hospital
Montreal, Quebec
Canada

Christopher E Kelly MD
Assistant Professor of Urology
Department of Urology
New York University School of Medicine
New York, NY
USA

Steven P Lapointe MD FRCSC
Assistant Professor of Urology
University of Montreal
Division of Urology
Hôpital Ste-Justine
Montreal, PQ
Canada

Gary E Lemack MD
Assistant Professor of Urology
Department of Urology
UT Southwestern Medical Center
Dallas, TX
USA

Sivert Lindström MD PhD
Professor, Department of Biomedicine and Surgery
University of Health Sciences
Linköping
Sweden

Shing-Hwa Lu MD PhD
Department of Urology
National Yang-Ming University
School of Medicine and Taipei-Veterans General Hospital
Taipei
Taiwan

Helmut G Madersbacher MD PhD
Associate Professor of Urology
Head of the Neurourology Unit
Landeskrankenhaus University Hospital
Innsbruck
Austria

Attila Majoros MD
Urologist
Department of Urology
Semmelweis University
Budapest
Hungary

Patrick Marquis MD MBA
Managing Director
Mapi Values
Boston, MA
USA

Anders Mattiasson MD PhD
Professor of Urology
Department of Urology
Lund University Hospital
Lund
Sweden

Victor W Nitti MD
Associate Professor of Urology and
Vice-Chairman
Department of Urology
New York University School of Medicine
New York, NY
USA

Joao Luiz Pippi Salle MD PhD
Associate Professor
The Hospital for Sick Children
Division of Urology
Toronto
Canada

Simon Podnar MD DSC
Institute of Clinical Neurophysiology
Division of Neurology
University Medical Center Ljubljana
Ljubljana
Slovenia

Imre Romics MD PhD DSC
Professor and Chairman
Department of Urology
Semmelweis University
Budapest
Hungary

Erik Schick MD (LOUVAIN) LMCC FRCSC
Clinical Professor of Urology
University of Montreal
Maisonneuve-Rosemont Hospital
Consultant at Ste-Justine Hospital for Children
Montreal
Quebec
Canada

Ulla Sillén MD DMSC
Professor of Pediatric Surgery/Urology
Göteborg University
Göteborg
Sweden

Carlos Silva MD
Department of Urology
Hospital de S. João
Porto, Portugal

Manfred Stöhrer MD PhD
Professor and Chairman
Department of Urology
BG-Unfallklinik Murnau
Murnau
Germany

Philip EV Van Kerrebroeck MD PhD FELLOW EBU
Professor of Urology
Chairman
Department of Urology
University Hospital
Maastricht
The Netherlands

Jean-Jacques Wyndaele MD DSC PhD FELLOW EBU
Professor of Urology
University of Antwerpen
Fellow of the International Spinal Cord Society
Registered Rehabilitation Doctor and
Chairman, Department of Urology
University Hospital
Antwerpen
Belgium

Philippe Zimmern MD FACS
Professor of Urology
Holder of the Helen J and S Strauss Professorship
in Urology
Director of Bladder and Incontinence Center
UT Southwestern Medical Center
Dallas, TX
USA

Preface

In order to publish a complete textbook on the neurogenic bladder we obtained the participation of about 90 contributors, each an expert in his or her own field. The result is a voluminous 780-page book that was published in March 2004[1]. In the last twenty years this is the only English textbook to appear on this subject. The physiology and functional pathology of the lower urinary tract are discussed in great detail. The various neurological pathologies that may lead to neurogenic bladder are reviewed extensively. Clinical evaluation, classification, complications, prognosis and treatment of neurogenic bladder are discussed at length. Unfortunately the completeness of this important publication is encumbered by its size, which is partly due to the hundreds of figures and illustrations it contains. Nevertheless, we hope the result of our efforts will remain a useful and definitive instrument of reference for teachers, students and practicing physicians.

It appeared after careful analysis that there existed a need for a more handy or practical book focusing mainly on evaluation and treatment of the neurogenic bladder. The result is the present volume, *Evaluation and Treatment of the Neurogenic Bladder*. It contains the sections on evaluation, classification, all available treatments, synthesis of the different therapeutic approaches, and complications from the original up-to-date textbook.

We hope that this guide, in its present format, will compliment its big brother with a more concise presentation with all the important information on this, sometimes life threatening condition.

Jacques Corcos
Erik Schick
November 2004

---

[1] Textbook of the Neurogenic Bladder – Adults and Children. Edited by Jacques Corcos and Erik Schick, London: Martin Dunitz/Taylor & Francis plc, 2004.

Part I

Evaluation of neurogenic bladder dysfunction

1

Clinical evaluation: history and physical examination

Gary E Lemack

Introduction

The starting point for any new patient with neurologic disease that is referred with lower urinary tract (LUT) complaints is a thorough history and physical examination. While more exact and specific means are often necessary to pinpoint the nature of bladder dysfunction in such patients, a directed, though thorough history and physical examination are essential to defining which patients require more costly and invasive testing, and which can be followed with alternative strategies. The ongoing refinement of urodynamic testing certainly has permitted the precise characterization of bladder dysfunction in patients with severe neurogenic disorders, but failing to know what questions to ask and what signs to observe can lead to erroneous diagnoses and inappropriate testing. The focus of this chapter will be on obtaining as much information as possible on the initial visit by directed questioning and a focused examination, so as to be able to discern what testing, if any, is necessary on future visits.

History

Nature of neurologic disease

Most, though not all patients, will come already with a known neurologic disease. In patients with progressive conditions, it is useful to establish the onset of symptoms – often not the same as the timing of diagnosis – as well as recent changes in symptom severity, as this information may clearly influence treatment recommendations. Even patients with a presumably fixed neurologic condition, such as spinal cord injury (SCI) or myelomeningocele, may have symptomatic deterioration (i.e. due to development of a syrinx), and therefore any recent changes in sensory or motor function should be directly questioned. Often, patients or their caregivers will have tremendous insight

into the medical condition and will, for example, know the Hoehn and Yahr stage of their Parkinson's disease, which can be useful in predicting the severity of bladder dysfunction and prospects for further deterioration.[1] Patients with multiple sclerosis may give a history of recurrent flares in conjunction with worsening urinary symptoms, which should signal an investigation for recurrent urinary infections as a possible source.

In patients with more recent acute events, such as cerebrovascular accident, information about the stroke location and the recovery since the event can be useful, since stroke location can impact on prognosis.[2] Patients with history of back surgery (often several procedures) should be questioned as to the vertebral level of the surgery, and for the presence of ongoing sensory deficit.

Current treatments should also be documented, with particular attention to medications. Medications with properties that can affect the bladder outlet (typically with either α-agonist or α-antagonist properties) or detrusor contractility (typically those with anticholinergic properties) should be recorded, along with narcotic and skeletal muscle relaxant use.

Nature of lower urinary tract symptoms

Duration of symptoms

The timing of onset of urinary symptoms is a crucial piece of information to obtain during history taking. In slowly progressive diseases, such as multiple sclerosis, a clear date of onset will be impossible to establish, though a general assessment of the time course over which the symptoms worsened is essential. In some patients, the date of onset will be quite clear, though often, as is the case in patients with cerebrovascular accidents, the presence of pre-existing symptoms may be difficult to discern. Still, the clear temporal relationship of a particular urinary symptom with an event is strong evidence of a causal relationship, which can be further supported by urodynamic testing. A patient with SCI and stable LUT function who suddenly develops new incontinence may need to have repeated spinal cord imaging, whereas a patient with slowly improving urinary urgency following a stroke can often be safely followed with noninvasive monitoring.

Previous urologic history

Patients will often come referred with a diagnosis of recurrent urinary tract infections, but precisely documenting the offending organism and its sensitivities is essential to discovering its source. Failure to clear an ongoing infection (persistence) and repeated bouts of new infections imply different etiologies. Clearly, the method of bladder management will affect the susceptibility to infection, and the use of indwelling or intermittent catheterization should be documented. Additionally, the duration of each catheter use before change, and cleaning technique used (intermittent catheterization) should be recorded, as well as a careful reassessment of catheterization technique. A history of previous bladder, prostate, or upper tract surgery must be carefully detailed, and operative notes of complex reconstructions reviewed.

Current urinary symptoms

Lower urinary tract symptoms (LUTS) should be carefully assessed at the time of initial presentation. Patients should be questioned for the presence or progression of urinary urgency, frequency, and nocturia, in addition to other symptoms typically associated with disorders of bladder filling. Often, a 2- or 3-day voiding diary (see Chapter 3) can be of tremendous help in establishing micturition frequency and voided volumes.[3,4] In general, greater than 8 voids per day is considered abnormal, though clearly this finding is nonspecific. Urinary frequency may represent detrusor overactivity, impaired bladder capacity, excessive urine production (polyuria), impaired bladder emptying, urinary infection, stone disease, inflammatory bladder conditions, as well as many other possible etiologies.

LUTS typically associated with the voiding such as urinary hesitancy, straining, loss of stream, and interrupted urine flow are also important to establish. A staccato type of voiding pattern (choppy, interrupted pattern) can be a warning sign indicating detrusor-sphincter dyssynergia, and should prompt a more thorough evaluation, including urodynamic testing. Excessive straining, too, is nonspecific and could represent detrusor failure or bladder outlet obstruction, and therefore should also prompt urodynamic testing in patients with known neurologic disease.

Incontinence, when present, should be characterized fully. Stress incontinence, occurring with increases in intra-abdominal pressure, and most frequently associated with physical activity, coughing, straining, and sneezing, should be assessed for severity, approximate time of onset, and degree of progression. During history taking, incontinence may be assessed by pad usage (nonspecific) and questionnaire response, although questionnaire response may not be a reliable indicator of severity of stress-related leakage.[5,6] Several validated questionnaires are available in men[7] and women,[8] though few were specifically designed for use in patients with neurogenic bladder conditions.[9]

Urge incontinence – which is thought to be due to detrusor overactivity, rather than pelvic floor hypermobility or intrinsic sphincteric weakness alone, as is the case with stress leakage – may be best assessed by a voiding diary and pad usage. Typical symptoms include the sudden, uncontrollable urge to urinate, nighttime leakage episodes, and, sometimes, leakage during intercourse. This is the most common pattern among patients with multiple sclerosis, cerebrovascular accident, and Parkinson's disease, among whom the urodynamic finding of neurogenic detrusor overactivity is quite common.

Patients with overflow incontinence may present with constant low-grade dribbling, recurrent urinary infections, or, at times, renal insufficiency due to the presence of significantly elevated post-void residuals. In most instances, overflow incontinence is due to detrusor failure or severe bladder outlet obstruction. Patients in the spinal shock phase of SCI will typically present with this pattern (due to detrusor areflexia), which will often persist in those with lower lumbar and sacral cord injuries. Patients with continuous incontinence – which may be due to ureteral ectopy, fistula formation, or occasionally a scarred, fixed urethra – will report constant urinary drainage, often with very infrequent voids due to the lack of urine accumulation in the bladder.

Non-genitourinary review of systems

An assessment of bowel function is imperative, as often bowel and bladder dysfunction parallel one another in patients with neurologic conditions. In patients with SCI, the nature of bowel program should be established (i.e. digital stimulation, suppository use, etc.). The presence of fecal incontinence, tenesmus, chronic constipation, or obstipation should also be recorded.

A sexual history is also quite important, as sexual dysfunction is also extremely common among men and women with neurologic conditions.[10,11] Women may report lack of desire (loss of libido) or inability to have intercourse secondary to vaginal pain or dryness, or due to enhanced vaginal sensitivity (hyperesthesia), particularly in the case of multiple sclerosis. Men may report erectile dysfunction often secondary to altered penile sensation. Ejaculatory disturbances due to these changes in sensation (leading to either premature or delayed ejaculation), or bladder neck dysfunction (retrograde ejaculation) are also not uncommon. Patients with sympathetic outflow interruption, such as those with complete spinal cord lesions, will often experience anejaculation. In such instances, vibratory stimulation to the penis or electrical stimulation applied transrectally can often result in successful ejaculation.

Physical examination

Neurologic assessment

A brief neurologic examination is essential when first evaluating patients with presumed neurovesical dysfunction. Mental status should be assessed, as significant cognitive dysfunction and memory disturbances have been independently associated with abnormal toileting behavior. An appreciation of past and present intellectual capacity may also provide insight into the progression of LUT disorders, as well as guide the degree of complexity of treatment strategies. Both motor strength and sensory level should be determined, as distribution of motor and sensory disturbances can often predict LUT dysfunction.[12]

There should also be a thorough evaluation of both cutaneous and motor reflexes at the time of the initial encounter. The bulbocavernosus reflex, which is elicited by gently squeezing the glans penis in men or gentle compression of the clitoris against the pubis in women and simultaneously feeling for an anal sphincter contraction (by placing a finger in the rectum), assesses the integrity of the S2–S4 reflex arc. The anal reflex, which assesses integrity of S2–S5, can be checked by applying a pinprick to the mucocutaneous junction of the anus and evaluating for anal sphincter contraction. The cremasteric reflex may be somewhat less reliable, but assesses sensory dermatomes supplied by L1–L2.

Muscle motor reflexes should also be routinely evaluated. The most common of these are the biceps reflex (assesses C5–C6), patellar reflex (L2–L4), and Achilles (ankle) reflex (L5–S2). Evidence of an upper motor neurologic injury would include spasticity of the involved skeletal muscle, heightened response to reflex testing, and an upgoing toe on gentle stroking of the plantar surface of the foot (positive Babinski's sign).

General issues

Mode of ambulation and recent progression of ambulatory disturbances should be assessed at the initial visit. Clearly, the degree of physical independence of the patient, particularly as it relates to the ability to get to the toilet, often affects the degree of urge-related leakage episodes. Additionally,

certain patients who are non-ambulatory may have great difficulty with self-urethral catheterization. Should that be the case, an abdominal catheterizable stoma may be a more reasonable option in the appropriately selected patient.

Hand function in patients with cervical SCI, and particularly the ability to grasp firmly between the thumb and index or middle finger, must be carefully judged in patients who may require intermittent catheterization following treatment. However, it is no longer mandatory that patients have use of both hands prior to such an intervention, as single-unit catheter/collection systems have become commercially available.

An evaluation of the skin, particularly in the gluteal region should be carried out, as localized skin and subcutaneous infections as well as more severe skin breakdown are not uncommon among patients with restricted mobility. Such issues will need to be addressed before major reconstructive procedures are considered. Some patients may also have intrathecal pumps in place and their location, as well as that of their tubing, should be assessed prior to surgical endeavors.

Pelvic examination

Pelvic examination should be carried out to assess for vaginal estrogenization (noting a loss of lubrication, rugation, and blanching of the mucosal surface), and pelvic prolapse. One should also observe for urine loss (either spontaneous or induced by Valsalva's maneuver or cough). An assessment of the urethra is essential in both men and women, particularly those with chronic indwelling catheters, as traumatic hypospadias in men and bladder neck erosion in women may require surgical repair. A careful examination of sensation of the genitalia may provide insight into the nature of sexual dysfunction, as both hypo- and hyperesthesia have been described among patients with neurologic conditions. A rectal examination should assess for sphincter tone and for stool impaction, as chronic constipation may aggravate voiding dysfunction. In men, the prostate should be examined for areas of tenderness or fluctuance, since prostatitis and prostatic abscesses are not uncommon among men with severe neurovesical dysfunction, particularly those with chronic indwelling catheters.

Conclusion

As a starting point to a complete assessment of the neurourologic patient, a thorough history and physical examination are essential. Data obtained during this initial interview will determine when more invasive testing is necessary, and provide guidance as to the most appropriate treatment strategies for any given patient.

References

1. Lemack GE, Dewey RB, Roehrborn CG, et al. Questionnaire-based assessment of bladder dysfunction in patients with mild to moderate Parkinson's disease. Urology 2000; 56:250–254.

2. Khan Z, Starer P, Yang YC, Bhola A. Analysis of voiding disorders in patients with cerebrovascular accidents. Urology 1990; 32:265–270.

3. Wyman JF, Choi SC, Harkins SW, et al. The urinary diary in evaluation of incontinent women: a test–retest analysis. Obstet Gynecol 1988; 71:812–817.

4. Groutz A, Blaivas JG, Chaikin DC, et al. Noninvasive outcome measures of urinary incontinence and lower urinary tract symptoms: a multicenter study of micturition diary and pad tests. J Urol 2000; 164:698–701.

5. Lemack GE, Zimmern PE. Predictability of urodynamic findings based on the Urogenital Distress Inventory questionnaire. Urology 1999; 54:461–466.

6. Harvey MA, Kristjansson B, Griffith D, Versi E. The Incontinence Impact Questionnaire and the Urogenital Distress Inventory: a revisit of their validity in women without a urodynamic diagnosis. Am J Obstet Gynecol 2001; 185:25–31.

7. Barry MJ, Fowler FJ Jr, O'Leary MP, et al., and the Measurement Committee of the American Urological Association. The American Urological Association symptom index for benign prostatic hyperplasia. J Urol 1992; 148:1549–1557.

8. Uebersax JS, Wyman FF, Shumaker SA, et al. Short forms to assess life quality and symptom distress for urinary incontinence in women: the incontinence impact questionnaire and urogenital distress inventory. Neurourol Urod 1995; 14:131–139.

9. Sakakibara R, Shinotoh H, Uchiyama T, et al. Questionnaire-based assessment of pelvic organ dysfunction in Parkinson's disease. Auton Neurosci Bas Clin 2001; 92:76–85.

10. Lundberg PO, Hutler B. Female sexual dysfunction in multiple sclerosis: a review. Sex Dis 1996; 14:65–72.

11. Aisen ML, Sanders AS. Sexual dysfunction in neurologic disease: mechanisms of disease and counseling approaches. Am Urolog Assoc Update Ser 1998: 17:274–279.

12. Betts CD, D'Mellow MT, Fowler CJ. Urinary symptoms and the neurological features of bladder dysfunction in multiple sclerosis. J Neurol Neurosurg Psychiatry 1993; 56(3):245–250.

2

Quality of life assessment in neurogenic bladder

Patrick Marquis

Introduction

Normal bladder function requires coordinated interaction of sensory and motor components of both the somatic and autonomic nervous systems. The micturition reflex is a finely tuned neurological event that requires integration of most levels of the nervous system to regulate voiding function, so that damage to any one of the many neurological mechanisms involved affects urination. In particular, bladder contraction and reflex control depends on an intact neural axis – specifically, an undamaged sacral spinal cord together with its afferent and efferent connections.[1] Spinal cord injury (SCI), by contrast, generally results in absent sensation below the level of the lesion and, although patients with upper motor neuron lesions can have a local reflex of bladder contraction, it is often opposed by smooth and striated muscle dyssynergia in the sphincters controlling bladder voiding. Neurogenic bladder problems are therefore a near universal feature of spinal cord injury.

In the United States alone, there are at present estimated to be 200,000 patients with SCI and the number increases by about 10,000 per year.[2] According to De Vivo et al[3] the commonest causes of SCI are road accidents (45%), falls (22%), acts of violence (16%), and sports trauma (13%); 82% of victims are male, with a mean age of 31 years. This, self-evidently, represents a dramatic loss of healthy productive years for the individuals and major adaptation for their families, as well as a significant socioeconomic burden.

Spinal cord injury is serious in all cases, but the degree of resultant disability depends on the site of the injury along the spine. Five decades ago, treatment was largely aimed at keeping patients alive during the immediate post-injury period. When acute SCI management had improved to the point where survival was likely, the focus of treatment shifted to preventing the long-term medical complications which subsequently appeared, with urinary disorders being reported in one 25-year prospective study as the leading cause of death in SCI patients up to the mid 1970s.[4] Two decades later, a 13-member Department of Health expert panel reported that diseases of the urinary system had become only the fifth most common primary or secondary cause of death in SCI patients but that 80% or patients reported a urinary tract infection by their 16th year post-injury.[5] Nowadays, respiratory problems are regarded as the major cause of death in SCI patients, together with accidents and suicide, but urinary disorders remain a significant secondary cause of death and a major cause of morbidity.[6–8]

In practice, the impact of traumatic SCI is even greater than the usually drastic functional and mobility effects on the patients themselves, since it normally extends to sudden and fundamental changes in roles and relationships which affect uninjured family members.[9–11] The outcome and resolution of the shift in relationships between the injured and uninjured family members can profoundly affect how the SCI person reacts to and comes to terms with their injury, which in turn can affect their rehabilitation and ultimate ongoing quality of life (QoL). It follows that successful SCI treatment may also provide benefits which extend beyond patients themselves, to alter the QoL of the affected family members.

Patient quality of life

SCI sufferers are affected both physically and psychologically during the acute injury phase, during the process of adjustment after injury, and by their ongoing life situation once their medical situation has stabilized. Siösteen et al assessed the quality of life of 56 SCI patients in three subgroups ranked according to functional ability:[12] C6 tetraplegics, wheelchair-dependent paraplegics and ambulant paraplegics were assessed according to various functional and emotional criteria to arrive at an estimate of sickness impact profile (SIP) in both physical and psychological dimensions, the hospital anxiety and depression scale (HAD), and a mood activity checklist (MACL). Quality of life was self-assessed on both a visual analogue scale (VAS) and by means of 18 specific questionnaire points.

Sweden has extensive social and legislative support structures for disabled persons which are probably superior to those available in many other countries, and which could be expected to improve the lot of SCI patients as a result. Nevertheless, the authors found that disability severity had particular impacts on home and kitchen management and on mobility in the neighborhood. In their view, however, these impacts were partly explained by patient choice in obtaining help with some aspects of daily living in order to concentrate their own energies on other aspects, such as self-care or socializing, plus external factors such as architectural impediments that curtailed outdoor mobility and access. This was borne out by the finding that engagement in social and recreational activities, physical training, and private transport were not restricted by more severe disability.

Mental well-being and perceived overall QoL seemed to be influenced much more by engagement in social activities and the ability to drive adapted cars than they were by the degree of physical dysfunction. However, a cause and effect relationship is much harder to establish, since it may be that either patients with little depression or high levels of satisfaction with their lives are more likely to engage in these activities, or participation in itself might benefit mental well-being and perceived quality of life. Age and age at injury were negatively correlated to activity levels in all areas – especially social activities – but again this may be due more to the possibility that older persons are generally less able to cope with major life changes than younger persons with more energy and the motivation to find new goals and interests.

Overall, in this Swedish study, despite considerable group differences in levels of physical functioning, over 80% of subjects were gainfully employed or engaged in studies, and most had active leisure time. They reported normal or close to normal mood states and QoL perceptions, which shows that despite their often profoundly changed physical circumstances, it is entirely possible for SCI patients to lead satisfying and productive lives in the community, if extensive societal support and stimulation are available. Few societies provide the level of support found in Sweden, however, and it may be that familial adaptation and QoL, as well as that of the patient, are compromised when such support is lacking.

Family influences

Since the impact of SCI normally extends beyond patients themselves, McGowan and Roth studied the relationships between functional independence, perceived family functioning, and duration of disability in 41 non-institutionalized post-traumatic SCI families.[13] How SCI patients relate to their families can influence the emotional effects of their injury[14,15] and, as a result, the extent and course of their rehabilitation.[16,17] In fact the family's ability to adjust successfully is critical, but sudden permanent disability in one member places great strain on the whole family unit[18] so that communication patterns can change,[19] along with levels of emotional intimacy[16,20] and role identification.[21] In cases of poor treatment outcomes in SCI rehabilitation, investigation of the family context may be vital for a proper understanding of what has happened and how best to improve matters.[22]

The nature of the SCI patient–family interaction changes over time, from the initial acute crisis through to the necessary longer-term adjustment. It seems reasonable to assume therefore that family QoL likewise varies over time and that the estimation of QoL needs to take the time course of the family process into account. Family members may eventually become resentful despite at first seeming supportive, especially if rehabilitation progresses less well than expected. Despite some evidence that duration of disability may be correlated to greater acceptance of SCI,[23] some patients may actually regress in their acceptance of SCI disability over time[24] and in any case it may take years for some patients and families to fully accept their altered circumstances. McGowan and Roth's study worked with post-rehabilitation SCI patients and families. They found that SCI patients with higher levels of self-initiation of activities, social involvement, and overall levels of independence (which are all associated with improved QoL) perceived their family environment as affectively responsive, openly communicative, and clear in the delineation of role responsibilities.

Quality of life measurement in spinal cord injury

Various authors have used a range of instruments in an attempt to measure QoL in SCI patients. The Short-Form 36-item questionnaire (SF-36)[25] is a widely used and validated instrument for assessing QoL in illnesses as varied as diabetes, migraine, and heart disease. It has been used to measure QoL in urinary disorders[26,27] but is not an SCI-specific instrument. Other instruments such as the SIP have been employed in related disorders[28] but it is also not an SCI-specific instrument and, in addition, these instruments are less sensitive to changes in single patients with a specific condition, having been developed for the study of whole populations.

A review of the general medical literature (Medline, 1997) and a QoL specialist database, OLGA[29] revealed that although 13,000 articles were identified using the keyword 'QoL', only 20 were on SCI and none were specifically on urinary disorders in SCI. A recent Medline literature research confirmed this finding, with less than 18 articles identified using 'urogenic bladder' and 'QoL' as key words from 1996 to 2002. Most of the researches studied the QoL related to the underlying conditions such as SCI or multiple sclerosis. Very few focus on the specific QoL issues related to urinary disorders.[30–44]

Several validated QoL questionnaires have been specifically developed for urinary disorders in both men and women, but these are specific for urgency and mixed incontinence. Questionnaires relevant to men only include examples such as the benign prostate hypertrophy (BPH) health-related quality of life.[45] But none of these questionnaires was developed to assess all types of urinary disorder in a way that is specific to SCI or multiple sclerosis populations. Indeed, these questionnaires, even though specific to urinary disorders are not relevant to assess the impact of neurogenic bladder on QoL. A meta-analysis of 3710 articles on QoL and SCI between 1983 and 1992 reported:[46] 'because of limited rigour of research design and poor validity of measurements, conclusion about the ability of rehabilitative care to improve the quality of life for spinal cord injured persons could not be drawn from the studies reviewed'. The authors concluded that 'QoL research with SCI persons needs to be better designed and should include more uniform and valid criteria'.

Furthermore, the challenge researchers have to face when attempting to assess the QoL of patients with neurogenic bladder is to understand the specific burden of the urinary disorders in relation to the overall QoL impact of the underlying condition such as SCI or multiple sclerosis.

In order to overcome some of these shortcomings and provide a highly relevant measurement instrument, Costa et al undertook a series of patient interviews which resulted in an extensive list of relevant concepts that were subsequently developed into a highly relevant questionnaire to assess urinary disorders in SCI.[47]

Development and validation of a specific quality of life questionnaire to assess the impact of urinary disorders in spinal cord injury patients

A multidisciplinary scientific committee, consisting of urologists, rehabilitators, epidemiologists, and QoL experts, was convened with the intention of developing and validating a questionnaire to evaluate the extent to which urinary disorders specifically affect the QoL of SCI patients. The questionnaire could be used in international multicenter studies or to monitor the patient's care. The group opted for the sequential development approach, in which the questionnaire would be developed and validated in one language, followed by translation into other languages, with further linguistic and psychometric validation. The questionnaire was developed and validated in French, before being translated into English.

By interviewing patients and reviewing the literature, a range of QoL problems and concerns relevant to SCI patients with urinary disorders were identified and phrased in patient-relevant wording. Paraplegic, tetraplegic, or conus medullaris syndrome patients were interviewed. The interviews consisted of one section on the impact of functional impairment and one section about specific problems related to urinary dysfunction. This double-component structure was aimed at identifying and separating problems due to functional impairment from those caused by urinary disorders.

The initial exhaustive list of concepts extracted from the interviews led to the generation of questions based on the exact patient speech wording. These questions were analyzed for content validity by the committee and through face-to-face interviews with patients. Patients were asked if the questions were easy to understand, relevant, and if any important questions were missing from the questionnaire. The resulting questionnaire contained 84 questions, which were grouped into four broad issues: limitations (26 items), constraints (27 items), fears (18 items), and feelings (13 items). The questionnaire was designed to be patient-administered or interviewer-administered, depending on the degree of handicap.

The questionnaire generated through patient interviews was used in a cross-sectional validation study in 300 French patients with varying degrees of disability. Patients also completed a 56-item generic questionnaire, the Subjective Quality of Life Profile (SQLP).[48,49] This questionnaire offers two advantages over the well-known generic instruments like the SF-36. First, the SQLP does not measure functional status related to normality or ability to perform physical activities like walking or climbing stairs (which are irrelevant in most SCI patients). Instead, it uses items related to functional status to ask about the quality and the extent to which subjects are satisfied, or not, with their ability to perform activities like going where they want when alone, moving around at home, or playing sports, if any. In addition, the SQLP allows the user to generate targeted questions to supplement the core questionnaire. These questions were generated using the same questionnaire format in the areas of autonomy, social interaction, material comfort, sexual relationships, and adaptation of living.

An item reduction was performed on each scale whereby, in order to be retained, an item had to satisfy several psychometric criteria, as well as passing scientific committee review of its perceived relevance and importance. This yielded a list of questions, which was subsequently reduced after iterative analysis to a final 30-item questionnaire, assessing the specific impact of urinary problems (Specific IUP) grouped into four scales: limitations

Table 2.1 *Abbreviated content of the specific section of the Qualiveen™ questionnaire*

Scale	Item	Abbreviated item content
Limitations (9 items)	1	Bothered by urine leaks during the day
	2	Bothered by urine leaks at night
	3	Bothered by incontinence pads
	4	Bothered by a set timetable to pass urine during activities
	5	Bothered by time spent passing urine
	6	Bothered because nights are disturbed
	7	Bothered when traveling
	8	Bothered by personal hygiene problems when away
	9	Bladder problems complicate life
Constraints (8 items)	10	Able to go out without planning in advance
	11	Give up going out
	12	Be more dependent due to bladder problems
	13	Life regulated by bladder problems
	14	Plan everything
	15	Think about taking a change (clothes/incontinence pads)
	16	Wear incontinence pads as a precaution
	17	Be careful about quantity of fluid you drink
Fears (8 items)	18	Smell of urine
	19	Have urinary infections
	20	Bladder problems worsening
	21	Disturb partner at night
	22	Urine leaks during sexual intercourse
	23	Side-effects from drugs
	24	Skin problems
	25	Money problems due to expenses related to bladder problems
Feelings (5 items)	26	Feel ashamed because of bladder problems
	27	Loss of self-respect because of bladder problems
	28	Conceal bladder problems
	29	Questioning looks from others regarding time spent in toilets
	30	Worry because of bladder problems

Qualiveen is a registered trade mark of Coloplast A/S, Humlebaek, DK-3050, Denmark.

(9 items), constraints (8 items), fears (8 items), and feelings (5 items). The abbreviated content is shown in Table 2.1.

The psychometric properties of the reduced questionnaire were then assessed, including internal consistency, test–retest reliability, and clinical validity. The clinical validity was confirmed by testing hypotheses about the behavior of scores of the QoL instrument in various clinical situations, such as the overall degree of difficulty urinating, the derived satisfaction or dissatisfaction with urination, and the time spent urinating.[50]

Key findings from a specific quality of life questionnaire

Perrouin-Verbe et al have collated data from 400 SCI patients.[51] They self-administered the 30-item specific impact of urinary problems (Specific IUP) questionnaire, plus an additional 9-item general quality of life (General QoL) section derived from the SQLP. The questionnaire was named Qualiveen™ (registered trade mark of Coloplast A/S, Humlebaek, DK-3050, Denmark).

Scores range from 0 to 4 for the Specific IUP questionnaire, with 0 indicating no impact of urinary disorders on QoL (no limitations, or constraints or fears or negative feelings) and 4 indicating a high specific impact on QoL (greatest limitation, constraints, fears or negative feelings) and from −2 to +2 for the General QoL index, with negative values indicating poor QoL, positive values indicating good QoL, and 0 indicating neutral position (neither bad nor good).

The relationship between the specific scales of the Specific IUP and the General QoL index were studied using the Pearson correlation coefficient. Values between 0.40 and 0.60 were expected to mean that deterioration of the Specific IUP could lead to impairment in the general QoL.

Clinical validity was assessed by a number of comparisons of QoL scores in subgroups according to different sociodemographic and clinical criteria (gender, age, type of lesion, concomitant pathology, total incontinence, help at home, treatment for urinary problems, urinary tract infections, time since injury, mode of urination, time taken to urinate, use of protective devices or collectors). Kruskal–Wallis or Wilcoxon tests were used for group comparisons.

Results

The 400 SCI patients consisted mainly of men (72.5%), with an average age of 40 years, most of whom were living with a partner (59.0%) and receiving help at home (57.5%). More than half (52.2%) of the participants in the reference group were paraplegic and more than one-quarter (27.2%) were tetraplegic. The most frequently encountered methods of urination were self-catheterization (41.2%), percussion (27.7%), and abdominal straining or Credé's maneuver (22.5%). More than half the population wore protective or urine collection devices (52.2%); 58.8% reported having had a urinary infection in the previous 30 days, 30.2% had undergone surgery for urinary problems, and 44.7% of respondents were on treatment for their urinary problems. Table 2.2 shows that the Specific IUP scales were negatively correlated with the General QoL index, indicating that the higher the impact of urinary problems, the lower the General QoL, which confirmed the hypotheses. Correlations were statistically significant ($p < 0.001$).

Similarly, an increase in the score of the Specific IUP leads to an impairment in the General QoL, as shown in Figure 2.1: patients reporting lower scores, indicating low impact of urinary disorders (quartile 1), had a higher General QoL than patients reporting moderate scores (quartiles 2 and 3). Patients reporting the highest impact of urinary disorders (quartile 4) had the lowest General QoL.

Other key findings were found:

- Differences were observed between men and women for each of the specific scores but not for the General QoL index (not statistically significant). Women had higher limitations, constraints, and negative feelings and higher Specific IUP than men, indicating more specific QoL impairment. Women therefore tended to be more concerned about the limitations imposed by their urinary disorder, such as having to wear protective devices, spending a long time urinating, and problems experienced with personal hygiene while away from home. Men, on the other hand, reported more fears, such as a higher tendency to be concerned about smelling of urine, having bladder infections, or urine leaks.

- The General QoL index decreased consistently with age ($p \leq 0.0001$) but age didn't seem to influence the specific impact of urinary disorder on QoL.

- Specific QoL scores didn't reveal significant differences between the types of lesion, although tetraplegic patients reported higher levels of constraints and fears. Quality of life was particularly impaired in the early years post-injury, as patients reported more limitations and negative feelings, as well as poorer general QoL compared with those with older injuries.

- Patients requiring help at home reported both lower Specific and General QoL.

- The existence of concomitant pathologies affected QoL and gave higher scores in all four dimensions of the Specific IUP, as well as lower General QoL scores.

- The time taken to urinate affected both Specific and General QoL greatly. Patients who spent more than 10 min urinating reported higher limitations, constraints, and negative feelings. No difference was observed for the level of fears. The General QoL was also most severely affected in patients taking more than 10 min to urinate.

- Concerning the mode of urination, patients catheterized by someone else presented significantly worse values for the limitations and the constraints dimensions. Thus, ability to self-catheterize as opposed to requiring catheterization by others had an important impact on the General QoL: the latter presenting the lowest General QoL scores.

Table 2.2 *Correlation of Specific IUP scores, Specific IUP index, and the General QoL*

	Limitations	Constraints	Fears	Feelings	SIUP index	GQoL index
Limitations	1.00					
Constraints	0.65	1.00				
Fears	0.58	0.52	1.00			
Feelings	0.63	0.53	0.50	1.00		
SIUP index	0.87	0.81	0.78	0.82	1.00	
GQoL index	−0.45	−0.48	−0.33	−0.51	−0.54	1.00

$p < 0.001$ (Pearson's correlation coefficients).

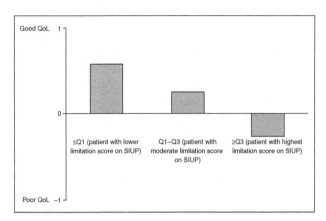

Figure 2.1
General QoL scores according to the level of Specific IUP.
Kruskal–Wallis test, $p = 0.0001$.

- Conversely, the use of protective devices or collectors had significant negative consequences on every dimension of the QoL.
- Patients who were completely incontinent had significantly higher constraints, feelings, and fears, indicating poorer Specific QoL although this itself did not reach significance.
- Patients undergoing treatment for urinary problems had significantly higher limitations, constraints, and fears than patients who were not being treated for urinary problems. For the feelings dimension the difference was non-significant. The difference in the General QoL index scores of these patients was not significant. Similarly, the effect of urinary tract infection was not reflected in the General QoL index score, although patients with urinary tract infections had significantly higher scores in all SIUP scales except for the feelings dimension.

Overall, the process followed to create the questionnaire has allowed the development of an instrument relevant to a broad range of SCI patients. It is the first specific instrument developed and shown to be reliable and valid in this population and has the added benefit of being supported by data generated in 400 SCI patients with varying degrees of disability, age, and gender.

These data can be considered as a reference which should be of great benefit to clinicians and health-related quality of life researchers. Knowing the baseline scores of a reference population should give a context to users of the questionnaire and allow them to interpret scores by comparison with those reference data – especially in judging whether scores are lower, higher, or similar to those in the same type of patients, and in judging the benefits of an intervention. This is particularly important in the case of disease-specific questionnaires, where comparison with normal data in a general population is inappropriate.

Summary

Most patients with a traumatic SCI subsequently develop urological problems, often due to bladder dysfunction brought about by the impaired nervous control caused by the spinal injury. Thankfully, today's improved urological care of neurogenic bladder means that life-threatening urinary tract complications leading to renal insufficiency or kidney failure now cause few deaths amongst SCI patients. It remains true, however, that SCI urological complications result in significant morbidity and can have drastic effects on the quality of life of SCI patients. Existing and emerging therapies need to be evaluated not simply in terms of their effect on bladder function or control per se but also in terms of any change in overall QoL that such therapeutic effects may bring about.

Treatment of neurogenic bladder may include one or more physical, neurological, behavioral, or pharmacological modalities, some of which can be difficult to compare directly. Consequently, the assessment of patient QoL is arguably one of the most relevant and perhaps reliable ways of measuring and comparing real-world clinical benefits. In order to fulfill this potential validation role, however, it is important to develop QoL instruments which are themselves robust, so that observed effects can safely be related to the treatment under investigation, rather than variability in the QoL measure employed.

Importantly, the occurrence of neurogenic bladder after SCI affects not only patients themselves but also their families or social contacts, who may find themselves suddenly thrust into an unexpected pseudo-nursing role, just as they and the patient are having to come to terms with the dramatic change in circumstances arising from the injury. An effective QoL instrument should help to quantify some of these effects and any changes brought about by existing or investigational therapies.

The SF-36 instrument and similar QoL measures have been used in many diseases, including SCI, but while they can quantify general health-related quality of life in SCI, they do not measure the specific impact of urological SCI problems such as neurogenic bladder. A reliable and validated specific questionnaire such as the Qualiveen, by contrast, can distinguish between patients with varying degrees of disability. References scores are available for a large population of SCI patients with different levels of urinary dysfunction, thus providing physicians and researchers with a context for the results from future studies.

This type of questionnaire is required to monitor patient QoL, providing a more comprehensive overview of patient's care, complementary to traditional clinical parameters. This questionnaire can also be used in clinical studies to assess the effect of interventions and treatments. The responsiveness of the questionnaire to change over time has not yet been investigated and this will be the subject of future research. Also, its validity in multiple sclerosis has to be assessed.

References

1. Wein AJ. Neuromuscular dysfunction of the lower urinary tract and its treatment. In: Campbell's urology, 7th edn. Philadelphia: WB Saunders, 1998:953–1006.

2. Stover SL, Fine PR, eds. Spinal cord injury: the facts and figures. Birmingham: University of Alabama at Birmingham, 1986.

3. De Vivo MJ, Richards JS, Stover SL, Go BK. Spinal cord injury: rehabilitation adds life to years. West J Med 1991; 154:602–606.

4. Hackler R. A 25 year prospective mortality in the spinal cord injured patient; comparison with the long term living paraplegia. J Urol 1977; 117:486–493.

5. Agency for Health Care Policy and Research. Prevention and management of urinary tract infections in paralyzed persons: summary, evidence report/technology assessment number 6. Silver Spring, MD: Agency for Health Care Policy and Research, US Department of Health and Human Services, 1999.

6. Stover SL, Fine PR. Epidemiology and economics of spinal cord injury. Paraplegia 1987; 25:225–231.

7. De Vivo MJ, Black KJ, Stover SL. Causes of death during the first 12 years after spinal cord injury. Arch Phys Med Rehabil 1993; 74:248–254.

8. Whiteneck GG, Charlifue SW, Frankel HL, et al. Mortality, morbidity and psychosocial outcomes of persons spinal cord injured more than 20 years ago. Paraplegia 1992; 30:617–630.

9. Bartol G. Psychological needs of the spinal cord injured person. J Neurosurg Nurs 1978; 10:171–175.

10. Bishop DS, Epstein NB, Baldwin LM. Disability: a family affair. In: Freeman DS, Trute B, eds. Treating families with special needs. Alberta, Canada: Alberta Association of Social Workers, 1982.

11. Hohman NGW. Psychological aspects of treatment and rehabilitation of the spinal cord injured person. Clin Orthop Rel Res 1975; 112:81–88.

12. Siösteen A, Lundqvist C, Blomstrand C, et al. The quality of life of three functional spinal cord injury subgroups in a Swedish community. Paraplegia 1990; 28:476–488.

13. McGowan MB, Roth S. Family functioning and functional independence in spinal cord injury adjustment. Paraplegia 1987; 25:357–365.

14. Harris P, Patel SS, Greer W, Naughton JAL. Psychological and social reactions to acute spinal paralysis. Paraplegia 1973; 2:132–136.

15. Klein RF, Dean A, Bogdonoff MD. The impact of illness upon the spouse. J Chronic Dis 1967; 20:241–248.

16. Bracken MB, Shepard MJ. Coping and adaptation following acute spinal cord injury: a theoretical analysis. Paraplegia 1980; 18:74–85.

17. Dinsdale SM, Lesser AL, Judd F. Critical psycho-social variables affecting outcome in a regional spinal cord center. Proc Vet Admin Spinal Cord Injury Conf 1971; 18:193–196.

18. Steinglass P, Temple S, Lisman SA, Reiss D. Coping with spinal cord injury: the family perspective. Gen Hosp Psych 1982; 4:259–264.

19. Rohrer K, Adelman B, Puchett J, et al. Rehabilitation in spinal cord injury: use of a patient–family group. Arch Phys Med Rehab 1980; 61:225–229.

20. Cleveland M. Family adaptation to the traumatic spinal cord injury of a son or daughter. Soc Wk in Health Care 1979; 4:459–471.

21. Shellhase LJ, Shellhase FE. Role of the family in rehabilitation. Soc Casework 1972; 11:544–550.

22. Trieschman RB. Spinal cord injuries: psychological, social and vocational adjustment. New York: Pergamon Press, 1980.

23. Woodrich F, Patterson JB. Variables related to acceptance of disability in persons with spinal cord injuries. J Rehab 1980; 3:26–39.

24. Rosensteil AK, Roth S. Relationship between cognitive activity and adjustment in four spinal-cord injured individuals: a longitudinal investigation. J Human Stress 1982; 3:35–43.

25. Ware JE, Snow KK, Kosinski M, Gandek M. SF-36 health survey. Manual and interpretation guide. Boston New England Medical Center: The Health Institute, 1993.

26. Sand PK, Staskin D, Miller J, et al. Effect of urinary control insert on quality of life incontinent women. Int Urogynecol J 1999; 10(2):100–105.

27. Fuhrer MJ, Rintala DH, Hart KA, et al. Relationship of life satisfaction to impairment, disability and handicap among persons with spinal cord injury living in the community. Arch Phys Med Rehab 1992; 73:552–557.

28. Schurmans JR, Weerman PC, Bosch JL, et al. Quality of life in heterotopic and orthotopic neobladder reconstruction: a comparison. Acta Urol Belg 1995; 63(3):55–58.

29. Erickson P, Scott J. The on-line guide to quality of life assessment (OLGA): resource for selecting quality of life assessments. In: Walker S, Rosser RM, eds. Quality of life assessments: key issues in the 1990s. Dordrecht: Kluwer Academic Publisers, 1993:221–232.

30. Lowe JB, Furness PD 3rd, Barqawi AZ, Koyle MA. Surgical management of the neuropathic bladder. Sem Pediatr Surg 2002; 11(2):120–127.

31. Fernandez O. Mechanisms and current treatments of urogenital dysfunction in multiple sclerosis. J Neurol 2002; 249(1):1–8.

32. Zorzon M, Zivadinov R, Monti Bragadin L, et al. Sexual dysfunction in multiple sclerosis: a 2-year follow-up study. J Neurol Sci 2001; 187(1–2):1–5.

33. Kachourbos MJ, Creasey GH. Health promotion in motion: improving quality of life for persons with neurogenic bladder and bowel using assistive technology. Sci Nursing 2000; 17(3):125–129.

34. Yavuzer G, Gok H, Tuncer S, et al. Compliance with bladder management in spinal cord injury patients. Spinal Cord 2000; 38(12):762–765.

35. Weld KJ, Dmochowski RR. Effect of bladder management on urological complications in spinal cord injured patients. J Urol 2000; 163(3):768–772.

36. Kumar H, Cauchi J, MacKinnon AE. Periurethral Goretex sling in lower urinary recontruction. Eur J Pediatr Surg 1999; 9(suppl 1):33–34.

37. Rashid TM, Hollander JB. Multiple sclerosis and the neurogenic bladder. Phys Med Rehab Clin N Am 1998; 9(3):615–629.

38. Westgren N, Levi R. Quality of life and traumatic spinal cord injury. Arch Phys Med Rehab 1998; 79(11):1433–1439.

39. Bakke A, Malt UF. Psychological predictors of symptoms of urinary tract infection and bacteriuria in patients treated with clean

intermittent catheterization: a prospective 7-year study. Eur Urol 1998; 34(1):30–36.

40. Vaidyananthan S, Soni BM, Brown E, et al. Effect of intermittent urethral catheterization and oxybutynin bladder instillation on urinary continence status and quality of life in a selected group of spinal cord injury patients with neuropathic bladder dysfunction. Spinal Cord 1998; 36(6):409–414.

41. Sutton MA, Hinson JL, Nickell KG, et al. Continent ileocecal augmentation cystoplasty. Spinal Cord 1998; 36(4):246–251.

42. Stohrer M, Kramer G, Goepel M, et al. Bladder autoaugmentation in adult patients with neurogenic voiding dysfunction. Spinal Cord 1997; 35(7):456–462.

43. Kuo HC. Clinical outcome and quality of life after enterocystoplasty for contracted bladders. Urolog Int 1997; 58(3):160–165.

44. Wielink G, Essink-Bot ML, van Kerrebroeck PE, et al. Sacral rhizotomies and electrical bladder stimulation in spinal cord injury. 2. Cost-effectiveness and quality of life analysis. Dutch Study Group on sacral anterior root stimulation. Eur Urol 1997; 31(4):441–446.

45. Lukacs B, Leplege A, MacCarthy C, Comet D. Construction and validation of a BPH-specific health-related quality of life scale including evaluation of sexuality. Proc Am Urol Ass 1995; 153(Suppl):320A.

46. Evans RL, Hendricks RD, Connis RT, et al. Quality of life after spinal cord injury: a literature critique and meta-analysis (1983–1992). J Am Paraplegia Soc 1994; 17:60–66.

47. Costa P, Perrouin-Verbe B, Colvez A, et al. Quality of life in spinal cord injury patients with urinary difficulties: development and validation of Qualiveen. Eur Urol 2001; 39:107–113.

48. Dazord A, Astolfl F, Guisti P, et al. Quality of life assessment in psychiatry: the Subjective Quality of Life Profile (SQLP) – first results of a new instrument. Community Ment Health J 1998; 34:525–535.

49. Guérin P, Dazord A, Cialdella Ph, et al. Le questionnaire "Profil de la Qualité de la Vie Subjective". Premiers éléments de validation. Thérapie 1991; 46:131–138.

50. Bergner M, Rothman ML. Health status measures: an overview and guide for selection. Ann Rev Public Health 1987; 8:191–210.

51. Perrouin-Verbe B, Amarenco G, Marquis P, et al. Quality of life related to urinary disorders in spinal cord injury patients. Use of the specific questionnaire Qualiveen: study of 400 patients. Submitted to Arch Phys Med Rehab.

3

The voiding diary

Martine Jolivet-Tremblay and Pierre E Bertrand

Introduction

Since the advent of urodynamic studies in clinical practice, urologists have tried to analyze voiding habits to better define lower urinary tract symptoms (LUTS). The bladder being an 'unreliable witness', diagnosis based solely on clinical symptoms was revealed to be inadequate.

The voiding diary is a well-known diagnostic tool for this purpose and it is now a component of every serious investigation. Unfortunately, it is still frequently overlooked by some, even if it is one of the simplest noninvasive tests to evaluate the function of the lower urinary tract (LUT). The patients complete it at home and/or at work, and it offers the advantage of assessing the severity of LUTS in their customary environment. By filling out the voiding diary, patients become active participants in the diagnostic process and their degree of motivation can be assessed.

The first studies published on voiding diaries concerned only urinary incontinence. However, since the end of the 1980s the voiding diary has become a widely accepted tool in the investigation of voiding dysfunctions, including obstructive uropathy, urinary tract infection, vesicoureteral reflux, and neurogenic bladder dysfunction.

The voiding diary is now a crucial part of most research protocols and has become an important criteria in the indication of treatments, such as injection of Botox (botulinum toxin A–hemagluttinin complex) or implantation of neurostimulation/neuromodulation devices.

Definition and terminology
The Abrams–Klevmark classification

Abrams and Klevmark[1] have described four different voiding diaries in a laudable effort to standardize the terminology. This classification is based on the type and amount of information contained in each of them (Table 3.1). The charts give objective information on the number of voidings, the distribution of voiding between daytime and nighttime, and each voided volume. The charts can also be used to record episodes of urgency and leakage and the number of incontinence pads used. The frequency–volume chart is not only useful in the assessment of voiding disorders but also in treatment follow-up.

Table 3.1 *Voiding diaries: the Abrams–Klevmark classification*			
Frequency chart	Frequency–severity chart	Frequency–volume chart	Urinary diary
Number of voidings + Number of incontinence episodes	Number of voidings + Number of incontinence episodes + Number of pads used	Time of each voiding + Volume of each voiding + Time of each incontinent episode	Time of each voiding + Volume of each voiding + Time of each incontinent episode + Types of drinks, foods, activities related to LUTS

Reproduced with modifications from Jolivet-Tremblay M, Schick E. The voiding diary. In: Corcos J, Schick E, eds. The urinary sphincter. New York: Marcel Dekker, 2001: 262.
LUTS, lower urinary tract symptoms.

The frequency chart

In this very simple chart only the number of micturitions and the number of incontinence episodes are registered per 24 hours. This limited information does not include urinary volume or the degree of incontinence.

The frequency–severity chart

In this chart, the number of micturitions and episodes of incontinence will be noted plus the number of pads used or cloths changed. This diary is a better evaluation of the severity of incontinence. However, it does not provide information on urinary volume or quantity of urine lost.

The frequency–volume chart

This type of voiding diary is the most widely used by urologists. It provides the maximum of information. Although it demands some effort on the part of the patient, it is an investment in his welfare. The time and the volume of urine voided at each micturition plus the number and the timing of each incontinent episode are registered on a chart. From this, the 24-hour diuresis, the frequency of micturition, the functional capacity of the bladder, and daytime diuresis, compared with nocturnal diuresis, etc., can be calculated. This type of voiding diary, however, does not provide information on fluid intake or its distribution through a 24-hour period.

The urinary diary

This is the most elaborate and complicated form of voiding diary. Besides its role as a frequency–volume chart, it also provides information on the types and number of beverages and foods taken every day. The patient also notes any activities related to LUTS. This type of chart is very onerous to the patient and is often difficult to analyze for the physician. It is mostly used in research protocols. Under normal circumstances, knowledge of fluid intake is not absolutely necessary since it generally parallels total diuresis.

The International Continence Society classification

In a recent report[2] a subcommittee of the International Continence Society suggested three types of diaries (Table 3.2):

1. *micturition time chart*, which records only the times of micturitions, day and night, for at least 24 h
2. *frequency–volume chart*, which records the volumes voided as well as the times of micturitions, day and night, for at least 24 h
3. *bladder diary*, which records the times of micturitions, voided volumes, incontinence episodes, pad usage, and other information such as fluid intake, the degree of urgency, and the degree of incontinence.

Rationale for the voiding diary

Routine use of the voiding diary in the investigation and follow-up of patients with LUTS will fulfill four objectives:

1. The voiding diary leads to an objective measurement of the patient's subjective complaints in a familiar environment. Patient perception of voiding habits may be misleading. For example, McCormack et al[3] studied 88 consecutive patients in whom urinary frequency was evaluated by a questionnaire at the first visit. This

Table 3.2 *Voiding diaries: the ICS classification*

Micturition time chart	Frequency–volume chart	Bladder diary
Times of micturition (minimum 24 hours)	Times of micturitions (minimum 24 hours) + Volumes voided at each micturition	Times of micturitions + Volumes voided at each micturition + Incontinence episodes + Pad usage, fluid intake, degree of urgency, degree of incontinence

was compared with the frequency obtained by analyzing the frequency–volume chart filled out by the patient for 7 consecutive days. A very wide discrepancy was noted between subjectively estimated frequency and chart-determined frequency.

2. It can help the physician to identify the etiology of the patient's LUTS.

3. As previously mentioned, when taking an active role in the elaboration of his voiding calendar, the patient becomes a participant to the diagnosis and treatment of the urological problem. This may serve as a measure of his motivation to get well.

4. The voiding diary is also an important tool in the follow-up of a medical treatment or a specific surgery. Siltberg et al[4] estimated that the voiding diary provided the best tool for follow-up in the treatment of the urge syndrome. It is now of common use in many clinical research protocols.

Data extracted from the voiding diary

Important parameters about the frequency of micturition and the number of episodes of incontinence can be extracted by careful examination of the data in the voiding diary. It also provides an accurate estimate of total diuresis in a 24-hour period. Nowadays, in the majority of urodynamic laboratories, all the parameters can be entered into a computer and, using a simple software program, a more precise and detailed analysis may be done. This kind of computer program, like the one developed in our laboratory, calculates the following parameters: the mean voided volume per micturition (ml), the frequency (units), the diuresis (ml/min), the mean interval between micturitions (min), and the voided volume during a specific period of the day (ml). All these parameters are calculated separately for daytime and nighttime. The rising micturition is the first daytime voiding registered in the software. This first voided volume is considered part of nocturnal diuresis and is treated as such by the computer program. It is assumed that daytime lasts 16 h (960 min) and nighttime 8 h (480 min). Therefore, the amount of urine voided during the day is divided by 960 and during the night by 480, to give the day and night diuresis in milliliters per minute. Further analysis produces two more parameters: output per 24 h (ml), which is the total voided volume during a 24-hour period, and the ratio between nighttime and daytime diuresis. In addition, the computer prints out the number of days analyzed, the number of incontinence episodes occurring during this period, and the number of micturitions for which volume was not measured by the patient. The computer program is designed to automatically correct daytime and nighttime diuresis as well as

Table 3.3 *Basic data provided by software*

Parameter	Normal	1 SD
Day:		
Mean voided volume (ml)	2.37	67
Frequency	5.63	1.26
Diuresis (ml/min)	1.11	0.35
Corrected diuresis (ml/min)	1.11	0.35
Interval between micturitions (min)	222	60
Output (ml)	1005	497
Corrected output (ml)	1005	497
Night:		
Mean voided volume (ml)	379	132
Frequency	0.08	0.16
Diuresis (ml/min)	0.84	0.27
Corrected diuresis (ml/min)	0.84	0.27
Interval between micturitions (min)	454	50
Output (ml)	409	130
Corrected output (ml)	409	130
Output in 24 hours (ml)	1473	386
Corrected output in 24 hours (ml)	1473	386
Diuresis ratio (night/day)	0.81	0.30

Reproduced with modifications from Jolivet-Tremblay M, Schick E. The voiding diary. In: Corcos J, Schick E, eds. The urinary sphincter. New York: Marcel Dekker, 2001: 264.

the total volume voided (output per day, output per night, output per 24 h) for micturitions when volume was not measured. The mean voided volume is calculated from all recorded volumes. This mean volume is then substituted for each missing micturition volume to give the corrected output. The diuresis ratio (night/day) is derived from this corrected diuresis.[5]

To facilitate interpretation of the patient's data, the computer will print out the normal value for each parameter, along with the standard deviation (SD) and the standard normal deviation (Z-value), which is the number of SDs an observation lies away from the mean. A Z-value of 2.00 or more suggests a significant deviation from the mean[6] (Table 3.3).

Furthermore, this software is able to print a graph of the mean voided volumes over a 24-hour period as a function of time.

We have used this computer program in our urodynamic laboratory for almost 20 years, analyzing more than 2000 frequency–volume diaries.

Normal values

To determine valuable information from the parameters of the voiding diary, it is essential to know normal values.

However, surprisingly, very little data are available concerning the normal values of voiding diaries. This is an important issue because baseline values are needed to compare data from patients with different LUTS.

Children

Normal values are difficult to obtain in children, and data in the literature are sparse. Bloom et al[7] analyzed the voiding habits of 1192 children without a history of urinary tract infection. They obtained a mean frequency of about 4–5 micturitions per day. Data were obtained by questionnaire, and no frequency–volume chart was filled out.

Mattsson[8] studied 206 children, aged 7–15 years, considered asymptomatic. All of them completed a 24-hour frequency–volume chart. They voided 2–10 times a day, but 95% of them had a voiding frequency of 3–8. About 10% voided once during the night. Voided volume varied greatly, the morning voiding being the largest, and the last voiding before bedtime, the smallest. Single voided volume varied between 20 and 800 ml, with total volumes over 24 h between 325 and 2100 ml. Wan et al[9] estimated that voiding frequency for normal children was approximately 6 times daily. They used a frequency chart on which urine volume could be measured, but this was not mandatory. They found the diary particularly useful in infrequent voiding. Hellström et al,[10] studying the micturition habits of 3556 7-year-old children, found that the frequency of micturition was 3–7 per day among those without symptoms of bladder disturbance and without previous urinary tract infection.

Esperanca and Gerrard[11] determined urinary frequency in 297 normal children aged 4–14 years. The average frequency for 4 year olds was 5.3 micturitions, whereas for 12 year olds it was 4.8.

Bower et al[12] constructed nomograms for mean maximum voided volume, mean voided volume, and mean minimum voided volume for specific age groups using data obtained from 322 incontinent children, aged 6–11 years, who completed a 2-day frequency–volume chart. They noted a wide variation of voided volumes, very much as Mattsson and Lindström did in normal children.[13] Based on all these findings, frequency–volume charts by themselves seem to be an unsuitable screening tool for children.

Females

There are abundant data published about normal values on the frequency–volume charts in women. Several authors[4,5,14–16] have established normal values for healthy women. Comparison of these data is given in Table 3.4.

Table 3.4   *Data obtained from frequency–volume charts of normal females*

	Boedker et al[42] (n = 123)	Larsson and Victor[14] (n = 151)	Siltberg et al[4] (n = 151)	Saito et al[15] (n = 20)[a]	Kassis and Schick[5] (n = 33)
Mean voided volume (day) in ml				179	237 (± 67)
Mean voided volume (night) in ml		} 250 (±79)	} 240	230	379 (± 132)
Mean frequency (day)				6.8	5.63 (± 1.26)
Mean frequency (night)	} 5.7	} 5.8 (± 1.41)	} 5.5	0.5	0.08 (± 0.16)
Diuresis in ml/min (day)					1.11 (± 0.35)
Diuresis in ml/min (night)					0.84 (± 0.27)
Excreta in ml (day)				1149	1.005 (± 497)
Excreta in ml (night)				234	409 (± 130)
Diuresis per 24 hours in ml	1350	1430 (± 487)	1350	1272	1473 (± 386)
Night diuresis					
Day diuresis					0.81 (± 0.30)
Functional capacity in ml		460 (± 174)	450		

Reproduced with permission from Jolivet-Tremblay M, Schick E. The voiding diary. In: Corcos J, Schick E, eds. The urinary sphincter. New York: Marcel Dekker, 2001:266.
[a]Also includes normal males.

It was in studies done on women that authors began to analyze diurnal and nocturnal data separately. The first results were obtained by Saito et al[15] and Kassis and Schick.[5] This distiction is important because nighttime diuresis may exceed daytime diuresis and be responsible for nocturia, especially in the elderly.

On this particular subject, according to Saito et al[15] an increase in urine volume during the night can be induced by three physiological events related to aging. First, the circadian rhythm of antidiuretic hormone or atrial natriuretic hormone secretion may be abnormal.[17] Second, the glomerular filtration rate or renal plasma flow may be altered because of a reduction in the concentrating ability of the distal tubules. Finally, an impaired cardiovascular system may not be able to supply sufficient amounts of blood to the kidneys during waking hours, creating edema in the lower extremities, which becomes mobilized in the supine position.

The calculated ratio of night over day diuresis can draw attention to one of these phenomena, which is important to recognize, because its logical consequence, nocturia, has nothing to do with a vesicourethral pathology (such as outflow obstruction, unstable bladder function, etc.).

Males

For men, no precise data concerning reference values for frequency–volume charts are published to our knowledge. The study already quoted by Saito et al[15] included males and females, but did not separate them in two subgroups. One reason for this lack of data may be the difficulty in defining the clinical characteristics of a normal male without LUTS. This 'normality' probably changes with age.

Recent data from the literature suggest that in men with LUTS suggestive of BPH, the urodynamically proven obstruction is the most important factor influencing voided volumes, cystometric capacity, and residual urine volume. By contrast, voiding frequency is not significantly influenced, because patients with small voided volumes minimize their fluid intake.[18] Using a 3-day frequency–volume chart Blanker et al[19] showed that the average volume per void declined with advancing age. Nocturnal voiding frequency seems to be indicative of nocturnal urine production, but nocturnal urine production is only a modest discriminator for increased nocturnal voiding frequency. These observations indicate that in daily practice the use of nocturnal urine production to explain nocturnal voiding frequency is of little value.[20] It should also be noted that in a recent large population-based study of 1688 men, circadian urine production could only be demonstrated in men younger than 65.[21]

Duration of the chart

There are no clear guidelines in the literature on the minimum number of days necessary to produce a reliable diary. A wide range of 1–14 days exists. The gold standard for now is probably 7 days. Abrams[22] recommended a 7-day chart, Barnick and Cardozo[23] a 5-day chart, Sommer et al[24] a 3-day chart, and Larsson and Victor[14] a 48-hour chart.

Barnick and Cardozo[23] compared a 5-day chart with a 1-day chart in a group of 150 women attending a urodynamic clinic. They found a significant correlation between the two sets of results with $p < 0.0001$.

Wyman et al[25] studied a 2-week diary in 55 incontinent women, and compared the first week with the second week. They concluded that a 1-week diary is sufficient to assess the frequency of micturition and incontinence episodes. The 7-day diary can consequently be considered as the gold standard for voiding diaries. This has recently been confirmed by Homma et al.[26]

Gisolf et al[27] reported on reliability of data obtained from the 24-hour frequency–volume charts of 160 men with LUTS secondary to BPH. Their study suggested that the 24-hour chart compared favorably to 3 days or more charts and concluded that the 1-day chart provided sufficient insight into voiding habits of this group of patients. According to Matthiessen et al,[28] nocturia secondary to nocturnal polyuria can be detected by a 3-day frequency–volume chart in men with LUTS suggestive of BPH. van Melick et al[29] analyzed 2- or 3-day charts of 98 females with urodynamically proven motor urge incontinence and concluded that a single 24-hour chart is sufficient to gain insight into these patients' voiding habits. Locher et al[30] focused on the number of incontinence episodes in a group of 214 community-dwelling women, aged 40–90 years. Based on the number of days necessary to obtain an internal consistency of 0.90 for Cronbach's alpha, they estimated that a 7-day frequency–volume chart is needed to provide a stable and reliable measurement of the frequency of incontinence episodes. Nygaard and Holcomb[31] compared two 7-day diaries completed at 4-week intervals by 138 stress urinary incontinent women. They observed a good correlation for the number of incontinence episodes between the two diaries (0.831), and the results of the first 3-day diaries correlated well with the last 4-day diaries. They concluded that a 3-day diary is an appropriate outcome measure for clinical trials evaluating treatments for stress incontinence, but a 7-day diary is preferable when the number of incontinence episodes is considered. Fitzgerald and Brubaker[32] introduced a new variable in the analysis of voiding diaries: the number of micturitions per liter of intake. They estimated that this represents the most stable measure to compare two 24-hour charts.

Recently Schick et al[33] compared the standard 7-day chart to various lengths of frequency–volume charts analyzing 14 parameters. Overall results showed that a 4-day diary is almost identical to the 7-day diary. However, when the number of incontinence episodes was considered of primary importance, a 5-day diary was preferable. This reduction in duration made compliance to the voiding diary easier for the patient.

How we do it

Patients are invited to fill out a 4-day frequency–volume chart in which diurnal and nocturnal voiding is clearly identified. The patient is specifically asked to register the time and volume of each voiding as well as the time of each incontinence episode. When, for some reason, the patient is unable to measure a voided volume, he notes only the time, and puts an 'X' instead of the volume. Volume can be expressed in milliliters (ml) or in fluid ounces (fl oz), but should remain uniform throughout the chart. The back of the chart offers simple instructions for completion, with examples for the patient.

It is clinically proven that patients easily understand the elaboration of the frequency–volume chart. More than 95% of our patients fill out the chart correctly. At the beginning we offered lenghty explanations to every patient. But, with time, written instructions proved to be clear enough to forego verbal explanations. The chart can be sent out by mail, fax, or even e-mailed, so that the patient arrives for a visit with complete frequency–volume information.

Reliability of the voiding diary

To be reliable, frequency–volume charts must be filled out correctly. In an effort to verify their accuracy, Palnaes Hansen and Klarskov[34] studied 18 subjects who noted their fluid intake and voided volumes and collected 24-hour urine samples for three consecutive days. They concluded that self-reported frequency–volume chart data are valid and useful for patients with voiding symptoms.

Barnick and Cardozo[23] studied 106 consecutive patients who received a 5-day frequency–volume chart by mail, to be filled out before their physical examination. Only 40% of them completed the chart correctly for the full 5 days.

Robinson et al[35] compared two 7-day diaries in 278 incontinent women. The first was completed with minimal instructions, the second after receiving extensive instructions. They concluded that a 7-day diary remained a reliable tool to assess urinary symptoms, even if patients received minimal instructions on filling out the chart.

According to our own experience, more that 1000 patients correctly completed the frequency–volume chart without extensive verbal instructions. The fact that we allow our patients to use milliliters or fluid ounces for volume measurements is probably helpful, because older people are less familiar with the metric system. Bailey et al[36] presented results similar to our own, with most patients completing the chart correctly before their first visit.

The frequency–volume chart as a diagnostic tool

The possibility of using the frequency–volume chart as a diagnostic tool is very tempting because of its simplicity and noninvasiveness. Several authors explored this possibility. Larsson and Victor[37] compared the frequency–volume charts of 81 stress-incontinent patients with those of 151 asymptomatic women. Interestingly, all three parameters (total voided volume, frequency, and largest single voided volume) differed statistically between the two groups; however, because of marked overlapping, the frequency–volume chart was judged an unreliable diagnostic tool for stress incontinence.

Larsson et al[38] analyzed the frequency–volume chart in bladder instability, compared it with a group of women without other LUTS, and related it to cystometric findings, to evaluate the quantitative aspects of urgency incontinence. A 2-day period on a 7-day chart was evaluated. None of the parameters of the frequency–volume chart (frequency of micturition, mean voided volume, largest single voided volume, and variability in voided volumes) were useful in differentiating between motor urgency and normal voiding habits. Moreover, no correlation was found between any of the data from the frequency–volume chart and the filling phase of urodynamic studies (first desire to void, bladder volume at first unstable contraction, bladder capacity, and bladder volume at first leakage). The authors concluded that frequency–volume charts didn't help in differential diagnosis, but that mean voided volume represented a good measure of the severity of detrusor instability symptoms.

In another study, Fink et al[39] compared the 24-hour frequency–volume chart in stress-incontinent and urge-incontinent women. When applying logistic regression to these two groups, the frequency of micturition during nighttime was the parameter that best discriminated between these medical conditions. Mean voided volume (over the 24-hour period) showed the highest differentiating power with $p < 0.0001$, but the large overlap between groups limited the value of the frequency–volume chart for differential diagnosis.

More recently, Siltberg et al[4] proposed a nomogram on which the frequency of micturition was plotted against the range of voided volumes. According to these authors, this plot could be used to select the degree of certainty (with 10% intervals for probability) of having motor urgency incontinence vs stress incontinence. Tincello and Richmond[40] tested this nomogram in 216 patients: for detrusor instability, it had a sensitivity of 52% and a specificity of 70%; for genuine stress incontinence, the sensitivity and specificity were 66% and 65%, respectively. They concluded that formal cystometric evaluation was necessary in incontinent females because the nomogram did not provide enough diagnostic information.

These observations are not really surprising. It seems simplistic to attempt characterization of such different complex physiopathological entities as continence and voiding with a single parameter: in this case, the frequency–volume chart. Nonetheless, this diagnostic tool remains an important element in our understanding of patient symptomatology and still one of the first tests to choose because it is easy to complete and it can be repeated later to assess the results of therapy.

Interpretation of frequency–volume charts

In our department, the computer software we described above analyzes every frequency–volume chart filled out by a patient. The most important parameters in the clinical setting are the frequency of micturition (day and night), 24-hour urinary output, the ratio of nighttime diuresis to daytime diuresis, and the mean voided volume (day and night). The hour-by-hour distribution is also very helpful.

Normal frequency–volume chart

Table 3.5 represents the results of a 3-day frequency–volume chart filled out by a 42-year-old lady who was referred because of incontinence. Three voided volumes were not recorded, representing 14.29% of the total number of micturitions during this 3-day period. The 24-hour corrected urinary output was within normal limits (1462 ml; Z-value: (0.03)), as well as the night/day diuresis ratio (0.73; Z-value: (0.28)). Daytime frequency (7.00; Z-value: 1.09) and nighttime frequency (0.00; Z-value: (0.50)) were almost within normal limits. Figure 3.1 illustrates the graphic representation of voidings and the mean voided volumes during a 24-hour period. The greatest single voided volume (480 ml), which represents in this example the daytime functional bladder capacity, was registered at 07:00 h. No micturition occurred between midnight and 07:00 h, and between 13:00 h and 16:00 h.

Table 3.5 *Normal frequency–volume chart (for details see text)*

Parameter	Patient's data (±1 SD)	Normal (±1 SD)	Z-value
Day:			
Mean voided volume (ml)	187 (72)	237 (±67)	(0.75)
Voiding frequency	7.00 (0.00)	5.63 (±1.26)	1.09
Diuresis (ml/min)	0.97	1.11 (±0.35)	(0.39)
Corrected diuresis (ml/min)	1.17	1.11 (±0.35)	0.17
Interval between micturitions (min)	192 (601)	222 (±60)	(0.50)
Output (ml)	935 (92)	1005 (±497)	(0.14)
Corrected output (ml)	1122 (92)	1005 (±497)	0.24
Maximal voided volume (ml)	480		
Night:			
Mean voided volume (ml)	340 (18)	379 (±132)	(0.30)
Voiding frequency	0.00	0.08 (±0.16)	(0.50)
Diuresis (ml/min)	0.71	0.84 (±0.27)	(0.49)
Corrected diuresis (ml/min)	0.71	0.84 (±0.27)	(0.49)
Interval between micturition (ml)	480 (0)	454 (±50)	0.52
Output (ml)	340 (102)	409 (±130)	(0.53)
Corrected output (ml)	340 (102)	409 (±130)	(0.53)
Maximal voided volume (ml)	0.00		
Output in 24 hours (ml)	1275	1473 (±386)	(0.51)
Corrected output in 24 hours (ml)	1462	1473 (±386)	(0.03)
Diuresis ratio (night/day)	0.73	0.81 (±0.3)	(0.28)

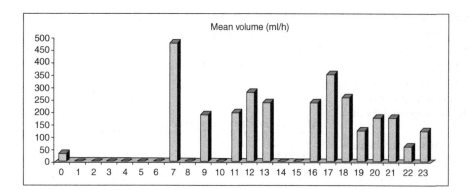

Figure 3.1
Graphic representation of a normal frequency–volume chart.

Increased 24-hour output (polyuria)

This type of voiding diary is relatively common and can be seen in patients with unbalanced diabetes or simple potomania of different magnitude.

This 45-year-old female consulted with symptoms suggestive of mixed urinary incontinence. She reported voiding about 20 times a day and 4–6 times at night. She complained of a sensation of incomplete emptying. Endoscopy revealed a bladder capacity of 300 ml and a post-void residual urine of 120 ml. The bladder wall was trabeculated, grade II. Gynecological examination showed a grade II anterior vaginal wall prolapse, resulting from a lateral defect. The Q-tip test demonstrated a 25° urethral mobility (normal <30°). No urinary incontinence could be observed during cough in the supine position. On multi-channel urodynamics, bladder capacity was 750 ml and the first desire to void occurred at 262 ml. Bladder wall compliance was normal. Maximum urethral closure pressure was 65 cmH$_2$O and the cough leak-point pressure was negative. No uninhibited detrusor contractions could be detected during the filling phase, but a strong post-void contraction was registered which, in view of the clinical symptoms, was considered as a manifestation of unstable bladder.

The frequency–volume chart (Table 3.6) showed a tremendous increase in the corrected 24-hour urinary output (12,591 ml!) with a normal night/day diuresis ratio (0.91; Z-value: 0.33). Daytime voiding frequency was 18.71, not because of a decrease in mean voided volumes (494 ml; Z-value: 3.83), but due to an important daytime diuresis (8746 ml; Z-value: 15.58). Nighttime diuresis was even more pronounced (3845 ml; Z-value: 26.43). In spite of this, voiding frequency was increased to a lesser degree (3.00; Z-value: 18.25), mainly because the mean nocturnal voided volume also increased (961 ml; Z-value: 4.41). The mean hourly voided volume (Figure 3.2) reflects the difference in mean voided volumes for nighttime and daytime.

Nocturnal polyuria

A 69-year-old female consulted because of urgency and increased frequency. She claimed hourly micturitions during the day and 5–6 voidings each night. She was enuretic until the age of 9. Endoscopy revealed grade II bladder trabeculation associated with a cystoscopic capacity of 400 ml. Urodynamic study demonstrated an unstable bladder with the first uninhibited contraction occurring at 60 ml. Cystometric capacity was 175 ml and the first desire to void occurred at 62 ml.

Her 7-day frequency–volume chart (Table 3.7) showed a slight increase in the 24-hour corrected output (1961 ml; Z-value: 1.15), but a significantly increased night/day ratio (4.66; Z-value: 12.84). Her daytime frequency was somewhat increased (7.43; Z-value: 1.43), but clearly less than the claimed frequency reported during the initial interview. Note that the decreased mean daytime voided volume (99 ml; Z-value: (2.06)) is not very different from the bladder volume at the first desire to void (62 ml) and the appearance of the first uninhibited detrusor contraction (60 ml). The chart confirms the significantly increased nighttime frequency (5.14; Z-value: 31.64), accompanied by a decreased mean voided volume (208 ml; Z-value: (1.29)).

On the graphical representation (Figure 3.3) one can easily see the predominantly nocturnal diuresis with the maximal functional capacity (325.31 ml) occurring during the second part of the night (04:00 h).

Sensory urgency

A 73-year-old female patient complained of stress urinary incontinence but also experienced incontinence episodes which were not associated with stress or urgency. Cystometric capacity was 800 ml with no post-void residual urine. Her bladder was stable on multichannel urodynamics. Abdominal leak-point pressure was estimated between

Table 3.6 *Increased 24-hour output (polyuria) (for details see text)*

Parameter	Patient's data (±1 SD)	Normal (±1 SD)	Z-value
Day:			
Mean voided volume (ml)	494 (205)	237 (±67)	3.83
Voiding frequency	18.71 (1075)	5.63 (±1.26)	10.38
Diuresis (ml/min)	8.82	1.11 (±0.35)	22.02
Corrected diuresis (ml/min)	9.11	1.11 (±0.35)	22.86
Interval between micturitions (min)	56 (222)	222 (±60)	(2.77)
Output (ml)	8464 (864)	1005 (±497)	15.01
Corrected output (ml)	8746 (1086)	1005 (±497)	15.58
Maximal voided volume (ml)	1350		
Night:			
Mean voided volume (ml)	961 (212)	379 (±132)	4.41
Voiding frequency	3.00 (0.00)	0.08 (±0.16)	18.25
Diuresis (ml/min)	8.01	0.84 (±0.27)	26.56
Corrected diuresis (ml/min)	8.01	0.84 (±0.27)	26.56
Interval between micturition (ml)	120 (185)	454 (±50)	(6.68)
Output (ml)	3845 (617)	409 (±130)	26.43
Corrected output (ml)	3845 (617)	409 (±130)	26.43
Maximal voided volume (ml)	1380		
Output in 24 hours (ml)	12,309	1473 (±386)	28.07
Corrected output in 24 hours (ml)	12,591	1473 (±386)	28.80
Diuresis ratio (night/day)	0.91	0.81 (±0.3)	0.33

Table 3.7 *Nocturnal polyuria (for details see text)*

Parameter	Patient's data (±1 SD)	Normal (±1 SD)	Z-value
Day:			
Mean voided volume (ml)	99 (48)	237 (±67)	(2.06)
Voiding frequency	7.43 (1.18)	5.63 (±1.26)	1.43
Diuresis (ml/min)	0.56	1.11 (±0.35)	(1.57)
Corrected diuresis (ml/min)	0.66	1.11 (±0.35)	(1.28)
Interval between micturitions (min)	177 (436)	222 (±60)	(0.75)
Output (ml)	537 (190)	1005 (±497)	(0.94)
Corrected output (ml)	635 (145)	1005 (±497)	(0.74)
Maximal voided volume (ml)	295.74		
Night:			
Mean voided volume (ml)	208 (64)	379 (±132)	(1.29)
Voiding frequency	5.14 (0.83)	0.08 (±0.16)	31.64
Diuresis (ml/min)	2.61	0.84 (±0.27)	6.54
Corrected diuresis (ml/min)	2.67	0.84 (±0.27)	6.77
Interval between micturition (ml)	80 (209)	454 (±50)	(7.48)
Output (ml)	1251 (103)	409 (±130)	6.47
Corrected output (ml)	1280 (156)	409 (±130)	6.70
Maximal voided volume (ml)	325.31		
Output in 24 hours (ml)	1787	1473 (±386)	0.81
Corrected output in 24 hours (ml)	1916	1473 (±386)	1.15
Diuresis ratio (night/day)	4.66	0.81 (±0.3)	12.84

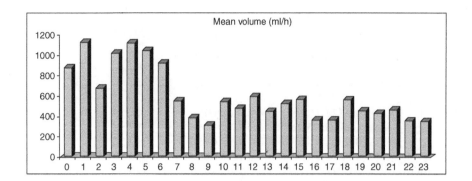

Figure 3.2
Graphic representation of the frequency–volume chart of a patient with an increased 24-hour output (polyuria).

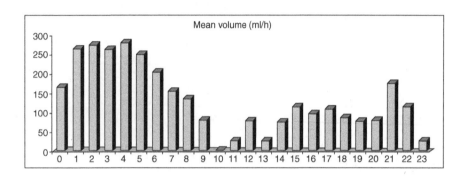

Figure 3.3
Graphic representation of the frequency–volume chart of a patient with significant nocturnal polyuria.

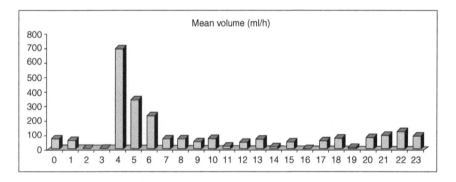

Figure 3.4
Graphic representation of the frequency–volume chart of a patient with sensory urgency.

100 and 150 cmH$_2$O, a grade III urethral incompetence,[41] explaining the clinical symptom of stress urinary incontinence.

Her 7-day frequency–volume chart (Table 3.8) demonstrated a 24-hour corrected urine output (1784 ml; Z-value 0.81) within normal limits. There was some degree of nocturnal polyuria (693 ml; Z-value: 2.18). Mean urinary frequency was 14.14 during daytime and 1.86 during nighttime, with mean voided volumes of 83 and 243 ml, respectively (Figure 3.4). The functional bladder capacity was 395.74 ml in daytime and 709.77 ml during the night. This significant difference between mean voided volumes in the absence of an unstable bladder suggested sensory urgency.

Effect of neuromodulation

A 29-year-old female was investigated because of significant increase in day and night urinary frequency,

associated with urgency, but she did not complain of incontinence. She claimed daytime voidings every 20 min and about 15 micturitions per night. Endoscopy was unremarkable, the cystoscopic capacity being 250 ml. Multichannel urodynamics failed to reveal uninhibited detrusor contractions during the filling phase. Cystometric capacity was 220 ml and the first desire to void occurred at a 42 ml volume in the bladder. The urethra was hypertonic (maximal urethral closing pressure: 104 cmH$_2$O).

The 7-day frequency–volume chart (Table 3.9) showed a normal 24-hour corrected urine output (1267 ml; Z-value: (0.53)) and a normal night/day diuresis ratio (0.50; Z-value: (1.04)). There was a very important decrease in the mean daytime (40 ml; Z-value: (2.94)) and nighttime (50 ml; Z-value: (2.49)) voided volumes. The voiding frequency was 25.57 during the day, and 4.71 during the night. The functional bladder capacity was 110.00 ml and 80.00 ml, respectively. Graphic representation exhibits almost constant mean voided volumes throughout the 24-hour period (Figure 3.5).

Table 3.8 *Sensory urgency (for details see text)*

Parameter	Patient's data (±1 SD)	Normal (±1 SD)	Z-value
Day:			
Mean voided volume (ml)	83 (63)	237 (±67)	(2.30)
Voiding frequency	14.14 (1.55)	5.63 (±1.26)	6.76
Diuresis (ml/min)	0.90	1.11 (±0.35)	(0.59)
Corrected diuresis (ml/min)	1.14	1.11 (±0.35)	0.08
Interval between micturitions (min)	92 (413)	222 (±60)	(2.17)
Output (ml)	866 (256)	1005 (±497)	(0.28)
Corrected output (ml)	1092 (237)	1005 (±497)	0.17
Maximal voided volume (ml)	295.74		
Night:			
Mean voided volume (ml)	243 (197)	379 (±132)	(1.03)
Voiding frequency	1.86 (0.35)	0.08 (±0.16)	11.11
Diuresis (ml/min)	1.44	0.84 (±0.27)	2.24
Corrected diuresis (ml/min)	1.44	0.84 (±0.27)	2.24
Interval between micturition (ml)	168 (203)	454 (±50)	(5.72)
Output (ml)	693 (243)	409 (±130)	2.18
Corrected output (ml)	693 (243)	409 (±130)	2.18
Maximal voided volume (ml)	709.77		
Output in 24 hours (ml)	1559	1473 (±386)	0.22
Corrected output in 24 hours (ml)	1784	1473 (±386)	0.81
Diuresis ratio (night/day)	1.60	0.81 (±0.3)	2.63

Table 3.9 *Pre-neuromodulation (for details see text)*

Parameter	Patient's data (±1 SD)	Normal (±1 SD)	Z-value
Day:			
Mean voided volume (ml)	40	237 (±67)	(2.94)
Voiding frequency	25.57	5.63 (±1.26)	15.83
Diuresis (ml/min)	0.98	1.11 (±0.35)	(0.37)
Corrected diuresis (ml/min)	1.02	1.11 (±0.35)	(0.25)
Interval between micturitions (min)	41	222 (±60)	(3.02)
Output (ml)	943	1005 (±497)	(0.13)
Corrected output (ml)	983	1005 (±497)	(0.04)
Maximal voided volume (ml)	110		
Night:			
Mean voided volume (ml)	50	379 (±132)	(2.49)
Voiding frequency	4.71	0.08 (±0.16)	28.96
Diuresis (ml/min)	0.49	0.84 (±0.27)	(1.30)
Corrected diuresis (ml/min)	0.59	0.84 (±0.27)	(0.92)
Interval between micturition (ml)	102	454 (±50)	(7.04)
Output (ml)	234	409 (±130)	(1.34)
Corrected output (ml)	284	409 (±130)	(0.96)
Maximal voided volume (ml)	80.00		
Output in 24 hours (ml)	1177	1473 (±386)	(0.77)
Corrected output in 24 hours (ml)	1267	1473 (±386)	(0.53)
Diuresis ratio (night/day)	0.50	0.81 (±0.3)	(1.04)

Dramatic changes were observed in the different parameters of the frequency–volume chart during percutaneous nerve stimulation (Table 3.10). Despite an increase in the corrected 24-hour urinary output (1623 ml; Z-value: 0.39), the night/day ratio did not change (0.43; Z-value: 0.39). The mean daytime voided volume increased significantly (184 ml; Z-value: (0.79)), as did the mean nighttime voided volume (219 ml; Z-value: (1.21)). Nocturia almost completely disappeared (0.29; Z-value: 1.29), as can also be seen in Figure 3.6. (Note the difference in the y-axis scale between Figures 3.5 and 3.6.) Daytime frequency was reduced by 60% (8.29;

Z-value: 2.11). Functional bladder capacity also increased significantly.

Conclusion

This overview of the literature on voiding diaries as well as our own experience leads us to the following conclusions.

Frequency–volume charts are an invaluable and indispensable tool in the investigation of LUTS patients and in understanding their symptoms. Interpretation of the

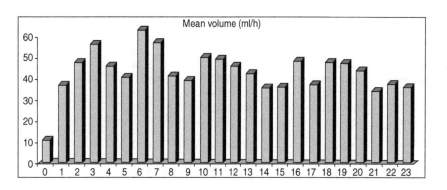

Figure 3.5
Graphic representation of the frequency–volume chart of a patient before testing for neuromodulation.

Table 3.10 *Per-neuromodulation (for details see text)*

Parameter	Patient's data (±1 SD)	Normal (±1 SD)	Z-value
Day:			
Mean voided volume (ml)	184 (73)	237 (±67)	(0.79)
Voiding frequency	8.29 (1.67)	5.63 (±1.26)	2.11
Diuresis (ml/min)	1.21	1.11 (±0.35)	0.27
Corrected diuresis (ml/min)	1.40	1.11 (±0.35)	0.82
Interval between micturitions (min)	153 (506)	222 (±60)	(1.15)
Output (ml)	1158 (371)	1005 (±497)	0.31
Corrected output (ml)	1342 (371)	1005 (±497)	0.68
Maximal voided volume (ml)	400.00		
Night:			
Mean voided volume (ml)	219 (15)	379 (±132)	(1.21)
Voiding frequency	0.29 (1.70)	0.08 (±0.16)	1.29
Diuresis (ml/min)	0.52	0.84 (±0.27)	(1.18)
Corrected diuresis (ml/min)	0.59	0.84 (±0.27)	(0.94)
Interval between micturition (ml)	420 (660)	454 (±50)	(0.68)
Output (ml)	250 (134)	409 (±130)	(1.22)
Corrected output (ml)	281 (199)	409 (±130)	(0.98)
Maximal voided volume (ml)	200.00		
Output in 24 hours (ml)	1408	1473 (±386)	(0.17)
Corrected output in 24 hours (ml)	1623	1473 (±386)	0.39
Diuresis ratio (night/day)	0.43	0.81 (±0.3)	(1.26)

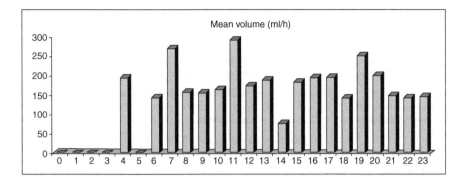

Figure 3.6
Graphic representation of the frequency–volume chart of the same patient as in figure 3.5, but during neuromodulation.

results is greatly simplified by simple computer software. The commercial unavailability of such software may explain why these charts are not more popular. Now, in many research protocols, small user-friendly computers are used to ease the completion of frequency–volume charts.

Normal values for women are well known. However, more research should be done to study voiding diaries in children. Reference values for men are desperately needed.

Although the 7-day diary is currently considered the gold standard, comparative studies have begun to determine whether the minimum number of days for a frequency–volume chart completion could be less than 7 and still maintain reliability.

The voiding diary is a precious diagnostic tool, but it cannot guarantee a precise diagnosis. Because of the complex nature of LUT dysfunction, it has become evident that frequency–volume charts will never replace urodynamic studies.

In addition to their value as a diagnostic tool, frequency–volume charts play an important role in evaluating the success of a surgical intervention (i.e. neuromodulation) or during follow-up of medical therapy.

In summary, the frequency–volume chart, although frequently overlooked, is a simple, objective, and noninvasive test for evaluating the function of the lower urinary tract.

References

1. Abrams P, Klevmark B. Frequency-volume charts: an indispensable part of lower urinary tract assessment. Scand J Urol Nephrol Suppl 1996; 179:47–53.

2. Abrams P, Cardozo L, Fall M, et al. The standardisation of terminology of lower urinary tract function: report from the standardisation sub-committee of the International Continence Society. Neurourol Urodyn 2002; 21:167–178.

3. McCormack M, Infante-Rivard C, Schick E. Agreement between clinical methods of measurement of frequency- and functional bladder capacity. Br J Urol 1992; 69:17–21.

4. Siltberg H, Larsson G, Victor A. Frequency/volume chart: the basic tool for investigating urinary symptoms. Acta Obstet Gynecol Scand 1997; 76(Suppl 166):24–27.

5. Kassis A, Schick E. Frequency-volume chart pattern in a healthy female population. Br J Urol 1993; 72:708–710.

6. Duncan RC, Knapp RG, Miller MC III. Introductory biostatistics for the health sciences. New York: John Wiley & Sons, 1977.

7. Bloom DA, Seeley WW, Ritchey ML, McGuire EJ. Toilet habits and continence in children: an opportunity sampling in search of normal parameters. J Urol 1993; 149:1087–1090.

8. Mattsson SH. Voiding frequency, volumes and intervals in healthy schoolchildren. Scand J Urol Nephrol 1994; 28:1–11.

9. Wan J, Kaplinsky R, Greenfield S. Toilet habits of children evaluated for urinary tract infection. J Urol 1995; 154:797–799.

10. Hellström AL, Hanson E, Hansson S, et al. Micturition habits and incontinence in 7-year-old Swedish school entrant. Eur J Pediatr 1990; 149:434–437.

11. Esperanca M, Gerrard JW. Nocturnal enuresis: studies in bladder function in normal children and enuretics. Can Med Ass J 1969; 101:324–327.

12. Bower WF, Moore KH, Adams RD, Shepherd RB. Frequency–volume chart data from incontinent children. Br J Urol 1997; 80:658–662.

13. Mattsson S, Lindström S. Diuresis and voiding pattern in healthy schoolchildren. Br J Urol 1995; 76:783–789.

14. Larsson G, Victor A. Micturition patterns in a healthy female population, studied with a frequency/volume chart. Scand J Urol Nephrol (Suppl 114) 1988; 114:53–57.

15. Saito M, Kondo A, Kato T, Yamada Y. Frequency-volume charts comparison of frequency between elderly and adult patients. Br J Urol 1993; 72:38–41.

16. Bodega A, Lendorf A, H-Nielsen A, Ghahn B. Micturition pattern assessed by the frequency/volume chart in a healthy population of men and women. Neurourol Urodynam 1989; 8:421–422.

17. Matthiesen TB, Rittig S, Norgaard JP, et al. Nocturnal polyuria and natriuresis in male patients with nocturia and lower urinary tract symptoms. J Urol 1996; 156:1292–1299.

18. Van Venrooij GE, Eckhardt MD, Boon TA. Data from frequency-volume charts versus maximum free flow rate, residual volume, and voiding cystometric estimated urethral obstruction grade and detrusor contractility in men with lower urinary tract symptoms suggestive of benign prostatic hyperplasia. Neurourol Urodyn 2002; 21:450–456.

19. Blanker MH, Groeneveld FP, Bohnen AM, et al. Voided volumes: normal values and relation to lower urinary tract symptoms in elderly men: a community-based study. Urology 2001; 57:1093–1098.

20. Blanker MH, Bernsen RM, Bosch JL, et al. Relation between nocturnal voiding frequency and nocturnal urine production in older men: a population-based study. Urology 2002; 60:612–616.

21. Blanker MH, Bernsen RM, Ruud Bosch JL, et al. Normal values and determinants of circadian urine production in older men: a population-based study. J Urol 2002; 168:1453–1457.

22. Abrams P. Urodynamics, 2nd edn. London: Springer-Verlag, 1997.

23. Barnick C, Cardozo L. Unpublished data quoted by Barnick C. In: Cardozo L, ed. Urogynecology. London: Churchill Livingstone, 1997:101–107.

24. Sommer P, Bauer T, Nielsen KK, et al. Voiding patterns and prevalence of incontinence in women. A questionnaire survey. Br J Urol 1990; 66:12–15.

25. Wyman JF, Choi SC, Harkins SW, et al. The urinary diary in evaluation of incontinent women. A test-retest analysis. Obstet Gynecol 1988; 71:812–817.

26. Homma Y, Ando T, Yoshida M, et al. Voiding and incontinence frequencies: variability of diary data and required diary length. Neurourol Urodyn 2002; 21:204–209.

27. Gisolf KW, van Venrooij GE, Eckhardt MD, Boon TA. Analysis and reliability of data from 24-hour frequency-volume charts in men with lower urinary tract symptoms due to benign prostatic hyperplasia. Eur Urol 2000; 38:45–52.

28. Matthiessen TB, Rittig S, Mortensen JT, Djurhuus JC. Nocturia and polyuria in men referred with lower urinary tract symptoms, assessed using a 7-day frequency-volume chart. BJU Int 1999; 83:1017–1022.

29. Van Melick HH, Gisolf KW, Ecjhardt MD, et al. One 24-hour frequency-volume chart in a woman with objective urinary motor urge incontinence is sufficient. Urology 2001; 58:188–192.

30. Locher JL, Goode PS, Roth DL, et al. Reliability assessment of the bladder diary for urinary incontinence in older women. J Gerontol A Biol Sci Med Sci 2001; 56:M32–M35.

31. Nygaard I, Holcomb R. Reproducibility of the seven-day voiding diary in women with stress urinary incontinence. Int Urogynecol J Pelvic Floor Dysfunc 2000; 11:15–17.

32. Fitzgerald MP, Brubaker L. Variability of 24-hour voiding diary variables among asymptomatic women. J Urol 2003; 169:207–209.

33. Schick E, Jolivet-Tremblay M, Dupont C, et al. Frequency-volume chart: the minimum number of days required to obtain reliable results. Neurourol Urodyn 2003; 22:92–96.

34. Palnaes Hansen C, Klarskov P. The accuracy of the frequency-volume chart: comparison of self-reported and measured volumes. Br J Urol 1998; 81:709–711.

35. Robinson D, McGlish DK, Wyman JF, et al. Comparison between urinary diaries completed with and without intensive patient instructions. Neurourol Urodynam 1996; 15:143–148.

36. Bailey R, Shepherd A, Trike B. How much information can be obtained from frequency-volume charts? Neurourol Urodynam 1990; 9:382–385.

37. Larsson G, Victor A. The frequency-volume chart in genuine stress incontinent women. Neurourol Urodynam 1992; 11:23–31.

38. Larsson G, Abrams P, Victor A. The frequency-volume chart in detrusor instability. Neurourol Urodynam 1991; 10:533–543.

39. Fink D, Perucchini D, Schaer GN, Haller U. The role of the frequency-volume chart in the differential diagnosis of female urinary incontinence. Acta Obstet Gynecol Scand 1999; 78:254–257.

40. Tincello DG, Richmond DH. The Larsson frequency/volume chart is not a substitute for cystometry in the investigation of women with urinary incontinence. Int Urogynecol J Pelvic Floor Dysfunct 1998; 9:391–396.

41. Schick E. The objective assessment of the resistance of the female urethra to stress: a scale to establish the degree of urethral incompetence. Urology 1985; 26:518–526.

42. Boedker A, Lendorf A, H-Nielsen A, Ghahn B. Micturition pattern assessed by the frequency/volume chart in a healthy population of men and women. Neurourol Urodyn 1989; 8:421–422.

4

The pad test

Martine Jolivet-Tremblay and Erik Schick

Introduction

Incontinence is not easy to quantify from patient interviews or clinical examinations.[1] Urinary incontinence, as defined by the International Continence Society (ICS) in 1988 is involuntary urine loss that is a social or hygienic problem.[2] This definition has been recently modified[3] to state simply that 'urinary incontinence is the complaint of any involuntary leakage of urine'. This modification became necessary because the previous definition related to a complaint on quality of life issues. Quality of life instruments have been and are being developed in order to assess the impact of both incontinence and other lower urinary tract symptoms on patients.[4] The importance of this condition, as perceived by the patient, differs widely from one individual to another. Some patients cannot accept the loss of a few drops of urine happening only during some specific, often limited, circumstance, whereas others wear diapers for years before seeking medical advice.

The role of the pad-weighing test is to quantify urine loss. It is the best available instrument for this purpose. However, it does not evaluate the impact a given degree of incontinence has on the patient's quality of life. The Urodynamic Society recommended the use of the pad-weighing test in the pre-treatment evaluation of incontinent patients as well as their post-treatment evaluation at each follow-up visit.[5] However, the Urodynamic Society did not specify the type of pad test to be used. On the other hand, the Agency for Health Care Policy and Research of the US Department of Health and Human Services did not mention the pad test for the identification and evaluation of urinary incontinence.[6] It is a tool that can be used for specific issues during the diagnostic process.

Discrimination between continence and incontinence

Because perineal pads absorb perspiration, vaginal discharge, etc., results should be interpreted with caution. It is important to determine an upper limit of weight gain by a pad in continent subjects before interpreting pad test results.

Many authors have investigated this issue (Table 4.1). Usually, the extra-urinary weight increase will be directly proportional to the length of the test. In the protocol described by Hahn and Fall,[7] the length of the exercise program is very brief. Each and every gram of increase in the pad weight is considered a urine loss. Continent patients show no pad weight increase at the end of the test. Conversely, Griffiths et al,[8] investigating elderly patients for 10 days, considered a diagnosis of urinary incontinence only if pad weight exceeded 10 g per 24 hours.

The majority of authors estimate that during a 1-hour test the upper limit of pad weight gain in continent subjects is close to 1 g, whereas during a 24-hour test it is between 4 and 10 g, with an upper limit of 15 g in 24 hours. According to these authors, a weight gain of more than 1 g in a single pad or 8 g in 24 hours may be considered significant. It should be remembered, nonetheless, that weight gains less than the above-mentioned limits do not exclude incontinence, and supplementary investigations may be necessary to confirm the diagnosis.[9]

Nygaard and Zmolek[10] carefully assessed the reproducibility of three comparable exercise protocols, their relationship with voided volume, and Pyridium® (phenazopyridine) staining in 14 continent volunteers. The average pad weight gain during these three sessions was 3.19 g ($\pm$ 3.16 g), with a range of 0.1–12.4 g. Because of the huge difference between subjects, they were unable to find a distinct cut-off value differentiating continence from incontinence. Similar experiences have been reported by others.[11] Adding Pyridium® (phenazopyridine) did not improve the specificity of the test.

Types of pad tests

Pad tests can primarily be divided into two groups: qualitative tests and quantitative tests.

Table 4.1 *Discrimination between continence and incontinence*

Length of test	Authors	Suggested value for continence	Comments
No time limit	Hahn and Fall[7]	0 g	–
40 min	Martin et al[53]	<2 g	(with 75% of cystometric capacity)
1 hour	Kroman-Andersen et al[43]	≤1 g	–
	Sutherst et al[1]	1 g	–
	Versi and Cardozo[54]	<0.94 g	–
	Ali et al[48]	<0.5 g	–
2 hours	Walsh and Mills[55]	1.2 g (∀1.35 g)/2 hours	
24 hours	Mouritzen et al[51]	<5 g/24 hours	
	Lose et al[49]	4 g/24 hours	(max: 8 g)
	Versi et al[47]	7.13 g (∀4.32 g)/24 hours	(95% upper confidence level <15)
	Griffiths et al[8]	≤10 g/24 hours	

Reproduced with permission from Schick E, Jolivet-Tremblay M. Detection and quantification of urine loss: the pad-weighing test. In: Corcos J, Schick E, eds. The urinary sphincter. New York: Marcel Dekker, 2001:276.

Qualitative tests

The qualitative test uses a substance to color urine orange: e.g. phenazopyridine (Pyridium), 200 mg three times a day. The patient is invited to wear hygienic pads and replace them periodically during normal daily activities. The degree of coloration on the pads is an assessment of incontinence.[12] This test is especially beneficial to document an insignificant urine loss which, however, may be quite bothersome for the patient, or when vaginal secretions cannot be differentiated easily from urinary incontinence.

A further approach has been suggested by Mayne and Hilton,[13] who compared the distal urethral electrical conductance test (DUEC) with weighed perineal pads and discovered that the DUEC was extremely sensitive at detecting leakage (sensitivity 97%). Janez et al[14] reported similar observations.

Quantitative tests

One of the initial efforts to quantify urine loss, interestingly, involved an electric device, the so-called Urilos system, designed by James et al.[15] It incorporates a pad containing dry electrodes. The urinary electrolytes alter the capacitance of the aluminum strip electrodes in the pad proportionally to the quantity of urine. Stanton and coworkers[16,17] investigated this device in greater detail. They noticed problems with reproducibility in different groups. In a group of 26 women exhibiting symptoms of urinary incontinence with a negative stress test 9 proved leakage. In a further group of 30 patients with symptoms of stress incontinence, one-third had a negative clinical stress test, but presented leakage with the Urilos system. Eadie et al[18]

concluded that the system was beneficial to confirm patient histories, in spite of the fact that it was laborious to achieve a quantitative measure of urine loss, particularly for volumes greater than 50 ml when the error range reached 35%. Presumably because of a lack of reliability, this device never gained wide acceptance.

A more efficient approach to the quantification of urine loss is to weigh perineal pads after different lengths of time during which patients are requested to execute standardized activities. This approach has resulted in a relatively large number of publications in which authors have experimented with various test durations, with or without different exercise protocols, in an attempt to define the optimal combination of reproducibility, reliability, and practicality.[19]

Patient populations
Children

Rare reports can be found in the literature on the use of pad tests in the pediatric population.

Hellström et al[20] compared a 2-hour pad test on the ward (with standardized activities and provoked diuresis) with a 12-hour pad test completed in the home environment. Both tests were similar in the detection of urine loss (68 and 70%, respectively), but the detection rate increased in about 10% of the 105 patients when fluid provocation was included in the home pad test.

Imada et al[21] studied 23 incontinent children with a 1-hour pad test, as recommended by the ICS,[1] and compared the results with an interval test during which the pad was utilized between three successive voidings and then weighed. They concluded that the interval test validates the clinical symptoms more appropriately than the 1-hour test. They advocated the former for the objective evaluation of urinary incontinence in children.

Adults

Many reports on the pad-weighing test for adults have been published in the literature: they vary mainly in the length of time the pad was employed. The short tests last 1 or 2 hours,[22–31] and are generally associated with a standardized exercise or activity program, but there can also be no time limit imposed with only an exercise protocol to follow.[7,32,33] The longer tests go from 12 hours up to 10 days.[8,34–38] Various authors compared tests of different lengths[29–31] or tests done in different environments.[39]

Exercise protocol without a fixed time schedule

The provocative pad test designed by Hahn and Fall[7] involved a sequence of exercises with the bladder filled to half of its cystometric capacity. The test–retest correlation was good ($r = 0.940$). The test takes about 20 min to complete. In control groups of clinically continent females, urine loss at the end of the exercise schedule was 0 g. They advocated the use of this test in incontinent females. However, because urge symptoms emerge at irregular intervals and sometimes in particular situations in patients with bladder instability, a test of longer duration, for example 24 hours, seems to be more reliable.

Mayne and Hilton,[32] after filling the bladder with 250 ml of normal saline solution, compared a short pad test program with a 1-hour test in the same population. They could not find a notable difference between the two protocols.

Miller et al[33] suggested the paper towel test to quantify urine loss associated with stress. After three deep coughs, the authors estimated the amount of urine loss by the wet area on a tri-folded paper towel placed on the perineal region. They found the test to be simple, with good test–retest reliability. They recommended its use for losses less than 10 ml because the paper towel becomes saturated with volumes exceeding 15 ml.

More recently, Persson et al[40] proposed a rapid perineal pad test with a standardized bladder volume (300 ml) and a standardized physical activity of only 1 min. They found the test reproducibility and feasibility acceptable, making it suitable for follow-up studies.

The 1-hour test

The 1-hour test is the most extensively studied, since it was recommended by the Standardisation Committee of the ICS.[1]

Several authors have examined the reproducibility and reliability of this test. Klarskov and Hald[25] found the test to be reproducible and reliable when compared with subjective daytime incontinence. Jorgensen et al[28] advocated its reproducibility, particularly when bladder volume at the beginning of the test and diuresis during the test were taken into consideration ($r = 0.93$; $p < 0.0001$). When the test was achieved with a standardized bladder volume, the test–retest results were even superior ($r = 0.97$; $p < 0.001$), although personal variations of up to ± 24 g were noted.[30]

Mayne and Hilton[32] accomplished the test with 250 ml of fluid in the bladder. Lose et al[26] filled the bladder up to 50% of its cystometric capacity, whereas Kinn and Larsson[41] favored 75%.

The sensitivity of the test (i.e. the proportion of patients with incontinence who have a positive result) varies between 58 and 81%. Its positive predictive values (i.e. the probability of a patient with a positive test being incontinent), which is more relevant to clinical practice, is over 90%. The false-negative rate (i.e. incontinent patients with a negative pad test), nonetheless, is quite high (19–56.8%) (Table 4.2).

More recently Simons et al[42] compared two 1-hour tests performed with natural diuresis, 1 week apart. They concluded that, with similar bladder volumes, the test–retest reliability was clinically inadequate, as the first and second pad test could differ by −44 to +66 g.

It appears that the 1-hour test proposed by the ICS is not optimal, and its reliability is weak.[43] This can be improved when bladder volume at the beginning and during the test is known and standardized.

The 2-hour test

Some authors proposed extending the test to 2 hours because they felt that its exactitude might be improved. The patient is asked to drink a given amount of water as quickly as feasible at the beginning of the first hour to induce a constant level of diuresis. The pad test itself starts at the second hour and involves a fixed exercise protocol. Richmond et al[31] studied two groups of incontinent patients who were submitted to the same protocol, except that the exercise sequence varied. They found that the sequence in which exercises were accomplished did not affect the overall identification of incontinent patients. They estimated that the ideal length of the test was 2 hours. Haylen et al[44] reached the same conclusions. Eadie et al,[45] comparing the 2-hour pad test with the Urilos system, demonstrated that the 2-hour test did not produce reproducible results, and confirmed that it was difficult to obtain quantitative measures of urine loss with the Urilos system.

The 12-hour test

When medium- or long-term pad tests are examined, it is important to ensure that no significant evaporation takes place between the end of the test and the time the

Table 4.2 *Short-term pad test*

Authors	Sensitivity (%)	False-negative rate (%)	PPV (%)	NPV (%)	Comments
Anand et al[56]	70	30	92	53	Patients with LUTS
	81	19	91	72	Patients with SUI
Janez et al[57]	–	39.4	–	–	No fixed bladder volume
Cardozo and Versi[58]	68	32	91	48	No fixed bladder volume
Schüssler et al[59]	–	56.8	–	–	Fixed bladder volume
Jorgensen et al[28]	68	32	–	–	–
Lose et al[49]	58	42	–	–	Fixed bladder volume

PPV, positive predictive value; NPV, negative predictive value; LUTS, lower urinary tract symptoms; SUI, stress urinary incontinence.
Reproduced with permission from Schick E, Jolivet-Tremblay M. Detection and quantification of urine loss: the pad-weighing test. In: Corcos J, Schick E, eds. The urinary sphincter. New York: Marcel Dekker, 2001:279.

pads are weighed. In an evaporation test, the mean weight loss of the pads, placed in a hermetically closed plastic container, is 0.2 g (0.1–0.3) after 24 hours, irrespective of the water volume in the pad. Mean weight loss after 48 hours and 6 days is 0.4 g (0.2–0.7 g) and 0.8 g (0.5–1.2 g), respectively.[46] Versi et al[47] noted no difference in weight after 1 week, and less than a 5% change in weight after 8 weeks (with the upper 95% confidence limit of less than a 10% loss).

The 12-hour test has not been investigated on its own, but has been compared with the 1-hour test by Ali et al,[48] who estimated that the 1-hour pad test on the ward was characteristic of the importance of urinary loss that patients encountered in their home environment. Thus, a 12-hour prolongation was not considered to add clinically relevant information to that obtained during the 1-hour test.

The 24-hour test

This test was examined in detail by Rasmussen et al[46] and found to be reproducible when there are only modest changes in physical activity and diuresis. With extreme reduction of fluid intake or excessive activity, differences in urine loss may be noted. Lose et al[49] compared this test with the 1-hour test. Among 31 stress or mixed incontinent women, 58% were categorized as incontinent with the 1-hour test and 90% with the 24-hour home test. They stated that the 24-hour test is effective as a discriminating tool for incontinence, but that its reproducibility is too low to be useful in scientific studies.

Versi et al[47] examined the 24- and 48-hour tests. Test–retest analysis demonstrated a strong correlation, with coefficients of 0.90 and 0.94, respectively. The reproducibility of the two time schedules was good, suggesting no additional benefit of a prolonged 48-hour test compared with a 24-hour schedule.

Assessing the test–retest reliability of 24-, 48-, and 72-hour pad tests, Groutz et al[50] found that the 24-hour pad test was a reliable instrument for defining the degree of urinary loss. Longer test duration increased reliability, but was associated with decreased patient compliance.

Similar conclusions were made by Mouritzen et al,[51] who compared the 1-, 24-, and 48-hour tests. They concluded that the 1-hour test underestimated the degree of incontinence and related less with clinical parameters than did the 24-hour test. On the other hand, the 24-hour test was as informative as the 48-hour test, making the latter obsolete.

Considering these studies, the 24-hour pad test is considered by many as the gold standard for the quantification of urinary incontinence.

The 48-hour test

The reproducibility of the 48-hour test appeared to be satisfactory ($r = 0.90$) and equivalent with the 1-hour test. Nevertheless, there was no relationship between these two tests ($r = 0.10$) according to Victor and Åsbrink.[52] Ekelund et al[37] showed this test can be successfully carried out in the patient's home, even with elderly women.

The elderly

Elderly patients represent a particular challenge to clinicians trying to quantify urine loss. There is a high incidence of urge incontinence among these patients. Also, some of them have notable mental impairment, making the completion of the test difficult. Finally, a number of these patients are unable to perform any formally designed exercise program.

Griffiths et al[8,34,35] studied the pad test thoroughly in the geriatric community. They established that physical examination often failed to show leakage in incontinent patients. The patient's voiding diary and the 1-hour pad weighing test were often discordant and impractical. In their hands, the 24-hour pad test proved to be the best method to demonstrate and quantify incontinence. Combining this noninvasive test with invasive urodynamics, these authors identified the type of urinary incontinence in 100 elderly patients. They found that the 24-hour test had sufficient reproducibility and good sensitivity (88%) for detecting urine loss, which was mainly nocturnal urge incontinence. Its quantity depended, however, on the preceding evening's fluid intake and on nocturia. They concluded that nocturnal toileting and evening liquid limitation could diminish nocturnal incontinence by a tiny, but profitable, proportion of older patients with extreme urge incontinence.

O'Donnell et al[38] described a procedure which helps nursing personnel to recognize, grade, and register incontinence severity while supervising several patients. This procedure, however, has not been verified for its reproducibility.

Conclusion

From a clinician's perspective, the pad-weighing test is beneficial when the quantity of urine loss is a significant element of management decisions. It is useful in distinguishing urinary incontinence from excessive perspiration or vaginal secretions. In this respect, a 1-hour test, or even a briefer one may be satisfactory. Under these circumstances, the test must be accomplished with a known bladder volume in order to provide reliable and objective information about the patient's condition.

For scientific and research purposes, the 24-hour pad test should be adopted, since it has good reproducibility, is simple to perform, and is done in the patient's own environment. It is better suited to detect and quantify urine loss secondary to urge incontinence than the 1-hour test. The 24-hour test should be used, along with other parameters, to assess success rates following various treatment modalities.

References

1. Sutherst JR, Brown MC, Richmond D. Analysis of the pattern of urine loss in women with incontinence as measured by weighing perineal pads. Br J Urol 1986; 58:272–278.

2. Abrams P, Blaivas JG, Stanton SL, Andersen JT. The standardisation of terminology of lower urinary tract function. Scand J Urol Nephrol (Suppl 114) 1988:5–19.

3. Abrams P, Cardozo L, Fall M, et al. The standardisation of terminology of lower urinary tract function: Report from the Standardisation sub-committee of the International Continence Society. Neurourol Urodyn 2002; 21:167–178.

4. Corcos J, Beaulieu S, Donovan J, et al., and members of the Symptom and Quality of Life Assessment Committee of the First International Consultation on Incontinence. Quality of life assessment in men and women with urinary incontinence. J Urol 2002; 168:896–905.

5. Blaivas JG, Appell RA, Fantl JA, et al. Standards of efficacy for evaluation of treatment outcomes in urinary incontinence: recommendations of the Urodynamic Society. Neurourol Urodyn 1997; 16:145–147.

6. Fantl JA, Newman DK, Colling J, et al. Urinary incontinence in adults: acute and chronic management. Clinical Practice Guideline No. 2, 1996 Update. Rockville, MD: Department of Health and Human Services. Public Health Service, Agency for Health Care Policy and Research. AHCPR Publication 96-0682, March 1996.

7. Hahn I, Fall M. Objective quantification of stress urinary incontinence: a short, reproducible, provocative pad-test. Neurourol Urodyn 1981; 10:475–481.

8. Griffiths DJ, McCracken PN, Harrison GM, Gormley EA. Relationship of fluid intake on voluntary micturition and urinary incontinence in geriatric patients. Neurourol Urodyn 1993; 12:1–7.

9. Siltberg H, Victor A, Larsson G. Pad weighing test, the best way to quantify urine loss in patients with incontinence. Acta Obstet Gynecol Scand (Suppl) 1997; 166:28–32.

10. Nygaard I, Zmolek G. Exercise pad testing test in continent exercisers: reproducibility and correlation with voided volume, pyridium staining and type of exercise. Neurourol Urodyn 1995; 14:125–129.

11. Ryhammer AM, Djurhuus JC, Laurberg S. Pad testing in incontinent women: a review. Int Urogynecol J Pelvic Floor Dysfunc 1999; 10:111–115.

12. Iselin CE, Webster GD. Office management of female urinary incontinence. Urol Clin N Am 1998; 25:625–645.

13. Mayne CJ, Hilton P. The distal urethral electric conductance test: standardization of method and clinical reliability. Neurourol Urodyn 1988; 7:55–60.

14. Janez J, Rudi Z, Mihelic M, et al. Ambulatory distal urethral electric conductance testing coupled to a modified pad test. Neurourol Urodyn 1993; 12:324–326.

15. James ED, Flack FC, Caldwell KP, Martin MR. Continuous measurement of urine loss and frequency in incontinent patient. Preliminary report. Br J Urol 1971; 43:233–237.

16. Stanton SL. Urilos: the practical detection of urine loss. Am J Obstet Gynecol 1977; 128:461–463.

17. Robinson H, Stanton SL. Detection of urinary incontinence. Br J Obstet Gynecol 1981; 88:59–61.

18. Eadie AS, Glen ES, Rowan D. The Urilos recording nappy system. Br J Urol 1983; 55:301–303.

19. Soroka D, Drutz HP, Glazener CM, et al. Perineal pad test in evaluating outcome of treatments for female incontinence: a systematic review. Int Urogynecol J Pelvic Floor Dysfunc 2002; 13:165–175.

20. Hellström AL, Andersen K, Hjälmås K, Jodal U. Pad test in children with incontinence. Scand J Urol 1986; 20:47–50.

21. Imada N, Kawauchi A, Tanaka Y, Watanabe H. The objective assessment of urinary incontinence in children. Br J Urol 1998; 81(Suppl 3):107–108.

22. Sutherst J, Brown M, Shawer M. Assessing the severity of urinary incontinence in women by weighing perineal pads. Lancet 1981; 1:1128–1129.

23. Murray A, Price R, Sutherst J, Brown M. Measurement of the quantity of urine lost in women by weighing perineal pads. Proc International Continence Society, Leiden, 1982:243–244.

24. Wood P, Murray A, Brown M, Sutherst J. Reproducibility of a one-hour urine loss test (pad test). Proc International Continence Society, Aachen, 1983; II:515–517.

25. Klarskov P, Hald T. Reproducibility and reliability of urinary incontinence assessment with a 60 min test. Scand J Urol Nephrol 1984; 18:293–298.

26. Lose G, Gammelgaard J, Jorgensen TJ. The one-hour pad-weighing test: reproducibility and the correlation between the test result, the start volume in the bladder and the diuresis. Neurourol Urodyn 1986; 5:17–21.

27. Christensen SJ, Colstrup H, Hertz JB, et al. Inter- and intra-departmental variations of the perineal weighing test. Neurourol Urodyn 1986; 5:23–28.

28. Jorgensen L, Lose G, Andersen JT. One-hour pad weighing test for objective assessment of female urinary incontinence. Obstet Gynecol 1987; 69:39–42.

29. Lose G, Rosenkilde P, Gammelgaard J, Schroeder T. Pad-weighing test performed with standardised bladder volume. Urology 1988; 32:78–80.

30. Donnellan SM, Duncan HJ, MacGregor RJ, Russel JM. Prospective assessment of incontinence after radical retropubic prostatectomy: objective and subjective analysis. Urology 1997; 49:225–230.

31. Richmond DH, Sutherst RJ, Brown MC. Quantification of urine loss by weighing perineal pads. Observations on the exercise regimen. Br J Urol 1987; 59:224–227.

32. Mayne CJ, Hilton P. Short pad test: method and comparison with 1-hour test. Neurourol Urodyn 1988; 7:443–445.

33. Miller J, Ashton-Miller JA, Delancey JOL. The quantitative paper towel test for measuring stress related urine loss. Proc International Continence Society, Yokohama, 1997:43–44.

34. Griffiths DJ, McCracken PN, Harrison GM. Incontinence in the elderly: objective demonstration and quantitative assessment. Br J Urol 1991; 67:467–471.

35. Griffiths DJ, McCracken PN, Harrison GM, Gormley EA. Characteristics of urinary incontinence in elderly patients studied by 24-hour monitoring and urodynamic testing. Age Aging 1992; 21:195–201.

36. Ryhammer AM, Laurberg S, Djurhuus JC, Hermann AP. No relationship between subjective assessment of urinary incontinence and pad test weight gain in a random population sample of menopausal women. J Urol 1998; 159(3):800–803.

37. Ekelund P, Bergstrom H, Milson I, et al. Quantification of urinary incontinence in elderly women with the 48-hour pad test. Arch Gerontol Geriatr 1988; 7:281–287.

38. O'Donnell PD, Finkbeiner AE, Beck C. Urinary incontinence volume measurement in elderly male inpatients. Urology 1990; 35:499–503.

39. Wilson PD, Mason MV, Herbison GP, Sutherst JR. Evaluation of the home pad test for quantitative incontinence. Br J Urol 1989; 64:155–157.

40. Persson J, Bergqvist CE, Wolner-Hanssen P. An ultra-short perineal pad-test for evaluation of female stress urinary incontinence treatment. Neurourol Urodyn 2001; 20:277–285.

41. Kinn A, Larsson B. Pad test with fixed bladder volume in urinary stress incontinence. Acta Obstet Gynecol Scand 1987; 66:369–372.

42. Simons AM, Yoong WC, Buckland S, Moore KH. Inadequate repeatability of the one-hour pad test: the need for a new incontinence outcome measure. Br J Obstet Gynecol 2001; 108:315–319.

43. Kroman-Andersen B, Jakobsen H, Andersen J. Pad-weighing tests: a literature survey on test accuracy and reproducibility. Neurourol Urodynam 1989; 8:237–242.

44. Haylen BT, Fraser MI, Sutherst JR. Diuretic response to fluid load in women with urinary incontinence; optimum duration of pad test. Br J Urol 1988; 62:331–333.

45. Eadie AS, Glen ES, Rowan D. Assessment of urinary loss over a two-hour test period: a comparison between Urilos recording nappy system and the weighed perineal pad method. Proc International Continence Society, Innsbruck, 1984:94–95.

46. Rasmussen A, Mouritzen L, Dalgaard A, Frimond-Moller C. Twenty-four hour pad weighing test: reproducibility and dependency activity level and fluid intake. Neurourol Urodynam 1994; 13:261–265.

47. Versi E, Orrego G, Hardy E, et al. Evaluation of the home pad test in the investigation of female urinary incontinence. Br J Obstet Gynaecol 1996; 103:162–167.

48. Ali K, Murray A, Sutherst J, Brown M. Perineal pad weighing test: comparison of one hour ward pad test with twelve-hour home pad test. Proc International Continence Society, Aachen, 1983; I:380–382.

49. Lose G, Jorgensen L, Thunedborg P. 24-hour home pad weighing test versus 1-hour ward test in the assessment of mild stress incontinence. Acta Obstet Gynecol Scand 1989; 68:211–215.

50. Groutz A, Blaivas JG, Chaikin DC, et al. Noninvasive outcome measures of urinary incontinence and lower urinary tract symptoms: a multicenter study of micturition diary and pad tests. J Urol 2000; 164:698–701.

51. Mouritzen L, Berild G, Hertz J. Comparison of different methods for quantification of urinary leakage in incontinent women. Neurourol Urodyn 1989; 8:579–587.

52. Victor A, Åsbrink AS. A simple 48-hour test for quantification of urinary leakage in incontinent women. Proc International Continence Society, London, 1985:507–508.

53. Martin A, Halaska M, Voigt R. Our experience with modified pad weighing test. Proc International Continence Society, Halifax, 1992:233–234.

54. Versi E, Cardozo L. One hour single pad test as a simple screening procedure. Proc International Continence Society, Innsbruck, 1984:92–93.

55. Walsh JB, Mills GL. Measurement of urinary loss in elderly incontinent patients. A simple and accurate method. Lancet 1981; 1:1130–1131.

56. Anand D, Versi E, Cardozo L. The predictive value of the pad test. Proc International Continence Society, London, 1985:290–291.

57. Janez J, Plevnik S, Vrtacnik P. Short pad test versus ICS pad test. Proc International Continence Society, London, 1985:386–387.

58. Cardozo L, Versi E. The use of a pad test to improve diagnostic accuracy. Proc International Continence Society, Boston, 1986:367–369.

59. Schüssler B, Hesse U, Horn J, Lentsch P. Comparison of two clinical methods for quantification of stress urinary incontinence. Proc International Continence Society, Boston, 1986:563–565.

5

Endoscopic evaluation of neurogenic bladder

Jacques Corcos and Erik Schick

Introduction

Urethrocystoscopy is not useful in the initial evaluation of neurogenic bladders, but becomes very instrumental in the assessment of lower urinary tract complications. Urethrocystoscopy cannot, by any means, give information on lower urinary tract function. For example, external sphincter contractions and relaxation observed during voluntary movement do not reflect the real functional value of this complex unit. Another classic example is the examination of endoscopic aspects of the bladder neck, which cannot replace functional studies for the evaluation of its opening and closing.

Urethrocystoscopy helps in the appraisal of urethral and bladder anatomical anomalies, most of the time secondary to complications such as urethral strictures, trabeculations, bladder stones, and diverticula. The aim of this chapter is to review these different aspects with some illustrations.

Equipment

Different companies offer different types and sizes of extremely well-designed, rigid urethrocystoscopes (Figure 5.1), some with fixed lens (12–70°), others with exchangeable lens (0°, 30°, 70°, 120°). The choice of lens depends on the segment of urinary tract that we want to study: 0 or 30° for the urethra and 70 or 120° for the bladder in general.

Since sensitivity is often not a problem in neurogenic bladder patients, rigid urethrocystoscopes are often preferred. They give a much better optical field than flexible cystoscopes (Figure 5.2) and allow various manipulations through a bigger working channel (irrigation, washing, small stone extraction, etc.). Flexible cystoscopes are extremely useful in men with preserved sensitivity, and the test is usually painless. In our experiences we do not use any local anesthetic, but only lubricating jelly. Others prefer to inject 2% Xylocaine (lidocaine (lignocaine)) jelly transurethrally 2–4 min before the procedure. One of the biggest advantages of these cystoscopes is the possibility of introducing them in a supine as well as in a sitting position. Because of their deflection abilities, they allow a retrograde view of the bladder neck as well as the complete exploration of diverticula, whatever the position.

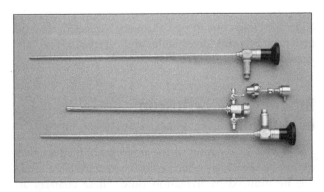

Figure 5.1
Rigid cystoscope.

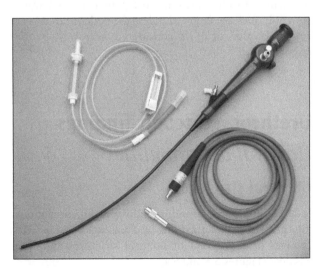

Figure 5.2
Flexible cystoscope.

Technique

Most of the time, the patient is installed in the lithotomy position, but, as mentioned earlier, a supine or a sitting position can be used with a flexible cystoscope.

After the usual disinfection of the genitalia with a non-alcoholic solution, draping creates a sterile field around the genitalia.

Once the patient is informed of the beginning of the examination, the cystoscope, lubricated with sterile jelly, is very gently introduced into the meatus. A global view of the urethra permits the confirmation of penile urethra integrity in men. The cystoscope is then pushed forward into the membranous urethra, making the external sphincter visible. This concentric muscle closes the urethra, and can usually be passed by gentle pressure on the cystoscope. The prostatic urethra is then observed, and the anatomy of the prostate noted, mainly the size of the lateral lobe and the presence or absence of a median lobe.

Once into the bladder, the technique is slightly different, depending on the type of cystoscope. With a rigid cystoscope, we normally use a 70° or 120° lens. The instrument will have only in–out and rotating motions, allowing a complete view of the bladder without bending the unit, which may cause unnecessary pain and discomfort. With a flexible cystoscope, the same in–out motion is applied, but the rotation motion is replaced by deflections of the instrument's tip, which gives a complete view of the bladder wall. Observation of the ureteral orifices, urine efflux from these orifices, and exploration of bladder diverticula may be necessary.

Washing, biopsies, etc., are performed at that time if indicated. Once the test is completed, the instrument is gently withdrawn after emptying of the bladder (when using a rigid instrument).

Drinking up to 6–8 glasses of water per day for 3 days is usually recommended and the patient is discharged. No antibiotics are required unless the patient has a heart artificial valve or it is considered necessary by the physician.

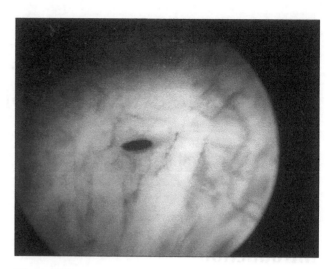

Figure 5.3
Urethral stricture.

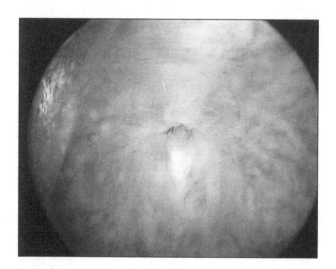

Figure 5.4
Urethral stricture.

Urethrocystoscopic findings
Urethral abnormalities

Urethral strictures

Indwelling catheters, multiple endoscopic manipulations, intermittent catheterizations, and neurogenic trophicity changes lead to frequent urethral strictures and false passages (Figures 5.3 and 5.4).

Strictures can be short and sometimes easy to break just with the cystoscope, or solid, long and tight enough to not allow the cystoscope to pass through. Neglected, they can generate urethral diverticula and urethroscrotal and urethrocutaneous fistulae.

Bladder neck cystoscopic evaluation

The degree of opening of the neurogenic bladder neck cannot be adequately evaluated by cystoscopy. False results can be induced by irrigation flow. These changes are dynamic and not anatomical. They should be evaluated by video urodynamic or simple voiding cystogram.

However, after bladder neck incision or resection to decrease bladder neck resistance, bladder neck strictures can be easily seen by cystoscopy, but, here again, their real impact on bladder function can be assessed only by voiding cystogram.

Endoscopic evaluation of urethral stents

Some specialized centers no longer perform incisional sphincterotomies, preferring endoluminal stents instead (i.e. Urolume – AMS). The techniques and results with these stents are detailed in Chapter 23.

It is usually easy to introduce a flexible cystoscope through these stents, which 'disappear' completely after a few months since the device is epithelialized through and in-between its pores: 90–100% of epithelialization of the stent has been demonstrated in 47.1% of cases 3 months after insertion, and in 87.7% of cases 12 months after insertion.

Mild epithelial hyperplasia can occur (34–44.4%) after stent insertion and may look like an obstructed urethra. Much less frequently, these strictures are severe (3.1%), requiring urethrotomy and sometimes insertion of a second stent at the same level as the first.[1]

Occasionally, however, and even several years later, part of the stent may remain visible, but usually does not cause any problems. Calcifications of the stents are rare. No stone formation has been reported.[1]

Structural bladder anomalies

The well-balanced bladder of a compliant patient looks normal (Figure 5.5) most of the time. However, it may show significant changes because of patient noncompliance with intermittent catheterization, medication, etc., or these treatments may have no effect.

Bladder wall abnormalities

Often associated with chronic infections but also often not related to any obvious disease, cystitis glandularis (Figure 5.6) and cystitis follicularis (Figure 5.7) can be found during systematic cystoscopic evaluation.

Bladder wall trabeculations

There is no consensus in the literature regarding the significance of bladder wall trabeculations (Figures 5.8–5.11).

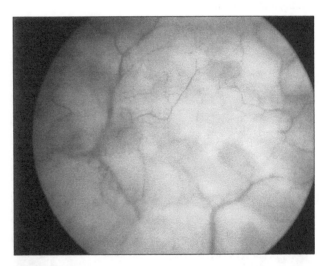

Figure 5.6
Cystitis glandularis.

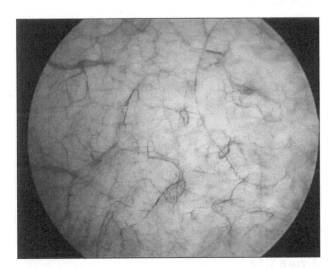

Figure 5.5
Normal bladder mucosa.

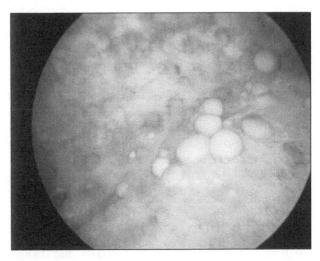

Figure 5.7
Cystitis follicularis.

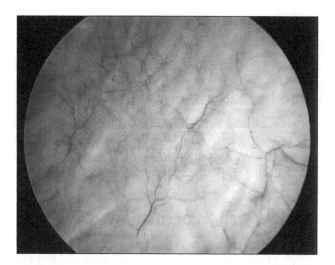

Figure 5.8
Trabeculation grade 1.

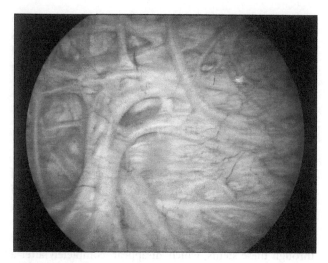

Figure 5.10
Trabeculation grade 3.

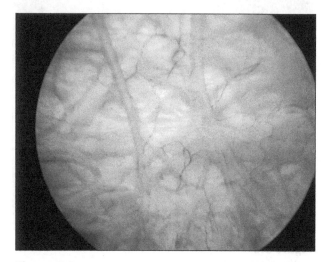

Figure 5.9
Trabeculation grade 2.

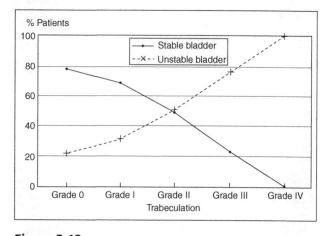

Figure 5.11
Trabeculation grade 4.

O'Donnell[2] suggested that they could be related to high bladder pressure.[1] To Brocklehurst,[3] McGuire,[4] Shah,[5] and O'Reilly[6] they are secondary to an infravesical obstruction. More authors believe that trabeculations reflect bladder overactivity and uninhibited contractions. Schick and Tessier[7] studied the correlation between endoscopic aspects of bladder walls and urodynamic parameters in 220 women. They concluded that there is a close correlation between trabeculation grade and the percentage of unstable bladders (Figure 5.12).

Ureteral orifices

High bladder pressure, recurrent infections, and changes in bladder wall thickness may provoke alterations in the shape of the ureteral orifices. In some cases, they can look

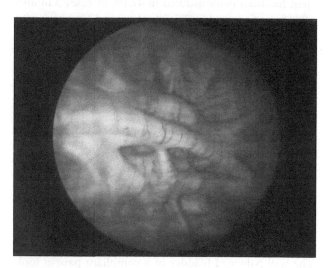

Figure 5.12
Correlation between the trabeculation grade and percentage of unstable bladders.

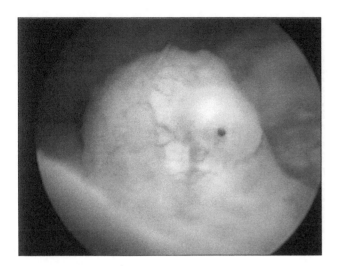

Figure 5.13
Ureterocele.

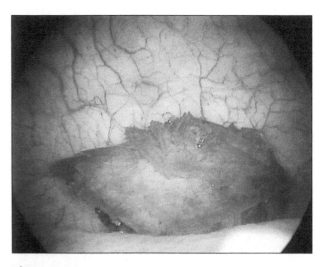

Figure 5.14
Bladder stone.

wide open. Their appearance cannot preclude the efficacy of the intramural ureteral valve mechanism and the presence of reflux. Reflux can be diagnosed only by cystogram with a contrast agent or a radioisotopic fluid. Ureterocele can have variable sizes (Figure 5.13).

Tumors, stones, and foreign bodies

Bladder stones

Usually secondary to infections, bladder stones are very frequent findings in neurogenic patients. They must be suspected in cases of recurrent *Proteus mirabilis* infections, increased spasticity or incontinence, elimination of small calcified fragments, etc. They are easy to diagnose by cystoscopy, and sometimes can be crushed for removal in the same set-up. Their aspects are extremely variable, from small, round, single or multiple stones to huge 'egg-like' stones (Figures 5.14 and 5.15).

Bladder tumors

Patients with chronic indwelling catheters must undergo annual cystoscopic bladder evaluation, which is the only way (with cytology) to detect suspicious lesions such as bladder carcinoma. Usually, these lesions start at the level of the trigone, where the catheter and the balloon lie down. In these patients, there is almost always a small reddish area which is difficult to differentiate from an early carcinoma (Figure 5.16). Biopsy of these lesions is a simple way of reassuring the physician and patient. Bladder tumors can

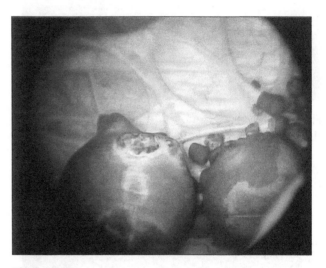

Figure 5.15
Bladder stone.

be located anywhere in the bladder and have different aspects, but most frequently papillary (Figure 5.17). Much less frequent are urethral tumors (Figure 5.18).

Foreign bodies

Foreign bodies are rare. Not infrequently, hairs can be found in patients with intermittent catheterization. Sometimes, they start to be calcified, and always have to be removed. Even less frequent are iatrogenic foreign bodies. Pieces of Foley catheter balloons or sutures from urological or non-urological procedures are eroded into the bladder (Figure 5.19 and 5.20).

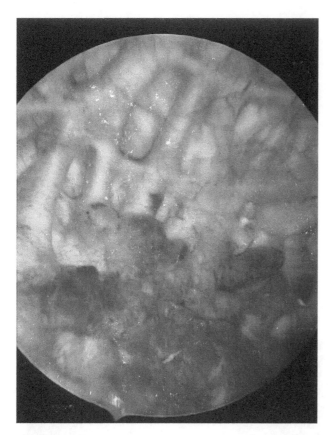

Figure 5.16
Mucosal catheter reaction.

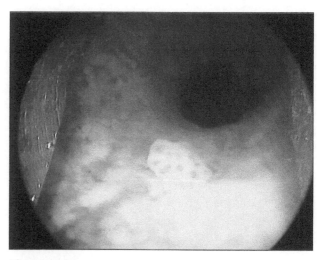

Figure 5.18
Urethral papillary tumor.

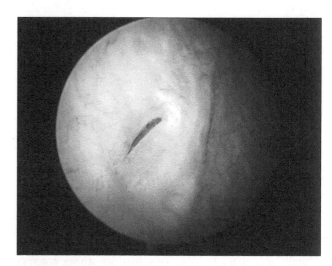

Figure 5.19
Stitch eroding the bladder wall.

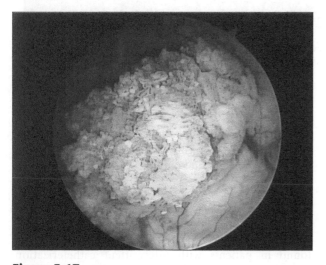

Figure 5.17
Bladder papillary tumor (partially calcified).

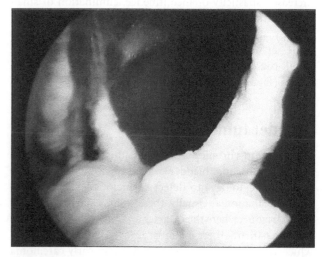

Figure 5.20
Calcified stitch into the bladder.

Conclusion

Urethrocystoscopy must be part of the regular evaluation of neurogenic bladders. It often allows us to understand the patient's worsening lower urinary tract function. Until now, and for most of the changes and abnormalities found by cystoscopy, no other test can replace it with the same accuracy and reliability.

References

1. Rivas DA, Chancelor MB. Sphincterotomy and sphincter stent prosthesis. In: Corcus J, Schick E, eds. The urinary sphincter. New York: Marcel Dekker, 2001:565–582.

2. O'Donnell P. Water endoscopy. In: Rax S, ed. Female urology. Philadelphia: WB Saunders, 1983:51–60.

3. Brocklehurst JC. The genito-urinary system. In: Brocklehurst JC, ed. Textbook of geriatric medicine and gerontology. New York: Churchill Livingstone, 1978:306–325.

4. McGuire EJ. Normal function of lower urinary tract and its relation to neurophysiology. In: Libertino IA, ed. Clinical evaluation and treatment of neurogenic vesical dysfunction. International perspectives in urology. Baltimore: Williams & Wilkins, 1984:1–15.

5. Shah PJR. Clinical presentation and differential diagnosis. In: Fitzpatrick JM, Krane RJ, eds. The prostate. Edinburgh: Churchill Livingstone, 1989:91–102.

6. O'Reilly PH. The effect of prostatic obstruction on the upper urinary tract. In: Fitzpatrick JM, Krane RJ, eds. The prostate. Edinburgh: Churchill Livingstone, 1989:111–118.

7. Schick E, Tessier J. Trabéculation de la paroi vésicale chez la femme: que signifie-t-elle? Presented at the 18th Annual Congress of the Association des Urologues du Québec, Montréal, November 1993.

6

Imaging techniques in the evaluation of neurogenic bladder dysfunction

Walter Artibani and Maria A Cerruto

In the evaluation of neurogenic bladder dysfunction, imaging techniques have the following goals and roles:

- they can suggest a neurogenic etiology in voiding disorders
- they can assess the central nervous system (CNS) in order to confirm and identify the neurogenic lesion, and to relate level and type of neurogenic lesion to bladder dysfunction
- they can evaluate the morphological status of the lower and upper urinary tract.

Imaging techniques suggesting a neurogenic etiology

Lumbosacral spine X-rays

Lower urinary tract (LUT) dysfunction in children, and more rarely in young adults, can be the expression of an underlying spinal dysraphism. In the majority of cases, abnormalities of the gluteosacral region and/or legs and foot are visible (e.g. small dimples, tufts of hair, subcutaneous lipoma, dermal vascular malformations, one leg shortness, high arched foot or feet). However, in some cases these abnormalities may be minimal or absent. A careful evaluation of the anteroposterior and lateral film of the lumbosacral spine can identify vertebral anomalies commonly associated with nervous system anomalies.[1–5]

Sacral agenesis involves the congenital absence of part or all of two or more sacral vertebrae. The absence of two or more sacral vertebrae always implies the presence of a neurogenic bladder dysfunction (Figures 6.1 and 6.2).[6,7]

The significance of spina bifida occulta can vary. Simple failure to fuse the laminae of the 4th and 5th lumbar vertebrae is unlikely to be important, but when the spinal canal

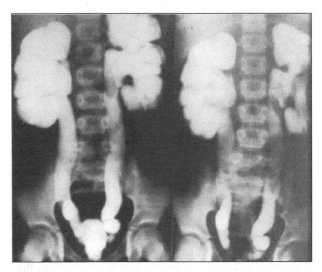

Figure 6.1
Sacral agenesis. Cystography: small retracted bladder and bilateral grade V vesicoureteric reflux.

is noticeably widened, there may be cord involvement (diastematomyelia, tethered cord syndrome).[8]

Open bladder neck and proximal urethra at rest

Open bladder neck and proximal urethra at rest, during the storage phase, can be observed during cystography, videourodynamics, or bladder ultrasonography, both in patients with and without neurologic diseases.

Distal spinal cord injury has been associated with an open smooth sphincter area, but whether this is due to sympathetic or parasympathetic decentralization or defunctionalization is still unclear.[9]

A relative incompetence of the smooth sphincter area may also result from interruption of the peripheral reflex

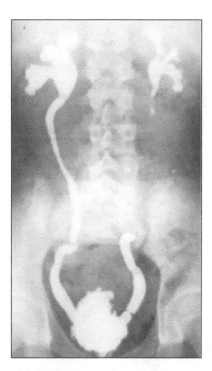

Figure 6.2
Sacral agenesis. Cystography: small sacculated bladder and bilateral grade III vesicoureteric reflux.

arc, which is very similar to the dysfunction observed in the distal spinal cord injury. Twenty-one out of 54 patients with spinal stenosis were found to have an open bladder neck at rest.[10,11]

In a review of 550 patients,[12] 29 out of 33 patients with an open bladder neck had neurologic diseases. Although the association was more commonly seen in patients with thoracic, lumbar, and sacral lesions, when compared to cervical and supraspinal lesions the difference was not significant. Damage of sympathetic innervation to the bladder was also frequently observed in patients undergoing major pelvic surgery, such as abdominal perineal resection of the rectum.

Patients with myelodysplasia showed an inordinately high incidence of open bladder neck (10 out of 18 patients, vs 19 out of 290 with different neurologic disorders).

Patients with sacral agenesis are included in the larger category of myelodysplastic patients and suffer from open bladder neck with areflexic bladder.

Shy–Drager syndrome is a Parkinson-like status with peripheral autonomic dysfunction. Detrusor hyperreflexia is usually found in association with an open bladder neck at rest and a denervated external sphincter.[13]

Peripheral sympathetic injury results in an open bladder neck and proximal urethra from damaged α-adrenergic innervation to the smooth muscle fibers of the bladder neck and proximal urethra.[14] Although it can occur as an isolated injury, this is usually associated with partial detrusor denervation and preservation of sphincter electromyographic (EMG) activity.

The loss of bladder neck closure suggests an autonomic neural deficit. The site and nature of the requisite deficit is unclear. Most authors agree on the importance of the sympathetic system in maintaining the integrity of the bladder neck,[15–19] although some authors have suggested the possible role of parasympathetic innervation.[20,21]

Open bladder neck at rest in children or in women with no neurologic diseases can represent a different disorder, either related to a congenital anomaly or secondary to an anatomical pelvic floor defect. Stanton and Williams[22] described an abnormality in girls with both diurnal incontinence and bed-wetting, based primarily on micturating cystourethrography, in which the bladder neck was wide open at rest. Murray et al[23] reported the 'wide bladder neck anomaly' in 24.5% of the girls (35) and 9.3% of the boys (10) amongst 251 children (143 girls and 108 boys) undergoing videourodynamics for the assessment of non-neuropathic bladder dysfunction (mainly daytime incontinence). The authors considered this anomaly as congenital and made the hypothesis that wide bladder neck anomaly in girls may provide a basis for the development of genuine stress incontinence in later life.

Chapple et al[24] reported that 21% of 25 totally asymptomatic women they investigated by transvaginal ultrasound had an open bladder neck at rest. Versi[25] found a 21% prevalence of open bladder neck at rest in 147 women visiting a urodynamic clinic and suggested that the finding is of little consequence.

Open bladder neck is a key point in defining type III stress incontinence according to the classification of Blaivas and Olsson.[26] This classification is based on history, imaging, and urodynamics, and distinguishes five diagnostic categories of stress incontinence. Incontinence type III is diagnosed by the presence of open bladder neck and proximal urethra at rest in the absence of any detrusor contraction suggesting an intrinsic sphincter deficiency. The proximal urethra no longer functions as a sphincter. There is obvious urinary leakage, which may be gravitational in nature or associated with minimal increase in intravesical pressure.

In pelvic fracture with membranous urethral distraction defects, when cystography (and/or cystoscopy) reveals an open bladder neck before urethroplasty, the probability of postoperative urinary incontinence may be significant, although the necessity of a simultaneous (or sequential) bladder neck reconstruction is controversial.[27–29]

In summary, when observing an open bladder neck and proximal urethra at rest, during the storage phase, whatever imaging technique is used, it may be worthwhile to evaluate the possibility of an underlying autonomic neural deficit (occult spinal dysraphism, sacral agenesia, postsurgery peripheral neural damage, Shy–Drager syndrome). Previous pelvic trauma or female gender can lead to a different perspective.

In the case of a manifest diagnosed neurogenic disease, open bladder neck and proximal urethra stand for various pathophysiologic situations and require a thorough urodynamic investigation in order to be correctly interpreted (e.g. sympathetic damage, associated detrusor-sphincter dyssynergia, previous endoscopic manipulation).

Imaging techniques assessing the central nervous system

Imaging of the central nervous system, otherwise known as neuroimaging, is a valuable aid in the diagnosis of a variety of CNS diseases which may cause LUT dysfunctions. Computed tomography (CT), magnetic resonance imaging (MRI), single-photon emission computed tomography (SPECT), and positron emission tomography (PET) have been used and reported.

When LUT symptoms are just part of the many symptoms caused by a CNS disease, the diagnosis is made on clinical grounds and neuroimaging is carried out only to confirm it. In rare cases, LUT symptoms are the only presenting symptoms of an underlying neurologic disorder and neuroimaging is instrumental in the diagnosis.

The literature shows an endless list of rare neurologic conditions presenting with different symptoms, including LUT symptoms, in which CT scan, MRI, SPECT, and PET imaging were carried out to identify the underlying CNS disease.

After a cerebrovascular accident, the urodynamic behavior of the lower urinary tract has been correlated to CT pictures of the brain.[30,31]

The presence of significant cerebral lesions has been clearly demonstrated by CT, MRI, or SPECT in the absence of clinical neurologic symptoms and signs in patients complaining of urge incontinence.[32] This can be particularly significant in elderly patients. Griffiths et al,[33] studying 48 patients with a median age of 80 years, reported that the presence of urge incontinence was strongly associated with depressed perfusion of the cerebral cortex and midbrain as determined from the SPECT scan.

Kitaba et al,[34] using MRI, reported subclinical lesions in the brain in 40 out of 43 men more than 60 years old who complained of urinary storage symptoms; of these 40 patients, 23 (57.5%) had detrusor hyperreflexia.

In spinal cord injured patients, CNS MRI can detect unsuspected cerebral or spinal lesions (ischemic and hemorrhagic areas, syringomyelia, spinal compression, spinal stenoses) which provide explanations for the possible discrepancy between the clinically assessed level of neurologic lesion and the urodynamically observed LUT dysfunction.

Spinal MRI is instrumental in diagnosing a tethered cord syndrome, as a primary disorder due to dural adhesions or as the outcome of previous surgical manipulation of the distal spinal cord.

PET studies provide information on specific brain structures involved in micturition in humans. In men and women who are able to micturate during scanning, an increase in regional blood flow was shown in the dorsomedial part of the pons close to the 4th ventricle, the pontine micturition center (PMC). PET studies carried out in both men and women also showed an activation of the mesencephalic periacqueductal gray (PAG) area during micturition. Based on experiments on cats, this area is known to project specifically to PMC and its stimulation elicits complete micturition. Experimental interruption of fibers from the PAG to the PMC results in a low-capacity bladder. PET studies during micturition in humans also showed an increased regional blood flow in the hypothalamus, including the preoptical area, which in cats can elicit bladder contractions.[35–37]

The present functional neuroimaging technology shows great potential to improve our knowledge of nervous functional anatomy in relation to vesicourethral function and dysfunction.

Imaging techniques of the lower and upper urinary tract in neurogenic bladder

Imaging of the lower urinary tract

Imaging of the lower urinary tract in neurogenic bladder dysfunctions aims at visualizing the morphology of the bladder and urethra, locating infravesical obstruction, vesicoureteric reflux, diverticula, fistula, and stones, providing a reasonable assessment of residual urine, and demonstrating leakage.

Bors and Comarr[38] described in detail the use of (video)-cystourethrography, with natural or retrograde filling, with or without ice-cooled contrast medium: the use of ice-cooled contrast medium – iced cystourethrography – can be useful in some suprasacral neurogenic patients in order to elicit detrusor reflex and voiding. Changes are detectable in the urethra (diverticula and fistulae at the level of penoscrotal junction, or a patulous urethra) and in the bladder (smooth overdistended bladder, trabeculation, wide open bladder neck, bladder asymmetry, 'Christmas Tree' bladder, thickened bladder wall, vesicoureteric reflux, paraureteric diverticula, bladder diverticula) (Figure 6.3). It is worthwhile to reread their description.

In expert hands ultrasonography can provide similar information. Color flow Doppler in combination with conventional B-mode sonography, has recently been

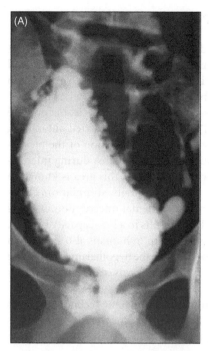

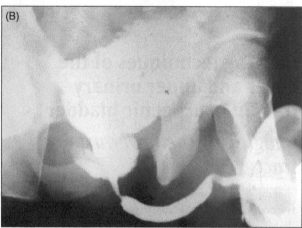

Figure 6.3
Myelomeningocele. Cystourethrography: (A) anteroposterior projection – 'Christmas tree' bladder, paraureteral diverticulum and grade I left vesicoureteric reflux, wide open bladder neck and proximal urethra, intraprostatic ducts visualization; (B) oblique projection during micturition – narrowed membranous urethra.

shown to be effective for detection and follow-up of vesicoureteric reflux in the neurogenic bladder, as an alternative to cystourethrography.[39]

LUT imaging by ultrasonography or cystourethrography can be performed as a separate test, but it is better performed at the time of urodynamic study (videourodynamics).[40] Videourodynamics is generally regarded as the 'gold standard' in the evaluation of LUT tract dysfunction. However, whether urodynamic and imaging testing should be performed simultaneously or on separate occasions is still controversial. Urodynamic examinations must be repeated several times to obtain reproducibility. The more parameters are studied, the more complicated the examination becomes, with a correspondingly higher risk of bias. Nevertheless, simultaneous videomonitoring along with tracings of detrusor pressure and possibly of EMG sphincter activity, are important means to make sure that the imaging is performed at the appropriate times so that the morphological features can be related to the various functional states.

Severe bladder trabeculation with diverticula and pseudodiverticula, vesicoureteric reflux, wide bladder neck, and proximal urethra, and narrowing at the level of the membranous urethra can suggest, mainly in children, the presence of neurogenic LUT dysfunction (occult spinal dysraphism, non-neurogenic neurogenic bladder) even in the absence of neurogenic symptoms and signs.[41–43] In these cases imaging abnormalities indicate the need for urodynamic evaluation, electrophysiological tests, and CNS imaging.

Residual urine evaluation can be worthwhile in neurogenic LUT dysfunctions. Residual urine is defined by the International Continence Society (ICS) as the volume of fluid remaining in the bladder immediately following completion of micturition.[44] Residual urine is usually referred to as an absolute value, but it can be measured also as a percentage of bladder capacity.

The measurement of post-void residual urine (PVR) can be performed by invasive or noninvasive means: invasive means are in-and-out catheterization and endoscopy; noninvasive means are transabdominal ultrasonography and radioisotope studies.

In-and-out catheterization is indicated as the gold standard for the measurement of PVR. Its invasiveness is not an issue in patients who are or will be in a regimen of intermittent catheterization. This method is subject to inaccuracies if the person performing the catheterization is not fully instructed as to the procedures and techniques to assure complete emptying (moving the catheter in and out slowly, twisting it, suctioning with syringe, suprapubic pressure), especially in cases of bladder diverticula and vesicoureteric reflux.[45] Stoller and Millard[46] showed inaccuracies in 30% of 515 male patients evaluated by full-time urological nurses with a mean difference between the initial and the actual residual volume of 76 ml in 30% of inaccurate assessments. After further training by the nurses, inaccurate assessments were reduced to 14%, with a mean difference of 85 ml.

Before the era of ultrasonography, PVR was measured noninvasively by the phenolsulfonphthalein excretion test[47] or with isotopes.[48] These tools have now been practically abandoned.

Ultrasonography is the least-invasive method of determining the PVR. There are several methods for this measurement, which are based on transverse and longitudinal ultrasound bladder imaging. Using either of three parameters (length, height, width) or the surface area in the transverse image and the length obtained in the longitudinal image, various volume formulae for a spherical or an ellipsoid body are utilized to estimate the bladder volume. Currently, no single formula can be indicated as the best to calculate bladder volume.

Several studies report sufficient accuracy in the ultrasound estimation of PVR.[49–55] The intra-individual variability of PVR is high from day to day and even within a 24-hour period. This was reported in men with benign prostatic hypertrophy (BPH) by Birch et al[56] and by Bruskevitz et al.[57] Griffiths et al[58] examined the variability of PVR among 14 geriatric patients (mean age 77 years), measured by ultrasound at three different times of the day during each of two visits at 2–4 week intervals. Within-patient variability was large (SD 128 ml) because of a large systematic variation with time of the day, with greatest volumes in early morning. The inherent random variability of the measurement was much smaller (SD 44 ml).

There are no data with regard to PVR variability in neurogenic bladders. The factors influencing the variability of PVR measurement are voiding in unfamiliar surroundings, voiding on command with a partially filled or overfilled bladder, the interval between voiding and the estimation of residual (it should be as short as possible), the presence of vesicoureteric reflux or bladder diverticula.

Recently, portable scanners have been introduced, with automatic measurement of bladder volume. In a prospective comparison,[59] where 100 measurements of PVR by portable ultrasound were compared with measurements by catheterization, the mean absolute error of the scanner was 52 ml. For volumes below 200 and 100 ml, the error was 36 and 24 ml, respectively. The portable scanner appears to be a valid alternative to in-and-out catheterization.

Imaging of the upper urinary tract

Neurogenic bladder dysfunction, primarily in the case of low bladder compliance or detrusor-sphincter dyssynergia or chronic retention with incontinence, can undermine urine transport through the ureterovesical junction from the kidneys to the bladder, resulting in hydronephrosis and renal damage. The relationship between high bladder storage pressure and renal deterioration has been well established by McGuire et al in a cohort of myelodysplastic children, showing that a detrusor leak point pressure >40 cmH$_2$O is detrimental to the upper urinary tract function.[60] Renal impairment is usually detectable at various stages by imaging of the kidneys and/or renal function tests.

Upper tract imaging is advisable at baseline and during follow-up in all cases of neurogenic bladder dysfunction,

and most of all in urodynamic situations with high risk of renal damage (high bladder pressure and inefficient voiding, with or without vesicoureteric reflux and infection).

The upper tract imaging modalities most commonly used include ultrasonography, intravenous urography (IVU), isotope scanning, CT scanning, and MRI.

Ultrasonography is an excellent tool for imaging of the upper urinary tract. It is noninvasive, and successful imaging of the kidneys is independent of renal function. Ultrasound can be used to assess many features of renal anatomy, including renal size and growth, hydronephrosis, segmental anomalies, stones, and tumors. In the evaluation of the patient with neurogenic LUT dysfunction, the detection of hydronephrosis is extremely important and may be a marker for a badly managed LUT. Because ultrasonography cannot predict function or degree of obstruction or reflux, other imaging modalities are often used after hydronephrosis is initially diagnosed by ultrasound. Ultrasound is an excellent tool to follow the degree of hydronephrosis or the response to treatment over time.

IVU is the original radiographic examination of the upper urinary (and lower) tract. Successful examination is dependent upon adequate renal function. Renal dysfunction, obstruction, congenital anomalies, fistula, stones, and tumors may be detected.

In some neurogenic patients, both kidney ultrasonography and IVU can be difficult to perform and interpret due to chronic constipation, excessive bowel gas, severe kyphoscoliosis or other spinal deformities, and the presence of internal fixation devices.

Isotopes are used primarily to examine functional characteristics of the upper urinary tract. Isotope scanning can be used to evaluate renal morphology and location. Renography is used to examine the differential function of the two kidneys as well as how they drain. There are many physiological factors and technical pitfalls that can influence the outcome, including the choice of radionuclide, timing of diuretic injection, state of hydration and diuresis, fullness or back pressure from the bladder, varying renal function, and compliance of the collecting system. Diuresis renography with bladder drainage is recommended when obstructive upper tract uropathy is suspected.[61–63]

CT scanning provides useful information about the anatomy of the upper urinary tract. Information can be independent of renal function; however, the addition of intravenous contrast can highlight specific anatomic characteristics (dependent upon renal function). CT scanning can be used as an alternative to ultrasonography or IVU, and in many cases provides additional information, although at a higher cost.

MRI offers some of the same benefits as CT in the evaluation of the upper urinary tract. Magnetic resonance urography is gaining popularity as an alternative to IVU, allowing multiplanar imaging and avoiding the intravenous injection of contrast media and the use of ionizing radiation. Its use in patients with neurogenic bladder due to spina dysraphism with gross spinal deformity has been shown to be valuable and effective, even in the presence of gross spinal deformity.[64]

Conclusions

Upper urinary tract imaging, by means of ultrasonography or MRI urography, is recommended at baseline and during follow-up, as needed, in neurogenic LUT dysfunctions. Their implementation is mandatory when low bladder compliance and chronic retention with/without incontinence indicate a high risk of renal impairment.

In the evaluation of the LUT, the simultaneous performance of imaging and urodynamics (videourodynamics) is the gold standard.

Some morphological findings at cystourethrography or ultrasonography – such as open bladder neck and proximal urethra at rest, heavily thickened sacculated and trabeculated asymmetric bladder, and membranous urethral narrowing – can have clinical and diagnostic relevance in raising the suspicion of a neurogenic disease, even in the absence of clear neurologic symptoms and signs.

Lumbosacral spine X-rays, followed when needed by MRI, have specific indications in children and young adults with suspected neurogenic LUT dysfunction, with or without gluteosacral stigmata.

CNS imaging should be considered when a neurologic disorder is suspected on the basis of clinical, imaging, and neurophysiological findings.

Functional neuroimaging by PET is going to provide new insight into the functional anatomy of CNS related to vesicourethral function and dysfunction. Neuroimaging can cover the gap between clinical neurologic level assessment and the type of vesicourethral dysfunction.

References

1. Anderson FM. Occult spinal dysraphism: a series of 73 cases. Pediatrics 1975; 55:826.

2. Flanigan RF, Russel DP, Walsh JW. Urologic aspects of tethered cord. Urology 1989; 33:80.

3. Kaplan WE, McLone DG, Richards I. The urologic manifestations of the tethered spinal cord. J Urol 1988; 140:1285.

4. Kondo A, Kato K, Kanai S, Sakakibara T. Bladder dysfunction secondary to tethered cord syndrome in adults: is it curable? J Urol 1986; 135:313.

5. Scheible W, James HE, Leopold GR, Hilton SW. Occult spinal dysraphism in infants: screening with high-resolution real-time ultrasound. Radiology 1983; 146:743.

6. Jacobson H, Holm-Bentzen M, Hage T. Neurogenic bladder dysfunction in sacral agenesis and dysgenesis. Neurol Urodyn 1985; 4:99.

7. Boemers TM, VanGool JD, DeJorg TPVM, Bax KMA. Urodynamic evaluation of children with caudal regression syndrome (caudal dysplasia sequence). J Urol 1994; 151:1038–1040.

8. Tarcey PT, Hanigan WC. Spinal dysraphism. Use of magnetic resonance imaging in evaluation. Clin Pediatr 1990; 29:228–233.

9. Artibani W, Andersen JT, Gaiewsky JB, et al. Imaging and other investigations. In: Abrams P, Cardozo L, Khoury S, Wein A, eds. Incontinence. 2nd International Consultation on Incontinence, 2001. Plymbridge Distributors, 2001:427–434.

10. Wein AJ. Pathophysiology and categorization of voiding dysfunction. In: Campbell's urology, 8th edn. Philadelphia: WB Saunders, 2002: 887–899.

11. Webster GD, Guralnick ML. The neurourologic evaluation. In: Campbell's urology, 8th edn. Philadelphia: WB Saunders, 2002: 900–930.

12. Barbalias GA, Blaivas JG. Neurologic implications of the pathologically open bladder neck. J Urol 1983; 129(4):780.

13. Salinas JM, Berger Y, De La Roche RE, Blaivas JG. Urological evaluation in the Shy–Drager syndrome. J Urol 1986; 135(4):741.

14. Blaivas JG, Barbalias GA. Characteristics of neural injury after abdominoperineal resection. J Urol 1983; 129(1):84.

15. de Groat WC, Steers WD. Autonomic regulation of the urinary bladder and sexual organs. In: Loewry AD, Spyers KM, eds. Central regulation of the autonomic functions, 1st edn. Oxford: Oxford University Press, 1990:313.

16. Nordling J. Influence of the sympathetic nervous system on lower urinary tract in man. Neurourol Urodyn 1983; 2:3.

17. Woodside JR, McGuire EJ. Urethral hypotonicity after suprasacral spinal cord injury. J Urol 1979; 121(6):783.

18. McGuire EJ. Combined radiographic and manometric assessment of urethral sphincter function. J Urol 1977; 118(4):632.

19. McGuire EJ. The effects of sacral denervation on bladder and urethral function. Surg Gynecol Obstet 1977; 144(3):343.

20. Nordling J, Meyhoff HH, Olesen KP. Cysto-urethrographic appearance of the bladder and posterior urethra in neuromuscular disorders of the lower urinary tract. Scand J Urol Nephrol 1982; 16(2):115.

21. Gosling JA, Dixon JS, Lendon RG. The autonomic innervation of the human male and female bladder neck and proximal urethra. J Urol 1977; 118(2):302.

22. Stanton SL, Williams D. The wide bladder neck in children. Br J Urol 1973; 45:60.

23. Murray K, Nurse D, Borzykowski M, Mundy AR. The congenital wide bladder neck anomaly: a common cause of incontinence in children. Br J Urol 1987; 59(6):533.

24. Chapple CR, Helm CW, Blease S, et al. Asymptomatic bladder neck incompetence in nulliparous females. Br J Urol 1989; 64(4):357.

25. Versi E. The significance of an open bladder neck in women. Br J Urol 1991; 68(1):42.

26. Blaivas JG, Olsson CA. Stress incontinence: classification and surgical approach. J Urol 1988; 139:737.

27. MacDiamis S, Rosario D, Chapple CR. The importance of accurate assessment and conservative management of the open bladder neck in patients with post-pelvic fracture membranous urethral distraction defects. Br J Urol 1995; 75:65.

28. Isekin CE, Webster GD. The significance of the open bladder neck associated with pelvic fracture urethral distraction defects. J Urol 1999; 162:347.

29. Shivde SR. The significance of the open bladder neck associated with pelvic fracture urethral distraction defects. J Urol 2000; 163:552.

30. Tsuchida S, Noto H, Yamaguchi O, Itoh M. Urodynamic studies in hemiplegic patients after cerebrovascular accidents. Urology 1983; 21:315.

31. Khan Z, Starer P, Yang WC, Bhola A. Analysis of voiding disorders in patients with cerebrovascular accidents. Urology 1990; 32:256.

32. Andrew J, Nathan PW. Lesions of the frontal lobes and disturbances of micturition and defecation. Brain 1964; 87:233–262.

33. Griffiths DJ, McCracken PN, Harrison GM, McEwan A. Geriatric urge incontinence: basic dysfunction and contributory factors. Neurourol Urodyn 1990; 9:406–407.

34. Kitada S, Ikel Y, Hasui Y, et al. Bladder function in elderly men with subclinical brain magnetic resonance imaging lesions. J Urol 1992; 147:1507–1509.

35. Blok BFM, Willemsen ATM, Holstege G. A PET study on brain control of micturition in human. Brain 1997; 120:111.

36. Blok BFM, Holdstege G. The central control of micturition and continence: implications for urology. Br J Urol Int 1999; 83(suppl 2):1.

37. Nour S, Svarer C, Kristensen JKL, et al. Cerebral activation during micturition in normal men. Brain 2000, 123:781–789.

38. Bors E, Comarr AE. Neurological urology, physiology of micturition, its neurological disorders and sequelae. Karger 1971:157.

39. Papadaki PJ, Vlychou MK, Zavras GM, et al. Investigation of vesicoureteral reflux with colour Doppler sonography in adult patients with spinal cord injury. Eur Radiol 2002; 12:366–370.

40. Webster DG, Kreder KJ. The neurourologic evaluation. In: Campbell's urology, 7th edn. Philadelphia: WB Saunders, 1998:927–952.

41. Hinman F. Urinary tract damage in children who wet. Pediatrics 1974; 54:142.

42. Allen TD. The non-neurogenic bladder. J Urol 1977; 117:232.

43. Williams DI, Hirst G, Doyle D. The occult neuropathic bladder. J Pediatr Surg 1975; 9:35.

44. ICS Standardization of terminology of lower urinary tract function. Neururol Urodyn 1998; 7:403.

45. Purkiss SF. Assessment of residual urine in men following catheterisation. Br J Urol 1990; 66(3):279.

46. Stoller ML, Millard RJ. The accuracy of a catheterized residual urine. J Urol 1989; 1741:15.

47. Ruikka I. Residual urine in aged women and its influence on the phenolsulfonphthaleine excretion test. Gerontol Clin 1963; 5:65–71.

48. Mulrow PJ, Huvos A, Buchanan DL. Measurement of residual urine with I-131-labeled Diodrast. J Lab Clin Med 1961; 57:

49. Piters K, Lapin S, Bessman AN. Ultrasonography in the detection of residual urine. Diabetes 1979; 28:320–323.

50. Pedersen JF, Batrum RJ, Grytter C. Residual urine detection by ultrasonic scanning. Am J Roentgenol Radium Ther Nucl Med 1975; 125:474–478.

51. Griffiths CJ, Muray A, Ramsden PD. Accuracy and repeatability of bladder volume measurement using ultrasonic imaging. J Urol 1986; 136:808.

52. Beacock CJM, Roberts EE, Rees RWM, Buck AC. Ultrasound assessment of residual urine. A quantitative method. Br J Urol 1985; 57:410–413.

53. West KA. Sonocystography. A method for measuring residual urine. Scand J Urol Nephrol 1967; 1:68.

54. McLean GK, Edell SL. Determination of bladder volumes by gray scale ultrasonography. Radiology 1978; 128:181–182.

55. Widder B, Kornhuber HH, Renner A. Restharnmessung in der ambulanten Versorgung mit einem Klein-Ultraschallgerat. Dtsch Med Wochen-schr 1983; 108:1552.

56. Birch NC, Hurst G, Doyle PT. Serial residual volumes in men with prostatic hypertrophy. Br J Urol 1998; 62:571.

57. Bruskewitz RC, Iversen P, Madsen PO. Value of post-void residual urine determination in evaluation of prostatism. Urology 1982; 20:602.

58. Griffiths DJ, Harrison G, Moore K, McCracken P. Variability of post-void residual urine volume in the elderly. Urol Res 1996; 24(1):23–26.

59. Ding YY, Sahadevan S, Pang WS, Choo PW. Clinical utility of a portable ultrasound scanner in the measurement of residual urine volume. Singapore Med J 1996; 37(4):365–368.

60. McGuire EM, Woodside JR, Borden TA. Prognostic value of urodynamic testing in myelodysplastic patients. J Urol 1981; 126:205–209.

61. Conway JJ. "Well-tempered" diuresis renography: it's historical development, physiological and technical pitfalls, and standardized technique protocol. Semin Nuclear Med 1992; 22:74–84.

62. Hvistendahl JJ, Pedersen TS, Schmidt F, et al. The vesico-renal reflex mechanism modulates urine output during elevated bladder pressure. Scand J Urol Nephrol 1997; 186(31 suppl):24.

63. O'Reilly PH. Diuresis renography. Recent advances and recommended protocols. Br J Urol 1992; 69:113–120.

64. Shipstone DP, Thomas DG, Darwent G, Morcos SK. Magnetic resonance urography in patients with neurogenic bladder dysfunction and spinal dysraphism. BJU Int 2002; 89:658–664.

7

Normal urodynamic parameters in children

Steven P Lapointe and Diego Barrieras

Introduction

Urodynamic examination yields invaluable information about lower urinary tract function in infants and children. First developed in adults, the techniques have been used in children extensively, using the same terminology and definitions as in adult urodynamics. The computers and devices used for evaluation of lower urinary tract function in children are similar to those used in adults, with appropriate catheter sizes according to age. Most importantly, these types of investigations are best performed by a physician or nurse who is specialized in the care of children. Caregivers must ensure that the results obtained do not reflect apprehension. The urodynamic team has to handle the child with care and patience, keeping a playful mood, distracting the child's attention from the surrounding environment, and following the pace set by the child to alleviate the pressure of performance. A center dedicated to children's care can accomplish this more easily, but with appropriate attention to these differences, children can be accommodated in an adult-oriented facility as well.

When evaluating a child with suspected lower urinary tract dysfunction, a detailed history should be obtained. The past medical history, especially previous urinary tract surgery or disease, and neurological status are relevant. The present medical history should include details about urinary tract infection, trauma, voiding pattern, incontinence, urgency, frequency, and urinary stream appearance; all are important. Bowel habits should be noted. To complete the history, we have found that recording a voiding diary gives objective data that can be repeated in the follow-up and involves the child and his parents in his care. Physical examination should include abdominal and genitalia examination, lumbosacral spine examination, and a brief neurological examination.

Because of the invasive and stressful nature of a complete urodynamics in children, uroflowmetry should be performed as an initial investigation of lower urinary tract dysfunction, except for children who present with diagnosed conditions such as spinal dysraphism or posterior valves. Uroflowmetry has been popularized as a study of lower urinary tract obstruction, mainly for benign prostatic hyperplasia (BPH).[1,2] Although the first reports on the use of uroflowmetry in children date back to the 1950s,[3] it had become a widespread tool by the 1980s.[4–7] Williot et al coupled measurement of uroflowmetry to post-void residual volume assessment using biplanar ultrasound.[7] They stated that the combination of dynamic flow analysis and accurate bladder residual volume assessment proved to be a simple yet comprehensive appraisal of the physiology of the lower urinary tract. These studies have several advantages that make them almost ideal for the pediatric population (see Table 7.1). They are noninvasive, physiological, and can be repeated as frequently as necessary.

Indications for uroflowmetry

Uroflowmetry has multiple applications in children of both sexes. It can be used in any clinical situation with suspected lower urinary tract dysfunction, even though it is not a highly specific diagnostic tool.[8] It has semiological value and gives important information as a screening method, helping diagnosis and/or leading to more elaborate testing (full urodynamics), particularly in evaluating voiding dysfunction and urinary tract infection. The studies can be used as a follow-up tool to assess the result of

Table 7.1 *Advantages and disadvantages of uroflowmetry in children*

Advantages	Disadvantages
Simple to perform	Not etiologic
Simple equipment	Less reproducible than in adults
Noninvasive	Children need to be toilet trained
Physiologic	
Can be repeated	
Low cost	

Table 7.2 *Indications for uroflowmetry in children*

- Urgency, frequency syndrome
- Urinary tract infection
- Incontinence (except isolated nighttime incontinence)
- Dysfunctional voiding syndrome
- Non-neurogenic neurogenic bladder (Hinman/Allen syndrome)
- Vesicoureteric reflux before and after surgical correction
- Neurogenic bladder
- Infravesical obstruction (urethral valves, urethral or meatal stenosis)
- Follow-up in hypospadias surgery and other urethral reconstruction
- Biofeedback method for bladder retraining

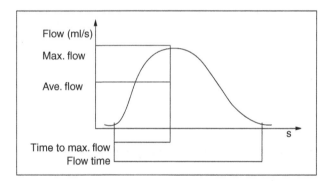

Figure 7.1
Normal uroflowmetry parameters.

surgical treatment, especially after hypospadias repair or in long-term follow-up of posterior urethral valve surgery. It is also very useful in following medical treatment, especially in bladder retraining for dysfunctional voiding and non-neurogenic neurogenic bladder.[9,10] In comparing multiple studies in the same patient, it is important to recognize that uroflowmetry in children is not as reproducible as in adults.[8,9] Consequently, the trend observed during successful studies has more diagnostic value.

Current indications for performing uroflowmetry in children are listed in Table 7.2.

The parameters obtained from uroflowmetry are identical to those in adults (Figure 7.1).

Technical aspects and pitfalls

To obtain optimal results from uroflowmetry, the voiding condition should be as close to normal as possible.

This is true in adults and it is even more important in children.[5,6] Children, especially under the age of 6, differ from older children and adults in the sense that they are usually less motivated, less patient, more apprehensive, and have limited understanding of what is going to happen.[6] The post-void residual volume can be determined by ultrasound using a mathematical model for calculation that considers the bladder to be a rectangular box. This equipment is readily available and cost-effective. Using a sagittal and a transverse view, two measures of bladder diameter are taken, and from these the volume in milliliters is generated. This technique is simple, noninvasive, accurate, and reproducible.[7] It should be noted that it has a slight tendency to overestimate the residual volume when compared to urethral catheterization.[8] Finally, like any ultrasonic technique it is operator-dependent, but this technique is easy to learn for those involved in urodynamic testing.

Interpretation of uroflowmetry

The availability of nomograms for analysis of uroflow data has been helpful in providing 'relative' data for size and weight, while recognizing that their absolute interpretation can be misleading.[4,10–13] However, there are general principles that guide the interpretation of the uroflowmetry data in children. As in adults, the results obtained are an integration of detrusor contractility and urethral resistance.[5] We believe that the shape of the flow curve is the most important feature of uroflowmetry, followed by maximal flow rate. Interestingly, the shape of the normal flow curve in children is the same as in adults and is a bell-shaped curve (Figure 7.2A) in more than 90% of normal children, even if the voided volume is under 100 ml.[5,10,11] With low or high voided volumes the shape of the curve has a tendency toward a more plateau appearance. There are three frequently encountered shapes. The staccato shape (Figure 7.2B) is indicative of either abnormal sphincter relaxation, and may be a reflection of dysfunctional voiding as in the non-neurogenic neurogenic bladder, unsustained bladder contraction, or abdominal straining. Children with dysfunctional voiding often benefit from bladder retraining, in which case uroflowmetry and nomograms can be used as a method of biofeedback. A plateau-shaped (Figure 7.2C) curve may be normal but can indicate infravesical obstruction, especially if associated with a low maximal and average flow rates. In such a case, depending on history and physical examination, further diagnostic tests may be indicated. For example, a voiding cystogram would permit diagnosing posterior urethral that sometimes is present at an older age. It should also be noted that after hypospadias surgery uroflowmetry curves are

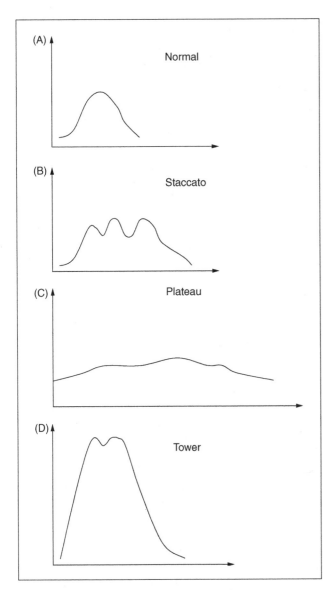

Figure 7.2
Normal and abnormal uroflowmetry curves.

references, and should be available in the laboratory.[4,10,11] From a practical standpoint, the maximal flow rate has more value than the average flow rate and has a linear relationship with the voided volume.[6] The maximal flow rate should equal the square root of the voided volume[6] (Q_{max} = square root of voided volume). For example, with a voided volume of 100 ml the maximal expected flow rate should be 10 ml/s and with a voided volume of 225 ml it should be 15 ml/s. Most often when these values are low, they are associated with a plateau-shaped curve.

Uroflowmetry and electromyography recordings

The residual volume estimate may provide conflicting results after uroflowmetry. When analyzing post-void residual volume in children, one should consider the fear and anxiety that might be involved on behalf of the child. However, we believe that, as a screening tool, a normal flow rate coupled with a complete emptying (0 ml) excludes the likelihood of serious underlying abnormalities.[2,7,13] On the contrary, defining what is a clinically significant residual volume is difficult in the face of an anxious child, and its value as a single diagnostic measure, grading of severity, or prognosis of urologic abnormality is poor. With young children, an isolated post-void residual volume measure without symptoms may merely reflect the child's apprehension. We would not ascribe any significance to it. Thus, we routinely use simultaneous electromyography (EMG) recordings with perineal patch electrodes to further discriminate normal children from patients with abnormal voiding pattern due to dysfunctional voiding or to underlying neurogenic bladder.

Treatment and further evaluation are then tailored according to the findings. If a child with no anatomical anomalies presents with clinical symptoms, high residual volume, or dyssynergia on cutaneous EMG recording, we would proceed with bladder and bowel management programs. Should the latter fail, despite simultaneous bladder-oriented pharmacotherapy, we would proceed with urodynamic studies. If a child presents with anatomical abnormalities during evaluation and an abnormal EMG–uroflowmetry, then we would proceed directly towards full urodynamic evaluation.

In summary, the noninvasive nature of EMG-coupled uroflowmetry and post-void residual assessment by ultrasound make them ideal in screening and follow-up of children. Their relative simplicity and ease of performance add to their wide application. The results of these studies are not highly specific but, when interpreted in the light of the clinical history, physical findings, and eventually other diagnostic studies, they give important

those of a plateau type with low maximal and average flow rates. The physician should only be concerned when there is a trend towards worsening over successive studies.[14] A tower-shape curve (Figure 7.2D) is usually associated with a high maximal flow rate and is believed to be reflective of dysfunctional voiding. It is more frequently encountered in girls and is often referred to as 'supervoiders'.

One has to be critical when looking at these results. Artifacts, mostly caused by misdirection of the stream, will change the shape of the curve, as well as the numerical values generated.[5]

The maximal and average flow rates closely correlate with voided volume, which is dependent on the age and size of the child. Again, the nomograms are helpful as information in establishing a diagnosis, especially in dysfunctional voiding or Hinman/Allen syndrome, and elaborating a treatment plan and following its results (e.g. during bladder retraining as a feedback, and following hypospadias surgery).

Some children require more extensive urodynamic studies. Indications include abnormal curve pattern associated with detrusor-sphincter dyssynergia (DSD) on cutaneous EMG, abnormal flow rate with daytime urinary incontinence, and chronic or recurrent bacteriuria that is refractory to bladder and bowel management. Clear indications for complete urodynamics as the initial test include patients with suspected infravesical obstruction such as posterior valves, overt or suspected neurogenic bladder dysfunction, and treatment failures of vesicoureteral reflux.

Only a few studies have looked at normal urodynamics in children. Sillen et al[15] evaluated bladder function in healthy neonates and infants using free voiding studies with a 4-hour voiding observation and subsequent urodynamics studies. They showed that voiding in the healthy neonate is characterized by small, frequent voids of varying volume. Thirty percent of the cases presented an interrupted voiding pattern, which seemed to be an immature phenomenon since it was seen in 60% of preterm neonates and disappeared completely before the age of toilet training. They theorized that there exists a physiological DSD, which may explain the frequent post-void residual observed in the young.[16,17] Along with the small caliber of the urethra, this can also explain the observed high voiding pressure. They observed some bladder hyperactivity on cystometric evaluation, as patients exhibited premature voiding contractions after only a few milliliters of filling volume with leakage of urine. Characteristics of the normal neonate micturition thus include physiological DSD, low bladder capacity, and high voiding pressure, associated with some detrusor hyperactivity.

Their findings are challenging the concept that neonates display simply a normal voiding reflex and that regulation of micturition in neonates involves higher neuronal pathways.

Another study from Sweden evaluated urodynamics in normal infants and children.[6] One of the most important statements of this study was that a tense and apprehensive child will not produce reliable urodynamic data. Studies should be done in an appropriate setting with an experienced urodynamicist. Their study also showed that inhibition of the detrusor improves during the first 5 years of life. Development of normal voiding pattern evolves as adequate proprioception of the bladder improves, allowing the child to have a better control on micturition. To this maturational process we should add the new concept of improvement of physiological DSD with age, as suggested by the study of Sillen et al.[15]

Urodynamic studies

Bladder capacity

Hjälmås observed that most urodynamic variables are age-dependent.[6] Several formulae have been proposed in the literature to assess normal bladder capacity in children (see Table 7.3). However, the most urodynamically sound formula was described by Houle et al,[20] as they evaluated 69 normal children, measuring total bladder capacity (ml), full resting pressure (cmH$_2$O), as well as the volume (ml) and the percentage of the total bladder capacity stored at detrusor pressures of less than 10, 20, 30, and 35 cmH$_2$O. According to their results, minimal acceptable total bladder capacity for age can be estimated by 16(age) + 70 in ml, which was derived using criteria for safe storage characteristics of the bladder in children. Table 7.3 summarizes some of these mathematical formulae.

Bladder compliance

Normal compliance in children has been established somewhat arbitrarily. The minimally acceptable value for bladder compliance during bladder filling has been set at 10 ml/cmH$_2$O.[21] Values above this level can be considered normal. Other researchers[22] have further stratified compliance as being poor <10 ml/cmH$_2$O, moderate between 10 and 20 ml/cmH$_2$O and mild between 21 and 30 ml/cmH$_2$O. The clinical relevance to such classification has yet to be determined.

It is important to remember that, as observed in adults, compliance may be influenced by the rate of bladder filling, which should be at a rate corresponding to 10% of the expected bladder capacity per minute. Compliance should be evaluated at regular intervals during cystometric recording (25–50–75%) as opposed to only at final capacity, since loss in compliance that occurs early in the filling phase puts the upper tract at higher risk than changes noted only near the end of the cystometric curve.[21]

Uninhibited contractions are recorded in the same way as in the adult; i.e. any appreciable detrusor contraction, especially if it causes urine leakage or urgency. (Since this chapter discusses only normal urodynamics in children, detrusor leak point pressure or abdominal leak point pressure will not be discussed, as they do not occur in the normal child.)

Voiding pressures

Hjälmås, in his study,[6] described intravesical pressures that are lower in girls than in boys, and lower in infants than in older children, but intravesical pressure does not vary with

Table 7.3 *Normal values for complete urodynamic studies in children*

Urodynamic characteristic	Normal value in children
Uroflow	Maximal flow rate = square root of the voided volume[6]
Bladder capacity (ml)	Houle et al:[20] 16 (age (years)) + 70 Koff:[18] (age (years) + 2) $\times$ 30 Kaefer et al:[19] (2 $\times$ age (years) + 2) $\times$ 30 (child <2 years old) (age (years) divided by 2 + 6) $\times$ 30 (child >2 years old) Hjälmås:[6] 30 + (age (years) $\times$ 30)
Uninhibited contractions	Any appreciable detrusor contraction
Bladder compliance	>10 ml/cmH$_2$O[21]
Voiding pressures	Infant male: median 100 cmH$_2$O[15] Infant female: median 70 cmH$_2$O[15] 1–3 years old child male: 70 cmH$_2$O[6] 1–3 years old child female: 60 cmH$_2$O[23] 7 years and older: similar to adult
Post-void residual (limited reliability)	Infant: 1 void/4 hour complete, median PVR 4–5 ml up to 2 years old: 4–5 ml[17] 3 years old and up: 0 ml

age. However, he mentioned that bladder pressure recordings represent the most important source of error when examining children. He strongly emphasized that the examination has to be performed in a kind, friendly, and relaxed atmosphere. Median pressure measurements in male infants of more then 100 cmH$_2$O and 60–70 cmH$_2$O in females have been observed. In children 1–3 years of age, voiding pressure can be 70 cmH$_2$O in males[6] and 60 cmH$_2$O in females.[23] After the age of 7, values tend toward those of adults.

Post-void residual

Post-void residual urine has been studied, but to date only a few studies have presented significant data as to what represents normal post-void residual urine. It is recognized that infants do not empty their bladder at each void,[17] but they seem to empty their bladder completely at least once during a 4-hour observation period.[15] Residual urine using a 4-hour observational protocol has been reported to be minimal (4–5 ml) up to age 2.[17,24] Residual urine should be 0 ml at 3 years and older.[24] Caution should be used when post-void residual urine is considered as a significant factor in diagnosis, as many children may present fear and anxiety at the time of observation.

A summary of normal urodynamic values in children is presented in Table 7.3.

References

1. Gleason DM, Lattimer JK. The pressure flow study: a method for measuring bladder neck resistance. J Urol 1962; 87:844.

2. Abrams PH, Griffiths DJ. The assessment of prostatic obstruction from urodynamics measurements and from residual urine. Br J Urol 1979; 51(2):129–134.

3. Scott RJ, McIlhaney JS. The voiding rates in normal children. J Urol 1959; 82:224.

4. Churchill BM, Gilmour RF, Williot P. Urodynamics. Pediatr Clin North Am 1987; 34:1133–1157.

5. Jorgensen JB, Jensen KM. Uroflowmetry. Urol Clin North Am 1996; 23:237–242.

6. Hjälmås K. Urodynamics in normal infants and children. Scand J Urol Nephrol Suppl 1988; 114:20–27.

7. Williot P, McLorie GA, Gilmour RF, Churchill BM. Accuracy of bladder volume determinations in children using a suprapubic ultrasonic bi-planar technique. J Urol 1989; 141:900–902.

8. Meunier P, Mollard P, Nemoz-Behncke C, Genet JP. [Urodynamic exploration in functional micturition disorders in children]. Arch Pediatr 1995; 2:483–491.

9. Ewalt DH, Bauer SB. Pediatric neurourology. Urol Clin N Am 1996; 23(3):501–509.

10. Segura CG. Urine flow in children: a study of flow chart parameters based on 1361 uroflowmetry tests. J Urol 1997; 157:1426–1428.

11. Jensen KM, Nielsen KK, Jensen H, et al. Urinary flow studies in normal kindergarten- and schoolchildren. Scand J Urol Nephrol 1983; 17:11–21.

12. Gaum LD, Wese FX, Liu TP, et al. Age related flow rate nomograms in a normal pediatric population. Acta Urol Belg 1989; 57:457–466.

13. Wese FX, Gaum LD, Liu TP, et al. Body surface related flow rate nomograms in a normal pediatric population. Acta Urol Belg 1989; 57:467–474.

14. Jayanthi VR, McLorie GA, Khoury AE, Churchill BM. Functional characteristics of the reconstructed neourethra after island flap urethroplasty. J Urol 1995; 153:1657–1659.

15. Sillen U. Bladder function in healthy neonates and its development during infancy. J Urol 2001; 166:2376–2381.

16. Roberts DS, Rendell B. Postmicturition residual bladder volumes in healthy babies. Arch Dis Child 1989; 64:825–828.

17. Sillen U, Solsnes E, Hellstrom AL, Sandberg K. The voiding pattern of healthy preterm neonates. J Urol 2000; 163:278–281.

18. Koff SA. Estimating bladder capacity in children. Urology 1983; 21:248.

19. Kaefer M, Zurakowski D, Bauer SB, et al. Estimating normal bladder capacity in children. J Urol 1997; 158:2261–2264.

20. Houle AM, Gilmour RF, Churchill BM, et al. What volume can a child normally store in the bladder at a safe pressure? J Urol 1993; 149:561–564.

21. Gilmour RF, Churchill BM, Steckler RE, et al. A new technique for dynamic analysis of bladder compliance. J Urol 1993; 150:1200–1203.

22. Horowitz M, Combs AJ, Shapiro E. Urodynamics in pediatric urology. In: Nitti VW, ed. Practical urodynamics. Philadelphia: WB Saunders, 1998:254–269.

23. Wen JG, Tong EC. Cystometry in infants and children with apparent voiding symptoms. Br J Urol 1998; 81:468–473.

24. Jansson UB, Hanson M, Hanson E, et al. Voiding pattern in healthy children 0 to 3 years old: a longitudinal study. J Urol 2000; 164:2050–2054.

Evaluation of neurogenic bladder dysfunction: basic urodynamics

Christopher E Kelly and Victor W Nitti

Classification of neurogenic voiding dysfunction

The main objective in assessing patients with suspected neurogenic lower urinary tract (LUT) dysfunction is to determine what effect the neurologic disease has on the entire urinary tract so that treatment can be implemented to relieve symptoms and prevent upper and lower urinary tract damage. The functional classification system described by Wein (Figure 8.1) is a useful framework with which to conceptualize neurogenic voiding dysfunction and provides a basis for the discussion of various diagnostic and treatment modalities.[1] This simple and practical system can be easily applied to our diagnostic criteria (e.g. urodynamics). Of equal importance is the fact that treatment options can be chosen based on this system. The functional classification system is based on the simple concept that the LUT has two basic functions: storage of adequate volumes of urine at low pressures, and voluntary and complete evacuation of urine from the bladder. For normal storage and emptying to occur there must be proper and coordinated functioning of the bladder and bladder outlet (bladder neck, urethra, external sphincter). Hence, neurogenic LUT dysfunction can be classified under the following rubrics: 'failure to store', 'failure to empty', or a combination thereof. Abnormalities in LUT function may be the result of bladder dysfunction, bladder outlet dysfunction, or a combined dysfunction. Figure 8.2 summarizes how neurologic disease can adversely affect the bladder and/or the bladder outlet, causing storage and emptying dysfunction.

Prior to our discussion, it is important to emphasize that symptoms do not always indicate the magnitude to which the disease is affecting the urinary tract, especially in neurologic disorders. Serious urinary tract damage can result in the absence of symptoms. It is also vital to realize that

---

Functional classification:

1. Emptying abnormality (failure to empty)
2. Storage abnormality (failure to store)
3. Emptying and storage abnormality

Anatomic abnormality:

1. Bladder dysfunction
2. Bladder outlet dysfunction
3. Bladder and bladder outlet dysfunction

Figure 8.1
Functional classification of voiding disorders.

Failure to store

A. Bladder dysfunction:
   - Neurogenic detrusor overactivity
   - Impaired compliance

B. Bladder outlet dysfunction:
   - Neurogenic intrinsic sphincter deficiency

Failure to empty

A. Bladder dysfunction:
   - Detrusor underactivity
   - Acontractile detrusor

B. Bladder outlet dysfunction:
   - Detrusor-external sphincter dyssynergia
   - Bladder neck dyssynergia

Figure 8.2
Effects of neurologic disease on storage and emptying function.

patients with neurologic disease are at risk for developing the same urologic and gynecologic problems as persons of the same age without neurologic disease.[2] For example, just because a women has had a cerebrovascular accident does not exclude her from having stress urinary incontinence. And, lastly, the clinician should remember that neurologic lesions may be 'complete' or 'incomplete'. Hence, urologic manifestations of neurologic disease may not always be predictable. A complete neuro-urologic evaluation of patients with neurogenic voiding dysfunction is therefore important.

In this chapter we will discuss the evaluation of patients with neurogenic LUT dysfunction with urodynamics. Prior to this discussion, a working knowledge of the neurophysiology of micturition is essential. Additionally, the effect of particular neurologic diseases on lower urinary tract function is covered elsewhere in the book.

Assessment of patients with neurogenic lower urinary tract dysfunction

History and physical examination

Any patient with obvious or suspected neurogenic voiding LUT dysfunction deserves a neurologic work-up. Controversy exists as to how often patients should be reassessed urologically. We recommend that patients be reviewed at least annually, and the complete work-up be repeated if significant changes occur in the neurologic status or LUT signs or symptoms.

Prior to urodynamic testing a complete history and physical examination are imperative. A thorough understanding of the patient's condition and symptoms are essential so that urodynamic investigations can be 'customized' to answer questions relevant to that particular patient. Initial evaluation of patients with suspected neurogenic LUT dysfunction should include a thorough history of the patient's general health and neurologic disease. It is important to understand how the neurologic disease affects daily activities, whether it affects other systems, and whether its course is stable or changing. In patients who do not have a history of neurologic disease (i.e. occult neurologic disease), it is important to carefully and directly question them even about their more subtle neurologic complaints.[2]

A standard and complete urologic examination should be performed on all patients with suspected neurogenic LUT dysfunction. A good general neurologic examination to assess sensation, strength, dexterity, and mobility is essential, as all of these can affect treatment of neurogenic LUT dysfunction. A specific and comprehensive evaluation of the sacral nerve (S2–S4) reflex arc is critical. A digital rectal examination will establish rectal tone and control. The bulbocavernosus reflex and perianal sensation should also be assessed. Finally, lower extremity spasticity along with patellar and ankle reflexes should be evaluated.

Laboratory studies

Basic serum and urine tests, including renal function tests and serum electrolytes, should be performed. Urinalysis and urine culture are essential, particularly in patients with an increased risk for developing urinary tract infections: those with chronic indwelling catheters, on intermittent self-catheterization, or those carrying high post-void residual volumes.

Noninvasive urodynamic assessment

Noninvasive studies such as uroflowmetry and measurement of post-void residual urine can be readily performed to give an initial assessment of the patient's ability to empty the bladder. While nonspecific for underlying dysfunction, uroflowmetry is often used as a screening test for voiding dysfunction and as a means for selecting patients for more sophisticated urodynamic studies. It also provides an objective way to monitor the emptying in patients who have specific diagnoses and are followed with observation or specific therapy.

Since the upper urinary tract in neurogenic voiding dysfunction can be adversely affected by secondary reflux, ascending infection, hydronephrosis, or stones, a baseline study is recommended. A renal ultrasound or intravenous pyelogram can be used to assess for hydronephrosis or stones. Bladder ultrasound provides an excellent modality to rule out bladder stones, which are reported in over 30% of patients with indwelling catheters.[3] When suspected, vesicoureteral reflux can be assessed by a voiding cystourethrogram or as part of a videourodynamic evaluation. When more detailed information on renal function is required, such as obstruction or cortical scarring, a nuclear renogram is obtained.

Although it is an invasive technique, a few words on cystourethroscopy are important. It is indicated in those with indwelling catheters on a yearly basis. Besides evaluating for bladder calculi, epithelial changes can be detected. These patients carry a 5% lifetime risk of developing squamous cell carcinoma of the bladder.[4-6]

Urodyamics

Multichannel urodynamic evaluation is the mainstay of evaluation in patients with neurogenic LUT dysfunction. The goals of urodynamic testing in patients with neurologic disease are:

1. To provide documentation of the effect of neurologic disease on the LUT.
2. To correlate the patient's symptoms with urodynamic events.
3. To assess for the presence of urologic risk factors associated with urologic complications: detrusor striated sphincter dyssynergia (DESD), impaired bladder compliance, sustained high-pressure detrusor contractions, and vesicoureteral reflux.

The urodynamic evaluation consists of several components, including the uroflowmetry, cystometrogram (CMG), abdominal pressure monitoring, electromyography (EMG), and voiding pressure–flow studies. Simultaneous fluoroscopic imaging of the entire urinary tract during urodynamics (i.e. videourodynamics) can be helpful in cases of known or suspected neurogenic voiding dysfunction. It is not unusual to repeat a study several times in order to fulfill the above goals.

Cystometrogram

The filling CMG is used to mimic the bladder's filling and storage of urine while the pressure–volume relationship within the bladder is recorded. It is best to fill the bladder at a rate of 30 ml/min or less. In our experience, faster filling rates can exaggerate urodynamic observations. Important bladder parameters with respect to neurologic disease are bladder sensation, the presence of involuntary detrusor contractions (IDC), compliance (storage pressures), and cystometric capacity. IDCs associated with neurologic disease are referred to as neurogenic detrusor overactivity according to the International Continence Society (Figure 8.3).[7] The magnitude, or pressure, of IDCs is often determined by the amount of resistance provided by the bladder outlet. For example, in cases of high outlet resistance such as DESD or anatomical obstruction, detrusor pressure with IDC can be quite high, whereas in cases of low outlet resistance, the IDC pressure is often low with subsequent incontinence. Neurogenic detrusor overactivity is caused by lesions above the sacral micturition center, including the spinal cord and brain. Simply stated, the inhibition of the spinal micturition reflex from suprapontine centers is blocked.

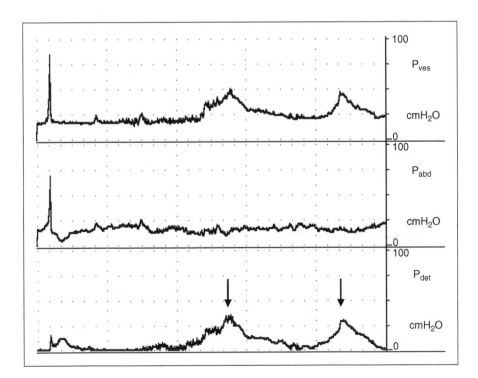

Figure 8.3
Filling phase of a urodynamic study in a 68-year-old woman with urge incontinence after cerebrovascular accident. Note the involuntary detrusor contractions (arrows). There is a rise in total bladder pressure (P_{ves}) and detrusor pressure (P_{det}), but no change in abdominal pressure (P_{abd}).

There are several very important points regarding involuntary contractions:

1. The clinician must be absolutely sure that the contraction is indeed involuntary. Sometimes a patient may become confused during the study and actually void as soon as he feels the desire.
2. It is extremely important to determine whether or not a patient's symptoms are reproduced during the involuntary contraction. However, in cases of neurologic disease, IDCs can occur with symptoms and should not be discounted.
3. The volume at which contractions occur and the pressure of the contractions should be recorded.
4. It is often worthwhile to repeat the CMG at a slower filling rate if the patient experiences uncharacteristic symptoms (e.g. incontinence or spasms) or detrusor activity.
5. If the patient experiences incontinence during an involuntary contraction (urge incontinence), this should be noted. Sometimes the involuntary contraction will bring on involuntary voiding to completion (precipitant micturition).[8]

Compliance is defined as the change of volume for a change in detrusor pressure and is calculated by dividing the volume change (ΔV) by the change in detrusor pressure (ΔP_{det}) during that change in bladder volume. It is expressed in milliliters per centimeter H_2O (ml/cmH_2O). The spherical shape of the bladder as well as the viscoelastic properties of its components contribute to its excellent compliance, allowing storage of progressive volumes of urine at low pressure. When the pressure begins to rise with increasing volumes, compliance is decreased or 'impaired'. Impaired compliance is not uncommon in neurogenic voiding dysfunction and is potentially hazardous. The degree of impaired compliance in neurogenic voiding dysfunction is often dependent on outlet resistance. However, poor compliance can also occur with chronically catheterized bladders. Impaired compliance leads to high bladder storage pressures. The calculated value of compliance is probably less important than the actual bladder pressure during filling. This is because the compliance value can change, depending on the volume over which it is calculated. This is probably why compliance, despite being a well-known and accepted parameter, is rarely reported in terms of a discrete or well-defined value in the urologic literature.

Normal compliance has been difficult to establish. Toppercer and Tetreault evaluated a group of normal asymptomatic women and women with stress incontinence and found mean compliance to be 55.71 ± 27.37.[9] If two standard deviations are used, normal would be between 1 and 110 ml/cmH_2O. When compliance is calculated as a single point on the pressure–volume curve it becomes a 'static' property. Gilmour et al point out that this oversimplifies the concept of compliance and may lead to potentially erroneous conclusions.[10] For example, an abrupt and potentially dangerous rise in pressure may occur as compliance rapidly decreases.

However, the value for compliance will be very different, depending on whether it is calculated over the entire filling volume or over the volume in which the change in pressure actually occurred. McGuire and associates have shown that sustained pressures of 40 cmH_2O or greater during storage can lead to upper tract damage.[11] Storage pressures in this

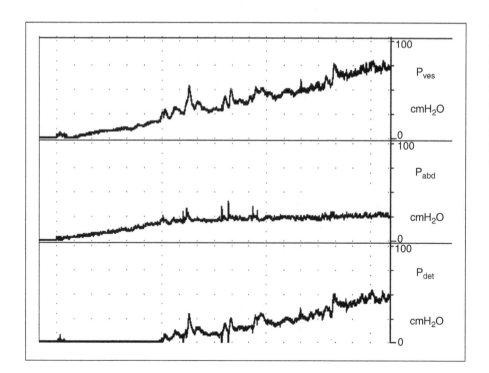

Figure 8.4

Impaired compliance in a 35-year-old male with a T8 spinal cord injury. Note that there is an initial rise in both total vesical pressure (P_{ves}) and abdominal pressure (P_{abd}), but the P_{ves} and, thus, the detrusor pressure (P_{det}) continue to rise to pressures exceeding 40 cmH_2O.

range are dangerous, regardless of the volume in the bladder or calculated compliance value (Figure 8.4). In poorly compliant bladders in children, Churchill and associates have suggested determining compliance between initial filling and the point at which detrusor pressure exceeds 35 cmH$_2$O.[10] More recently, these investigators have applied the concept of dynamic compliance and argue that the amount of time spent with bladder compliance less than 10 ml/cmH$_2$O (an empirically derived value) will strongly influence upper tract deterioration.[12]

We would certainly agree that prolonged high-pressure storage is an ominous urodynamic finding, independent of any discrete value of compliance. One must remember that compliance may be dependent on filling rate during a urodynamic study; overly rapid filling rates may produce erroneously lower compliance values. Lastly, neurogenic detrusor overactivity can mimic impaired compliance. Two methods of differentiating these two entities are (1) stopping the infusion rate and, if necessary, (2) having the patient perform a sustained Kegel maneuver to suppress possible involuntary contractions. Involuntary detrusor contractions can also occur in the face of impaired compliance (Figure 8.5).

Storage parameters – leak point pressures

During the filling portion of the cystometrogram, urinary storage can also be assessed. Assessment of storage is important because patients with neurogenic bladders often have issues pertaining to urinary incontinence and/or storage pressures. Urinary leakage can be secondary to a bladder dysfunction (neurogenic detrusor overactivity or impaired compliance) and/or a sphincteric dysfunction (e.g. intrinsic sphincter deficiency). The bladder, or detrusor,

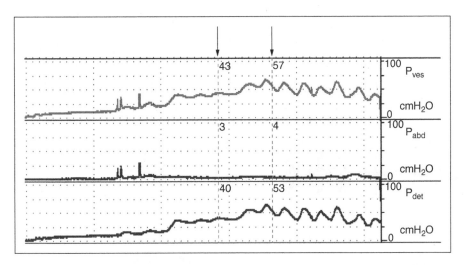

Figure 8.5
Involuntary detrusor contractions occurring in the face of impaired compliance in a teenage girl with myelomeningocele. The left arrow indicates where detrusor pressure equals and then exceeds 40 cmH$_2$O. The right arrow indicates where leakage occurs – at a bladder leak point pressure of 53 cmH$_2$O. P_{ves}, total vesical pressure; P_{det}, detrusor pressure; P_{abd}, abdominal pressure.

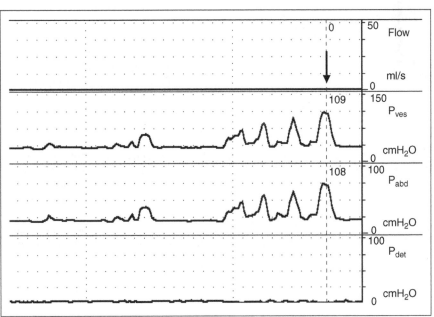

Figure 8.6
Urodynamic tracing of a female patient with stress incontinence. Tracing shows progressive Valsalva maneuvers until leakage occurs (arrow) at an abdominal pressure of 109 cmH$_2$O, which is the abdominal leak point pressure (ALPP). Note that there is no rise in detrusor pressure. P_{ves}, total vesical pressure; P_{det}, detrusor pressure; P_{abd}, abdominal pressure.

leak point pressure (DLPP) test measures the detrusor pressure required to cause urinary incontinence in the absence of increased abdominal pressure. The DLPP is a direct reflection of the amount of resistance provided by the external sphincter. The higher the bladder outlet resistance (e.g. as in detrusor-sphincter dyssynergia), the higher the DLPP. High storage pressures and high DLPP are potentially dangerous to upper urinary tracts (Figure 8.5). Knowledge of the DLPP is useful because it allows the clinician to determine the volume at which detrusor pressure reaches dangerous levels.

Urinary leakage secondary to sphincteric dysfunction can be measured by the abdominal or Valsalva leak point pressure (ALPP).[13] The ALPP is an indirect measure of the ability of the urethra to resist changes in abdominal pressure as an expulsive force.[14] Clinically, it is used to determine the

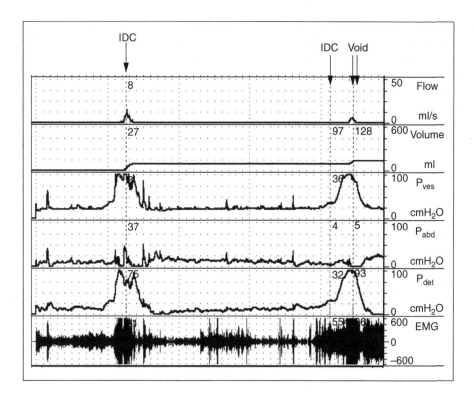

Figure 8.7
Urodynamic tracing of an 18-year-old woman with frequency, urgency, and urge incontinence who was diagnosed with a tethered cord. Note the involuntary detrusor contraction (IDC, arrow) associated with high-volume urine loss as registered in the flow meter. There is increased sphincter activity, as demonstrated by increased electromyograph (EMG) activity consistent with detrusor-external sphincter dyssynergia (DESD). On the second fill there is again an IDC, but this time the patient is instructed to void (double void). Note that there is increased EMG activity throughout the IC and 'voluntary void'. Detrusor pressures with IDCs are quite high because of the resistance of the contracting striated sphincter. P_{ves}, total vesical pressure; P_{det}, detrusor pressure; P_{abd}, abdominal pressure.

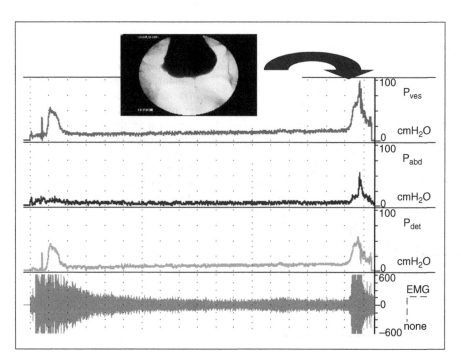

Figure 8.8
Detrusor-external sphincter dyssynergia (DESD) and detrusor-internal sphincter dyssynergia in a 35-year-old male with a high cervical spinal cord injury. There are two IDCs with associated increased electromyograph (EMG) activity consistent with DESD. However, the fluoroscopic picture taken at the time of the second IDC shows an incompletely opened bladder neck consistent with detrusor-internal sphincter dyssynergia. This patient underwent a striated sphincterotomy as well as a bladder neck incision to facilitate emptying and lower pressures. P_{ves}, total vesical pressure; P_{det}, detrusor pressure; P_{abd}, abdominal pressure.

presence of stress urinary incontinence and the degree of sphincter incompetence (Figure 8.6). Normally, there is no physiologic abdominal pressure that should cause incontinence, and therefore there is no 'normal ALPP'. Unlike the DLPP, an elevated ALPP does not indicate potential danger to the kidneys.

Voiding phase

As important as filling and storage is the voiding or emptying phase, known as micturition. Prior to urodynamic assessment, one must determine how the patient voids. If voiding is voluntary, the strength and duration of the detrusor contraction is assessed. Detrusor contractility may be impaired in particular types of neurologic disease, particularly with lower motor neuron or denervating lesions. This can cause impaired contractility or areflexia.

Aside from detrusor contraction, outlet resistance can be measured while voiding. Although the most common cause of outlet resistance in neurogenic voiding dysfunction is DESD, bladder outlet obstruction can occur anywhere distal to the bladder. Several nomograms and formulas exist to categorize pressure–flow relationships in terms of non-obstructed, obstructed, or equivocal.[15–19] It is important to

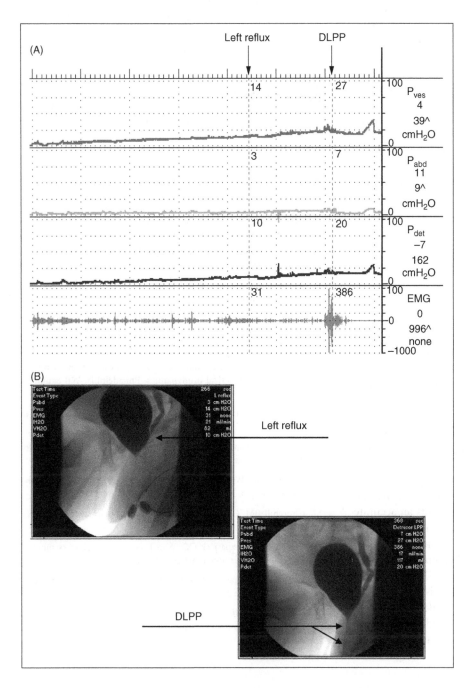

Figure 8.9
Videourodynamic study in a 3-year-old boy with myelomeningocele who is on anticholinergic medication but remains wet between catheterizations. There is mild left hydronephrosis on renal ultrasound. P_{ves}, total vesical pressure; P_{det}, detrusor pressure; P_{abd}, abdominal pressure. EMG, electromyography. (A) This study shows that leakage occurs as a result of impaired compliance: bladder leak point pressure (DLPP) = 20 cmH$_2$O. (B) Video portion shows left vesicoureteral reflux occurring at a relative low detrusor pressure of 10 cmH$_2$O (upper left arrow), and confirms the DLPP of 20 cmH$_2$O (lower right arrow).

note that interpretation of bladder outlet obstruction during urodynamics should be performed at the point at which the patient was told to void. If the patient has an involuntary bladder contraction and empties the bladder prematurely, this pressure–flow relationship should not be misinterpreted as being equivalent to normal physiologic voiding.

Electromyography during urodynamics permits the urologist to evaluate the striated sphincter function during micturition. Often, surface patch electrodes are used, but needle electrodes permit more accurate placement and more accurate recording. Normally, voluntary voiding is preceded by a complete relaxation of the striated sphincter. Detrusor-external sphincter dyssynergia refers to obstruction to the outflow of urine during bladder contraction caused by involuntary contraction of the striated sphincter during an IDC.[20,21] It is secondary to a neurologic lesion and is not associated with a learned voiding dysfunction such as dysfunctional voiding. DESD results in a functional obstruction that usually affects emptying, and ultimately leads to high storage pressures secondary to impaired compliance and incomplete emptying. True DESD is seen in patients with suprasacral spinal lesions (Figure 8.7). Depending on the level of the lesion, patients also may develop detrusor-internal sphincter dyssynergia. In such cases the bladder fails to open appropriately with a bladder contraction due to autonomic dysfunction. It typically occurs in lesions above T10. Detrusor-internal sphincter dyssynergia is best diagnosed by videourodynamics (Figure 8.8).

Videourodynamics

Videourodynamics, or simultaneous fluoroscopic monitoring of the urinary tract during urodynamics, is the most comprehensive and accurate way of assessing neurogenic lower urinary tract dysfunction (Figures 8.8 and 8.9).[22] During the evaluation of filling and storage, videourodynamics allows for the determination of vesicoureteral reflux and the pressure at which this occurs. Moreover, assessment of the DLPP or ALPP is facilitated as fluoroscopy is often more sensitive than direct observation in determining urinary leakage. Videourodynamics also permits the radiographic evaluation of the bladder neck during filling and anatomic abnormalities such as bladder and urethral diverticula and fistula. During the voiding phase, fluoroscopy permits an accurate determination of the site of obstruction when high-pressure/low-flow states exist. Videourodynamics also provides an excellent way of evaluating sphincter behavior during voiding, especially in cases where EMG tracing is imperfect or equivocal. Videourodynamics is the definitive test to determine the presence of detrusor-internal sphincter dyssynergia by the lack of opening of the bladder neck on fluoroscopy during a detrusor contraction. Using fluoroscopy

with EMG can help make the diagnosis of detrusor-internal and detrusor-external sphincter dyssynergia.[23]

Conclusion

In patients with known neurologic disease, careful urodynamic evaluation may be necessary to gauge any deleterious effect on the urinary tract, to determine the etiology of LUT symptoms, and to screen for any urologic risk factors. Often times, urodynamics are necessary for the asymptomatic patient because the effects of the disease on the urinary tract can be 'silent'. Patients without a history of neurologic disease whose urologic evaluation is suspicious for neurogenic LUT dysfunction should be evaluated for occult neurologic disease.

References

1. Wein AJ. Classification of neurogenic voiding dysfunction. J Urol 1981; 125:605.

2. Nitti VW. Evaluation of the female with neurogenic voiding dysfunction. Int Urogynecol J 1999; 10:119–129.

3. Bunts RC. Management of urological complications in 100 paraplegics. J Urol 1958; 79:733–736.

4. Bejany BE, Lockhart JL, Rhamy RK. Malignant vesical tumors following spinal cord injury. J Urol 1987; 138:1390–1392.

5. Bickel A, Culkin J, Wheeler J. Bladder cancer in spinal cord injury patients. J Urol 1991; 146:1240–1241.

6. Broecker BH, Klein FA, Hackler RH. Cancer of the bladder in spinal cord injury patients. J Urol 1981; 125:196–197.

7. Abrams P, Cardozo L, Fall M, et al. The standardization of terminology of lower urinary tract function. Neurourol Urodynam 2002; 21:167–178.

8. Nitti VW. Cystometry and abdominal pressure monitoring. In: Nitti VW, ed. Practical urodynamics. Philadelphia: WB Saunders, 1998:38–51.

9. Toppercer A, Tetreault JP. Compliance of the bladder: an attempt to establish normal values. Urology 1979; 14:204.

10. Gilmour RF, Churchill BM, Steckler RE, et al. A new technique for dynamic analysis of bladder compliance. J Urol 1993; 150:1200.

11. McGuire EM, Woodside JR, Borden TA. Prognostic value of urodynamic testing in meylodysplastic children. J Urol 1981; 126: 205.

12. Churchill BM, Gilmour PE, Williot P. Urodynamics. Ped Clin NA 1987; 34:1133.

13. McGuire EJ, Fitzpatrick CC, Wan J, et al. Clinical assessment of urethral sphincter function. J Urol 1993; 150:1452–1454.

14. McGuire EJ, Cespedes RD, O'Connell HE. Leak point pressures. Urol Clin N Am 1996; 23:253–262.

15. Abrams PH, Griffiths DJ. Assessment of prostate obstruction from urodynamic measurements and from residual urine. Br J Urol 1979; 51:129–134.

16. Schafer W. Principles and clinical application of advanced urodynamic analysis of voiding function. Urol Clin N Am 1990; 17:553–566.

17. Abrams P. Bladder outlet obstruction index, bladder contractility index and bladder voiding efficiency; three simple indices to define bladder voiding function. BJU Int 1999; 84:14–15.

18. Blaivas JG, Groutz A. Bladder outlet obstruction nomogram for women with lower urinary tract symptomatology. Neurourol Urodyn 2000; 19:553–564.

19. Lemack GE, Zimmern PE. Pressure flow analysis may aid in identifying women with outflow obstruction. J Urol 2000; 163(6):1823–1828.

20. Blaivas JG, Singa HP, Zayed AAH, Labib KB. Detrusor-external sphincter dyssynergia. J Urol 1981; 125:541–544.

21. Blaivas JG, Singa HP, Zayed AAH, Labib KB. Detrusor-external sphincter dyssynergia: a detailed EMG study. J Urol 1981; 125:545–548.

22. Blavais JG. Videourodynamic studies. In: Nitti VW, ed. Practical urodynamics. Philadelphia: WB Saunders, 1998:78–93.

23. Watanabe T, Chancellor MB, Rivas DA. Neurogenic voiding dysfunction. In: Nitti VW, ed. Practical urodynamics. Philadelphia: WB Saunders, 1998:142–155.

9

Urodynamics in infants and children

Kelm Hjälmås and Ulla Sillén

Introduction

Urodynamics in infants and children is basically the same procedure as in adults and shares the same techniques and objectives. There is, however, one fundamental difference: *the patient is a child*. Essentially, this means two things. First, a child harbors intuitive fear for any unknown procedure but is, at the same time, largely unresponsive to rational argumentation about the nature of and the need for the examination. Second, the child is a growing individual, increasing in weight 20-fold from infancy to puberty. This means that for children there exists no single set of 'normal' urodynamic variables but rather a continuum of each variable, depending on and correlating to the age and the body size of the individual.

This chapter will concentrate on those two aspects: first, on how to prepare, inform, reassure, encourage, and comfort the child before and during the urodynamic examination; second, how to report the expected range of 'normal' values for urodynamic variables from infancy to adolescence.

Historical notes on urodynamics in infants and children

It is hard to understand why bladder function in children did not receive any attention from medical scientists until the mid-20th century. Before that time, it seems to have been understood, without a trace of critical thinking, that almost all children had bladders that worked perfectly well, regarding both storage and evacuation of urine. If a functional disturbance such as incontinence was indeed noted, traditional wisdom suggested that it was due to psychological problems within the child and/or the family. In contrast, we are now aware that non-neurogenic bladder-sphincter dysfunction in children is caused by delayed maturation (most often genetically determined)

of the central nervous system (CNS) bladder control. Psychological problems in an incontinent child are a consequence of the bladder dysfunction, not the other way round, with few exceptions.

From 1959 onwards, the first urodynamic studies on normal and pathological bladder function in infants and children came into print.[1-9] A rapidly increasing number of studies followed, once it became clear that at age 7 years as many as 10% of children have non-neurogenic disturbance of bladder/sphincter function. Knowledge surfaced that bladder dysfunction plays a major role not only for urinary incontinence but also, even more importantly, for the creation and persistence of vesicoureteral reflux (VUR) and urinary tract infection (UTI), with the accompanying risk for deterioration of renal function.[10] Children with *neurogenic* bladder dysfunction (NBD) due to myelodysplasia and other disorders of the CNS were exposed to the same risk to an even larger degree. Surprisingly, however, this fact did not become obvious until the late 1960s, when it was finally understood that the devastating UTIs and the frequent progress of bacterial resistance during antibiotic therapy in myelomeningocele children was caused by inadequate bladder emptying, leaving post-void residual behind. Regular and low-pressure bladder evacuation with the aid of clean intermittent catheterization (CIC), introduced by Jack Lapides in 1972, led to a dramatic reduction in the rate and severity of UTIs in this patient group and even resulted in disappearance of reflux in many patients.[11]

Development of bladder function

The normal development of lower urinary tract function from infancy to adolescence has to be reviewed before describing the urodynamic procedures and techniques used in children and what results to expect. This is necessary in order to understand the dynamic nature of the urodynamic variables in the growing individual.

Bladder function during infancy has previously been regarded as automatic, with voiding induced by a constant volume in the bladder[12] and without cerebral influence. During the last decade it has been shown convincingly that the brain is already involved in the voiding reflex from birth. This is best illustrated by the finding that in the majority of cases newborn babies wake up or show signs of arousal before voiding.[13,14] This means that the reflex pathway connection to the cerebral cortex is anatomically already developed in this age group; however, voiding is neither conscious nor voluntary – the infant is only disturbed by the signal. Both maturation and probably training are needed for the voidings to be conscious and voluntary.

Neonates and infants void at varying bladder volumes during infancy and this is contrary to the belief that the voiding reflex is a simple spinal reflex elicited by a constant bladder volume. This has been shown in free voiding studies of both pre-term[15] and full-term infants[13] in whom bladder volume initiating voiding varies from 30% to 100% of functional bladder capacity. The reason for this variation is unknown, but the bladder volume initiating micturition is higher after a period of sleep.

The infant's voiding is also characterized by a physiological form of detrusor-sphincter dyscoordination, which has been shown in free voiding studies as interrupted voidings and increase in post-void residual urine (Figure 9.1).[16] This phenomenon has also been observed in urodynamic studies as an intermittent increase in the electromyographic (EMG) activity of the pelvic floor during voiding, concomitant with fluctuations in voiding detrusor pressure (Figure 9.2).[14,17] A longitudinal study of free voidings from birth to age 3 years revealed that the suggested dyscoordination disappears successively, and is not seen after potty-training age.[13] Another important observation in the study by Jansson et al[13] is the increase in post-void residual urine during the first couple of years of life. The reason for the incomplete emptying in infancy is probably the physiological form of dyscoordination discussed above, with interruption of the urine stream before the bladder is empty. However, with the acquisition of continence the residual volume decreased in this group of healthy children and the ability to empty the bladder was complete at the age of 3.

In the longitudinal study of free voidings by Jansson et al[13] it was also observed that bladder capacity was almost unchanged during the first two years of life but showed a steep increase at the time the child gets dry (see Figure 9.6). A similar accelerated increase in bladder capacity which is age related has also been noted in other studies.[12,18] This increased bladder capacity has been considered as a prerequisite for both day- and nighttime continence. Conversely, continence during night has been considered to be obtained only after achievement of day dryness.[19,20] The reason for this increase in bladder capacity has previously only been discussed in terms of general maturation.

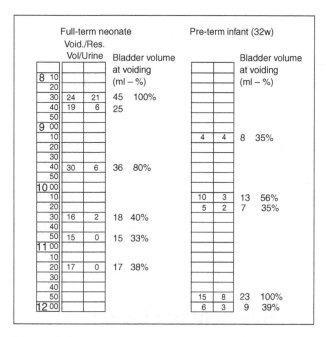

Figure 9.1
Four-hour voiding observation in a full-term neonate and a pre-term infant (gestation age 32 weeks) showing varying bladder volumes initiating voiding (the sum of voided volume and residual urine). The volumes vary between 33% and 100% of the highest volume in the bladder (= the bladder capacity) during the observation. Note the interrupted voiding seen once in the full-term and twice in the pre-term infant.

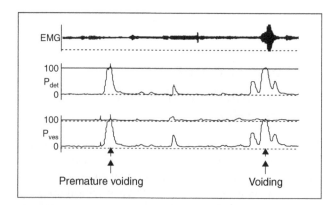

Figure 9.2
Cystometric recording in a non-refluxing newborn sibling of a child with vesicoureteral reflux (VUR). Note the premature voiding contraction after infusion of 5 ml with leakage of urine. Voiding after a total filling of 30 ml of saline shows an increase of electromyographic (EMG) activity of the pelvic floor and concomitant fluctuation in detrusor voiding pressure.

Acquisition of bladder control

Development of bladder control was earlier supposed to begin at 1 year of age and often to be fully developed by age 4.5 years. It was described by Muellner as 'a maturation which could not be influenced by training'. Another factor which was considered important was the doubling of bladder capacity between 2 and 4.5 years of age.[12,21] These statements about maturation, combined with the improvement in the quality of disposable napkins, have contributed to a more liberal view about what age potty-training should be started. In fact, during the last decades, potty-training has been regarded as unnecessary due to the belief that physical maturation should dictate when a child becomes dry. It is quite clear from other areas, however, that training can accelerate maturation.

Potty-training was instituted early before the era of disposable napkins. Some authors have reported bladder control much earlier than nowadays,[19,20] whereas others have not been able to show such a connection.[22]

If bladder control only means to void on the potty when the child is put there by the parent regularly or when the child indicates a need to void, it can be obtained early. The degree of maturation needed for such basic training is probably already present during the first year of life.[23] The goal of potty-training, to obtain full social bladder control, cannot be achieved solely with the early potty-training dicussed above. The prerequisites for success are influenced both by physical maturation and the child's interest in this task as well as by support from adults, routines, and parental expectations. Most children may stay dry in their usual milieu around the age of 2. However, the child has to reach at least 3.5–4 years of age to become mature enough to be able to cope with every aspect of their own toileting (including taking off and on clothes, flushing the toilet, closing the door, etc.).

The markedly improved emptying after potty-training, discussed above, is very interesting, since it is something that can be used in the treatment of incomplete emptying in this age group, through institution of potty-training earlier than what is common.

Indications for urodynamics in children

The indications for urodynamics in infants and children are the same as for adults: namely, suspicion of neurogenic or non-neurogenic bladder dysfunction or structural outflow obstruction. Thus, they include neurogenic bladder, gross vesicoureteral reflux (particularly in infants), recurrent UTIs, uroflow/residual measurement suggesting infravesical obstruction, and urinary incontinence (including nocturnal enuresis) that has been refractory to conventional treatment (urotherapy and drugs) for at least 1 year.

Neurogenic bladder dysfunction, whether suspected or established, is the most important of these indications. It should be said up front that cystometry in a patient with neurogenic bladder has to be repeated regularly during the patient's lifetime. In a child, cystometry should be performed at least once yearly because neurogenic bladder in the child is a dynamic disorder that is prone to change and then most often deterioration. The common cause is tethering of the spinal cord, which occurs in 75% of myelomeningoceles and in 100% of lipomyelomeningoceles.[24]

Age-related aspects

The investigation must be adapted to the child's needs!

In urology textbooks in the past, it could be read that 'cystometry cannot be performed in children younger than 7 years of age'. In one circumstance this statement was true: namely, when a young child was referred to a urodynamic laboratory that was used to examine adult patients only. Non-prepared children who hesitated to enter the laboratory and thereby upset the time schedule were looked upon as disturbing and irrational patients – which children certainly are if not treated according to their own needs! Children *are* irrational, sensitive, and skeptical towards all kinds of medical technology. Thus their need for information, patience, and loving care cannot be emphasized too much. The stress felt by a tense child during a urodynamic examination may very well generate results suggesting bladder dysfunction (overactive bladder and/or sphincter) even if that same child in a safe and relaxed mood would have shown completely normal urodynamic findings.

Ideally, the child should be prepared for what will be coming by being shown around the laboratory the day before the examination and given a summary in everyday language of what is going to happen (Figure 9.3). Several of these children have already undergone voiding cystography and may have unpleasant memories of the catheterization, so this topic has to be touched upon with great care.

During the examination, the child is handled in a relaxed and patient way. Even young children should be handled with respect for their personal integrity. As much as possible, the procedure should be performed 'as in play'. A video with popular cartoons has been a great asset in our laboratory and has helped children to overlook frightening equipment in the room (Figure 9.4). However, nothing can substitute for an experienced nurse or laboratory assistant who loves to take care of children.[25,26]

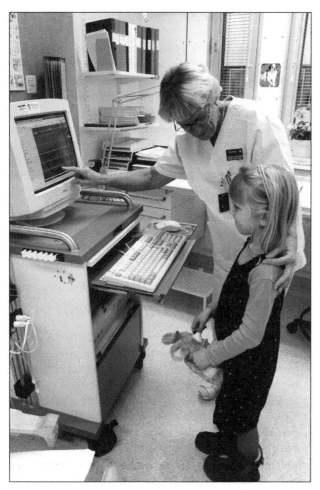

Figure 9.3
Child familiarizing herself with the urodynamic laboratory while receiving information from the laboratory assistant the day before the actual investigation.

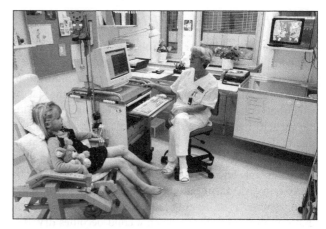

Figure 9.4
Cystometry is not necessarily a distressful experience, especially when an interesting video is running.

Sedation

Exceptionally, when a child expresses outspoken anxiety for the procedure, in particular the catheterization, sedation with midazolam may be an option.[27] We have no experience with using midazolam (Dormicum®, Roche) in urodynamic studies but have used the drug for several years when performing voiding cystourethrography (VCUG).[28] In these studies the drug does not seem to affect bladder/sphincter function in any way, but placebo-controlled, randomized studies have not yet been performed. The sedation is satisfactory and side-effects very rare. The drug company only offers Dormicum for intravenous use. However, in our practise, we use the intravenous preparation for oral or rectal administration and have noticed the same sedative efficacy without added side-effects. For *oral administration*, Dormicum 5 mg/ml is used in the dosage 0.3–0.5 mg per kg body weight, max. 7.5 mg, mixed in a small amount of juice or cola. Effective sedation occurs within 15–30 min and the duration of sedation is 30–50 min. Dormicum 1 mg/ml is used for *rectal administration* in the dosage 0.2–0.3 mg per kg body weight, max. 5 mg. Effective sedation occurs within 10–20 min and duration of sedation is 30–50 min. Observe that pulse oximeter, suction apparatus, and equipment for ventilation should be at hand. If the child falls asleep, secure free airways. The child should be supervised for at least 1 h 30 min before leaving for home.[28] Midazolam for sedation of a child going through a urodynamic investigation may be a good option in the future once placebo-controlled, randomized studies have been performed.

Age

Infants below 1 year of age pose very few problems during urodynamic investigation. They are simply too young to be afraid of the procedure. The most problematic age group are children aged 2–4 years who are old enough to feel scared but too young to understand the reasons for the examination.

Children with neurogenic bladder generally accept the urodynamic investigation without much problems. It is easier for these children to accept and for the staff to perform the procedure than is the case for children with intact lower urinary tract sensation.

Urodynamic methodology
Noninvasive urodynamics
Uroflow

Measurement of the urinary flow rate, including assessment of the shape of the flow curve, is a very useful investigative tool in children with non-neurogenic bladder/sphincter dysfunction but has a very limited value in neurogenic bladder patients. The simple reason is that a child with neurogenic bladder is only exceptionally able to perform a formal micturition.

Post-void residual urine (assessed with ultrasound)

This procedure is mandatory and should be repeated frequently in all children with neurogenic bladder. In infants and small children, who are not treated with CIC, the 4-hour voiding observation is used to investigate emptying ability.[16] The child uses a napkin during the test and voidings are indicated by a gossip strip or a light signal. Voided volume is measured by weighing the napkin after each voiding and post-void residual urine is checked by ultrasonography. Since post-void residual urine varies also in healthy babies with complete emptying only occasionally, the investigation has to include a 4-hour period and not only isolated voidings.

Post-void residual urine should also be checked in patients on CIC to make sure that the catheterization is performed in a correct and efficient way. Some children tend to withdraw the catheter too early. Others may get a dislocation of the bladder when growing up, necessitating a change of body position during CIC in order to achieve complete emptying.

Pad test

To estimate and follow urinary leakage between voidings or catheterizations during daily activity, the pad test is the most appropriate investigation, including hourly change of pads that are weighed to get the leakage volume. The leakage volume and frequency are important parameters to follow at least once a year, since changes can indicate tethering. It is also important as an indicator of the efficacy of treatment with anticholinergic medication.

Pelvic electromyography using cutaneous electrodes

Pelvic EMG for registration of pelvic floor activity during cystometry will sometimes detect neuromuscular activity even in patients with neurogenic bladder, but it will be difficult or impossible to find out from which portion of the pelvic floor muscles the signals emanate. Therefore, in many instances, the EMG will not deliver any clinically useful information. Nevertheless, cutaneous EMG should be performed as routine in order to keep up the competence of the urodynamic laboratory.

Invasive urodynamics: traditional cystometry

Invasive urodynamics is synonymous with cystometry (with the possible addition of EMG using needle electrodes).

Frequently asked questions (FAQs) regarding cystometric techniques

At which points of time should infants and children with neurogenic bladder dysfunction be examined with cystometry? The literature provides strong evidence that CIC in congenital NBD should be started as soon as possible in infancy,[29,30] because there is an obvious risk of deterioration of bladder function already in infancy as well as later in childhood.[31,32] Frequent and regular follow-up of bladder function (cystometry at least once a year) is mandatory, in particular during the first 6 years of life.[33]

Gas or fluid filling of the bladder? Gas should not be used.

Fluid-filled or transducer tip catheters for pressure measurement? For obvious reasons, transducer tip catheters must be used for natural fill (ambulatory) cystometry. When traditional cystometry is performed in the laboratory, however, they are too fragile, too expensive, and too difficult to calibrate for regular use. A fluid-filled pressure measurement system should be the standard here.

Transurethral or suprapubic catheters? Double-lumen transurethral catheters are ideal for infants and children with neurogenic bladder. Most of these patients have limited or absent urethral sensation. Moreover, the possible obstruction caused by the transurethral catheter is of minor importance in this patient group, since it is hardly ever possible to perform a formal pressure–flow measurement.

What filling rate should be used? The rate at which fluid is instilled in the bladder influences bladder wall dynamics, thus capacity, intravesical pressure, and compliance.[34] High filling rates create an artificial situation, with continuous pressure rise. Therefore, filling rates have to be standardized and not allowed to exceed physiological filling rates during maximal diuresis. The recommended rate is 1/20 (5%) of the patient's expected bladder capacity per minute, since in a healthy individual the bladder will be filled to capacity in 20 min during maximal diuresis. The patient's expected bladder capacity can be assessed from a diary in which the parents note the CIC volumes for a couple of days. The largest volume should be chosen (excluding the first morning voiding). Alternatively (particularly in severe incontinence with small CIC volumes), the expected bladder capacity in children 3 years of age and above can be calculated from the simple rule-of-thumb equation:

$$\text{Expected bladder capacity (ml)} = 30 + (\text{age in years} \times 30)$$

An alternative rule of thumb is that 1% of the body weight approximately predicts a child's bladder capacity. A 3-year-old would be expected to have a bladder capacity around 120 ml, so a filling rate of 6 ml/min should be used.

How many filling cycles are needed? In non-neurogenic cases, two. Even if the child seems to be at ease during the examination, the first filling is experienced by the child as more stressful than the following ones. Detrusor and/or sphincter overactivity is therefore more commonly seen during the first filling. The second filling will already reflect the urodynamic status of the bladder in a reliable way. Additional fillings don't need to be done because they produce similar findings to the second one.[9] However, in children with neurogenic bladder a single filling may be sufficient because lower urinary tract sensation is impaired and psychological mechanisms hardly influence bladder/sphincter function.

When to stop filling in a patient unable to feel a desire to void? This is the common situation in patients with NBD. The infusion should be finished when any of the following occurs:

1. strong urgency
2. micturition
3. feeling of discomfort
4. high basic detrusor pressure (>40 cmH$_2$O)
5. large infused volume ($>150\%$ of the expected bladder capacity unless the CIC diary has shown larger volumes at CIC)
6. rate of urinary leakage $\geq$ rate of infusion.

When is the bladder cooling test (formerly Bors ice water test) indicated in the urodynamic investigation of infants and children with established or suspected NBD? In every case, as a general rule. It has been shown that neurologically normal infants and children exhibit a positive bladder cooling test (BCT) during the first 4 years of life, whereas the test is negative in children older than 6 years.[35] In infants and children with NBD, a negative BCT before age 4 demonstrates a lesion of the sacral reflex arch, whereas a positive BCT in children older than 6 years indicates a lesion of inhibiting suprasacral spinal pathways.[36] The BCT is performed after finishing the traditional cystometry. The reactivity of the detrusor is first checked with body-warm saline infused rapidly in an amount corresponding to one-third of the cystometric bladder capacity. If this infusion does not elicit any significant detrusor contraction, the bladder is emptied and the same amount (one-third of bladder capacity) of cold (around 4°C) saline is infused rapidly. A positive test is defined as a detrusor contraction within 1 min with detrusor pressure ≥ 30 cmH$_2$O.

How to measure leak point pressure – and what is its value? The ideal way of measuring leak point pressure (LPP) is to note the detrusor pressure at the moment when leakage of urine is observed, during cystometry. This means that the laboratory assistant would have to monitor the patient's genital area continuously, which is seldom possible. Instead, the flowmeter is often used to indicate leakage; but it is then important to make adjustments for the time delay between pressure registration and the flowmeter deflection, in particular when leakage occurs in connection with a phasic detrusor contraction. It is assumed that LPP >40 cmH$_2$O in children with NBD suggests an increased risk for development of renal damage. This assumption makes sense, because maintained *intravesical* pressure above 30–40 cmH$_2$O is certainly associated with an increased incidence of VUR and upper tract dilatation.[37] Thus, an assessment of LPP should be routinely included in the urodynamic evaluation of a child with NBD.

What is the role of electromyography in the urodynamic evaluation of children with neurogenic bladder dysfunction? 'Quantitative' EMG using perineal surface electrodes (Ag/AgCl) will not always produce clinically valuable information in this patient group. It can be argued, however, that the EMG activity should be registered routinely in order to maintain competence in the urodynamic laboratory.

How should intra-abdominal pressure be measured? Ideally, with a transducer tip catheter inserted into the left fossa of the abdominal cavity, a method which does not cause any complications even during extended use for natural fill cystometry.[38] The second-best choice is to measure *prevesical* pressure in a minute pool of saline in the cavum Retzii between the bladder and the abdominal wall.[39] The common method, though, is to measure *intrarectal* pressure, hoping that it will represent intra-abdominal pressure. It does not, of course; at best, it gives a general idea about the extravesical pressure environment in which the bladder is working. However, the intrarectal pressure is easily accessible with a catheter passed through the anus. This fact – together with a solid chunk of urodynamic tradition – and, additionally, the invasive nature of the two first-mentioned options, helps to propagate intrarectal pressure as the standard for assessing perivesical pressure. The rectal catheter should be open-ended and continuously and slowly (3 ml/h) perfused with saline to prevent blocking by feces. It is important to check pressure transmission by asking the patient to strain or cough or by applying pressure on the suprapubic area. Be aware that the rectal catheter will sometimes transmit pressure peaks generated by spontaneous rectal contractions, something that may result in false-negative detrusor pressure readings. Thus, detrusor pressure calculated as intravesical minus intrarectal pressure is not always a reliable urodynamic variable.

Invasive urodynamics: videocystometry

Performing cystometry and fluoroscopic monitoring of the bladder and urethra at the same time no doubt increases the diagnostic accuracy of the urodynamic procedure, e.g. by allowing determination of bladder pressure at the moment when VUR occurs. The combined examination is also of value in patients with high-grade VUR where a common problem is to decide how much of the infused volume corresponds to bladder capacity and how much is stored in the refluxing systems. It can thus be said that some clinical questions will not be possible to answer without concurrent use of cystometry and X-ray. Therefore, videocystometry has become a standard urodynamic procedure for children with NBD (and other diagnoses) in many centers. However, videocystometry has its disadvantages. The most important of these is that videocystometry makes the examination even more complex by introducing additional machinery face to face to the (possibly) bewildered child. Even well-prepared and cooperative children may have difficulties in adapting to a highly sophisticated procedure. Since the child patient needs significant modification of the cystometric techniques compared to the adult, it can be questioned whether increasing the level of investigative sophistication is the right way to go. In our institution we have, so far, limited the use of videocystometry to clinical research (e.g. congenital reflux, posterior urethral valves) and to the occasional child with difficult-to-understand bladder problems where the combination of cystometry and imaging has sometimes helped us to arrive at the correct diagnosis.

Invasive urodynamics: natural fill (ambulatory) cystometry

Natural fill cystometry differs from traditional laboratory cystometry by (1) allowing the patient to be mobile, i.e. not restricting him to the laboratory chair, and (2) using the patient's own diuresis as the filling medium of the bladder. In both adults and children significant differences have been found between values obtained by artificial and

natural filling urodynamics, respectively. Especially, steeper pressure rise and larger voided volumes were observed during and after artificial filling, whereas voiding pressures were found to be higher after natural filling. The natural fill cystometry also seems to be more sensitive in detecting detrusor instability than the traditional, artificial filling method.[40] The lower incidence of detrusor instability and the greater voided volumes found on traditional cystometry probably reflect an inhibition of detrusor function because of the relatively fast artificial filling.

In neurogenic bladders in adults, important differences were noted between conventional and natural fill cystometry. High increases in pressure registered during artificial filling, interpreted as low compliance of the bladder wall, were not reproduced during natural fill cystometry but rather replaced by phasic detrusor activity. Natural filling disclosed a combination of greater residual urine volumes, greater resting pressures, and greater phasic activity in patients with upper tract dilatation.[41]

In infants and children, results obtained by conventional cystometry and natural fill cystometry have shown the same differences as in adults regarding both non-neurogenic and neurogenic bladder dysfunction. The two methods were compared in a group of 17 children (mean age 6.8 years) with various urological disorders.[42] As in adults, the natural fill study yielded lower voided volumes, a less steep pressure rise on filling, and higher detrusor pressures during micturition. Additionally, natural fill urodynamics revealed detrusor instability in more patients than did the conventional cystometry.

The studies cited recorded bladder and rectal pressure for time periods ranging between 4 and 6 hours. In a study from our institution[38] we took full advantage of the ambulatory, natural fill method by extending the recording time to a mean of 20 hours. It was thus possible to compare the bladder behavior between day and night, which yielded interesting results. Also, the small patients were truly ambulatory since they were carrying the recording device in a backpack. There was no disruption of the child's normal activities and the children seemed almost completely unaware that they were subjected to a sophisticated investigation of their bladder function. Sixteen boys aged 1.4–6 years (mean age 3.4) with endoscopically resected posterior urethral valves (at a mean age of 3.6 months) were studied. All the boys had detrusor instability in the daytime but the bladders became stable during sleeping hours. At natural fill cystometry, voiding detrusor pressure was higher and functional bladder capacity much lower during the day than at night. Dissimilarities noted between natural fill and conventional cystometry were the same as found in all other studies.

A couple of studies have compared natural fill with conventional cystometry in children with neurogenic bladder. In 2 of 11 children with myelodysplasia (mean age 10 years) more phasic detrusor activity and higher pressure amplitudes were found during 6 h of natural fill cystometry.[43] In another study of 20 children (age 6–11 years) with neurogenic bladder, natural fill cystometry (mean duration 12 hours) discovered detrusor overactivity in 45% of the children in contrast to traditional cystometry in the same children where half had been judged to have normal bladder function and the other half low-compliance bladders.[44]

In conclusion, natural fill cystometry in infants, children, and adults shows a lower pressure rise during filling, a higher incidence of detrusor overactivity, a higher detrusor pressure on micturition, and a lower voided volume than is found at conventional cystometry. It cannot be excluded that 'low compliance neurogenic bladder' might sometimes turn out to be an investigational artifact due to the unphysiological high rate of artificial bladder filling, since studies in both children and adults have shown the rapid rise of pressure during artificial filling being replaced by phasic detrusor overactivity.[41,44] Natural fill urodynamics does not use artificial filling, and it causes minimal psychological trauma, especially important for the pediatric patient, so it no doubt delivers the more authentic reflection of true bladder physiology. However, data on natural fill cystometry in children with neurogenic bladder are still sparse, and, before replacing traditional with natural fill urodynamics, additional studies are needed. In particular, it will be necessary to find out how decreased distensibility of the bladder wall is presenting itself in the natural fill studies. Increase of basal detrusor pressure above 20–30 cmH$_2$O is seldom seen during natural fill but has been interpreted as an important sign of poor compliance when seen in traditional cystometry and found to be associated with dilatation of the upper tracts and deterioration of renal function. Since the rapid rise of basal detrusor pressure may be looked upon as a significant finding, it is still too early to appoint natural fill urodynamics to be the future golden standard in the investigation of neurogenic bladders in children, even if the possibility remains that natural fill may lead to profound reassessment of the urodynamic neurogenic pathophysiology.

Evaluation of urodynamic results

What are we looking for?

As in adult urodynamics, *the four C's:*

- capacity (of the bladder reservoir)
- contractility (of the detrusor and sphincter)
- compliance (of the bladder wall)
- continence.

And, in addition:

- lower urinary tract sensation
- evacuation (as reflected by absence or presence of post-void residual).

Normal urodynamic variables in infants and children

In infants and children, it goes without saying that normal values differ widely from the adult ones; and that, in growing individuals, variables such as bladder capacity vary according to the age and size of the child.

Bladder capacity

Increase of bladder capacity is not linear to age or weight during the first years of life. There are two periods when the increase is accelerated. The first is during the first months of life. In free voiding studies of pre-term infants in gestation week 32, median bladder capacity was 12 ml[15] (Figure 9.5) and in similar studies of full-term babies 3 months of age median capacity was 52 ml[13] (Figure 9.6). The capacity is almost unchanged at 1 and 2 years of age (67 and 68 ml, respectively). At 3 years of age, on the other hand, the median capacity is 123 ml, meaning a doubling during the third year of life (see Figure 9.6).[13]

The first step in increase of bladder capacity is thus around birth and is a fourfold increase, which should be compared with the increase in body weight, which is only three-fold. The second step is at the age of toilet-training when gaining control over voidings. The main stimulant for this second increase in bladder capacity can be suggested to be due to the fact that the child starts to get dry at

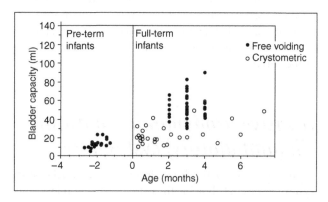

Figure 9.5
Age vs bladder capacity as measured in free voiding studies in both pre-term[15] and full-term[13] infants, and at cystometry in full-term infants.[17]

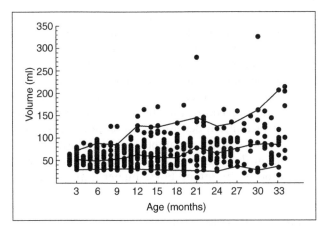

Figure 9.6
Bladder capacity vs age in a longitudinal study of free voidings in infants and children aged 0–3 years, investigated every 3rd month. The lines indicate the 5th, 50th, and 95th percentiles.[13]

night, which means higher overnight bladder volumes. Indications for such a connection are the finding that high overnight bladder volumes have been shown to be responsible for development of high bladder capacity in patients with VUR[45] and also in boys with posterior urethral valves.[38] Overnight bladder volume has also been shown to be the determinant for functional bladder capacity in healthy children after potty-training.[46]

The relationship between free voiding and cystometric capacity changes during the first years of life. In the neonatal period, cystometric capacity[17] is lower as compared to free voiding capacity[13] (see Figure 9.5), whereas after the infant year the opposite is seen. This can be partly attributed to the fact that older children postpone voiding at cystometry due to fear of voiding with a catheter in the bladder and of the unfamiliar situation of the assessment. This fear cannot be expected in the neonatal child and voiding is thus not postponed for this reason. Another possible explanation for the low cystometric capacity in the neonatal period might be the overactivity suggested by Bachelard et al, shown as an ease to induce detrusor contractions prematurely in catheter investigations.[17]

Even if development of bladder capacity during the first years of life is not linear, we suggest that a linear formula is used for calculation of expected bladder capacity for age as a simple rule of thumb. We have chosen to use:

Expected bladder capacity (ml) = 30 + (age in years × 30)[25]

since this linear increase in capacity is very similar to the nonlinear increase in capacity as described by Jansson et al[13] investigating children longitudinally from birth to age 3 years in free voiding studies (see Figure 9.6).

According to the International Continence Society (ICS), the term 'functional bladder capacity' should no

longer be used because of difficulties of definition, and it should be replaced with 'voided volume'. Children void widely different volumes during the same day, sometimes when they feel a desire to void but quite often because their mothers tell them to go to the toilet.[46] The common way to decide a child's bladder capacity is to keep a voiding diary (frequency–volume chart) for 2 days and select the largest voiding volume, excluding the first morning voidings that rather represent nocturnal bladder capacity. For children on CIC, the same method is used to define the child's approximate bladder volume.

Measured capacity less than 65% of the calculated value is believed to denote a bladder which is *small for age*, whereas a measured volume that is more than 150% of the calculated value may denote a bladder that is *large for age*.[25]

Detrusor contractility

Storage phase. It has been shown during recent years that instability is rarely seen in infants[14,17] which is contrary to the earlier concept of instability as a normal phenomenon in this age group.[9] The lack of unstable contractions during filling has been shown in natural fill cystometry,[14] which is an investigation that is sensitive when it comes to identification of instability. This lack of instability during filling has also been observed in standard cystometric investigations of healthy infants, including a study of siblings of children with reflux.[17]

In infants with bladder dysfunction, on the other hand, instability during filling is common, such as those with posterior urethral valves[38] and neurogenic bladder.[31] Therefore, instability can probably be used to diagnose bladder dysfunction in this age group just like in older children.

During the first months of life, on the other hand, there seems to be another form of overactivity, which was observed in 20% of the children as an isolated detrusor contraction after only a few milliliters of filling at cystometry and, with leakage of urine, looked at as a premature voiding contraction.[17] Bladder capacity in these age groups urodynamically registered was also low,[17] and was much lower than that seen after free voidings.[13] These findings taken together indicate that the voiding reflex can easily be elicited in this age group, in the cystometric investigations, by a catheter in the bladder and infusion of saline (see Figure 9.2). This overactivity vanishes after a few months and, simultaneously, bladder capacity increases. The phenomenon does not seem to have anything to do with instability, since instability is seldom seen in infants,[14,17] but rather be looked upon as an immature behavior of the detrusor muscle.[47,48]

Voiding phase. Voiding detrusor pressure is probably higher during early infancy compared to that seen in older children. Bachelard et al[17] and Wen and Tong[49] investigated infants considered to have normal low urinary tract with conventional cystometry using a urethral catheter. The pressure levels registered in these studies were very different; median 127 vs mean 75 cmH$_2$O. One explanation of the different results may be the age of the infants studied, which was median 1 month and 6 months, respectively. Yeung et al also found high voiding pressure levels in small infants.[42] However, it should be noted that they used natural fill cystometry, which gives higher pressure levels than standard cystometry.

Female infants have significantly lower pressures at voiding compared with males and only slightly higher than those of older girls (Table 9.1).

This difference in voiding detrusor pressure between males and females must be attributed to the difference in anatomy, with the long narrow urethra in male infants allowing higher outflow resistance and inducing higher voiding pressure. Thus, the standards for voiding pressure in healthy infants are imprecise and can be a median of more than 100 cmH$_2$O in males and 60–70 cmH$_2$O in females (see Table 9.1). In children 1–3 years of age median voiding pressures have been reported to be 70 cmH$_2$O in males[9] and 60 in females.[49]

High voiding pressure in infants is correlated with low bladder capacity. This further explains the above-described differences in voiding pressure levels in the studies by Wen and Tong[49] and Bachelard et al.[17] In the latter study, the infants were younger and thus had lower capacity.

Any discernible peak in the detrusor pressure recording during the filling phase is a pathological finding, but in order to avoid recording artifacts it may be prudent to allow only for peaks with a duration of >10 s and amplitude of >10 cmH$_2$O. In neurogenic bladder urodynamics, one should keep in mind that traditional cystometry seems to suppress phasic detrusor activity and exaggerate the rise of basic pressure (giving the impression of low compliance) compared with natural fill cystometry.[41,44]

Variables to register. Variables to register comprise the following:

- Number of phasic contractions and their duration and amplitude together with the infused volume when they occurred. Note subjective reaction, if any.

- Basic detrusor pressure at start and end of filling (excluding a possible sharp terminal rise of pressure). Avoid to include phasic contractions.
- Detrusor pressure at start of significant leakage (LPP) and the infused volume when leakage occurred.
- Absence or presence of a coordinated detrusor micturition contraction. In the case of a micturition contraction, any detrusor pressure above 100 cmH$_2$O is to be regarded as pathological in children, denoting outflow obstruction or detrusor overactivity, or both. In infant boys, higher values may be normal.

Bladder cooling test. Variables to register are:

- outcome: positive (detrusor contraction >30 cmH$_2$O) or negative (30 cmH$_2$O)
- maximal detrusor pressure, registered in cmH$_2$O.

Sphincter contractility

In children with neurogenic bladders, EMG registration will not always produce any information about urethral sphincter activity. When the EMG recording seems unreliable, indirect evidence will have to do. Leak point pressure >40 cmH$_2$O denotes either neurogenic sphincter overactivity or a sphincter with intact innervation. Likewise, the finding of intravesical pressures well above 40 cmH$_2$O without any detectable leakage of urine suggests detrusor-sphincter dyssynergia or, alternatively, a normal sphincter contracting to prevent leakage (guarding reflex).

Compliance of the bladder wall

The concept of compliance characterizes the distensibility of the bladder wall during the reservoir phase. A subnormal compliance value denotes increase of bladder wall stiffness due to change of wall structure or a tonic detrusor contraction and is a risk factor for development of upper tract damage. Compliance is expressed as the volume (ml) that the bladder can accommodate with a resulting pressure increase of 1 cmH$_2$O. It is calculated from a middle segment of the detrusor pressure registration up to 30 cmH$_2$O, avoiding phasic contractions. A 'normal' value for compliance in adults has not been validated but it is generally felt that it should be more than 20 ml/cmH$_2$O, e.g. that basic pressure increase up to an adult bladder volume of 400 ml should be 20 cmH$_2$O or less from empty to full bladder. But we will encounter problems trying to apply this value of compliance to the wide range of bladder volumes in children. For example, a child with a bladder capacity of 100 ml (which would be normal in a 3-year-old child) and a 20 cmH$_2$O pressure

Table 9.1 *Voiding detrusor pressure in infants*

References	Mean voiding detrusor pressure (cmH$_2$O)	
	Males	Females
Yeung et al[42]	117	75
Bachelard et al[17]	127	72
Wen and Tong[49]	75	60

increase from empty to full bladder will give a compliance value of 5 ml/cmH$_2$O, a value which would be clearly pathological in an adult. An adjustment must be done to make values comparable between children and adults. It has been suggested that the lowest acceptable value of compliance in a child should be 1/20 (5%) of the child's normal capacity per cmH$_2$O, a calculation that would be compatible with the lowest limit of 'normal' compliance, 20 ml/cmH$_2$O, in adults. Then, a compliance of 5 ml/cmH$_2$O at a bladder capacity of 100 ml would be within the normal range.

Safe capacity. Instead of calculating compliance in order to characterize the reservoir properties of the bladder wall, we use the concept of 'safe capacity' at our institution. The bladder volumes at 20 cmH$_2$O and 30 cmH$_2$O base line detrusor pressure are registered. The 20 cmH$_2$O value stands for a truly safe and the 30 cmH$_2$O a borderline value for compliance at reservoir capacity.

Continence

Cystometry of a child is not only a laboratory investigation but also allows for a careful and prolonged clinical observation of the child. In addition to the urodynamic results produced by the cystometry, this observation provides important information regarding the child's reactions to bladder filling and, not least, in which situations and at which bladder volumes leakage of urine can be noted.

Lower urinary tract sensation

From age 4 onwards, it is possible to extend the clinical observation during cystometry by asking the child whether he feels the catheter being introduced and if he experiences any sensation from the bladder during filling. Some degree of urethral sensation is not seldom present in children with neurogenic bladder, whereas bladder sensation is most often absent or very weak. Discomfort or pain at end filling when the bladder has become filled to capacity is probably elicited from functional sensory nerve endings in the peritoneum partly covering the bladder. When the child signals discomfort (in small children seldom verbally, but rather by being anxious, crying, or moving restlessly), infusion should be discontinued. The cystometry protocol should include the soft data obtained regarding sensation.

Bladder evacuation

Infants do not empty the bladder at every voiding,[13,15,16,49,51] but, characteristically one voiding during 4 hours is complete, according to results from the 4-hour observations. This is seen both in pre-term infants (gestation week 32)[15] and neonates, and during the first years of life.[13] The residual urine during 4 hours is more or less constant from the neonatal period until just before the age of 2 years; median 4–5 ml.[13,15,16] During the third year, when gaining control over voidings, on the other hand, the emptying of the bladder becomes complete, so that the median residual urine is 0 ml.[13]

In healthy children above 3–4 years of age, the bladder empties completely at each voiding. Five milliliters in post-void residual may be accepted due to the unavoidable time delay from the end of voiding until the bladder can be examined with ultrasound; 5–20 ml is borderline and is an indication for repeating the ultrasound. In schoolgirls treated for bacteriuria, recurrence was significantly more common in those with post-void residual urine greater than 5 ml.[52] In children with NBD, assessing post-void residual urine by aspiring through the bladder catheter may not always yield reliable results due to the common dislocation of the base of the neurogenic bladder, so a check with ultrasound is strongly recommended. Ultrasound to determine residual urine should also be performed frequently on all children on CIC for the same reason.

Conclusions

The free voiding pattern in the neonatal period is characterized by small, frequent voidings (one voiding per hour) with volumes that vary intra-individually and leave residual urine most of the time. The incomplete emptying is suggested to be due to a physiological form of dyscoordination. Towards potty-training age the emptying improves, and, at that time (third year), the bladder capacity also doubles. Voiding during quiet sleep is rarely seen, even in the neonatal infant, meaning that the child shows signs of arousal at voiding.

Bladder instability is rarely seen in urodynamic studies of young infants, although premature voiding contractions are seen in the neonatal period, with leakage of urine after only a few milliliters of filling. This latter increased reactivity of the detrusor muscle is also suggested to be responsible for the cystometric small bladder capacity in this age group and the high voiding pressure levels.

Classification of neurogenic bladder dysfunction in infants and children

A classification of neurogenic bladder in spina bifida children was suggested by van Gool.[53] As can be seen in Table 9.2, a simple but clinically useful classification can be created from the urodynamic data. Detrusor and sphincter are classified as underactive or overactive, so the neurogenic dysfunction can be categorized in four main groups. Two of these display underactive sphincter with incontinence as the major clinical problem, and the two others have overactive sphincter with outflow obstruction and deficient bladder emptying as their main clinical characteristics. It should be added, however, that about 5% of children with myelomeningocele display normal bladder function at cystometry, in particular those who have their spinal cord anomaly in a high position (cervical, thoracic, or high thoracolumbar) (Figure 9.7).

Table 9.2 *Four patterns of bladder-sphincter dysfunction in children with myelomeningocele*[53]

Sphincter	Detrusor		Clinical correlate
	Underactive	Overactive	
Underactive	35	42	Incontinence
Overactive	13	42	Outflow obstruction

Examples of common urodynamic patterns in neurogenic bladder dysfunction in children

The most ominous urodynamic pattern, threatening the integrity of the kidneys, is dyssynergia between detrusor and sphincter. The micturition detrusor contraction is counteracted by sphincter contractions, leading to poor evacuation of the bladder, as seen in a 4-year-old boy with lumbosacral myelomeningocele (Figure 9.8).

Almost equally dangerous for the renal health is the pattern with an underactive or paretic detrusor, low compliant bladder wall, and overactive sphincter (Figure 9.9). The child attempts, without much success, to empty the bladder by forceful contractions of the abdominal muscles. As in the previous case, a regular, carefully performed CIC program is absolutely essential in order to avoid UTIs, reflux, and renal damage in this 4-year-old boy with lumbosacral myelomeningocele.

The pattern is often not as clear-cut as in the two previous cases. In the next example, the detrusor is overactive and there is borderline compliance (Figure 9.10).

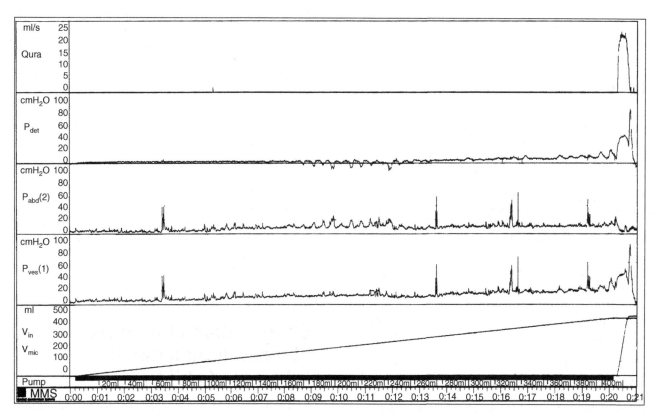

Figure 9.7
Normal cystometry in a 4-year-old boy with high thoracolumbar myelomeningocele.

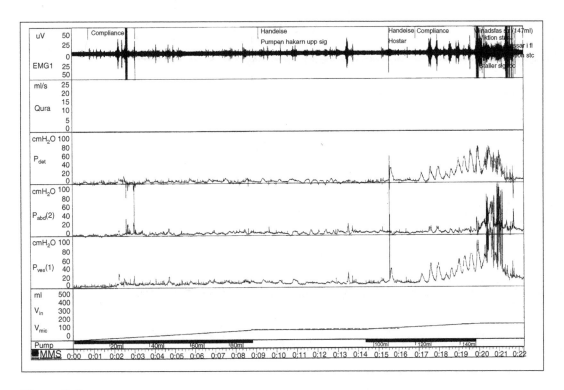

Figure 9.8
Normal compliance, discrete detrusor overactivity, and micturition contraction forcefully counteracted by sphincter contraction, thus pronounced dyssynergia, in a 4-year-old boy with lumbosacral myelomeningocele.

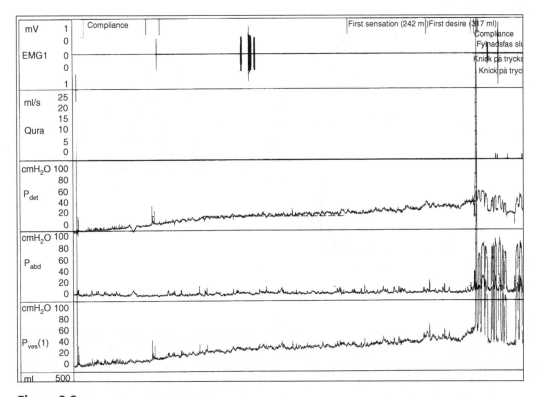

Figure 9.9
Detrusor underactivity, low bladder wall compliance, and poor effect of straining, suggesting sphincter overactivity, in a 4-year-old boy with lumbosacral myelomeningocele.

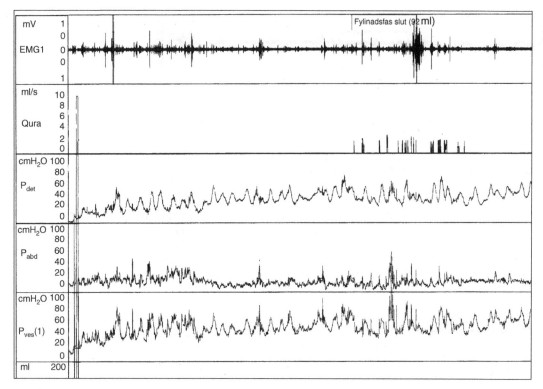

Figure 9.10

Example of cystometry which is not readily elucidated in a 9-month-old boy with lumbosacral myelomeningocele. Detrusor overactivity and borderline bladder wall compliance, but what about the sphincter behavior? Electromyography (EMG) may indicate a somewhat overactive pelvic floor, but there are, on the other hand, rather frequent mini-micturitions and a larger one at the end of the registration ('START MIKT').

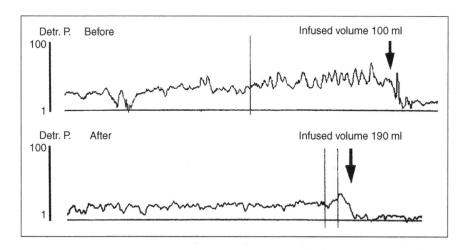

Figure 9.11

Intravesical oxybutynin may efficiently inhibit detrusor overactivity in a 5-year-old girl with lumbosacral myelomeningocele. Detrusor pressure and compliance become normal and capacity nearly doubles after intravesical instillation of 5 mg of oxybutynin.

The sphincter may also be somewhat overactive, as judged from the EMG; but, on the other hand, there are several small micturitions and a larger one at the end of the registration. This patient, with lumbosacral myelomeningocele, is only 9 months old, so there may remain an element of physiological immaturity in the urodynamic pattern.

The final example, a 5-year-old girl with lumbosacral myelomeningocele (Figure 9.11), depicts the beneficial effect on detrusor overactivity that is often attained with the use of detrusor-relaxing drugs (in this case, oxybutynin 5 mg twice daily administered intravesically). As can be seen, both phasic and tonic (compliance!) detrusor contractility normalizes.

References

1. Scott R Jr, McIlhaney JS. The voiding rates in normal male children. J Urol 1959; 82:244.

2. Zatz LM. Combined physiologic and radiologic studies of bladder function in female children with recurrent urinary tract infections. Invest Urol 1965; 3:278.

3. Whitaker J, Johnston GS. Estimation of urinary outflow resistance in children: simultaneous measurement of bladder pressure, flow rate and exit pressure. Invest Urol 1969; 7:127.

4. Palm L, Nielsen OH. Evaluation of bladder function in children. J Pediatr Surg 1967; 2:529.

5. Starfield B. Functional bladder capacity in enuretic and non-enuretic children. J Pediatr 1967; 70:777.

6. Gierup HJW. Micturition studies in infants and children. Intravesical pressure, urinary flow and urethral resistance in boys without infravesical obstruction. Scand J Urol Nephrol 1970; 3:217.

7. Kroigaard N. The lower urinary tract in infancy and childhood. Micturition cinematography with simultaneous pressure-flow measurement. Acta Radiol 1970; (suppl):300:3–175.

8. O'Donnell B, O'Connor TP. Bladder function in infants and children. Br J Urol 1971; 43:25.

9. Hjalmas K. Micturition in infants and children with normal lower urinary tract. A urodynamic study. Scand J Urol Nephrol 1976; (suppl)37.

10. Gool JD van, Kuijter RH, Donckerwolcke RA, et al. Bladder-sphincter dysfunction, urinary infection and vesico-ureteral reflux with special reference to cognitive bladder training. Contrib Nephrol 1985; 39:190.

11. Lindehall B, Claesson I, Hjalmas K, Jodal U. Effect of clean intermittent catheterisation on radiological appearance of the upper urinary tract in children with myelomeningocele. Br J Urol 1991; 67:415–419.

12. Muellner SR. Development of urinary control in children. JAMA 1960; 172:1256–1260.

13. Jansson UB, Hanson M, Hanson E, et al. Voiding pattern in healthy children 0 to 3 years old: a longitudinal study. J Urol 2000; 164:2050–2054.

14. Yeung C, Godley M, Ho C, et al. Some new insights into bladder function in infancy. Br J Urol 1995; 76:235–240.

15. Sillén U, Sölsnes E, Hellström A-L, Sandberg K. The voiding pattern of healthy preterm neonates. J Urol 2000; 163:278.

16. Holmdahl G, Hanson E, Hanson M, et al. Four-hour voiding observation in healthy infants. J Urol 1996; 156:1809–1812.

17. Bachelard M, Sillén U, Hansson S, et al. Urodynamic pattern in asymptomatic infants: siblings of children with vesicoureteral reflux. J Urol 1999; 162:1733.

18. Zerin M, Chen E, Ritchey M, Bloom D. Bladder capacity as measured at voiding cystourethrography in children: relationship to toilet training and frequency of micturition. J Urol 1993; 187:803.

19. Bakker E, Wyndaele JJ. Change in the toilet-training of children during the last 60 years: the cause of an increase in lower urinary tract dysfunction? BJU Int 2000; 86:248.

20. Brazelton TB. A child-oriented approach to toilet training. Pediatrics 1962; 29:121.

21. Klackenberg G. A prospective longitudinal study of children. Data on psychic health and development up to 8 years of age. Acta Paediatr Scand Suppl. 1971; 224:1–239.

22. Largo R, Molinari L, von Siebenthal K, Wolfensberge U. Does a profound change in toilet-training affect development of bowel and bladder control? Dev Med Child Neurol 1996; 38:1106–1116.

23. Marten W, deVries MD, deVries PNP. Cultural relativity of toilet training readiness: a perspective from East Africa. Pediatrics 1977; 60:170–177.

24. Shurtleff DB. 44 years experience with management of myelomeningocele: presidential address, Society for Research into Hydrocephalus and Spina Bifida. Eur J Pediatr Surg 2000; 10 (suppl 1):5–8.

25. Hjälmås K. Urodynamics in normal infants and children. Scand J Urol Nephrol 1988; (suppl) 114:20–27.

26. Swithinbank L, O'Brien M, Frank D, et al. The role of paediatric urodynamics revisited. Neurourol Urodyn 2002; 21:439–440.

27. Bozkurt P, Kilic N, Kaya G, et al. The effects of intranasal midazolam on urodynamic studies in children. Br J Urol 1996; 78:282–286.

28. Stokland E, Andreasson S, Jacobsson B, Jodal U, Ljung B. Sedation with midazolam for voiding cystourethrography in children: a randomized double-blind study. Pediatr Radiol 2003; 33(4):247–249.

29. Tanikaze S, Sugita Y. Cystometric examination for neurogenic bladder of neonates and infants. Hinyokika Kiyo 1991; 37:1403–1405.

30. Agarwal SK, McLorie GA, Grewal D, et al. Urodynamic correlates or resolution of reflux in meningomyelocele patients. J Urol 1997; 158:580–582.

31. Sillén U, Hanson E, Hermansson G, et al. Development of the urodynamic pattern in infants with myelomeningocele. Br J Urol 1996; 78:596–601.

32. Bauer SB. The argument for early assessment and treatment of infants with spina bifida. Dialog Pediatr Urol 2000; 23(11):2–3.

33. Tarcan T, Bauer S, Olmedo E, et al. Long-term follow up of newborns with myelodysplasia and normal urodynamic findings: is follow up necessary? J Urol 2001; 165:564–567.

34. Klevmark B. Natural pressure-volume curves and conventional cystometry. Scand J Urol Nephrol 1999; (suppl 201):1–4.

35. Geirsson G, Lindstrom S, Fall M, et al. Positive bladder cooling test in neurologically normal young children. J Urol 1994; 151:446–448.

36. Gladh G, Lindstrom S. Outcome of the bladder cooling test in children with neurogenic bladder dysfunction. J Urol 1999; 161:254–258.

37. Flood HD, Ritchey ML, Bloom DA, et al. Outcome of reflux in children with myelodysplasia managed by bladder pressure monitoring. J Urol 1994; 152:1574–1577.

38. Holmdahl G, Sillen U, Bertilsson M, et al. Natural filling cystometry in small boys with posterior urethral valves: unstable bladders become stable during sleep. J Urol 1997; 158:1017–1021.

39. Bjerle P. Relationship between perivesical and intravesical urinary bladder pressures and intragastric pressure. Acta Physiol Scand 1974; 92:465–473.

40. Robertson A, Griffiths C, Ramsden P, Neal D. Bladder function in healthy volunteers: ambulatory monitoring and conventional urodynamic studies. Br J Urol 1994; 73:242–249.

41. Webb RJ, Griffiths CJ, Ramsden PD, Neal DE. Ambulatory monitoring of bladder pressure in low compliance neurogenic bladder dysfunction. J Urol 1992; 148:1477–1481.

42. Yeung C, Godley M, Duffy P, Ransley P. Natural filling cystometry in infants and children. Br J Urol 1995; 75:531–537.

43. De Gennaro M, Capitanucci ML, Silveri M, et al. Continuous (6 hour) urodynamic monitoring in children with neuropathic bladder. Eur J Pediatr Surg 1996; 6(suppl 1):21–24.

44. Zermann DH, Lindner H, Huschke T, Schubert J. Diagnostic value of natural fill cystometry in neurogenic bladder in children. Eur Urol 1997; 32:223–228.

45. Sillén U, Hellström A-L, Sölsnes E, Jansson U-B. Control of voidings means better emptying of the bladder in children with congenital dilating VUR. BJU Int 2000; 85(suppl 4):13.

46. Mattsson SH. Voiding frequency, volumes and intervals in healthy school children. Scand J Urol Nephrol 1994; 28:1–11.

47. Sugaya K, de Groat WC. Influence of temperature on activity of the isolated whole bladder preparation of neonatal and adult rats. Am J Physiol Regul Integr Comp Physiol 2000; 278:238.

48. Zderic SA, Sillén U, Liu G-H, et al. Developmental aspects of bladder contractile function: evidence for an intracellular calcium pool. J Urol 1993; 150:623.

49. Wen JG, Tong EC. Cystometry in infants and children with no apparent voiding symptoms. Br J Urol 1998; 81:468.

50. Roberts DS, Rendell B. Postmicturition residual bladder volumes in healthy babies. Arch Dis Child 1989; 64:825–828.

51. Gladh G, Persson D, Mattsson S, Lindstrom S. Voiding patterns in healthy newborns. Neurourol Urodyn 2000; 19:177–184.

52. Lindberg U, Bjure J, Haugstvedt S, Jodal U. Asymptomatic bacteriuria in schoolgirls. III. Relation between residual urine volume and recurrence. Acta Paediatr Scand 1975; 64:437–440.

53. Van Gool J. Spina bifida and neurogenic bladder dysfunction: a urodynamic study. Thesis. Utrecht: Uitgeverij Impress, 1986:154.

10

Electrophysiological evaluation: basic principles and clinical applications

Simon Podnar and Clare J Fowler

Introduction

Electrophysiological methods record bioelectrical potentials generated by excitable cell membranes. When applied in a clinical setting to recordings from nerves and skeletal muscle these tests are often referred to as clinical neurophysiological investigations. Clinical neurophysiological methods are well-established, and have been used in clinical practice for almost half a century.

Neurophysiological techniques have so far been applied in the pelvic floor mostly for research purposes, but they have also been proposed for everyday diagnostics in selected groups of patients. The WHO Consensus on Incontinence stated that electrophysiological assessment is useful in selected patients with suspected peripheral nervous system lesions such as lower motor neuron (LMN) lesions, patients with multiple system atrophy (MSA), and also in women with urinary retention.[1]

The emphasis of this chapter is on clinically useful and 'established' electrophysiological tests, which are of diagnostic value in individual patients with neurogenic bladders. Concentric needle electromyography (CNEMG) and bulbocavernosus reflex (BCR) testing will be discussed in detail. Other tests not considered to be of clinical value in the diagnosis of individual patients will be only briefly described. For more detailed description of these research-type clinical uroneurophysiological tests,[1] reference to other reviews is recommended.[1,2]

Electrophysiological tests in assessment of patients

General remarks

A particular diagnostic test should be considered in a patient when the information it may provide will significantly affect further treatment and/or clarify prognosis. Clinical neurophysiological findings consistent with the diagnosis of

'a neurogenic bladder' can be found in patients with established diagnosis of neurological disease but in these circumstances add little to the case. However, in patients being investigated for bladder symptoms of suspected neurological origin, neurophysiological tests may reveal evidence of neural damage and thus point to neurological diagnosis.[3]

Basically, in neurological disease affecting the bladder, two main patterns of abnormalities can be found: the LMN and the upper motor neuron (UMN) pattern (see below), which are, respectively, due to lesions of the anterior horn cell or alpha motor neuron, spinal root, and peripheral nerve in the case of an LMN lesion (Figure 10.1) or due to

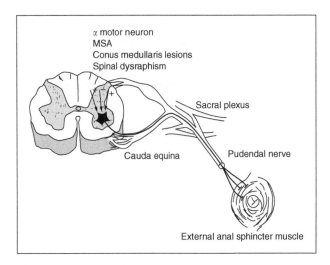

Figure 10.1

The sacral reflex arc. The sacral spinal cord, with sensory (afferent) root entering posteriorly, and motor (efferent) root leaving anteriorly, is shown. Although not shown here, below the lower end of the spinal cord (conus medullaris) lumbar and sacral spinal roots travel for several segments within the spinal canal before leaving it (cauda equina). An enlarged alpha motor neuron with facilitatory (+) and inhibitory (−) suprasegmental influences is also shown. MSA, multiple system atrophy.

damage of suprasegmental pathways in the central nervous system in the case of UMN lesions. Neurological examination is very valuable in helping to make the distinction between these two conditions. In very general terms a UMN lesion would be expected to be associated with detrusor overactivity, whereas an LMN lesion would be associated with bladder atonia (hyporeflexia), although this rule is by no means hard and fast.

Electrophysiological tests can be understood as an extension of the clinical neurological examination. The tests are seldom useful in patients with a completely normal neurological examination, and are helpful only in patients in whom specific neurological lesions are suspected.[3] In general, neurophysiological tests may be used to elucidate those findings summarized in Table 10.1. Some of these properties are relevant when applied to the striated muscle of the pelvic floor.

Other physiological tests to evaluate bladder disorders (measurement of post-void residual, uroflow, cystometry, etc.) are different in that they test function and, as a consequence, can be regarded as complementary. Similarly, neurophysiological tests are complementary to imaging studies – such as ultrasound, computer tomography (CT), and magnetic resonance imaging (MRI) – of the lower urinary tract. Neurophysiological tests, however, have limitations (Table 10.2).

Clinical assessment before electrophysiological evaluation

Selected patients with urinary disorders should be referred to specialists, who will perform a focused clinical examination of the lower urinary tract and anogenital region. To document and quantify patients' complaints, and obtain additional data, functional investigations (measurement of post-void residual, uroflow, cystometry) and imaging studies might be considered. A neural lesion would be suspected, particularly when bowel and sexual dysfunction accompany urinary dysfunction, and it

Table 10.1 *Unique information provided by electrophysiological tests. Normal clinical neurological examination and appropriate electrophysiological testing (see Method column) document preserved neural integrity, and other causes for the pelvic floor dysfunction should be sought. On the other hand, the electrophysiological test abnormality in appropriate clinical setting supports and documents the clinical diagnosis of a neurogenic lesion. The electrophysiological tests can then often help to provide information about severity, localization, and type (mechanism) of the lesion. These factors are crucial for the assessment of prognosis.*

Information	Structure	Method	Finding
Integrity preserved	The lower motor neuron	CNEMG	Absent spontaneous denervation activity; continuous MUP firing during relaxation
	Lower and upper motor neuron	CNEMG	Dense IP on voluntary activation
	Sacral reflex arc	CNEMG	Dense IP on reflex activation (touch)
		Sacral reflex response	Brisk BCR of normal latency
	Somatosensory pathways	Pudendal SEP	Normal shape and latency of responses
Localization of lesions	Root vs plexus/nerve	CNEMG	Paravertebral denervation activity in neighboring myotomes
		SNAP	Normal (penile) SNAP with impaired (penile) skin sensation
Severity of lesions	Complete vs partial	CNEMG	Profuse spontaneous denervation activity; absent MUPs
	Severe vs moderate	Sacral reflex response	BCR absent
Type of lesion	Conduction block vs axonotmesis	CNEMG	Absent/sparse spontaneous denervation activity
	Axonotmesis vs neurotmesis	CNEMG	Appearance of nascent MUPs after complete muscle denervation

BCR, bulbocavernosus reflex; CNEMG, concentric needle electromyography; IP, interference pattern; MUP, motor unit potential; SEP, somatosensory evoked potentials; SNAP, sensory nerve action potential.

Table 10.2 *The limitations of electrodiagnostic tests*

Limitations	Reason	Comments
Uncomfortable		Without significant risks
Difficult localization	• Multiple lesions • Proximal peripheral sacral lesions	Proximal lesion 'masks' distal on CNEMG, and distal lesion masks proximal on SNAP testing Paravertebral muscles are absent in the lower sacral segments
Timing of investigation	• Few abnormalities before several weeks post injury • Less pronounced pathological signs after a few months	
Tests do not reflect the function of the whole structure studied	Low correlation with function	No electrophysiological parameter validated to measure weakness

CNEMG, concentric needle electromyography; SNAP, sensory nerve action potential.

is then that uroneurophysiological evaluation would be considered.[3]

At the beginning of each uroneurophysiological evaluation, a focused history of the patient's complaints needs to be taken, including questions about urinary, anorectal, and sexual (dys)function. History of low back pain irradiating to legs, and numbness and tingling on the posterior part of thighs, buttocks, and in the perineal region will point to a cauda equina lesion. In older patients, inquiry about general slowness, disordered gait, tremor, and autonomic dysfunction (orthostatic hypotension, etc.) should be made to reveal extrapyramidal disorders such as Parkinson's disease. Dissemination of neurological symptoms in time and in neurological location (blurred vision, difficult gait, urinary and fecal urgency, etc.) suggests a diagnosis of demyelinating disease of the central nervous system (multiple sclerosis). For research purposes the use of standardized questionnaires for anorectal,[4,5] urinary,[6,7] and sexual[8,9] (dys)function is recommended.

As a minimum, at the beginning of each electrophysiological evaluation a brief neurological examination should also be performed, looking for signs of pyramidal (UMN) and peripheral nervous system (LMN) lesions (particularly in lower limbs), and also for extrapyramidal and cerebellar signs. Examination of the anogenital region should in this setting include assessment of anal sphincter tone during rest, squeeze, and push, sensation of touch and pinprick in the perineal/perianal area, and eliciting of the BCR and anal

reflex (bilaterally). If uroneurophysiological tests are to be performed, a detailed explanation of the aims and methods of the electrodiagnostic evaluation should be given to the patient.

Innervation of the pelvic structures

The nervous system is divided into two motor systems (the somatic and the autonomic), and the (somato)sensory system (Figure 10.2). Within a particular anatomical system we can distinguish central and peripheral parts. The central part includes the motor and sensory pathways contained within the brain and spinal cord (the central nervous system). The central nervous system also contains, at different levels, interneuronal systems, which are important in neural 'integrative functions' (e.g. sacral spinal interneurons in the BCR arc[10]).

The motor system comprises a UMN (i.e. all neurons participating in the supraspinal motor control), an LMN (innervating muscles and glands), and muscle. Cell bodies of the UMN lie in the motor cortex and other gray matter (nuclei) of the brain (including some brainstem nuclei) and connect directly or via interneurons to the LMNs of the spinal cord (and cranial motor nerve nuclei in the brainstem). The LMNs lie either in the anterior horns of

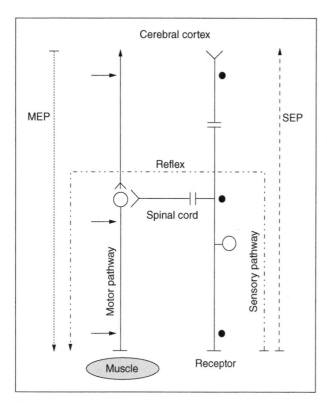

Figure 10.2
Components of the somatic sensory and somatic motor systems and the electrophysiological tests that evaluate them. Arrows on the motor (left) side indicate different stimulation sites (from above) of motor cortex, spinal roots, and peripheral nerves (terminal motor latency test). Small circles on the sensory (right) side indicate different recording sites (from below) from peripheral nerve (sensory nerve action potential, SNAP), spinal roots/cord, and somatosensory cortex. (Note that for SNAP recording both distal stimulation and proximal recording[82] or reverse[83] could be employed.) In addition, concentric needle electromyography (CNEMG) and single fiber electromyography (SFEMG) assess the lower motor neuron and muscle. Kinesiological EMG evaluates the integrity of upper motor neuron and neurocontrol reflex arcs. MEP, motor evoked potential; SEP, somatosensory evoked potential. (Redrawn with permission from Vodušek DB.)[58]

the gray matter of the spinal cord (the somato-motor nuclei) or in the lateral horns of the spinal cord (the autonomic nuclei): the first innervate skeletal muscle, and the latter smooth muscle and glands.

The somatosensory system can be divided into a peripheral part (receptors and the sensory input into the spinal cord) and a central part (ascending pathways in the spinal cord and above). Sensory fibers from the skin and those accompanying axons from α motor neurons are called somatic afferents. Those accompanying autonomic (parasympathetic or sympathetic) fibers are called visceral afferents.

Somatic lower motor neurons of the sacral spinal cord

The α motor neurons of the sphincter (Onuf's) nucleus are somewhat smaller than those innervating limb and trunk skeletal muscles. Like other motor neurons, which innervate striated muscle, they lie in the anterior horn of the spinal cord. Their axons are of large diameter and myelinated to allow rapid conduction of impulses and travel to the periphery in the cauda equina, the sacral plexus, and the pudendal nerves (see Figure 10.1). Within the muscle, the motor axon tapers and then branches to innervate muscle fibers. Each motor neuron innervates a number of muscle fibers – this constitutes the motor unit (MU). The innervation of healthy muscle is such that fibers that are part of the same MU are unlikely to be adjacent to one another but are scattered in checkerboard pattern. The diameter of the muscle area innervated by each lower sacral α motor neuron (MU territory) is probably smaller than the corresponding area in limb or trunk muscles.

Primary sensory neuron

Sensory receptors are the most peripheral part of the somatic and autonomic sensory neurons. Receptors code mechanical or chemical stimuli into bioelectrical activity – i.e. nerve action potentials which traverse the peripheral axon (within peripheral nerves and the sacral plexus), cell body within the spinal ganglion, and the central axon of the peripheral sensory neuron (within the cauda equina). In the spinal cord the central axon branches, with segmental branches contributing in the reflex arc, and central branches (within dorsal column) conveying sensory information to the brain. Both somatic and visceral parts of the sensory system are organized in this way.

The simplified model of the neuromuscular system includes also the autonomic system, which is divided into sympathetic and parasympathetic parts.

Physiological principles of electrophysiological testing

An excitable membrane and transmission of traveling action potentials are characteristic of nerve and muscle cells. This bioelectrical activity is the substrate for function of the nervous tissue (i.e. transmission of information) and precedes the function of the muscle (i.e. contraction). It is this bioelectrical activity which makes possible the application of electrodiagnostic methods.

To obtain the information about the bioelectrical activity of muscle, nerve, spinal roots, spinal cord, and brain, recordings from these structures are necessary. All clinical neurophysiological recordings are extracellular. The electrodes may be near (i.e. intramuscular needle or wire electrodes), or distant from the source of bioelectrical activity (i.e. surface electrodes applied over the skin). The spread of the electrical field through tissues from the generators obeys physical laws of volume conduction. From muscle, both the ongoing (spontaneous) and elicited (willfully, reflexly, by nerve depolarization) activity can be recorded. From most of the other nervous structures (nerves, spinal roots, spinal cord), recording of the spontaneous bioelectrical activity can not be measured. To explore these structures, electrical (and less often magnetic or mechanical) stimulation is applied, and the propagated bioelectrical activity recorded at some distance along the nervous pathways. The electrophysiological responses obtained on stimulation are compound action potentials produced by simultaneous activation of populations of biological units (neurons, axons, muscle fibers of MUs).

Classification of electrophysiological tests

A functional classification of the electrophysiological tests consists of (see Figure 10.2):

- tests evaluating the somatic motor system (electromyography, EMG; terminal motor latency measurements, and motor evoked potentials, MEP)
- tests evaluating the sensory system (sensory neurography, somatosensory evoked potentials, SEP)
- methods assessing reflexes (BCR)
- tests assessing functioning of the sympathetic (sympathetic skin response, SSR) and parasympathetic autonomic nervous systems.

Such a 'logical' classification is preferable to a historical classification.

Uroneurophysiological tests that are of diagnostic value in individual patients with neurogenic bladder

Electromyography

Kinesiological electromyography

The aim of the kinesiological EMG is to assess patterns of individual muscle activity during various maneuvers (i.e. EMG activity patterns of pelvic floor muscle during bladder filling and voiding). It is usually not called kinesiological EMG, although this would be preferable to distinguish it from other EMG methods.

Various types of surface or intramuscular (needle or wire) electrodes can be used for recording of the kinesiological EMG signal. Bioelectrical activity will typically be sampled from a single intramuscular detection site. As motor unit potential (MUP) parameters are not analyzed, it can be recorded with a less-sophisticated apparatus than other types of EMG, even if intramuscular electrodes are used for recording. There is no commonly accepted standardized technique. When using surface electrodes there are problems related to the validity of the signal (e.g. artifacts and also contamination from other muscles). In contrast, with intramuscular electrodes in large pelvic floor muscles, there are questions as to whether the whole muscle is properly represented by the measured signal. Little is known about the normal activity patterns of different pelvic floor and sphincter muscles: urethral sphincter (US), urethrovaginal sphincter, the external anal sphincter (EAS) muscle, different parts of the levator ani, etc. It is generally assumed that they all act in a coordinated fashion (as one muscle), but differences have been demonstrated even between the intra- and peri-US in normal women.[11] Coordinated behavior is frequently lost in abnormal conditions, as has been shown for the levator ani, the US, and the EAS.[21]

The normal (kinesiological) sphincter EMG shows continuous activity of MUPs at rest, which may be increased voluntarily or reflexly. Such activity of low-threshold MUs[13] has been recorded for up to 2 hours[14] and even after subjects have fallen asleep during the examination.[15] Such activity can also be recorded in many but not all detection sites of the levator ani[16] and of the deeper EAS muscle.[17,18] The US and the EAS as well as the pubococcygeus muscles can sustain voluntary activation for only about 1 min.[16] On voiding, disappearance of all EMG activity in the US precedes detrusor contraction. In the central nervous system disorders, however, detrusor contractions may be associated with increase of sphincter EMG activity.[19,20] Detrusor-sphincter dyssynergia can be easily demonstrated by kinesiological EMG performed as a part of cystometric measurement.[12]

Neurogenic incoordinated sphincter behavior has to be differentiated from voluntary contractions that may occur in poorly compliant patients. The pelvic floor muscle contractions of the so-called non-neurogenic voiding disorder may be a learned abnormal behavior, and can be encountered in some women with dysfunctional voiding.[22]

In health the pubococcygeus in woman reveals similar activity patterns to the USs and the EAS at most detection sites: i.e. continuous activity at rest, some (but not invariable) increase of activity during bladder filling, and reflex increases in activity during any activation maneuver performed by the subject (talking, deep breathing, coughing).

The pubococcygeus also relaxes during voiding.[16] However, in disease, the patterns of activation and the coordination between the two sides may be lost.[23]

Any diagnostic value of kinesiological EMG apart from polygraph cystometric recordings to assess detrusor/sphincter coordination has yet to be established.

The demonstration of voluntary and reflex activation of pelvic floor muscles is indirect proof of the integrity of the respective neural pathways and should also be a part of a CNEMG examination, although the latter is performed primarily to diagnose an LMN lesion (see below). In contrast, kinesiological EMG is used mainly for diagnosis of the central nervous system, i.e. UMN lesions.

Concentric needle electromyography

The aim of CNEMG testing is to differentiate abnormal from normally innervated striated muscle. Although EMG abnormalities are detected as a result of a host of different lesions and diseases, there are in principle only two standard manifestations which can occur: disease of the muscle fibers themselves and changes in their innervation.

The concentric needle electrode consists of a central insulated platinum wire that is inserted through a steel cannula. This type of electrode records activity from muscle tissue up to 2.5 mm from the electrode tip.

For the CNEMG examination, an advanced EMG system, that has the facility for quantitative template-based MUP analysis (multi-MUP) is ideal.[24] The commonly used amplifier filter's setting for CNEMG is 5 Hz to 10 kHz. This must be identical to those set when reference values were compiled, and needs to be checked if MUP parameters are to be measured.

Because of easy access, sufficient muscle bulk, and relative ease of examination, the EAS is the most practical muscle for CNEMG testing of the lower sacral segments.[17,25] To examine the subcutaneous EAS muscle the needle is inserted about 1 cm from the anal orifice, to a depth of a 3–6 mm. For the deeper EAS muscle, 1–3 cm deep insertions are made at the anal orifice, at an angle of about 30° to the anal canal axis.[25] For MUP analysis, both EAS muscles can be sampled and the data pooled.[17] For kinesiological assessment, however, the subcutaneous and the deep muscles must be examined separately.[17]

Both left and right EAS muscles should almost always be examined, by needle insertions into the middle of the anterior and posterior halves. The needle is angled backwards and forwards in a systematic manner (through two insertion sites on each side).[26]

CNEMG examination of the EAS muscle can be divided into observation of insertion activity and of spontaneous denervation activity, and assessment of MUPs and of interference pattern (IP). In addition, it is suggested that the number of continuously active MUPs during relaxation be

observed,[18] as well as MUP recruitment on reflex and voluntary activation.[26]

In normal muscle, needle movement elicits a short burst of 'insertion activity,' which is due to mechanical stimulation of excitable membranes. This is recorded at a gain of 50 μV per division, which is also used to record spontaneous denervation activity (sweep speed 5–10 ms/division). Absence of insertion activity with appropriately placed needle electrode[25] usually means complete atrophy of the muscle. Such complete atrophy of all EAS muscles on both sides was found in 9% of men after cauda equina lesions.[27]

Immediately after an acute complete denervation, all MU activity ceases, and (apart from insertion activity) no electrical activity can be recorded. Ten to twenty days later insertion activity becomes more prominent and prolonged and abnormal spontaneous activity appears in the form of short biphasic spikes (fibrillation potentials) and biphasic potentials with prominent positive deflections (positive sharp waves) (Figure 10.3A). This type of activity is referred to as 'spontaneous denervation activity' and originates from denervated single muscle fibers.

In partially denervated muscle, some MUPs remain and mingle eventually with spontaneous denervation activity. As the MUPs in sphincter muscles are also short and mostly bi- or triphasic, as are fibrillation potentials, it takes considerable EMG experience to differentiate one from another. In this situation, examination of the bulbocavernosus muscle is particularly useful because in contrast to sphincter muscles it lacks ongoing activity of low-threshold MU during relaxation (see Figure 10.3A).[26]

In longstanding partially denervated muscles, peculiar abnormal activity called simple or complex repetitive discharges appears, caused by repetitive firing of groups of potentials. This activity may be provoked by needle movement, muscle contraction, etc., or may occur spontaneously, rhythmically. This activity may sometimes be found in USs of patients without any other evidence of neuromuscular disease, and indeed without lower urinary tract problems, although in such cases it is not prominent. A type of repetitive discharge activity called 'decelerating bursts (DB) and complex repetitive discharges (CRD)' can be found in the external US muscles of some young women. The DBs produce the myotonic-like sound similar to underwater recordings of whales. The CRDs, however, sound like a helicopter over the loudspeaker on the EMG system. This activity may be so abundant that it is thought to cause involuntary muscle contraction and urinary retention.[28]

In contrast to limb muscles, where electrical silence is present on relaxation, in sphincter muscles some MUPs are continuously firing. Additional sphincter MUPs can be activated reflexly or voluntarily, and it has been shown that there are two MUP populations with different characteristics: reflexly or voluntarily activated high-threshold MUPs,

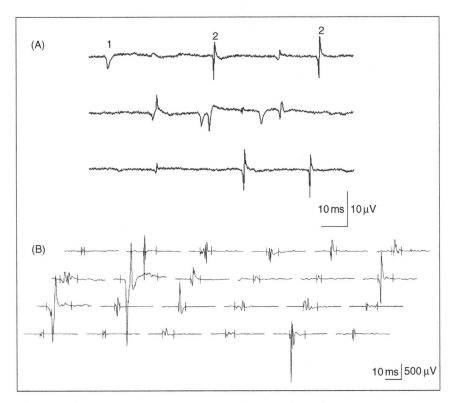

Figure 10.3

Findings of electromyographic (EMG) examination using a standard concentric EMG needle in a 36-year-old man after surgical decompression of the cauda equina due to central herniation of the intervertebral disc L4–L5. The patient had long-term sacral dysfunctions: atonic bladder (emptied by abdominal straining), severe constipation, and severe erectile dysfunction. (A) The EMG activity during relaxation in the left bulbocavernosus muscle 2 months after surgical decompression of the cauda equina. Note the distinct spontaneous denervation activity in the form of biphasic potentials with prominent positive deflections: positive sharp waves (1) and short biphasic spikes (fibrillation potentials (2)): No motor unit potentials (MUPs) could be recruited in that muscle reflexly or voluntarily, which pointed to complete denervation of the muscle. (B) The MUPs sampled (by multi-MUP analysis) from the left subcutaneous external anal sphincter (EAS) muscle during a control uroneurophysiological examination 7 months later. Mean duration was 7.3 ms (Z = +0.7 − SD above the mean), mean area was 808 µVms (Z = +4.2), and the mean number of turns was 4.3 (Z = +1.5). Good reinnervation of the muscle after (probably) complete denervation, pointed to a combination of neurapraxia (block in nerve transmission) and axonotmesis (degeneration of the nerve fibers with preserved continuity of nerve roots) as opposed to neurotmesis (nerve roots severed) as a mechanism of the cauda equina injury.

which are larger than continuously active low-threshold MUPs. As a consequence, to increase accuracy of MUP analysis, for a template-based multi-MUP analysis, standardization of activity level during sampling at which 3–5 MUPs are sampled on a single muscle site is recommended.[13]

In partially denervated sphincter muscle there is a loss of MUs. To quantify this exactly, use of multi-MUP analysis was proposed.[18] By this approach, apart from the number of remaining MUs after partial denervation (i.e. in cauda equina lesions), the segmental and suprasegmental inputs to motor neurons within the anterior spinal horns as well as the excitation level of the motor neurons can be assessed. This approach was found particularly useful in patients with idiopathic fecal incontinence, but has not been studied in patients with neurogenic bladders.[18]

With axonal reinnervation after complete denervation, nascent MUPs appear first, being short-duration, low-amplitude, bi- and triphasic potentials, soon becoming polyphasic, serrated, and of prolonged duration.

Changes due to collateral reinnervation are reflected by prolongation of the waveform of the MUPs (Figure 10.4), which may have small, late components (satellites). In newly formed axon sprouts endplates, neuromuscular transmission is insecure, resulting in MUPs instability (jitter and blocking of individual components). Over a period of time, provided there is no further denervation, the reinnervating axonal sprouts increase in diameter, so that activation of all parts of the reinnervated MU becomes nearly synchronous, which increases the amplitude and reduces the duration of the MUPs (see Figure 10.4). This phenomenon may be different in sphincter muscles in ongoing

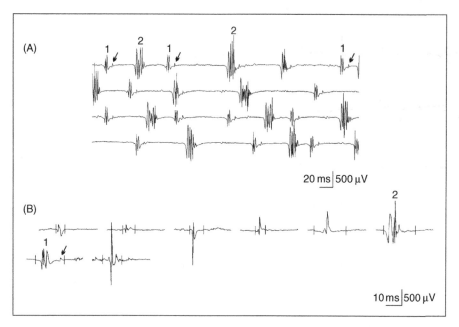

Figure 10.4

Findings of electromyographic (EMG) examination using a standard concentric EMG needle in a 36-year-old man with myelitis of the conus medullaris. The patient had several episodes of urinary and fecal incontinence, impaired sensation of bladder and rectum fullness, and moderate erectile dysfunction, all of which resolved spontaneously after a few months. (A) The EMG activity in the right deeper external anal sphincter (EAS) muscle during voluntary activation 2 months after the beginning of the disease. Note the extremely polyphasic motor unit potentials (MUPs) of increased duration, and late potential (arrows). Consecutive firing of the same MUP slightly changed, which points to MUP instability. No spontaneous denervation activity, and no low threshold MUPs continuously firing during relaxation were present. Reflex recruitment of MUPs was severely reduced but present in the same muscle. All these findings indicated subacute partial (moderately severe) denervation of the muscle. (B) During the same EMG examination only 8 MUPs needed to be sampled (by multi-MUP analysis) from the same muscle to obtain 3 MUPs with values of duration, area, and the number of turns above the upper outlier limit. To declare muscle pathological (neurogenic) using outlier criterion this number (3 out of 20 or less MUPs) is needed. Although at the same time mean values for duration, area, and the number of turns were also all pathological ($Z > 2.0$), they cannot be used in this situation to declare muscle neuropathic, because less than 20 MUPs were sampled. Two MUPs from (A) are also presented below (Nos 1 and 2). Note that averaging used by multi-MUP analysis changed the shape of unstable MUPs (reduced number of phases and turns).

degenerative disorders such as MSA, where long-duration MUPs seem to remain a prominent feature of MUs.[29] Less-pronounced increase in MUP amplitude on reinnervation in sphincter muscles might also be due to a less-efficient fusion of individual muscle fiber potentials in muscles with short spike components of MUPs (also in facial muscles).

Three techniques are available to systematically examine individual MUPs. The first MUP analysis technique follows an algorithm similar to that used by the early electromyographers of Buchthal and his school, who carried out the first quantitative MUP assessments.[30] They measured MUP duration and amplitude from paper records of EMG activity, whereas nowadays the MUPs are automatically analyzed on the screen. Using this modified manual-MUP analysis the highest number of MUPs (up to 10) can be obtained from the muscle site at low levels of activity (at higher levels of activation the baseline becomes unsteady). It takes 2–3 min for each site to be analyzed. This technique is demanding for the operator, because reproducible MUPs have to be identified, the one with the smoothest

baseline chosen, and, in most cases, the duration cursors set manually, which inevitably introduces personal bias.[24]

The introduction of the trigger and delay unit led to its widespread use in analysis of individual MUPs.[31] On applying this technique, during a constant level of EMG activity, the trigger unit is set on a steadily firing MUP. This approach is particularly useful for detection of late MUP components, and then inclusion into MUP duration measurement. The number of MUPs at each site depends on the version of the technique used. In some systems only the highest amplitude MUP can be triggered, which enables sampling of only 1–3 MUPs from each examination site. Single-MUP analysis is time consuming, provides fewer MUPs than the other two described techniques, and is biased towards high amplitude and high threshold MUPs. Furthermore, it is also prone to personal bias.[24]

The recent and sophisticated CNEMG techniques are available only on advanced EMG systems; such is the template operated multi-MUP analysis (Figures 10.3 and 10.4).[32] The needle must be located so that a 'crisp' sounding pattern of EMG activity can be heard over the loudspeaker, indicating that the needle electrode is near to muscle fibers. Then, during an appropriate level of EMG activity, the operator starts the analysis and the computer takes the previous (last) 4.8 s period of the signal. From that signal MUPs are automatically extracted, quantified, and sorted into up to six classes. MUP classes, representing consecutive discharges of a particular MUP, are then averaged and presented (see Figures 10.3 and 10.4). Cursors are set automatically using a computer algorithm that, in addition to certain amplitude deflection, demands the minimum angle of the MUP trace towards the baseline.[32] After acquisition, the operator has to edit the MUPs. Thus, from each examination site up to six different MUPs can be obtained.[24,32,33] Multi-MUP analysis is the fastest and the easiest to apply of the three quantitative MUP analysis techniques mentioned. It can be applied at continuous activity during sphincter muscle relaxation, as well as at slight to moderate levels of activation.[13,24] The multi-MUP technique has (like single-MUP analysis) difficulties with highly unstable and/or polyphasic MUPs. It often fails to sample them, sorts the same MUP to several classes (recognizes it as different MUPs – duplicates), cuts prolonged MUPs into two, or distorts them by averaging. The MUPs with unsteady baseline (unclear beginning or end) need to be recognized and deleted.[29] The multi-MUP technique samples a slightly lower number of MUPs per muscle compared with the manual-MUP technique.[24]

In the small half of the sphincter muscle, collecting 10 different MUPs has been said to be a minimal requirement on using single-MUP analysis. Using manual-MUP and multi-MUP techniques, sampling of 20 MUPs (standard number in limb muscles) from each EAS muscle presents no problem in healthy controls and most patients (see Figures 10.3B).[24] Normative data obtained from the EAS muscle by standardized EMG technique using all these three MUP analyses have been published.[24] Analysis made from the same taped EMG signal, using reference data for mean values and outliers[34] (see Figure 10.4), revealed similar sensitivity of manual-MUP, single-MUP, and multi-MUP analysis for detecting neuropathic changes in the EAS muscle of patients with chronic cauda equina lesions.[24]

A number of MUP parameters are used in the diagnosis of neuromuscular disease (see Figure 10.5). Traditionally, MUP amplitude and duration were measured, and the number of phases was counted.[30] In a study comparing the sensitivity of individual MUP parameters for differentiating normal from neuropathic sphincter muscles of patients with chronic lesion to the cauda equina, area was the most sensitive, followed by the number of turns, and size index. A high correlation between MUP parameters was also shown in the same study, which points to probable redundancy of using all available MUP parameters.[35]

Indeed, a recent study performed in the EAS muscle revealed that probably only the parameters of area, duration,

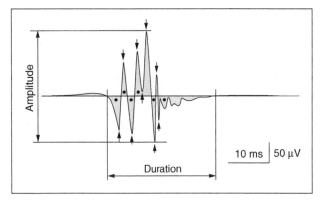

Figure 10.5
The motor unit potential (MUP) parameters. Amplitude is the voltage difference (μV) between the most positive and most negative point of the MUP trace. The MUP duration is the time (ms) between the first deflection and the point when the MUP waveform finally returns to the baseline. The number of MUP phases (small circles) is defined by the number of MUP areas (see below) alternately below and above the baseline, and can be counted as the 'number of baseline crossings plus one'. Turns (arrows) are defined as changes in direction of the MUP trace that are larger than the specified amplitude (100 μV). The MUP area measures the integrated surface of the MUP waveform (shaded).

and the number of turns are needed in MUP analysis. Other MUP parameters (amplitude, the number of phases, duration of the negative peak, thickness, size index) appear to be redundant, and their use might reduce specificity of MUP analysis.[36]

The MUP area is measured as the total surface between the MUP trace and the baseline of the EMG signal (msμV) (see Figure 10.5). It is largely determined by the activity of muscle fibers within a 2.0 mm radius to the recording concentric needle electrode.[37]

The MUP duration is the time (ms) between the first deflection and the point when the MUP waveform finally returns to the baseline (see Figure 10.5). It depends on the number of muscle fibers of a particular MU within 2.5 mm diameter and is little affected by the proximity of the recording electrode to the nearest fiber.[37] The difficulty with the duration measurement is in defining the beginning and end of the MUP. During manual positioning of duration cursors, amplifier gain is crucial: at higher gain, MUPs seem longer.[38] It is unclear whether to include late components (satellite potentials) into MUP duration or not. Late components are defined as the part of MUP starting at least 3 ms after the end of the main spike of the MUP.[38] Although it was agreed not to include them into MUP duration measurement,[38,39] it seems that their exclusion might reduce the sensitivity of MUP analysis, at least in MSA.[40] However, no valid normative data for MUP parameters with inclusion of late components have been published.

A turn is defined as a change in direction of the MUP trace, which is larger than specified amplitude (100 μV) (Figure 10.5). The number of MUP turns cannot distinguish between neuropathic and myopathic muscles, but this is not relevant in the EAS muscle since myopathy confined exclusively to the striated sphincter muscles is unknown.

In addition to continuous firing of low-threshold MUPs in sphincters, additional high-threshold MUPs[13] are recruited voluntarily and reflexly (see Figure 10.4B). By such maneuvers, the amount of recruitable MUs is estimated. Normally, MUPs should intermingle to produce a dense IP on the oscilloscope screen when muscle is contracted well, and during a strong cough.

The IP can be assessed using a number of automatic quantitative analyses, the turn/amplitude analysis being the most popular.[41] However, quantitative IP analysis was shown to be only half as sensitive as the MUP analysis techniques[24] in distinguishing between normal and neuropathic muscles.[24] However, with the needle electrode in focus, qualitative assessment of IP during voluntary or reflex muscle contraction by coughing is recommended.

In summary, template-based multi-MUP analysis is as sensitive as the traditional MUP analysis techniques,[24] fast (5–10 min per muscle), easy to apply, less prone to personal bias, and is a clinically useful technique.[27] In the EAS muscle its use is further facilitated by the availability of common normative data, which are unaffected by age, gender,[42] number and characteristics of vaginal deliveries,[33] mild chronic constipation,[43] or EAS muscle examined (the subcutaneous or the deeper).[17] All these make multi-MUP analysis the technique of choice for quantitative analysis of the EAS reinnervation.

Single fiber electromyography

The aim of single fiber electromyography (SFEMG) testing is similar to CNEMG – to differentiate normal from abnormal striated muscle. The SFEMG electrode has similar external proportions to a concentric needle electrode, but instead of having the recording surface at the tip, a fine insulated platinum or silver wire embedded in epoxy resin is exposed through an aperture on the side 1–5 mm behind the tip. The platinum wire forms the recording surface, and has a diameter of 25 μm. It will pick up activity from within a hemispherical volume of 0.3 mm in diameter. This is very much smaller than the volume of muscle tissue from which a concentric needle electrode records, which has an uptake area of 2.5 mm diameter. Because of the arrangement of muscle fibers in a normal MU, an SFEMG needle will record only 1–3 single muscle fibers from the same MU. When recording with an SFEMG needle, the amplifier filters are set so that low-frequency activity is eliminated (500 Hz to 10 kHz). Thus, the contribution of each muscle fiber appears as a short biphasic positive–negative action potential.

The SFEMG parameter that reflects MU morphology is the fiber density, which is defined as the mean number of muscle fibers belonging to an individual MU per detection site. To assemble these data, recordings from 20 different intramuscular detection sites are necessary.[44] The normal fiber density for the EAS is below 2.0.[45,46] Changes with age have been reported,[47] showing women to have significantly greater fiber density than men.[46]

The fiber density is increased in reinnervated muscle. The technique has been particularly applied to sphincter muscles in order to correlate increased fiber density findings to incontinence.[48] Due to its technical characteristics, SFEMG electrode is able to record even small changes that occur in MUs due to reinnervation, but is less suitable to detect changes due to denervation itself (i.e. abnormal insertion and spontaneous denervation activity).

The SFEMG electrode is also most suitable to record any instability of MUPs, although this is not routinely assessed in pelvic floor muscles for diagnostic purposes. The instability is revealed as jitter, which is defined as the variability with consecutive discharges of the interpotential interval between two muscle fiber action potentials belonging to the same MU. It may be increased not only in diseases affecting neuromuscular transmission but also by recent reinnervation.

Single fiber electromyography vs concentric needle electromyography

Quantified CNEMG provides the same information on reinnervation changes in muscle as the SFEMG parameter of fiber density,[49,50] but, in addition, CNEMG will reveal spontaneous denervation activity. In muscle after severe partial denervation, the areas of fibrosis are silent to EMG exploration, and the results are based only on the remaining MUP activity. The remaining innervated muscle is easier to establish with CNEMG, which records from a larger volume of tissue. Furthermore, a CNEMG examination can be extended in the same diagnostic session from, for example, lumbar and upper sacral myotomes to the lower sacral myotomes, after a cauda equina lesion. A concentric electrode can also be employed at the same diagnostic session for recording evoked direct and reflex muscle responses. SFEMG electrodes are more sophisticated, and as a consequence much more expensive. In contrast to CNEMG electrodes, no disposable SFEMG electrodes are available.

Use of CNEMG is the method of choice in routine examination of skeletal muscle, and is generally available in clinical neurophysiology laboratories, whereas SFEMG is not so widely used. As a consequence, SFEMG, although an established electrodiagnostic technique, is not recommended for clinical electrophysiological evaluation of patients with neurogenic bladders.

Sacral reflexes

The term sacral reflex refers to electrophysiologically recordable responses of pelvic floor muscles to (electrical) stimulation of sensory fibers in the uro-genito-anal region. In the lower sacral segments there are two common clinically elicited reflexes, the anal and the BCR. Both have the afferent and the efferent limb of their reflex arc in the pudendal nerve, and are centrally integrated at the S2 to S4 cord levels. Electrophysiological correlates of these reflexes have been described.

Measurements of latencies and amplitudes of reflex responses and evoked potentials, including sympathetic skin responses, relate not only to conduction in peripheral and central neural pathways but also to transmission across synapses and within networks of central nervous system interneurons. Therefore, conduction may be influenced by factors that are not apparent from a simplified anatomical model (see Figure 10.1). For example, changes in the threshold, amplitude, and latency of the BCR occur as a consequence of changes in the physiological state of the bladder,[51,52] and differ in pathological conditions (i.e. suprasacral spinal cord lesions).[53]

The aim of electrophysiological testing of sacral reflexes is to assess integrity of the sacral (S2–S4) spinal reflex arc, and to evaluate excitation levels of sacral spinal cord motor neurons.

It is possible to use electrical,[54,55] mechanical,[56,57] or magnetic[58] stimulation. Whereas the latter two modalities have only been applied to the penis and clitoris, electrical stimulation can be applied at various sites: to the dorsal penile/clitoral nerve, perianally, and (using a catheter-mounted ring electrode) at bladder neck/proximal urethra.[59] In clinical practice, electrical and mechanical stimulation of the penis or clitoris can be used (Figure 10.6), so this will be discussed in some detail.

The sacral reflex evoked on the dorsal penile or the clitoral nerve stimulation was shown to be a complex response, often comprising two components (Figure 10.7). The first component, with latency of about 33 ms, is the response that has been most often called the BCR. It is stable, does not habituate, and is based on variability of single motor neuron latency reflex discharges; it is thought to be an oligosynaptic reflex. The second component has a similar latency to the sacral reflexes evoked by stimulation perianally or from the proximal urethra. The variability of single motor neuron reflex responses within this component is much larger, as is typical for a polysynaptic reflex.[10] The second component is not always demonstrable as a discrete response. Double electrical stimuli may be used to facilitate the reflex response when both components cannot be elicited using single electrical pulses.[60]

Sacral reflex responses recorded with needle or wire electrodes can be analyzed separately for each side of the

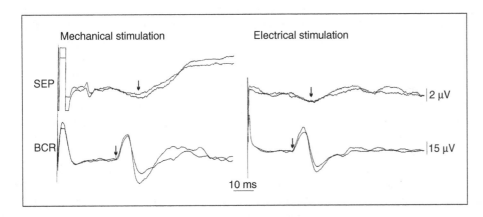

Figure 10.6

Bulbocavernosus reflex (BCR) responses and pudendal somatosensory evoked potentials (SEP) recorded simultaneously in a 9-year-old boy (body height 140 cm), without uroneurological abnormalities. Responses were elicited by consecutive (left) mechanical stimulation (nonpainful squeeze of the penis by the electromechanical hammer) and (right) electrical stimulation (single 20 V stimuli over the dorsal penile nerves). Responses were detected by bifocal montage of the surface electrodes (BCR, active electrode over the external anal sphincter muscle/reference electrode over the bulbocavernosus muscle; SEP, active electrode 2 cm behind Cz/reference electrode on Fz both over the scalp according to the International 10–20 electroencephalography (EEG) System).[68] Measurements were obtained by averaging 100 responses. Latencies to the beginning of the BCR responses (arrows) were 33.4 ms and 25.2 ms; latencies to the first positive peak (P40) (arrowheads) were 47.0 ms and 36.7 ms on mechanical and electrical stimulation, respectively. Peak-to-peak amplitudes of the BCR responses were 69 μV and 63 μV; amplitude of P40 measured 2.0 μV and 1.8 μV on mechanical and electrical stimulation, respectively. Note similar amplitudes but pronounced differences in latency measurements caused by mechanical characteristics of electromechanical hammer used in this study. Latency of the pudendal SEP on electrical stimulation in this child was already within (Z = −1.9) normative limits for adults (41 ± 2.3 ms).[69]

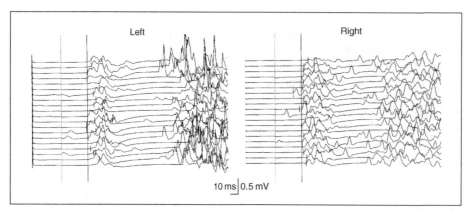

Figure 10.7

Findings of uroneurophysiological examination in a 32-year-old man 2 months after traumatic fracture of pubic bones and urethral rupture. After surgical repair of urethra, the patient continued to leak urine and complained of moderate erectile dysfunction. His bowel function was normal. On concentric needle electromyography (CNEMG) during relaxation some spontaneous denervation activity was detected in the left, but not the right bulbocavernosus muscle. On reflex and voluntary activation, normal motor unit potentials (MUPs) were recruited. In addition, normal bulbocavernosus reflex (BCR) responses were elicited by electrical stimulation (single 80 mA stimuli over dorsal penile nerves), and CNEMG electrode detection in the left and right bulbocavernosus muscles. Left and right latency of the first component of the BCR: 29 ms (marked by solid vertical line). Note also the second component of the BCR. Electrophysiological examination thus confirmed the integrity of the neural structures, and revealed only very slight axonal damage to the left pudendal nerve. Such mild damage could not result in prominent urinary incontinence reported by patient. This was probably due to direct damage to the bladder neck, urethra, or possibly urethral sphincter or its terminal innervation. Similarly, erectile dysfunction was most probably caused by local injury and not by more proximal nervous lesion.

EAS or each bulbocavernosus muscle (see Figure 10.7). Using unilateral dorsal penile nerve blocks, the existence of two unilateral BCR arcs has been demonstrated.[61] Thus, by detection from the left and right bulbocavernosus (and probably also the EAS) muscles, separate testing of both BCR arcs can be performed. Sensitivity of the test can be increased also by use of the inter-side latency difference (normative limits in case of simultaneous bilateral detection: <3 ms).[61] This is important, because in cases of unilateral (sacral plexopathy, pudendal neuropathy) or asymmetrical lesions (cauda equina), which are common, a healthy BCR arc may obscure a pathological one. Similarly, using mechanical stimulation (light touch or pinprick) of the perianal area on each side, with needle detection from the subcutaneous EAS muscles of each side (left and right) during the CNEMG, a separate testing of both reflex arcs can be performed. In the authors' laboratories, testing of BCR on electrical stimulation is performed in conjunction with a CNEMG if no brisk reflex response is present on mechanical stimulation of the perianal/perineal region and recording from the EAS muscle.[26]

Standardization of the technique has been proposed.[1] It was recommended that surface stimulation electrodes be placed on the penis/clitoris, and 10 single, 0.2 ms long stimuli be applied at supramaximal intensity at time intervals of 2 s (=0.5 Hz). Recording is by concentric needle or surface electrodes placed into/over the EAS, or bulbocavernosus muscle in men, using filters: 10 Hz to 10 kHz; sweep speed, 10 ms/div; and gain, 50–1000 μV/div. Onset latency is the only parameter measured.[1]

Sacral reflex responses on stimulation of the dorsal penile and clitoral nerve have been said to be of value in patients with cauda equina and other LMN lesions, although it is recognized that a reflex with a normal latency does not exclude the possibility of an axonal lesion in its reflex arc (see Figure 10.7). The sensitivity and specificity of sacral reflex responses in patients with conditions associated with neurogenic bladders are not known. In diabetics the nerve conduction studies performed in limbs are more sensitive in revealing peripheral neuropathy than sacral reflex latencies.

Abnormally short latency of BCR has been claimed to suggest either the abnormally low position of conus medullaris in tethered cord syndrome[62] or a suprasacral cord lesion.[63]

Mechanical stimulation has been used to elicit BCR in both sexes[56] and has been found to be a robust technique. Either a standard commercially available reflex hammer or a customized electromechanical hammer can be employed. Such stimulation is painless and can be used in children.[57] The latency of the mechanically elicited BCR is comparable to that elicited electrically. Differences are caused by the somewhat longer pathway for mechanically evoked stimulation (stimulates receptors instead of peripheral nerve) as well as by the variability in the time course of the mechanical stimulation device (see Figure 10.6).[57]

Recently, responses of the bulbocavernosus muscle after mechanical suprapubic stimulation were also described.[64] It was hypothesized that this is a polysynaptic reflex elicited by the stimulation of the bladder wall tensoreceptors, which could be involved in pathogenesis of detrusor-sphincter dyssynergia in some patients with neurogenic bladders.[64]

Sacral reflex testing should be a part of the diagnostic battery of which CNEMG exploration of the pelvic floor muscles is the most important part. Electrophysiological assessment of sacral reflexes is a more quantitative, sensitive, and reproducible way of assessing the S2–S4 reflex arcs than any of the clinical methods.[65] The results, however, should be interpreted with caution, always being mindful of the clinical context.

Pudendal somatosensory evoked potentials

The pudendal SEP is easily recorded following electrical stimulation of the dorsal penile or clitoral nerve.[66,67] This response is, as a rule, of highest amplitudes at the central recording site (Cz − 2 cm: Fz of the International 10–20 electroencephalography (EEG) System)[68] and is highly reproducible (see Figure 10.6). Amplitudes of the P40 measure 0.5–12 μV. The first positive peak at 41 ± 2.3 ms (called P1 or P40) is usually clearly defined in healthy subjects using a stimulus 2–4 times stronger than sensory threshold current strength.[69] Later negative (at around 55 ms) and then further positive waves are interindividually quite variable in amplitude and expression and, furthermore, have little known clinical relevance.

Pudendal SEP recordings on penile/clitoral stimulation are sometimes useful in patients with sensory loss in the lower sacral dermatomes, and brisk BCR on clinical examination such that an UMN lesion is suspected.[26] Pudendal SEPs were recorded in patients with neurogenic bladder dysfunction due to multiple sclerosis but it is now known that in this clinical situation the tibial cerebral SEPs are more often abnormal than the pudendal SEP, and only in exceptional cases is the pudendal SEP abnormal but the tibial normal, suggesting an isolated conus involvement.[70] Pudendal SEP measurements were also measured in patients with neurogenic bladders due to spinal cord lesions and diabetes. Pathological pudendal SEPs seemed to predict poor surgical outcomes after resection of a tight filum terminale.[71]

A study that looked at the value of the pudendal SEP for detecting relevant neurological disease when investigating urogenital symptoms found it to be of lesser value than a clinical examination looking for signs of spinal cord disease in the lower limbs (i.e. lower limb hyper-reflexia and extensor plantar responses).[72] However, there may be circumstances, such as when a patient is complaining of loss of bladder or vaginal sensation, where it is reassuring to be able to record a normal pudendal SEP. The method as such is valid and robust, but its clinical value, particularly in the investigation of incontinence, is minimal.

Uroneurophysiological tests that are not of diagnostic value in individual patients with neurogenic bladders

Neurophysiology of the sacral motor system

Motor nerve conduction studies

Recording of the muscle response (compound motor action potential or M-wave)[39] on electrical stimulation of its motor nerve is the routine method of electrophysiological evaluation of limb nerves. By stimulating the nerve at two levels, motor nerve conduction velocity can be calculated, which distinguishes between lesions of myelin and axons causing motor weakness. For this purpose, however, the technique requires access to the nerve at two well-separated points for stimulation and measurement of the distance between them, a requirement which cannot be easily met in the pelvis. Thus, the only electrophysiological parameter of motor conduction that can be measured also in the pelvic floor is the pudendal nerve terminal motor latency (PNTML).

Latency measures the fastest-conducting fibers, but give little or no information about the loss of biological units generating electrical currents (axons, etc.), which is the determinant of functional importance. However, latencies depend less on irrelevant biological and technical factors, and are therefore more robust measurements than evoked potentials or reflex studies. On the other hand, the amplitude of the compound potential correlates with the number of activated biological units. (A conduction block and pathological dispersion of conduction velocities within a neural pathway also affect amplitudes.) Amplitudes are thus the more relevant physiological parameter, but M-wave amplitudes of the EAS, US, or other pelvic floor muscles on stimulation of the pudendal nerves have unfortunately not yet proved contributory.

PNTML is usually measured by stimulation with a special surface electrode assembly fixed on a gloved index finger – the St Mark's electrode.[73] This consists of a bipolar stimulating electrode fixed to the tip of the gloved finger, with the recording electrode pair placed 8 cm proximally on the base of the finger. The finger is inserted into the rectum. Stimulation of the pudendal nerve is performed close to the ischial spine and the recording is performed from the EAS muscle. Using this stimulator, the PNTML for the anal sphincter MEP is typically around 2 ms.

Prolongation of the PNTML measured by the St Mark's electrode was found in a variety of patient groups, and was taken as a sign of damage to the pudendal nerve. This has led to the term pudendal neuropathy, which is used particularly by coloproctologists. Some workers less familiar with theoretical principles of clinical neurophysiology equate a prolongation of PNTML with pelvic floor denervation. This, however, is mistaken, as prolongation of latency is a poor measure of denervation, as already explained. What type of abnormality this latency prolongation indicates is unclear, as there have not been any relevant morphological studies.

Delays of PNTML in patient groups, even when present, were short – approximately 0.1–0.3 ms – and it is unlikely that these represent a functionally relevant change.

In practice, the PNTML is unhelpful for diagnosis in individual patients with sacral dysfunction.[74–76] Elicitability of a compound motor action potential in pelvic floor muscles (using the perianal stimulation) may be helpful in patients with combined UMN and LMN lesions in whom no MUP activity can be recorded. In this situation the presence of compound motor action potential rules out complete peripheral (axonal) lesion.

Anterior sacral root (cauda equina) stimulation

Transcutaneous stimulation of deeply situated nervous tissue became possible with the development of special electrical and magnetic stimulators. When applied over the spine at the exit from the vertebral canal, spinal roots can be stimulated, and there have been reports of these techniques applied to the sacral roots.[59,77,78]

Electrical or magnetic stimulation depolarizes underlying neural structures in a nonselective fashion, and concomitant activation of several muscles innervated by lumbosacral segments occurs. It has been shown that responses from gluteal muscles may contaminate attempts to record from the sphincters and lead to error.[79] Thus, surface recordings from sphincter muscles are inadvisable.

Recording of MEP with magnetic stimulation has been less successful than with electrical stimulation, at least with standard coils, and there are often large stimulus artifacts. Positioning of the ground electrode between the recording electrodes and the stimulating coil may decrease the artifact.[80]

Demonstrating the presence of a perineal MEP on stimulation over lumbosacral spine and recording with a CNEMG electrode may occasionally be helpful, but an absent response has to be evaluated with caution. The clinical value of the test has yet to be established.

Assessment of central motor pathways

Using the same magnetic or electrical stimulation it has been shown to be possible to stimulate the motor cortex and record a response from the pelvic floor. Magnetic stimulation is not painful and cortical electrical stimulation is nowadays only used for intraoperative monitoring. The aim of these techniques is to assess conduction in the central motor pathways.

By electrical stimulation over the motor cortex of healthy subjects, MEPs in the EAS,[79,80] the US,[81] and the bulbocavernosus[79] muscles were reported. The mean latencies were 30–35 ms if no facilitatory maneuver was used. If, however, stimulation is performed during a period of slight voluntary contraction of the muscle of interest, the latencies of MEPs shortened significantly (for up to 8 ms), as has been shown in limb muscles.

By applying stimulation both over the scalp and in the back (at level L1), and subtracting the latency of the respective MEPs, a central conduction time (i.e. time of conduction in central motor pathways from the motor cortex) could be obtained. Central conduction times of approximately 22 ms without, and about 15 ms with, the facilitation (i.e. slight voluntary contraction) have been reported.[77]

Substantially longer central conduction time in patients with multiple sclerosis and spinal cord lesions as compared to healthy controls have been found,[78] but as all those patients had clinically recognizable cord disease, the diagnostic contribution of the technique remains doubtful.

A well-formed sphincter MEP with a normal latency in a patient with a functional disorder or a medicolegal case may occasionally be helpful, but there is no established clinical use for this type of testing.

Neurophysiology of the sacral sensory system

Electroneurography of the dorsal penile nerve

Electroneurography of the dorsal penile nerve is used to assess sensory nerve conduction of lower sacral segments. Theoretically, normal amplitude sensory nerve action potential (SNAP) of dorsal penile nerves in an insensitive penis distinguishes a lesion of sensory pathways proximal to the dorsal spinal ganglion (central pathways, cauda equina) from a lesion of and distal to ganglion (sacral plexus, pudendal nerves). By placing a pair of stimulating electrodes across the penile glans and a pair of recording electrodes across the base of the penis a SNAP can be recorded (with amplitude of about 10 μV). The sensory conduction velocity of the dorsal penile nerve has been reported as 27 m/s. The method was claimed to be helpful in diagnosing neurogenic erectile dysfunction as a consequence of sensory penile neuropathy,[82] but the problems of measuring the conduction distance pose considerable practical difficulties and the test is rarely used.

More practical seems to be the method of stimulating the pudendal nerve by the St Mark's electrode transrectally, and recording from the penis.[83]

Electroneurography of dorsal sacral roots

SNAPs on stimulation of dorsal penile and clitoral nerves may be recorded intraoperatively when the sacral roots are exposed. This has been found helpful in preserving roots relevant for perineal sensation in spastic children undergoing dorsal rhizotomy and possibly decreasing the incidence of postoperative voiding dysfunction.[84] At the level of lower thoracic and upper lumbar vertebrae a low-amplitude (<1 μV) spinal SEP can be recorded with surface electrodes. It is a monophasic negative potential with a mean peak latency of about 12.5 ms[69] and is probably due to postsynaptic activity in the spinal cord. Responses using surface electrodes are often unrecordable in obese healthy men[77] and in many women.

With epidural electrodes, sacral root potentials on stimulation of the dorsal penile nerve could only be recorded in 13, and cord potentials in 9 out of 22 subjects; latencies of these spinal SEPs were 11.9 ± 1.8 ms,[85] substantiating the results obtained by surface recording.[69]

No use of such recordings out of the operating room has been established.

Cerebral somatosensory evoked potentials on electrical stimulation of urethra, bladder, and anal canal

These responses are claimed to be more relevant to neurogenic bladder dysfunction than the pudendal SEP, as the Aδ sensory afferents from bladder and proximal urethra, which convey impulses from these regions, accompany the autonomic fibers in the pelvic nerves (see above).

Cerebral SEP can be obtained on stimulation of the bladder urothelium. When making such measurements, it is of utmost importance to use bipolar stimulation in the bladder or proximal urethra, because otherwise

somatic afferents are depolarized due to spread of electrical current. These cerebral SEPs have been shown to have maximum amplitude over the midline (Cz – 2 cm: Fz) but even so may be of low amplitude (1 μV and less) and variable configuration, making it difficult to identify the response in some control subjects. The typical latency of the most prominent negative potential (N1) is about 100 ms.[86]

However, clinical usefulness of such recordings has not been established.

Autonomic nervous system tests

All of the neurophysiological methods for evaluation of the neurogenic bladder discussed so far assess the thicker myelinated fibers only, whereas it is the autonomic nervous system, the parasympathetic part in particular, which is the most relevant for bladder function. Although in most instances local involvement of the sacral nervous system (such as due to trauma or compression) will usually involve both somatic and autonomic fibers together, there are some local pathological conditions that cause isolated lesions of the autonomic nervous system, such as mesorectal excision of carcinoma[87] or prostatectomy.[88] In addition, several types of peripheral neuropathy preferentially affect thin autonomic fibers. Methods assessing the parasympathetic and sympathetic systems directly would thus be very helpful. Information on parasympathetic bladder innervation can to some extent be obtained by cystometry, which, however, is a test of overall organ function and usually cannot locate the lesion. Although not strictly an electrophysiological test, thermal sensory testing was found useful in assessment of the thin sensory nerve fibers from sacral segments,[88,89] which are often affected concomitantly with thin autonomic fibers.

Sympathetic skin response

The sympathetic nervous system mediates sweat gland activity in the skin. On stressful stimulation a potential shift can be recorded with surface electrodes from the skin of palms and soles, and has been reported to be a useful parameter in assessment of neuropathy involving unmyelinated nerve fibers. The response, SSR, can also be recorded from perineal skin and from the penis. The SSR is a reflex that consists of myelinated sensory fibers, a complex central integrative mechanism, and a sympathetic efferent limb (with postganglionic nonmyelinated C fibers).[90] The stimulus used in clinical practice is usually an electrical pulse delivered to the upper or lower limb (to mixed nerves), but the genital organs can also be stimulated. The latencies of SSR on the penis following stimulation of a median nerve at the wrist have been reported as between 1.5[91] and 2.3 s[92] and could be obtained in all normal subjects with a large variability. The responses rapidly habituate, and depend on a number of endogenous and exogenous factors, including skin temperature, which should be above 28°C. Only an absent SSR can be taken as abnormal.

There is no consensus on the clinical value of SSR testing in sacral dysfunction.

Corpus cavernosum electromyography

Electrodiagnostic tests of sacral parasympathetic nerve function, as for instance corpus cavernosum EMG, also called spontaneous cavernosal activity,[93] would in principle constitute the most definitive indicator of neurogenic sacral organ involvement. Further research to validate this and other potentially useful methods such as detrusor EMG will clarify their place in both research and diagnostics; currently, these tests cannot be suggested for patient diagnosis.

Patient groups with neurogenic bladders in whom uroneurophysiological tests are of clinical value

Parkinsonism

Neuropathic changes can be recorded in sphincter muscles of patients with multiple system atrophy (MSA).[19,29,50,94–97] Multiple system atrophy is a progressive neurodegenerative disease, which is often (particularly in its early stages) mistaken for Parkinson's disease. Urinary incontinence in both genders, and erectile dysfunction in men are early features of the condition, often present for some years before the onset of typical neurological features.[96] Autonomic failure causing postural hypotension and cerebellar ataxia causing unsteadiness and clumsiness may be additional features. The disease is usually (in 80% of patients) unresponsive to antiparkinsonian treatment. As a part of the neurodegenerative process, loss of motor neurons occurs in Onuf's nucleus, so that partial but progressive denervation of the sphincter and the bulbocavernosus muscles occurs[19] and recorded MUPs show changes of reinnervation.[29,95]

Sphincter EMG has been demonstrated to be of value in distinguishing between idiopathic Parkinson's disease and MSA,[29,95] but may not be sensitive in the early phase of the

disease,[19] and not specific after 5 years of parkinsonism.[97] Prolonged duration of MUPs[29,95] abnormal spontaneous activity,[94] as well as diminished number of continuously active low-threshold MUs and IP abnormalities[98] have been described EMG markers for degeneration of Onuf's nucleus occurring in patients with MSA. The changes of chronic reinnervation may be found in other parkinsonian syndromes such as progressive supranuclear palsy (PSP),[99] in whom neuronal loss in Onuf's nucleus was also demonstrated histologically.[100] Chronic reinnervation changes can also be demonstrated as an increase in fiber density on SFEMG.[50] In contrast to previous reports, a recent study failed to demonstrate significant differences between two small groups of MSA and Parkinson disease patients.[98] This might be a consequence of excluding late components from MUP duration, which was made also in another study that did not find MUP analysis useful.[94] In a small number of patients with MSA or primary autonomic failure, the EAS muscle CNEMG was reported sensitive and specific for men, but nonspecific for women, in supporting a diagnosis of MSA.[101] Kinesiological EMG performed during urodynamics can also be valuable in Parkinson's disease[19] and in MSA[20] patients documenting loss of coordination between detrusor and US muscles (detrusor-sphincter dyssynergia).

CNEMG includes observation of denervation activity[94] and quantitative MUP analysis,[29,95] and is clearly indicated in patients with suspected MSA, particularly in the early stages of the disease.[97] If the test is normal early in the disease, but suspicion of the disease persists, it might be of value to repeat the test at some later date.[19]

Cauda equina and conus medullaris lesions and spinal dysrhaphisms

Lesions to the cauda equina and/or conus medullaris are an important cause of pelvic floor dysfunction. Usually the neural tissue damage is caused by compression within the spinal canal due to disc protrusion, spinal fractures, epidural hematomas, tumors, congenital malformations, etc. Unfortunately, accidental damage to cauda equina may occur during surgical interventions, mainly on lumbar discs.

Patient presentation depends very much on the etiology of the lesion. In cases of disc protrusion, spinal fractures, and epidural hematomas, presentation is often dramatic. Acute severe back pain radiating to legs, associated by numbness and tingling in legs (particularly posterior aspects of thighs), buttocks, and perineal region are noted first. Urinary retention with overflow incontinence and, later, severe constipation follow. When damage is due to disc protrusion, history of previous back pain with sciatica, in spinal fractures the history of trauma, and in epidural hematomas of coagulation disorder, anticoagulation therapy, or recent spinal surgery is usually present. With tumors, the presentation of the cauda equina lesion is much more insidious.

After detailed clinical examination of the perineal region (with particular emphasis on perianal sensation), CNEMG of the EAS muscle (and sometimes bulbocavernosus muscle – see below) and electrophysiological evaluation of BCR (when absent clinically) need to be considered.[26]

Generally stated, detection of pathological spontaneous activity by CNEMG has good sensitivity and specificity to reveal moderate and severe partial denervation, and complete denervation, of pelvic floor muscles 3 weeks or more after injury to the cauda equina and/or conus medullaris (see Figure 10.3A). Traumatic lesions to the lumbosacral spine or particularly to the pelvis are probably the only acquired condition where complete denervation of the perineal muscles can be observed. (Complete denervation of all EAS muscles was present in 9% of men with cauda equina/conus medullaris lesions.)[27] Most other lesions will, by contrast, cause partial denervation. CNEMG of the bulbocavernosus muscles is of particular importance a few weeks after partial denervation in the lower sacral myotomes to detect spontaneous denervation activity.[26]

CNEMG (MUP analysis) can show changes of reinnervation, which appear months after injury.[24] Following a cauda equina lesion, the MUPs are likely to be prolonged and polyphasic,[102] and other MUP parameters are also increased (see Figures 10.3A and 10.4B).[24,27] Similar marked changes are seen in patients with lumbosacral myelomeningocele. EMG was found to contribute to prediction of functional outcome in children with spina bifida.[103]

BCR is useful in evaluation of subjects with cauda equina and/or conus medullaris lesions to assess the integrity of the reflex arc. In patients with a tethered cord syndrome measurement of BCR latency can be of additional value, as a very short reflex latency in this clinical situation supports the possibility of the abnormally low position of the conus medullaris.[62] Although in patients with a normal position of conus medullaris urodynamic studies better predicted occurrence of a tight filum terminale, pathological pudendal SEPs correlated with poor surgical outcomes.[71]

Electrophysiological assessment is useful to determine the sequels of the lesion, and in insidious cases for reaching the diagnosis.

Sacral plexus and pudendal nerve lesions

Neurological lesions located in the sacral plexus and pudendal nerves are less common than lesions of the cauda equina or conus medullaris. They can be caused by pelvic fractures,[104] hip surgery,[104] complicated deliveries,[105] malignant infiltration, local radiotherapy,[106] and by use of orthopedic traction tables.[107] They are more often unilateral. In principle, one can distinguish between such a lesion and a cauda equina or the conus medullaris lesions by unilateral absence of dorsal penile SNAP, and absent spontaneous denervation activity in the paravertebral muscles. However, both of these tests are difficult to perform (due to difficult unilateral dorsal penile/clitoral nerve stimulation, and absent paravertebral muscles in the lower sacral segments, respectively), so localization of the lesion will usually be made clinically, or in the case of extensive sacral plexus lesions, by examination of the first sacral and lower lumbar segments.

Urinary retention in women

For many years it was said that isolated urinary retention in young women was due either to psychogenic factors or was the first symptom of onset of multiple sclerosis. However, CNEMG in this group has demonstrated that many such patients have profuse complex repetitive discharges (CRDs) and decelerating burst (DB) activity in the US muscle.[108]

Why this activity should occur is not known but in the syndrome described by one of the authors, it was associated with polycystic ovaries.[109] Most commonly, the initial episode of urinary retention is precipitated by a gynecological surgical procedure using general anesthesia, at the mean age of 28, and the condition does not progress to a general neurological disorder.[110] It was shown that this pathological spontaneous activity endures during micturition and may cause interrupted flow.[22] The disorder of sphincter relaxation appears to lead to secondary changes in detrusor function – either instability or failure of contractility.

Because CNEMG will detect both changes of denervation and reinnervation as occur with a cauda equina lesion (see above), as well as this peculiar abnormal spontaneous activity, it can be argued that this test is mandatory in women with urinary retention.[22,108] It should certainly be carried out before stigmatizing a woman as having psychogenic urinary retention.

Patient groups with neurogenic bladders in whom uroneurophysiological tests are of research interest

Uroneurophysiological techniques have been important in research, substantiated hypotheses that a proportion of patients with sacral dysfunction, such as stress urinary and idiopathic fecal incontinence, have involvement of the nervous system,[73,111] established the function of the sacral nervous system in patients with suprasacral spinal cord injury,[112] and revealed the consequences of particular surgeries.[113] However, in individual patients from these groups, uroneurophysiological tests are unlikely to be contributory.

Generalized peripheral neuropathies

Generalized peripheral neuropathies, particularly those that affect thin nerve fibers, can also cause neurogenic bladder. Most important causes of such neuropathies are diabetes mellitus and acute inflammatory demyelinating polyneuropathy (AIDP or Guillain–Barré syndrome). Most of these neuropathies are length-dependent, with longer fibers first and more severely affected. As a consequence, electrophysiological tests applied on distal lower limb nerves will usually be more sensitive than when applied to nerves that innervate the perineal area/pelvic floor (see above).

Diseases of the central nervous system

Kinesiological tests, performed as a part of cystometric measurements, are often useful in patients with CNS signs having diagnosis of neurogenic bladder. Electrodiagnostic tests of conduction performed in patients with central lesions are only very occasionally indicated. PSEP were found to provide information of diagnostic relevance in the initial diagnostic evaluation of patients with multiple sclerosis, and was also suggested as a screening test for cystometric evaluation in this population.[114] CNEMG is not indicated in central lesions unless segmental spinal cord (conus medullaris) involvement[70] is suspected (see above).[1]

Conclusion

Several electrophysiological tests have been proposed for evaluation of the pelvic floor, the sphincter muscles, and their motor and sensory innervation. Although all tests mentioned in this chapter continue to be of research interest, it is particularly the CNEMG, which is of definite usefulness in everyday routine diagnostic evaluation of selected groups of patients with pelvic floor dysfunction, those with atypical parkinsonism, those with traumatic spinal and pelvic lesions, or young women with urinary retention.

It is expected that new computer-assisted techniques of CNEMG analysis will improve the usefulness of the test as

a diagnostic method to reveal neuropathic pelvic floor muscle involvement.

Further research into and experience with other discussed neurophysiological tests will reveal their contribution to clinical assessment of individual patients, which is presently unknown.

References

1. Fowler CJ, Benson JT, Craggs MD, Vodušek DB, Yang CC, Podnar S. Clinical neurophysiology. In: Abrams P, Cardozo L, Khoury S, Wein A, eds. Incontinence. Plymouth (UK) Health Publication Ltd., 2002; 8b:389–424.

2. Vodušek DB, Fowler CJ. Clinical neurophysiology. In Fowler CJ, ed. Neurology of bladder, bowel and sexual dysfunction. Boston: Butterworth-Heinemann, 1999: 109–143.

3. Fowler CJ, Sakakibara R, Frohman EM, et al, eds. Neurologic bladder, bowel and sexual dysfunction. Amsterdam: Elsevier Science, 2001.

4. Jorge JM, Wexner SD. Etiology and management of fecal incontinence. Dis Colon Rectum 1993; 36:77–97.

5. Agachan F, Chen T, Pfeifer J, et al. A constipation scoring system to simplify evaluation and management of constipated patients. Dis Colon Rectum 1996; 39:681–685.

6. Jackson S, Donovan J, Brookes S, et al. The Bristol Female Lower Urinary Tract Symptoms questionnaire: development and psychometric testing. Br J Urol 1996; 77:805–812.

7. Donovan JL, Peters TJ, Abrams P, et al. Scoring the short form ICSmaleSF questionnaire. International Continence Society. J Urol 2000; 164:1948–1955.

8. Rosen RC, Riley A, Wagner G, et al. An international index of erectile function (IIEF): a multidimensional scale for assessment of erectile dysfunction. Urology 1997; 49:822–830.

9. Quirk FH, Heiman JR, Rosen RC, et al. Development of a sexual function questionnaire for clinical trials of female sexual dysfunction. J Womens Health Gend Based Med 2002; 11:277–289.

10. Vodušek DB, Janko M. The bulbocavernosus reflex. A single motor neuron study. Brain 1990; 113:813–820.

11. Chantraine A, De Leval J, Depireux P. Adult female intra- and periurethral sphincter-electromyographic study. Neurourol Urodynam 1990; 9:139–144.

12. Mathers SE, Kempster PA, Swash M, Lees AJ. Constipation and paradoxical puborectalis contractions in anismus and Parkinson's disease; a dystonic phenomenon? J Neurol Neurosurg Psychiatry 1988; 51:1503–1507.

13. Podnar S, Vodušek DB. Standardization of anal sphincter EMG: low and high threshold motor units. Clin Neurophysiol 1999; 110:1488–1491.

14. Chantraine A, Leval J, Onkelinx A. Motor conduction velocity in the internal pudendal nerves. In: Desmedt JE, ed. New developments in electromyography and clinical neurophysiology, Vol. 2. Basel: Karger, 1973:433–438.

15. Jesel M, Isch-Treussard C, Isch F. Electromyography of striated muscle of anal urethral sphincters. In: Desmedt JE, ed. New developments in electromyography and clinical neurophysiology, Vol. 2. Basel: Karger, 1973:406–420.

16. Deindl FM, Vodušek DB, Hesse U, Schussler B. Activity patterns of pubococcygeal muscles in nulliparous continent women. Br J Urol 1993; 72:46–51.

17. Podnar S, Vodušek DB. Standardization of anal sphincter electromyography: uniformity of the muscle. Muscle Nerve 2000; 23:122–125.

18. Podnar S, Mrkaić M, Vodušek DB. Standardization of anal sphincter electromyography: quantification of continuous activity during relaxation. Neurourol Urodyn 2002; 21:540–545.

19. Stocchi F, Carbone A, Inghilleri M, et al. Urodynamic and neurophysiological evaluation in Parkinson's disease and multiple system atrophy. J Neurol Neurosurg Psychiatry 1997; 62:507–511.

20. Sakakibara R, Hattori T, Uchiyama T, et al. Urinary dysfunction and orthostatic hypotension in multiple system atrophy: which is the more common and earlier manifestation? J Neurol Neurosurg Psychiatry 2000; 68:65–69.

21. Chancellor MB, Kaplan SA, Blaivas JG. Detrusor-external sphincter dyssynergia. In: Bock G, Whelan J, eds. Neurobiology of incontinence. Chichester: John Wiley, 1990:195–213.

22. Deindl FM, Vodušek DB, Bischoff C, et al. Dysfunctional voiding in women: which muscles are responsible? Br J Urol 1998; 82:814–819.

23. Deindl FM, Vodušek DB, Hesse U, Schussler B. Pelvic floor activity patterns: comparison of nulliparous continent and parous urinary stress incontinent women. A kinesiological EMG study. Br J Urol 1994; 73:413–417.

24. Podnar S, Vodušek DB, Stålberg E. Comparison of quantitative techniques in anal sphincter electromyography. Muscle Nerve 2002; 25:83–92.

25. Podnar S, Rodi Z, Lukanovič A, Vodušek DB. Standardization of anal sphincter EMG: technique of needle examination. Muscle Nerve 1999; 22:400–403.

26. Podnar S, Vodušek DB. Protocol for clinical neurophysiologic examination of pelvic floor. Neurourol Urodyn 2001; 20:669–682.

27. Podnar S, Oblak C, Vodušek DB. Sexual function in men with cauda equina lesions: a clinical and electromyographic study. J Neurol Neurosurg Psychiatry 2002; 73:715–720.

28. Fowler CJ, Kirby RS, Harrison MJG. Decelerating bursts and complex repetitive discharges in the striated muscle of the urethral sphincter associated with urinary retention in women. J Neurol Neurosurg Psychiatry 1985; 48:1004–1009.

29. Palace J, Chandiramani VA, Fowler CJ. Value of sphincter EMG in the diagnosis of Multiple System Atrophy. Muscle Nerve 1997; 20:1396–1403.

30. Buchthal F. Introduction to electromyography. Copenhagen: Scandinavian University Press, 1957.

31. Czekajewski J, Ekstedt J, Stålberg E. Oscilloscopic recording of muscle fiber action potentials. The window trigger and delay unit. Electroenceph Clin Neurophysiol 1969; 27:536–539.

32. Stålberg E, Falck B, Sonoo M, et al. Multi-MUP EMG analysis – a two year experience in daily clinical work. Electroenceph Clin Neurophysiol 1995; 97:145–154.

33. Podnar S, Lukanovič A, Vodušek DB. Anal sphincter electromyography after vaginal delivery: neuropathic insufficiency or normal wear and tear? Neurourol Urodyn 2000; 19:249–257.

34. Stålberg E, Bischoff C, Falck B. Outliers, a way to detect abnormality in quantitative EMG. Muscle Nerve 1994; 17:392–399.

35. Podnar S, Vodušek DB. Standardization of anal sphincter electromyography: utility of motor unit potential parameters. Muscle Nerve 2001; 24:946–951.

36. Podnar S, Mrkaić M. Predictive power of different motor unit potential parameters in anal sphincter electromyography. Muscle Nerve 2002; 26:389–394.

37. Nandedkar S, Sanders D, Stålberg E, Andreassen S. Simulation of concentric needle EMG motor unit action potentials. Muscle Nerve 1988; 11:151–159.

38. Stålberg E, Andreassen S, Falck B, et al. Quantitative analysis of individual motor unit potentials: a proposition for standardized terminology and criteria for measurement. J Clin Neurophysiol 1986; 3:313–348.

39. Anon. AAEE glossary of terms used in clinical electromyography. Muscle Nerve 1987; 10(8 Suppl):G1–G60.

40. Podnar S, Fowler CJ. Sphincter electromyography in diagnosis of multiple system atrophy: technical issues. Muscle Nerve 2004.

41. Nandedkar SD, Sanders DB, Stålberg EV. Automatic analysis of the electromyographic interference pattern. Part II: Findings in control subjects and in some neuromuscular diseases. Muscle Nerve 1986; 9:491–500.

42. Podnar S, Vodušek DB, Stålberg E. Standardization of anal sphincter electromyography: normative data. Clin Neurophysiol 2000; 111:2200–2207.

43. Podnar S, Vodušek DB. Standardization of anal sphincter electromyography: effect of chronic constipation. Muscle Nerve 2000; 23:1748–1751.

44. Stålberg E, Trontelj JV. Single fiber electromyography: studies in healthy and diseased muscle, 2nd edn. New York: Raven Press, 1994.

45. Neill ME, Swash M. Increased motor unit fiber density in the external anal sphincter muscle in ano-rectal incontinence: a single fiber EMG study. J Neurol Neurosurg Psychiatry 1980; 43:343–347.

46. Jameson JS, Chia YW, Kamm MA, et al. Effect of age, sex and parity on anorectal function. Br J Surg 1994; 81:1689–1692.

47. Laurberg S, Swash M. Effects of aging on the anorectal sphincters and their innervation. Dis Colon Rectum 1989; 32:737–742.

48. Snooks SJ, Badenoch DF, Tiptaft RC, Swash M. Perineal nerve damage in genuine stress incontinence. Br J Urol 1985; 57:422–426.

49. Vodušek DB, Janko M, Lokar J. EMG, single fiber EMG and sacral reflexes in assessment of sacral nervous system lesions. J Neurol Neurosurg Psychiatry 1982; 45:1064–1066.

50. Rodi Z, Vodušek DB, Denišlič M. External anal sphincter electromyography in the differential diagnosis of parkinsonism. J Neurol Neurosurg Psychiatry 1996; 60:460–461.

51. Dyro FM, Yalla SV. Refractoriness of striated sphincter during voiding: studies with afferent pudendal reflex arc stimulation in male subjects. J Urol 1986; 135:732–736.

52. Kaiho Y, Namima T, Uchi K, et al. Electromyographic study of the striated urethral sphincter by using the bulbocavernosus reflex: study on change of sacral reflex activity caused by bladder filling. Nippon Hinyokika Gakkai Zasshi 2000; 91:715–722.

53. Sethi RK, Bauer SB, Dyro FM, Krarup C. Modulation of the bulbocavernosus reflex during voiding: loss of inhibition in upper motor neuron lesions. Muscle Nerve 1989; 12:892–897.

54. Ertekin Ç, Reel F. Bulbocavernosus reflex in normal men and patients with neurogenic bladder and/or impotence. J Neurol Sci 1976; 28:1–15.

55. Vodušek DB, Janko M, Lokar J. Direct and reflex responses in perineal muscles on electrical stimulation. J Neurol Neurosurg Psychiatry 1983; 46:67–71.

56. Dykstra D, Sidi A, Cameron J, et al. The use of mechanical stimulation to obtain the sacral reflex latency: a new technique. J Urol 1987; 137:77–79.

57. Podnar S, Vodušek DB, Tršinar B, Rodi Z. A method of uroneurophysiological investigation in children. Electroenceph Clin Neurophysiol 1997; 104:389–392.

58. Loening-Baucke V, Read NW, Yamada T, Barker AT. Evaluation of the motor and sensory components of the pudendal nerve. Electroenceph Clin Neurophysiol 1994; 93:35–41.

59. Vodušek DB. Evoked potential testing. Urol Clin N Am 1996; 23:427–446.

60. Rodi Z, Vodušek DB. The sacral reflex studies: single versus double pulse stimulation. Neurourol Urodynam 1995; 14:496–497(abs).

61. Amarenco G, Kerdraon J. Clinical value of ipsi- and contralateral sacral reflex latency measurement: a normative data study in man. Neurourol Urodyn 2000; 19:565–576.

62. Hanson P, Rigaux P, Gilliard C, Biset E. Sacral reflex latencies in tethered cord syndrome. Am J Phys Med Rehabil 1993; 72:39–43.

63. Bilkey WJ, Awad EA, Smith AD. Clinical application of sacral reflex latency. J Urol 1983; 129:1187–1189.

64. Amarenco G, Bayle B, Ismael SS, Kerdraon J. Bulbocavernosus muscle responses after suprapubic stimulation: analysis and measurement of suprapubic bulbocavernosus reflex latency. Neurourol Urodyn 2002; 21:210–213.

65. Blaivas JG, Zayed AA, Labib KB. The bulbocavernosus reflex in urology: a prospective study of 299 patients. J Urol 1981; 126:197–199.

66. Haldeman S, Bradley WE, Bhatia N. Evoked responses from the pudendal nerve. J Urol 1982; 128:974–980.

67. Haldeman S, Bradley WE, Bhatia N, et al. Cortical evoked potentials on stimulation of pudendal nerve in women. Urology 1983; 6:590–593.

68. Guérit JM, Opsomer RJ. Bit-mapped images of somatosensory evoked potentials after stimulation of the posterior tibial nerves and dorsal nerve of the penis/clitoris. Electroenceph Clin Neurophysiol (EP) 1991; 80:228–237.

69. Vodušek DB. Pudendal somatosensory evoked potential and bulbocavernosus reflex in women. Electroenceph Clin Neurophysiol 1990; 77:134–136.

70. Rodi Z, Vodušek DB, Denišlič M. Clinical uro-neurophysiological investigation in multiple sclerosis. Eur J Neurol 1996; 3:574–580.

71. Selcuki M, Coskun K. Management of tight filum terminale syndrome with special emphasis on normal level conus medullaris (NLCM). Surg Neurol 1998; 50:318–322.

72. Delodovici ML, Fowler CJ. Clinical value of the pudendal somatosensory evoked potential. Electroenceph Clin Neurophysiol 1995; 96:509–515.

73. Kiff ES, Swash M. Normal proximal and delayed distal conduction in the pudendal nerves of patients with idiopathic (neurogenic) faecal incontinence. J Neurol Neurosurg Psychiatry 1984; 47:820–823.

74. Barnett JL, Hasler WL, Camilleri M. American Gastroenterological Association medical position statement on anorectal testing techniques. American Gastroenterological Association. Gastroenterology 1999; 116:732–760.

75. Osterberg A, Graf W, Edebol Eeg-Olofsson K, et al. Results of neurophysiologic evaluation in fecal incontinence. Dis Colon Rectum 2000; 43:1256–1261.

76. Suilleabhain CB, Horgan AF, McEnroe L, et al. The relationship of pudendal nerve terminal motor latency to squeeze pressure in patients with idiopathic fecal incontinence. Dis Colon Rectum 2001; 44:666–671.

77. Opsomer RJ, Caramia MD, Zarola F, et al. Neurophysiological evaluation of central-peripheral sensory and motor pudendal fibers. Electroenceph Clin Neurophysiol 1989; 74:260–270.

78. Eardley I, Nagendran K, Lecky B, et al. The neurophysiology of the striated urethral sphincter in multiple sclerosis. Br J Urol 1991; 67:81–88.

79. Vodušek DB, Zidar J. Perineal motor evoked responses. Neurourol Urodynam 1988; 7:236–237(abs).

80. Jost WH, Schimrigk K. A new method to determine pudendal nerve motor latency and central motor conduction time to the external anal sphincter. Electroenceph Clin Neurophysiol 1994; 93:237–239.

81. Thiry AJ, Deltenre PF. Neurophysiological assessment of the central motor pathway to the external urethral sphincter in man. Br J Urol 1989; 63:515–519.

82. Bradley WE, Lin JT, Johnson B. Measurement of the conduction velocity of the dorsal nerve of the penis. J Urol 1984; 131:1127–1129.

83. Amarenco G, Kerdraon J. Pudendal nerve terminal sensitive latency: technique and normal values. J Urol 1999; 161:103–106.

84. Deletis V, Vodušek DB, Abbott R, et al. Intraoperative monitoring of dorsal sacral roots: minimizing the risk of iatrogenic micturition disorders. Neurosurgery 1992; 30:72–75.

85. Ertekin Ç, Mungan B. Sacral spinal cord and root potentials evoked by the stimulation of the dorsal nerve of penis and cord conduction delay for the bulbocavernosus reflex. Neurourol Urodynam 1993; 12:9–22.

86. Hansen MV, Ertekin Ç, Larsson LE. Cerebral evoked potentials after stimulation of the posterior urethra in man. Electroenceph Clin Neurophysiol 1990; 77:52–58.

87. Pietrangeli A, Bove L, Innocenti P, et al. Neurophysiological evaluation of sexual dysfunction in patients operated for colorectal cancer. Clin Auton Res 1998; 8:353–357.

88. Lefaucheur JP, Yiou R, Salomon L, et al. Assessment of penile small nerve fiber damage after transurethral resection of the prostate by measurement of penile thermal sensation. J Urol 2000; 164:1416–1419.

89. Lee JC, Yang CC, Kromm BG, Berger RE. Neurophysiologic testing in chronic pelvic pain syndrome: a pilot study. Urology 2001; 58:246–250.

90. Arunodaya GR, Taly AB. Sympathetic skin response: a decade later. J Neurol Sci 1995; 129:81–89.

91. Opsomer RJ, Pesce F, Abi Aad A, et al. Electrophysiologic testing of motor sympathetic pathways: normative data and clinical contribution in neurourological disorders. Neurourol Urodynam 1993; 12:336–338(abs).

92. Daffertshofer M, Linden D, Syren M, et al. Assessment of local sympathetic function in patients with erectile dysfunction. Int J Impotence Res 1994; 6:213–225.

93. Colakoglu Z, Kutluay E, Ertekin Ç. The nature of spontaneous cavernosal activity. BJU Int 1999; 83:449–452.

94. Schwarz J, Kornhuber M, Bischoff C, Straube A. Electromyography of the external anal sphincter in patients with Parkinson's disease and multiple system atrophy: frequency of abnormal spontaneous activity and polyphasic motor unit potentials. Muscle Nerve 1997; 20:1167–1172.

95. Eardley I, Quinn NP, Fowler CJ, et al. The value of urethral sphincter electromyography in the differential diagnosis of parkinsonism. Br J Urol 1989; 64:360–362.

96. Beck RO, Betts CD, Fowler CJ. Genitourinary dysfunction in multiple system atrophy: clinical features and treatment in 62 cases. J Urol 1994; 151:1336–1341.

97. Libelius R, Johansson F. Quantitative electromyography of the external anal sphincter in Parkinson's disease and multiple system atrophy. Muscle Nerve 2000; 23:1250–1256.

98. Giladi N, Simon ES, Korczyn AD, et al. Anal sphincter EMG does not distinguish between multiple system atrophy and Parkinson's disease. Muscle Nerve 2000; 23:731–734.

99. Valldeoriola F, Valls-Sole J, Tolosa ES, Marti MJ. Striated anal sphincter denervation in patients with progressive supranuclear palsy. Mov Disord 1995; 10:550–555.

100. Scaravilli T, Pramstaller PP, Salerno A, et al. Neuronal loss in Onuf's nucleus in three patients with progressive supranuclear palsy. Ann Neurol 2000; 48:97–101.

101. Ravits J, Hallett M, Nilsson J, et al. Electrophysiological tests of autonomic function in patients with idiopathic autonomic failure syndromes. Muscle Nerve 1996; 19:758–763.

102. Fowler CJ, Kirby RS, Harrison MJ, et al. Individual motor unit analysis in the diagnosis of disorders of urethral sphincter innervation. J Neurol Neurosurg Psychiatry 1984; 47:637–641.

103. Tsai PY, Cha RC, Yang TF, et al. Electromyographic evaluation in children with spina bifida. Zhonghua Yi Xue Za Zhi (Taipei) 2001; 64:509–515.

104. Stoehr M. Traumatic and postoperative lesions of the lumbosacral plexus. Arch Neurol 1978; 35:757–760.

105. Feasby TE, Burton SR, Hahn AF. Obstetrical lumbosacral plexus injury. Muscle Nerve 1992; 15:937–940.

106. Vock P, Mattle H, Studer M, Mumenthaler M. Lumbosacral plexus lesions: correlation of clinical signs and computed tomography. J Neurol Neurosurg Psychiatry 1988; 51:72–79.

107. Amarenco G, Ismael SS, Bayle B, et al. Electrophysiological analysis of pudendal neuropathy following traction. Muscle Nerve 2001; 24:116–119.

108. Fowler CJ, Kirby RS. Electromyography of the urethral sphincter in women with urinary retention. Lancet 1986; 1(8496):1455–1457.

109. Fowler CJ, Christmas TJ, Chapple CR, et al. Abnormal electromyographic activity of the urethral sphincter, voiding dysfunction, and polycystic ovaries: a new syndrome? BMJ 1988; 297(6661): 1436–1438.

110. Swinn MJ, Wiseman OJ, Lowe E, Fowler CJ. The cause and natural history of isolated urinary retention in young women. J Urol 2002; 167:151–156.

111. Snooks SJ, Barnes PR, Swash M, Henry MM. Damage to the innervation of the pelvic floor musculature in chronic constipation. Gastroenterology 1985; 89:977–981.

112. Koldewijn EL, Van Kerrebroeck PE, Bemelmans BL, et al. Use of sacral reflex latency measurements in the evaluation of neural function of spinal cord injury patients: a comparison of neurourophysiological testing and urodynamic investigations. J Urol 1994; 152:463–467.

113. Liu S, Christmas TJ, Nagendran K, Kirby RS. Sphincter electromyography in patients after radical prostatectomy and cystoprostatectomy. Br J Urol 1992; 69:397–403.

114. Sau G, Siracusano S, Aiello I, et al. The usefulness of the somatosensory evoked potentials of the pudendal nerve in diagnosis of probable multiple sclerosis. Spinal Cord 1999; 37:258–263.

11

Practical guide to diagnosis and follow-up of patients with neurogenic bladder dysfunction

Erik Schick and Jacques Corcos

Introduction

Many traumatic, congenital, tumoral, or degenerative neurological pathologies have direct consequences on vesicourethral function. Imaging techniques will give information on the anatomical and morphological status of the urinary tract. Endoscopy will provide further information, such as mucosal appearance, small tumors, urethral stenosis, the degree of prostatic enlargement, and urethrovesical mobility in females. Urodynamics is the only diagnostic tool that allows functional evaluation of the urinary tract. It does not replace any of the other diagnostic modalities, but rather complements them. It plays a major role in therapeutic decisions and during follow-up.

Neurogenic bladder dysfunction after trauma

Traumatic injury to the central nervous system (cerebral or spinal) is often followed by the so-called spinal shock phase. The bladder is areflexic during this phase, which may last from 2 weeks up to 8 weeks,[1,2] but sometimes up to 1 year.[3,4] Complete urodynamic evaluation during this period is useless.[5] Intermittent catheterization is the best treatment modality.

In the case of an incomplete spinal cord lesion, the reappearance of bladder sensation will indicate the end of the spinal shock phase. In the case of a complete lesion, the reappearance of osteotendinous reflexes, urine spillage around the urethral catheter if it was left in place, and incontinence episodes between intermittent catheterizations will suggest the presence of some kind of bladder activity. The first urodynamic evaluation is made at this time.

The site of the neurological lesion will give some indication as to the type of neurogenic bladder function to expect. Lesion above T7 results in hyperreflexic bladder, whereas lesion at T11 or below results in areflexic bladder. Lesion between T8 and T10 constitutes the 'gray zone', and can result either in hyperreflexic or areflexic bladder.[4] Vesico-sphincteric dyssynergia is more difficult to predict because only two-thirds of hyperreflexic bladders will be accompanied by dyssynergic voiding.[4]

Neurogenic bladder dysfunction after non-traumatic neurological pathology

Usually, the urologist will see these patients with a well-defined neurological diagnosis when urinary symptoms are already present. In this case, immediate urodynamic evaluation is indicated, together with other diagnostic modalities such as urine culture, ultrasonographic imaging of the upper urinary tract, and free flowmetry, if possible.

Autonomic dysreflexia

Autonomic dysreflexia is an exaggerated sympathetic response to afferent stimulation when spinal cord injury (SCI) is at the level of T6 or above. Acute, life-threatening autonomic dysreflexic episodes can be controlled by chlorpromazine (1 mg) or phentolamine (5 mg), given intravenously.[6] On a long-term basis, chronic α-adrenergic blockade in small doses, such as prazosin (1 mg daily), will be helpful.[7] Our practice is to administer nifedipine (10 mg), a calcium channel blocking agent, sublingually to patients with a potential risk of developing acute autonomic dysreflexia during urological manipulations (e.g. endoscopy, urodynamics), 30 min before these procedures (Figure 11.1).

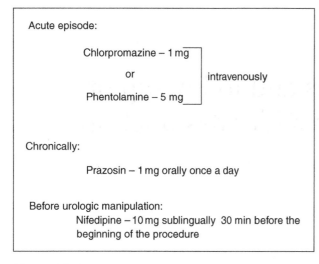

Figure 11.1
Treatment of autonomic dysreflexia.

Renal surveillance

In a follow-up study by Donelly et al of paraplegics from World War II, renal disease was the most common cause of death in the first 20 years after the injury, accounting for 40% of all deaths.[8] More recently, in a series of 406 consecutive SCI patients followed for 15 years, Webb et al[9] reported a death-rate of 0.5% (2/406) secondary from renal complications. This highlights the importance of dedicated follow-up to significantly reduce kidney-related mortality in these patients.

Renal ultrasound[10] combined with plain radiography of the abdomen[11] tends to replace intravenous pyelography (IVP) in upper urinary tract evaluation.[12] Color flow Doppler sonography could eventually replace retrograde cystography in the detection of vesicoureteral reflux. In a recent study, Papadaki et al[13] reported that color Doppler ultrasonography diagnosed all grade IV and V, 87.5% of grade III, 83.3% of grade II, and 57.4% of grade I refluxes. There were 6 false-positive and 5 false-negative findings among 187 SCI adults.

In many major SCI centers, radionuclide renograms are used for routine follow-up of renal function, instead of IVP.[6] A study by Phillips et al[14] showed that a decline in effective plasma flow was the best predictor for therapeutic intervention.

It has been our practice to obtain a renal ultrasonogram and a plain abdominal X-ray in all patients with neurogenic bladder dysfunction as part of their initial evaluation, together with urodynamic studies. The results of the latter give information on pressure conditions in the bladder. With a high-pressure system, the upper urinary tract is at high risk for deterioration, and upper tract monitoring

should be more frequent (every 6–12 months). In the case of a low-pressure system, this danger is only relative, and we undertake renal ultrasound study approximately every 3–5 years if no change in clinical symptoms suggests modification of the bladder's pressure status. However, if clinical symptoms change, ultrasonography of the kidneys and urodynamic studies are repeated promptly. Figure 11.2 summarizes, in a schematic way, our initial evaluation and follow-up of patients with neurogenic bladder dysfunction.

Urodynamics

Urodynamics are cornerstones in the diagnosis and management of neurogenic bladder dysfunction. In this respect, the main parameters that require special attention are high detrusor pressure during the filling or storage phase of the bladder (decreased bladder wall compliance and/or sustained detrusor contraction), and detrusor-external sphincter dyssynergia during micturition. Well-conducted, multichannel (video)urodynamic evaluation will highlight these conditions and consequently allow the initiation of appropriate therapeutic measures that should ultimately transform a high-pressure system to a low-pressure system.

Endoscopy

Cystourethroscopy is an essential part of the initial evaluation of all patients with neurogenic bladder dysfunction. It allows visualization of anatomic urethral occlusion, especially in the male. It should be emphasized that there is a fundamental difference between occlusion and obstruction. Urethral occlusion means a more or less pronounced change in urethral caliber, such as a fibrotic stricture. This can be diagnosed endoscopically. In contrast, obstruction is a dynamic concept, which, from the hydrodynamic point of view and simplified to some extent,[15] essentially means a 'high-pressure–low-flow' relationship. This can be diagnosed by urodynamics. Benign prostatic enlargement illustrates the relationship between the two concepts. Endoscopically, one can observe a protrusion of the lateral lobes of the prostate into the urethral lumen, joining each other on the midline. From this picture, however, it is not possible to extrapolate how the detrusor will contract, and how the urethra will relax to allow voiding to take place. In other words, one cannot estimate to what extent this prostatic enlargement will interfere with flow and be responsible for an eventual obstruction.

In the female, the best chance to visualize stress incontinence is to ask the patient to cough when the bladder

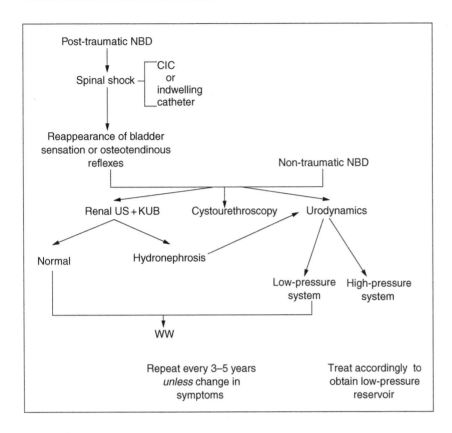

Figure 11.2

Diagnosis and follow-up of patients with neurogenic bladder dysfunction. US, ultrasound; CIC, clean intermittent catheterization; KUB, plain abdominal X-ray; NBD, neurogenic bladder dysfunction; WW, watchful waiting.

has reached its cystometric capacity, at the end of the cystoscopic examination. Also, the best condition to evaluate the bladder neck hypermobility is when the bladder is completely empty.

In both sexes, bladder wall trabeculation suggests an overactive bladder, rather than outlet obstruction (see also Chapter 5).

References

1. Light JK, Faganel J, Beric A. Detrusor areflexia in suprasacral spinal cord injuries. J Urol 1985; 134:295–297.

2. Chancellor MB, Kiilholma P. Urodynamic evaluation of patients following spinal cord injury. Sem Urol 1992; 10:83–94.

3. Wheeler JS Jr, Walter JW. Acute urologic management of the patient with spinal cord injury: initial hospitalisation. Urol Clin N Am 1993; 20:403–411.

4. Perlow DL, Diokno AC. Predicting lower urinary tract dysfunctions in patients with spinal cord injury. Urology 1981; 18:531–535.

5. Chancellor MB. Urodynamic evaluation after spinal cord injury. Phys Med Rehab Clin N Am 1993; 4:273–298.

6. Chancellor MB, Blaivas JG. Spinal cord injury. In: Chancellor MB, Blaivas JG, eds. Practical neurourology. Boston: Butterworth-Heinemann, 1995:99–118.

7. McGuire EJ. Immediate management of the inability to void. In: Parsons FK, Fitzpatrick JM, eds. Practical urology in spinal cord injury. London: Springer Verlag, 1991:5–10.

8. Donelly J, Hackler RH, Bunts RC. Present urologic status of the World War II paraplegic: 25-year follow-up. Comparison with status of the 20-year Korean War paraplegic and the 5-year Vietnam paraplegic. J Urol 1972; 108:558–562.

9. Webb DR, Fitzpatrick JM, O'Flynn JD. A 15-year follow-up of 406 consecutive spinal cord injuries. Br J Urol 1984; 56:614–617.

10. Bodley R. Imaging in chronic spinal cord injury – indications and benefits. Eur J Radiol 2002; 42:135–153.

11. Morcos SK, Thomas DG. A comparison of real-time ultrasonography with intravenous urography in the follow-up of patients with spinal cord injury. Clin Radiol 1988; 39:49–50.

12. Chagnon S, Vallée C, Laissy JP, Blery M. Ultrasonographic evaluation of the urinary tract in patients with spinal cord injuries. Systematic comparison with intravenous urography in 50 cases. J Radiol (Paris) 1985; 66:801–806.

13. Papdaki PJ, Vlychou MK, Zavras GM, et al. Investigation of vesico-ureteral reflux with colour Doppler sonography in adult patients with spinal cord injury. Eur Radiol 2002; 12:366–370.

14. Phillips JP, Jadvar H, Sullivan G, et al. Effect of radionuclide renograms on treatment of patients with spinal cord injury. Am J Roentgenol 1997; 169:1045–1047.

15. Kranse R, van Mastrigt R. Relative bladder outlet obstruction. J Urol 2002; 168:565–570.

Part II

Classification

12

Classification of lower urinary tract dysfunction

Anders Mattiasson

Introduction

A system of classification lives only as long as it is generally perceived to correspond to the reality it is intended to describe. The need to revise it is thus present on a continuous basis. The current classification system for disorders and terminology in the lower urinary tract[1–3] needs to be revised.[4] The new approach described herein does not represent any generally accepted system, but rather is a proposal for a new manner in which to view the reality. It is rooted in disorder/illness processes and injuries being described in terms of structure and function and not, as previously (and presently), primarily in terms of consequential effects such as symptoms. Actually, we should be speaking of lower urinary tract disorders. Dysfunction in fact describes only one half of the structure + function pair. We should also be quite aware that a classification that we use as researchers due to, among other things, pedagogical reasons, must ultimately be separated from the one which we in the capacity of caregivers use in contact with, for example, the patients.

In this chapter the general classification of lower urinary tract disorders comprises the subject matter. A consistent and uniform way of looking at things comprises the basis of a functioning classification system. What one chooses as the basis for the system is in fact of crucial significance. In most of the other fields of medicine, illnesses and injuries are described in pathophysiological terms. So the case ought to be the same on the part of the lower urinary tract. Hence, it is difficult to maintain a system that is based upon a description of the circumstances for the genesis of different forms of urinary incontinence. In certain cases it is the patient's experiences that are the point of departure, such as with urge and so-called overactive bladder, whereas physical exertion or stress is the point of departure in other cases. It is more constructive to describe how the tissues and organs are engaged on different levels in terms of structure and function (S + F) right down to the cell and molecular biology level, and to then describe what the consequences are that give rise to symptoms and difficulties

and other conceivable consequential effects.[4] This can be illustrated as in Figure 12.1.

By deciding to use S + F as a basis for a classification system, a decision has been made once and for all as far as it concerns this system precisely. All divisions and categorizations must then, in its continuation, also fit in with each other in the holistic spirit described above. Structure and function are different ways of regarding and expressing the same thing. Complete covariance can be presumed to exist in a well-balanced situation. Structural changes do not occur without altered functionality and vice versa.

This is how the situation appears in a simple system (Figure 12.2). When multiple tissues and multiple organs are connected together, as in the lower urinary tract, new conditions arise, where the different parts come to influence each other. In reality, they are all part of a balanced situation

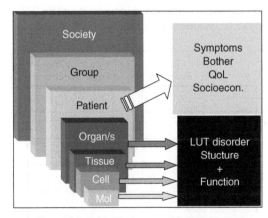

Figure 12.1
Lower urinary tract disorders are best described in pathophysiological terms of structure and function. Symptoms and bother are secondary phenomena, and therefore not as suitable for the primary classification. QoL, quality of life; Socioecon., socioeconomics; Mol, molecule.

intended to fulfill the task of storing and evacuating urine, and an imbalance in one of the parts inexorably comes to have an effect on the other component parts. The lower urinary tract acts as a single functional unit.

All of the different parts of the micturition cycle and the different components of the lower urinary tract cannot, however, be included in a fully comprehensive classification system without them being represented at all levels. This is especially important as the lower urinary tract contains within itself functions that are diametrically opposed in every individual part, i.e. in a part of the micturition cycle optimized for storage and in a different part for emptying. In such a case it is important to capture all these parts as well as the transition forms between them. Hence not only should the bladder, trigone/bladder neck, and urethra be included but also the vagina, prostate, pelvic floor, as well as all the different types of supporting structures. Vessels and nerves have not been mentioned, but are included of course, and strictly speaking the parts of the nervous system involved must also be included in order to form a whole (Figure 12.3).

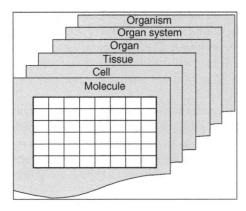

Figure 12.2
All levels and all parts of the lower urinary tract and its innervation can be included in one matrix.

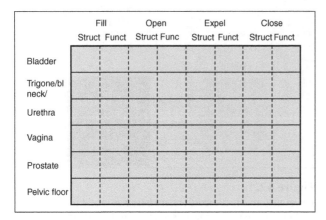

Figure 12.3
When all parts of the lower urinary tract and the whole micturition cycle are characterized regarding both structure and function, the result will be a complete recognition pattern.

The micturition cycle

The classification and thus the description of lower urinary tract disturbances is directly dependent on where one finds oneself in the micturition cycle. Due to the filling and discharge functions being so intimately intertwined, it is often difficult to distinguish which signals are related to what parts of the urinary tract. For example, during filling of the bladder, activity including detrusor contractions can arise too early. This is in fact activity that is characteristic of emptying that appears here during filling. How should this be classified? To do this, the initial point of departure must be fixed. Since the functional status of the lower urinary tract changes in step with the filling and emptying, we must have multiple well-defined points of departure. These actually differ from one another, and collectively represent the entire micturition cycle. The activity that belongs in the different phases can be represented graphically with a simple sketch (Figure 12.4) that depicts the pressure conditions in the bladder and urethra during the different parts of the micturition cycle.

It is logical to make a new division of the micturition cycle in such a manner that the emptying also encompasses the short transitions between storage and evacuation. It is of course precisely at their beginning and ending, respectively, that the storage pattern is broken. The commencement of micturition concerns the direct preparations for emptying, such as the pressure drop in the urethra that takes place during the flow of urine itself. This also applies for the cessation of micturition when the pressure conditions are restored after the flow has ended. The entire storage phase is then governed by a picture that in itself is dynamic, but which in terms of pressure is essentially constant. It is an important and critical point in the micturition cycle when diametrically opposed functions, in contrast to those that have been prevailing, normally for a number of hours, need to be established

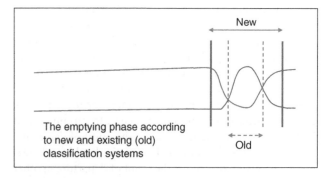

Figure 12.4
When the pressure changes of the bladder and the urethra before and after the expulsion of urine are both included in the emptying phase, this also means that the storage and the emptying phases of the micturition cycle have been redefined.

in order to perform the emptying. The storage-to-emptying turning point is quite important and it has been proposed that it be given an identity of its own, namely the 'SE turn'.

The balance between the lower urinary tract and the nervous system

The lower urinary tract and the parts of the nervous system involved in the micturition cycle balance each other in a purposeful manner independently of the functional phase (Figure 12.5). They are so intimately associated that they can be regarded as the partners in a marriage, i.e. a unit in which both parts are needed to a similar degree. The fact that a large part of the nervous system is situated functionally and anatomically between the lower urinary tract and that part of the nervous system where important coordination and perception are located also makes it easy to view the lower urinary tract as being in a position of dependence. In the classification system that is based upon structure and function, no distinction is drawn between the lower urinary tract and the nervous structures involved.

During the storage phase, an adjustment occurs in the bladder wall for the increasing volume without any

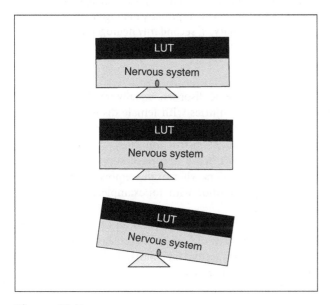

Figure 12.5
The lower urinary tract (LUT) and the nervous system are balancing each other. All parts influence each other. The system becomes more lable with increasing filling of the bladder (triangle). A disturbance can be balanced out, i.e. a disorder can be present without causing any symptoms.

appreciable rise in pressure. Nevertheless, the afferent input increases and gradually increasing activity can be read in, for example, the external sphincter in step with the filling of the bladder. Continence is preserved at the bladder neck level, i.e. a low-pressure system for closure. Somatic and adrenergic innervation of striated and smooth musculature are the most influential neuromuscular mechanisms of the closure function. In connection with exertion, activation of the pelvic floor and compression of the urethra become significant factors in the maintenance of continence. Cholinergic innervation via the pelvic nerves is regarded as being inhibited during the bladder's filling phase.

Upon initiation of emptying, a significant change occurs in the nervous and muscular activity. The outflow tract and the urethra must be opened and bladder contraction initiated. Positive feedback must be established and maintained all the way to complete bladder emptying. In order to cause the opening of the intermediate segment and the external sphincter, the stimulation of the smooth and striated muscle contraction that participates in the closure is minimized, i.e. adrenergic and somatic nervous activity is inhibited. At the same time, a contraction probably occurs of certain muscle fibers in order for the funnelling of the outflow tract to be able to take place. In addition, relaxation-mediating substances are released to ensure an open outflow tract and the least possible resistance. The bladder contraction is certainly effectuated primarily under cholinergic influence; however, other substances do seem to be of significance, particularly with functional disorders. We also know that altered activity in C fibers in the bladder is significant in the genesis of increased activation of the entire system for emptying preparedness. This is perhaps also significant for normal functioning, even though the perception has long been that they are normally tacit.

This switching between diametrically different functional states has spawned the 'on-and-off' concept. For individual structures and functions, it works well for describing a course of events. However, the whole is comprised of a number of on-and-off pairs, which do not operate in step with each other; hence, the designation ceases to be appropriate. When one adds that simultaneously exciting and inhibiting influences on nerves and/or muscles seem to be typical for different parts of the lower urinary tract during both filling and emptying, one understands why on-and-off can only be used to describe the occurrence of reciprocity in itself, not the course of events in the lower urinary tract.

A special situation exists in the lower urinary tract in the manner in which mechanisms are activated to guarantee the shutting off of the outflow and urethra, and thus continence, at the same rate as which a preparedness is also built up to be able to open up precisely these structures instantaneously. One cannot rule out the possibility that the activation of the continence-preserving external urethral sphincter leads to an activation of afferent pathways which have an inhibitory effect in the spinal cord and on the pelvic nerves. When the contraction in the sphincter is voluntarily released on command from higher centers, inhibitory influence that prevents the activation of the micturition reflex disappears, and activation with accompanying opening of the outflow tract can occur. With such an arrangement, the apparently paradoxical arrangement with the simultaneous building up of activity that promotes both filling and emptying would appear to be both possible and easily explained.

It is possible to say, as shown in Figure 12.5, that the degree of instability in the system increases with an increasing degree of bladder filling. Under normal circumstances the system is of course in balance; however, in the event of illness/injury the main focus is displaced, albeit with retained balance, i.e. without any signs of any disorder. When the process proceeds or when the system is provoked, e.g. through an increasing degree of bladder filling, an imbalance arises, i.e. symptoms appear. It is not always the case that this imbalance is synonymous with symptoms presenting themselves. For example, with a bladder outlet obstruction, reduced detrusor functionality can arise secondarily to the outlet obstruction without the individual experiencing any symptoms. The same applies of course with other types of disruptions.

Classification according to involvement of the nervous system

In principle it can be said that all disruptions that give rise to symptoms have a neurogenic component by definition, since the center for the perception of the illness/injury is located in the same nervous system on a slightly higher level, and there, among other things, it contains the consciousness (Figure 12.6).

If the disorder/injury has its origin purely in the nervous system (**1**), the disruption can be regarded as primarily neurogenic; however, as soon as the lower urinary tract becomes involved it then contains both a neurogenic as well as a LUT component. The situation is the same with illnesses and injuries that engage the lower urinary tract itself, i.e. most often they are both neurogenic and LUT primarily at the same time (**2**). However, one can say that they are partly neurogenic and partly LUT. Conditions such as benign prostatic hyperplasia (BPH) without an effect on the lower urinary tract or changes in, for example, ligaments, can probably be said to be non-neurogenic (**4**). However, this applies only as long as they do not give rise to symptoms; otherwise, they must be classified as secondarily neurogenic (**3**) (Figure 12.7).

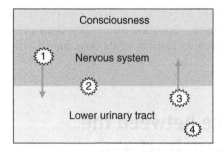

Figure 12.6
Different types of lower urinary tract disorders and their relation to the nervous system (see also Figure 12.7).

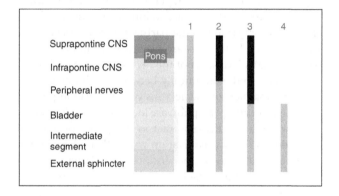

Figure 12.7
Different types of lower urinary tract disorders and their relation to the nervous system (see also Figure 12.6). Light bars refer to primary site of disorder/lesion, dark bars to secondary involvement. 1, primary neurogenic; 2, partly neurogenic, primary; 3, secondarily neurogenic; 4, non-neurogenic, LUT.

Partly neurogenic disorders usually involve a loss – e.g. neuromuscular injuries with female disorders – whereas secondary neurogenic usually means compensation – e.g. with BPH and outlet obstruction. Hence, as a consequence, the treatment is often a nature of supplemental factors with female disorders, whereas the removal of that which is in excess is the solution with, for example, BPH with outlet obstruction.

If we were to turn it all around and proceed from the lower urinary tract, the classification should, from top to bottom, be 'LUT, secondary', 'partly LUT, primary', 'LUT, primary', and LUT instead.

Disorder, consequences, and comorbidity

Primary LUT disorders can thus be partly non-neurogenic, partly secondary, or partly neurogenic. The non-neurogenic conditions, which do not provide symptoms, will not be taken up for further discussion here. Those that are partly neurogenic encompass a pathophysiological process/lesion which probably rarely stops with this, but rather due to the presence of the disease process changes will appear both in it and in the tissues/organ that is affected, in this case the lower urinary tract. This in turn involves changes in structure and innervation in the area that is primarily encompassed, which becomes the object of a process of change. This can in turn naturally lead to symptoms in the same manner as the original disorder or injury.

Precisely because the lower urinary tract is so close-knit functionally and morphologically, processes which injure a part of it will often ultimately also damage the whole. Figure 12.8 shows how different factors can be related in an entire chain, and that an individual symptom can be difficult to connect clinically to a certain factor.

Complicating factors are often logically intertwined with the disorder, even if the link may be latent. With comorbidity, the situation is however slightly different. Many of the changes which are a property of the organism as a whole or of other organ systems can affect the lower urinary tract and either initiate dysfunctional conditions on their own, or in conjunction with other causes, or affect a previously existing illness process (Figure 12.9). An example of a situation where difficulties can exist in reading what contributes to an illness picture is an outflow obstruction with BPH as well as simultaneous metabolic factors, possibly with an influence on the autonomous innervation of the lower urinary tract.

Patterns of recognition

In theory, one can collect information on structure and functionality as measurements of different types in all parts of the lower urinary tract during all parts of the micturition cycle (Figure 12.10).

By illustrating this graphically on a simulated three-dimensional display, different disorder conditions are recognizable by their distinctive features, i.e. as patterns of recognition. Information on completely normal individuals of both genders and at different ages would serve as a reference. An example of a pattern of recognition is shown in Figure 12.10. At present it is not possible to work with such an abundance of detail; however, the largest and most important of the parts must represent the whole. It then is advantageous to seek to attain a degree of representation

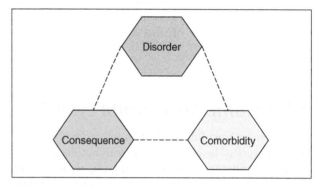

Figure 12.9
The interdependence of the disorder, its consequences, and the influence from other disease processes.

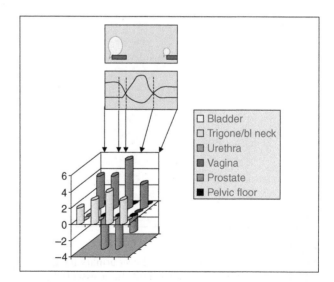

Figure 12.10
A simulated three-dimensional recognition pattern can reflect the influence of the disorder and its consequences, i.e. the impact on the lower urinary tract in different parts of the micturition cycle. Arbitrary scale.

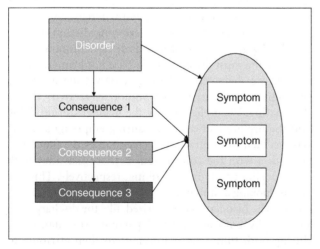

Figure 12.8
In a given clinical situation it is often unclear from what part of the pathophysiological process that symptoms emanate.

for different levels in the lower urinary tract and its functions. To include the bladder and external sphincter seems quite natural, but so does including the parts that play a central role in the pressure-changing phases, i.e. the trigone, bladder neck, and proximal urethra. Since we do not know precisely the details of the functional contributions of these structures to low-pressure shutting during storage and funnelling as well as pressure decreases during emptying, we can amalgamate them into an intermediate segment with intermediate functionality.

Figure 12.11 illustrates three parts – the external sphincter, the intermediate segment, and the bladder – for a normal man (A) and woman (C) as well as during emptying with the unisex picture A′C′. Figure 12.11B shows how the prostate has a negative influence on the dynamics of the intermediate segment and also how the lumen is restricted by adenomas with a reduced flow of urine as a consequence, whereas Figure 12.11D shows how it can appear with incontinent women, i.e. with a higher flow than normal. Both are examples of what one could call harmonic disorders.

A harmonic micturition cycle?

Lower urinary tract functionality in women with incontinence appears to be characterized by diminished outflow resistance and more efficient emptying than normal, whereas increased resistance and more difficult emptying as well as a changed voiding pattern seem to be typical for men with an outlet obstruction. One could say that it is easier for women to trigger emptying as a consequence of

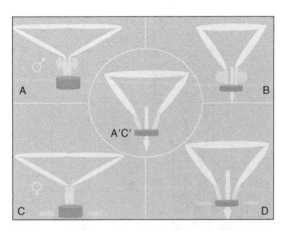

Figure 12.11
A simplified, reduced model of the lower urinary tract, introducing the intermediate segment. Three essential components – the bladder, the intermediate segment, and the external sphincter – of the lower urinary tract in both men and women are in this model. To this can be added the pelvic floor in the female and the prostate in the male. Further explanations are given in the text.

the decline in neuromuscular functionality, whereas for men it is easier to trigger and more difficult to empty due to the appearance of an obstruction. Even if both men and women show altered innervation as an element of these changes, the synchronization between the different component parts is still preserved. With such harmonic disorders the fundamental pattern of the micturition cycle is actually preserved. Even if overactivity, obstructions, or dislocations – via, for example, provocations – occur, the synchronization still continues to be maintained.

However, with disharmonic conditions, this pattern is broken such that simultaneously occurring activities in different parts of the lower urinary tract functionally oppose each other, resulting for example in an unsettled filling phase or more difficult emptying with an obstruction. This is first and foremost characteristic of primarily neurogenic disturbances, and what is especially characteristic are the occurrences of contractions for the purposes of producing a closing of the musculature on the outflow tract simultaneously with the bladder contracting and showing a pressure increase.

With central neurogenic disruptions, the picture is dominated by mass motor behavior, dyssynergy, and overactivity. With peripheral neurogenic and mixed disruptions there is usually a lower degree of activity, synergy more often than not, and both overactivity and underactivity are common occurrences. Disharmonic disruptions can arise without any form of micturition reflex, with pathological reflexes, and range to being with normal reflexes. The activity can thus at times be aberrant, i.e. arise unexpectedly during a part of the micturition cycle where it should normally not occur, such as overactivity. If this is synchronized with other parts so that the result, for example, becomes a premature micturition reflex, then it has a completely different clinical significance than if it were to appear to be unsynchronized and a bladder contraction takes place for a discharge that does not participate in the opening up, or which even actively shuts, as with detrusor-sphincter dyssynergy. Harmonic and disharmonic disruptions can thus be designated as synchronous or asynchronous.

By far the most disruptions that are not primarily neurogenic are characterized by overactivity. Even if sensory overactivity is occurring, it is motor overactivity that is dominating. We prefer to view the bladder during filling and the urethra and discharge during emptying as being passive; then we contrast our perception of the functional condition with the conspicuous activity that they both show during emptying and filling, respectively. This is a way of looking at it that leads to errors in terms of classification. The bladder is characterized, like the discharge and urethra, by both activity and passivity simultaneously during both filling and emptying. To then attribute to solely the more obvious and visible parts of these many different activities the epithet 'active' or 'overactive' does not lead to a firm foundation for classification: that not only excitation and contraction but also an inhibitory nervous influence can be designated to be an activity is in a way easy to comprehend.

Time-related changes

When a disorder process finds a foothold, completely regardless of whether it is spreading itself or not, it leads to changes in other parts of the lower urinary tract by affecting the balance. As time goes on, this imbalance grows if new balancing factors do not counterbalance the changes. Step by step those parts which are situated at the levels above the illness/injury become involved. Usually it is chronic conditions with a time scale spanning decades (Figure 12.12).

Trophic-structural changes are the rule, and are usually most pronounced in individuals who have higher degrees of obstruction and/or overactivity.[5] With women, it primarily involves, simply put, what is being lost; with men, what is being added; and with neurogenic disturbances, what is being reorganized. So, in addition to effects on the dynamics of the intermediate segment, a mechanical effect on the lumen of the urethra, and a certain flow limitation, a changed prostate also has effects on the bladder and therewith the nervous system. If no progress occurs in the primary process, growth in the secondarily arising changes will probably still occur. When remedying a problem in the lower urinary tract it is thus important that one can take hold of the problem by the root: i.e. don't treat problems that are related to the influence of the bladder first of all, but remedy the negative influence of the prostate on the urethra and the intermediate segment as the first priority. Although this is probably self-evident, it nevertheless deserves to be mentioned in this context.

The process that leads to female incontinence, and which probably began with trauma in connection with childbirth, is chronic and progressive in its nature, bringing post-polio syndrome to mind. Functional disturbances in the lower urinary tract are nearly always chronic conditions that cannot always be reversed, just compensated for, and naturally in the best case can even be prevented. Changes conditioned by the age of the organism must also be added to the pathophysiological process. It is therefore important to classify all age groups among both genders.

Bladder outlet obstruction

Bladder outlet obstruction (BOO) usually develops slowly, i.e. over many years.[5,6] It is much more common among men and mainly involves an impediment in the bladder neck and/or prostate.[7] An altered micturition pattern typically occurs, both with regard to the distribution of the instances of micturition during the day as well as to the characteristics of the individual instance of emptying in terms of how quickly and efficiently the emptying is initiated and carried out. We can also see how a pattern in the development of the obstruction picture grows over time as being to a large extent dependent upon the reaction to the impediment and not necessarily involving the impediment itself by looking at the lower urinary tract above the impediment and the nervous system reacting to the occurrence of a downstream impediment to emptying.[8] The impediment may be constant, but the reaction may become variable over time. Using current obstruction classification techniques, a clear discrepancy exists between the symptom picture that the patient reports and the findings of examinations we make with, for example, urodynamics in the form of pressure–flow measurements,[9,10] probably because our formula for obstruction is far too simplified. Factors that are related to an elevated urethral resistance ought to be complemented with a number of additional factors, as set out below.

The development of an obstruction of the lower urinary tract is most often a slow process taking many years. It usually involves successively more difficult emptying. The point in time of establishment is difficult to determine, as is obvious in an illustration of obstruction as a process besides the static condition we use for classification of obstruction today (Figure 12.13). In the typical case, an obstruction is a progressive process, and the development itself of an impediment is part of this process, i.e. a part of the obstruction; therefore, we must also include these circumstances in the new equation in order to describe impediments to evacuation of the bladder.

The obstruction can be characterized in different ways, depending upon where in the development cycle of the reaction to this change one finds oneself (Figure 12.14). An additional argument is that the obstruction concept is composed of and also encompasses all types of impediments to the emptying phase, not only increased urethra resistance as with prostate adenoma or the like but also

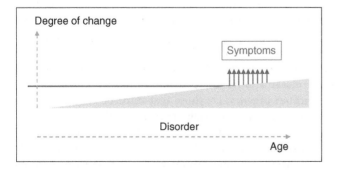

Figure 12.12
Non-malignant disorders of the lower urinary tract often develop slowly over considerable periods of time.

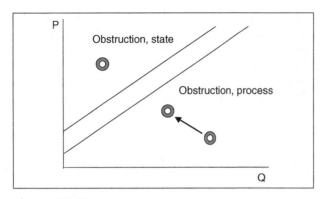

Figure 12.13
Obstruction is presently defined as illustrated in the upper left part of this nomogram from the International Continence Society (ICS). Obstruction can, however, also be a process over time, with a change in the direction of recognized obstruction.

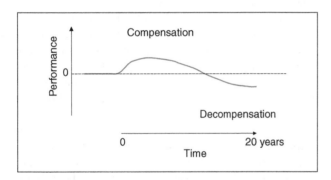

Figure 12.14
Given a certain increased, but over time unchanged, urethral outlet resistance, changes that are induced in the bladder, the nervous system, and in vessels can contribute to compensation with detrusor pressure increase during contraction, etc., in an early phase. One of the consequences of this changed function and the following remodeling of the bladder wall will be a decreased performance at comparable levels later during this process, and thus a decompensation.

changes in the level of the bladder neck, which in such cases can either be isolated or occur together with, for example, BPH (Figure 12.15).

An obstruction below the external sphincter as with, for example, a urethral stricture gives a different clinical picture than the one which appears when the bladder outflow and external sphincter are engaged. With a stricture, features of irritative difficulty such as urges, etc. are seldom seen, whereas this is common with more proximal obstructive processes.

Female incontinence

That the relationships between different female incontinence groups using the currently prevailing classification

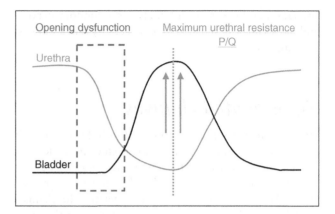

Figure 12.15
The increased detrusor pressure and the decreased urinary flow rate (not shown) used to reflect an outlet obstruction is only representing the moment of maximum performance, which means that an impediment of the opening function might only be caught and classified as an obstruction when we have included any hindrance to the emptying phase (shown as 'New' in Figure 12.4) in our definition of obstruction.

system, which of course builds upon the stress, urge, mixed, and overactivity terminology, have not become clearer over the years is certainly related to an insufficient knowledge of the structure and functionality of the underlying disorder processes, and thus the possibility of making comparisons.[11]

Neuromuscular insufficiency, triggering of normal or pathological reflex activity with or without sensations of urgency, and possible occurrences of incontinence can be described with the simple schedule illustrated in Figure 12.16. More detailed investigations of the different groups, particularly of the urethra and the pelvic floor, have in recent years only managed to move the different incontinence groups closer to each other.[12,13] Changes which they share include a weakness in the musculature of the urethra, pelvic floor, and vaginal wall, which should have a closing effect during stress, and a – possibly of reactive origin – faster establishment of the opening phase and more effective emptying pattern during micturition. A swift activation of emptying seems to be present, which involves a lowering of the pressure in the urethra. This pattern seems to be just as common in incontinent women without urgency, i.e. those that must be classified under stress incontinence using the current terminology.

What could such observations then mean for the classification of disorder(s) eventually leading to female incontinence? One cannot rule out that such opening activity comprises one, and perhaps the foremost, of the least common denominators for different types of female incontinence.[14] Stress incontinence would then not only be

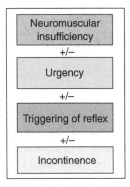

Figure 12.16
A neuromuscular insufficiency in the lower urinary tract might be present in many more women than those being incontinent. Urgency, overactivity, and incontinence might or might not be present. The relation between different types of female incontinence might be better understood.

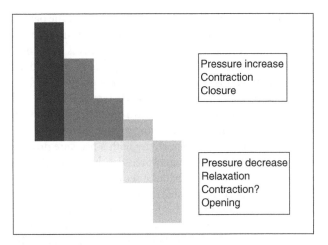

Figure 12.17
The ability to increase the urethral pressure during squeeze seems to also prevent pressure fall and urethral relaxation, whereas incontinent women who often have a reduced ability to increase the intraurethral pressure also present with a urethral relaxation. (Reproduced with permission from Teleman and Mattiasson 2002.)

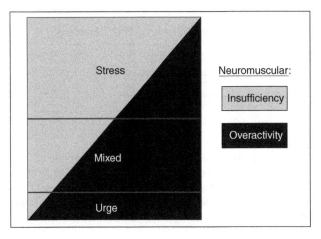

Figure 12.18
A combination of neuromuscular insufficiency and overactive behavior of the lower urinary tract could be a better way than stress, urge, and mixed to describe the condition giving rise to incontinence in women.

comprised of a passive component with insufficient closure due to imperfect contraction during stress but also have an active component in the form of a relaxation, a pressure drop, and opening of the urethra in the same situations. Such easily triggered relaxation activity that is associated with urgency would become classified in our present system as overactive bladder or mixed and urge incontinence, depending upon whether the leakage needs to be triggered with physical exertion and whether urge sensations are present or not. In contrast, using the pathophysiological process for classification would in its functional part instead be characterized by a loss of the functionality in closing abilities of the musculature and instead reveal the penetration of a relaxation-mediating component in a manner that is illustrated by a movement from left to right in Figure 12.17.

To bring together a new model that builds upon the simultaneous occurrence of neuromuscular insufficiency and an increased tendency for activation of emptying-encouraging mechanisms with the traditional stress, mixed, and urge model would give a result that looks like Figure 12.18.

Increased lower urinary tract activity

There are many different types of overactivity.[15] All possible nervous activity and a set of different transmitters or so-called neuromodulators can play important roles in the genesis of overactivity. Solely afferent overactivity with a sensory experience connected to it does exist. Solely efferent overactivity is somewhat more difficult to imagine; however, we certainly all believe that it is possible that purely efferential mechanisms can have an influence on, for example, reflex arches and cause overactivity to arise.

Combinations are common. Afferent overactivity is probably the driver in by far the most cases. A lower urinary tract that is disconnected from a functional context, i.e. without the passage of urine, does not make a nuisance of itself if complicating factors such as infections do not arise.

One often speaks of the significance of neurogenic and myogenic factors. It is important to map out both nerves and muscles; however, without the presence and contribution of both, there will not be much coordinated activity. Isolated myogenic activity with tonus and tension effects on the walls of the lower urinary tract can be found despite this.

Significant trophic changes are often a part of the pathophysiological process, with illnesses and disruptions to the functionality of the lower urinary tract. This is quite natural since structure and functionality go hand-in-hand. At the same time, it is worth noting that the prerequisites for pliability in this case seem particularly large, as nerves and muscles appear to interact: e.g. through the production and influence of nerve-stimulating growth factors.

Since the pattern of overactivity with a pressure drop in the urethra which immediately precedes the rise in bladder pressure is the same as what one sees at the onset of micturition, it appears reasonable to presume that the sequence of events is the same in both situations (Figure 12.19). If such is the case, then one can also characterize the overactivity as LUT instead of detrusor, since all parts of the lower urinary tract seem to be engaged. In addition, it is certainly more precise to call overactivity of this type emptying-related instead of filling-related, as is currently the case with the classification of symptoms related to so-called overactive bladder (Figure 12.20).

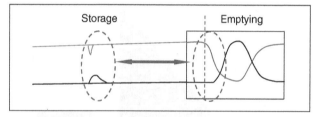

Figure 12.19
The same sequence of events with a urethral pressure fall that precedes the detrusor pressure increase is found in both overactivity and at the start of a normal micturition cycle. It seems reasonable to see this overactivity as emptying-related in nature rather than storage-related.

A simplified structure and function based classification of lower urinary tract disorders

Since it is not possible to map out all parts of every patient, there is a strong desire to be able to limit one's observations with respect to structure and functionality to a reasonable number. A simplified model that allows this should be able to include observations from the bladder and the outlet/urethra at an early point during bladder filling, at a late point in the filling phase, and with a provocation at the latter or both, as well as also having observations relating to the emptying of the bladder. With this, we must be able to move the focus from the bladder to also encompassing the outlet, urethra, prostate/pelvic floor, as well as including an evaluation of nervous functions as a part of our routine status. In doing so, we will be able to see the pathophysiological process and the disorder or injury as forming a basis for our classification. The symptom picture and other consequences should be added in order to describe manifestations which the patient experiences of the changes that have arisen. In a simplified model we cannot handle anything other than those structures and functions that we regard as being most essential in the micturition cycle. Among these, we count the bladder and the external sphincter, and then we should include the function that is responsible for shutting and opening at the bladder neck level and in the proximal urethra. Along these lines we probably would include the trigone, bladder neck, with men the preprostatic urethra, smooth musculature in the proximal urethra, and the mucous membrane in this area. It is more practical to regard these in their interrelationships and quite simply call them the intermediate segment and the intermediate function (Figure 12.21).

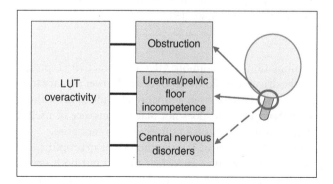

Figure 12.20
The proximal urethra is a probable trigger zone for LUT overactivity in both men and women. Another zone is comprised by the bladder.

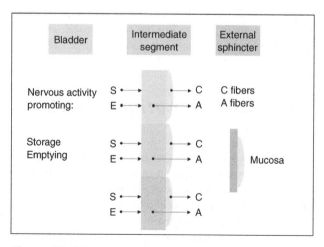

Figure 12.21
A simplified representation of the lower urinary tract and its innervation. S and E denote storage and emptying, respectively, whereas A and C refer to afferent nerve fibers.

For women one can add the pelvic floor to these and, for men, the prostate (Figure 12.22). Activity or morphology concerning efferent nerves that promote filling and emptying can be added, as well as different modalities of afferent innervation, Aδ and C fibers, respectively (Figure 12.23). Figure 12.22 illustrates how BPH can be envisioned to affect both the intermediate segment and the urethra lumen. This is a theoretical model, which, if true, would explain in a simple manner why a prostate enlargement can be of significance for both the urethra resistance with an established flow as well as for the capability to open the urethra during the initiation of the emptying.

How comprehensive in the sense of how widespread and how intensive a change is and how large an engagement it creates in the surrounding tissues and structures is important to include in a good classification. In addition, one should have a picture of whether afferent and efferent innervation in the three different fundamental parts displays normal characteristics or whether signs of altered innervation/functionality exist. This appears to be knowledge of increasing importance. Placing an extra emphasis on nerves and nervous activity is in line with the fundamental classification model, which proceeds from the neurogenic component in a disruption of the LUT. How this should be carried out and the means by which one should procure this information are of course important questions, but are not covered here. A theoretical model to describe LUT neuromuscular activity might have an appearance similar to that shown in Figure 12.23. After sufficient experience has been built up, one can probably content oneself with a few of the parameters mentioned. A simplified pattern of recognition could then look like Figure 12.24 in its basic structure.

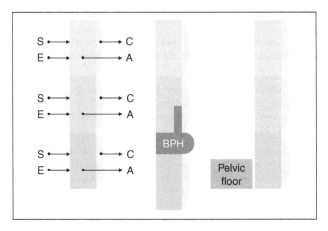

Figure 12.22
Benign prostatic hyperplasia (BPH) might influence not only the urethral lumen but also have a negative impact on the intermediate segment and, for example, bladder neck function. In the female, changes in the pelvic floor might be significant for the whole of the lower urinary tract. S and E denote storage and emptying, respectively, whereas A and C refer to afferent nerve fibers.

Consequences of disorders

The symptoms and the difficulties that an individual feels and experiences are of course completely central for how one should regard the illness/injury. However, they are

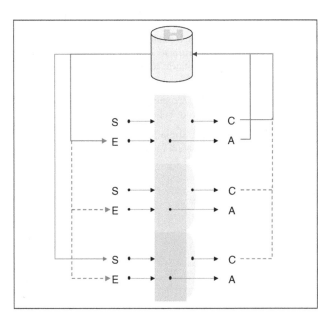

Figure 12.23
Representation of how both A- and C-fiber mediated activity can induce motor events in all parts of the LUT.

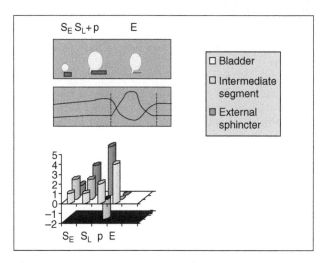

Figure 12.24
A simplified pattern of recognition can be based on a reduced number of observations, and thus provide a framework for clinical use. S_E = storage, early; S_L = storage, late; p = provocation; E = emptying. Arbitrary scale.

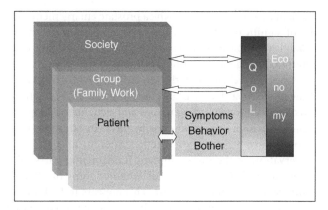

Figure 12.25

Important consequences of the patient's disorder are symptoms, behavior, bother, consequences for quality of life (QoL), and the socioeconomic situation. With increasing consequences, an increased interest should be expected from different groups and from society at large.

consequences of what has been incurred, and thus are secondary to their nature in a classification context (Figure 12.25). That the quality of life is affected to a significant degree by disruptions to the functionality of the lower urinary tract is clear, and likewise that the financial consequences for both the individual and society are most often significant. Their mutual interrelationship can be illustrated by Figure 12.25. A number of different confirming instruments has already been prepared in order to estimate the scope and significance of these consequences, and continued developmental work will provide us with still better measuring instruments.

References

1. Abrams P, Blaivas JG, Stanton SL, Andersen JT. The standardisation of terminology of lower urinary tract function. Scand J Urol Nephrol Suppl 1988; 114(5):5–19.

2. Abrams P, Cardozo L, Fall M, et al. The standardisation of terminology of lower urinary tract function: report from the Standardisation Sub-committee of the International Continence Society. Neurourol Urodyn 2002; 21(2):167–178.

3. Blaivas JG, Appell RA, Fantl JA, et al. Definition and classification of urinary incontinence: recommendations of the Urodynamic Society. Neurourol Urodyn 1997; 16:149–151.

4. Mattiasson A. Characterisation of lower urinary tract disorders: a new view. Neurourol Urodyn 2001; 20:601–621.

5. Hald T, Brading AF, Horn T, et al. Pathophysiology of the urinary bladder in obstruction and ageing. In: Denis, Griffiths, Khoury, et al, eds. Proceedings of the 4th International Consultation on Benign Prostatic Hyperplasia (BPH), 1997:129–178.

6. Patel M, Tewari A, Furman J. Prostatic obstruction and effects on the urinary tract. In: Narayan P, ed. Benign prostatic hyperplasia. Edinburgh: Churchill Livingstone, 2000:139–150.

7. Abrams P, Griffiths D. The assessment of prostatic obstruction from urodynamic measurements and from residual urine. Br J Urol 1979; 51:129–134.

8. Griffiths D, Höfner K, van Mastrigt R, et al. Standardisation of terminology of lower urinary tract function: pressure-flow studies of voiding, urethral resistance, and urethral obstruction. Neurourol Urodyn 1997; 16:1–18.

9. Bates P, Bradley WE, Glen E, et al. Third report on the standardisation of terminology of lower urinary tract function. Procedures related to the evaluation of micturition: pressure flow relationships, residual urine: Br J Urol 1980; 52:348–359; Euro Urol 6:170–171; Acta Urol Jpn 27:1566–1568; Scand J Urol Nephrol 1981; 12:191–193.

10. Bates P, Bradley WE, Glen E, et al. Fourth report on the standardisation of terminology of lower urinary tract function. Terminology related to neuromuscular dysfunction of lower urinary tract. Br J Urol 1981; 52:233–235; Urology 17:618–620; Scand J Urol Nephrol 15:169–171; Acta Urol Jpn 27:1568–1571.

11. Koelbl H, Mostwin J, Boiteeux JP, et al. Pathophysiology. In: Abrams, Cardozo, Khoury, Wein, eds. Proceedings from the 2nd International Consultation on Incontinence, 2001:202–241.

12. Petros PE, Ulmsten UI. An integral theory and its method for the diagnosis and management of female urinary incontinence. Scand J Nephrol Suppl 1993; 153:1–93.

13. Teleman P, Gunnarsson M, Lidfeldt J, et al. Urodynamic characterisation of women with naïve urinary incontinence – a population based study in subjectively incontinent and healthy 53–63 years old women. Eur Urol 2002; 42:583–589.

14. Mattiasson A, Teleman P. A common urethral motor disorder in all types of female incontinence. Submitted to publisher.

15. Fall M, Geirsson G, Lindström S. Toward a new classification of overactive bladders. Neurourol Urodyn 1995; 14:635.

Part III

Treatment

13

Conservative treatment

Jean-Jacques Wyndaele

Introduction

Conservative treatment is the most applied treatment modality in neurogenic bladder. The reasons for this are clear: most conservative therapeutic methods are cheap, available to the vast majority of patients around the world and, within the limits of proper application, complications are rare.

In this chapter we will give an overview of most techniques used in conservative treatment, including behavioral techniques, physiotherapy, and catheterization.

Behavioral techniques

The philosophy behind behavioral techniques is that one can only have a reasonable chance of acquiring a balanced bladder if daily life adjustments are made to the new situation of the lower urinary tract function caused by the neuropathy. Adjustments can be:

- Scheduled voiding at fixed times during the day when sensation is pathological.
- Voiding several times consecutively in order to lower a residual.
- Increasing the voiding interval to treat frequency. This includes 'bladder drill', aimed at retraining the bladder to hold more urine and inhibit inappropriate detrusor contractions during the filling phase of the micturition cycle.
- Adapting drinking habits, which includes balanced spread of fluid intake and advice on avoiding caffeinated beverages and identifying individual bladder irritants.
- Making the toilet more accessible and improving the patient's mobility.
- Changing drugs intake if these influence diuresis and/or bladder function.
- Treatment of other physical or psychological problems such as constipation and depression.[1]

Hadley divided scheduling regimens into four conceptual categories: bladder training, habit retraining, timed voiding, and prompted voiding.[2]

Keeping a voiding diary can offer information on functional bladder capacity, leakage, and sensation, which are important data for adjusting treatment and for a better understanding by patient and physician. Keeping a voiding diary can also have a therapeutic effect and, by itself, can lead to greater comfort.[3]

Behavioral adaptation and advice is important in all patients.

Physiotherapy

Detrusor overactivity from defective central inhibition or increased detrusor afferent activity can be improved by reinforcing inhibitory pathways. In the storage phase a number of detrusor inhibitory reflexes have been described as emanating from the detrusor via the sympathetic nerves and from the pelvic floor and external urethral sphincter via pudendal afferents.[4] The latter reflex implies that the resting tone in the pelvic floor and external urethral sphincter (supplied by branches of the pudendal nerve: S2–4) has an inhibitory effect on the detrusor. Furthermore, active contraction of these muscle fibers is said to enhance this inhibitory effect. Consequently, pelvic floor training should benefit those patients with weak pelvic musculature. The nerve roots of S2–4 are also involved in some muscles of the lower limb, and there is evidence that activation of S2–4 myotomes may have an inhibitory effect on the detrusor. These muscles include the gluteus maximus, the plantar flexors, and some small muscles of the foot. Hence, one can observe young children activating these myotomes, standing on tiptoes to suppress urgency, and there is no reason why adults cannot use this 'trick'.[5,6]

The sacral dermatomes include the saddle area and the back of the thighs and legs. In particular, the anus, clitoris, and glans penis are well supplied with sensory nerves, and activation of these afferents can inhibit the detrusor.[6]

Centrally, when these afferents are activated by electrical stimulation, they have at least two effects: (1) by provoking the inhibitory sympathetic neurons to the ganglia and the detrusor and (2) by providing central inhibition of the pre-ganglionic bladder motor neurons through a direct route in the sacral cord. Some young girls have been observed to 'curtsy' to control urgency. The pressure of the heel on the perineum presumably activates the sacral dermatomes, in addition to possibly elevating the bladder neck and supporting the proximal urethra. When learning bladder drill for urgency and urge incontinence, patients can be taught to sit down (on a rolled-up towel is best) and press on/squeeze the clitoris/glans penis and so activate the appropriate dermatomes. This reduces urgency, inhibits/reduces unwanted bladder contractions, and helps the patient to defer voiding, aiming to increase the functional bladder capacity. The daily use of transcutaneous electrical nerve stimulation (TENS) over S2–4 dermatomes has also been shown to have a beneficial effect on reducing urgency and urge incontinence. Self-adhesive electrodes delivering 2 Hz stimulation placed bilaterally over S3 in 40 children showed 67.5% response.[7] Sacral stimulation at 10 Hz over S3 in 71 adults with chronic sensory urgency, detrusor instability, or detrusor hyperreflexia during urodynamics showed a significant improvement in cystometric volumes with a concomitant reduction in detrusor pressure compared with pre-stimulation cystometry.[8] TENS applied over the peroneal or posterior tibial nerve is another option for activating sacral afferents.

There is abundant evidence to support the use of maximal electrical stimulation to activate the detrusor inhibitory reflexes from the anal and vaginal regions using electrodes specially designed for this purpose. Optimum electrical parameters include low-frequency (5–10 Hz) alternating rectangular pulses at maximum intensity. This activates the sympathetic inhibitory system to the bladder and the central inhibitory pathway to parasympathetic motor neurons, which have all been shown to operate at low frequencies.[9] In a group of 74 patients with detrusor instability and urge incontinence treated with maximal electrical stimulation, 51 were subjectively cured or significantly improved. Objectively, a significant decrease in frequency and significant increase in bladder volume were demonstrated.[10] A further study by Eriksen et al[11] demonstrated initial clinical and urodynamic cures in 50% of 48 women suffering from idiopathic detrusor instability following seven 20-min treatments of maximal stimulation using a vaginal and an anal electrode simultaneously. In addition, a significant improvement was observed in a further 33%. At 1 year follow-up, a persisting therapeutic effect was found in 77% and no serious side-effects were reported.[11] Also, maximal stimulation on the thigh muscles gave such effect.[12]

Detrusor hypoactivity may also respond to physiotherapy in the form of techniques to facilitate detrusor activity.

Activation of stretch receptors in the bladder wall can instigate a detrusor contraction, and so pressing or tapping over the bladder may set off a detrusor contraction. Likewise, bending forward and straining may help to initiate detrusor activity. However, suprapubic tapping and straining are risky techniques, as described below. Bladder emptying may be further enhanced by ensuring relaxation of the pelvic floor.

Furthermore, using maximal electrical stimulation of the pelvic floor muscles, Plevnik et al[13] treated six patients with spinal cord lesions from C5 to T4, all demonstrating detrusor-sphincter dyssynergia, in whom urinary retention developed. After two to four 20-min treatments over 4 weeks, using vaginal or anal electrodes and monophasic square pulses of 1 ms, frequency of 20 Hz and 50–90 mA, a reduction in maximal urethral pressure was reported. In addition, uninhibited detrusor contractions were reduced in four patients and reflex voiding by tapping was successful in all patients.

Intravesical transurethral bladder stimulation is used to rehabilitate the neurogenic bladder.[14] Its therapeutic goals are to achieve a sensation of bladder filling, to initiate a detrusor contraction, and to achieve conscious urinary control. The procedure combines direct stimulation of the bladder receptors with visual feedback using patient observance of cystometric pressure changes. The effects are technique-dependent.[15]

Several other techniques of pelvic floor physiotherapy can be successfully used in patients with neurogenic bladder: Biofeedback and relaxation can have indications in patients with partly preserved voluntary and/or sensory function.

Intravesical biofeedback has been used successfully in improving the sensation of bladder fullness and control of involuntary contractions.[16]

Triggered reflex voiding is much less applied than a decade ago, but nevertheless it is still used. Bladder reflex triggering comprises various maneuvers performed by the patient in order to elicit reflex detrusor contractions by exteroceptive stimuli.[17] The pathophysiological background is unphysiological in suprasacral lesions for which the technique is mostly used: it comprises C-fiber activation, bladder contraction involuntary and not sustained, detrusor-striated sphincter dyssynergia or detrusor-bladder neck dyssynergia, and autonomic dysreflexia.[18] Only in the minority of patients will triggering lead to balanced voiding. Complications such as infection,[19,20] upper urinary tract alterations/deterioration, and incontinence are frequent. If applied, patients should be encouraged to find the best individual trigger zone and points: suprapubic tapping, thigh scratching, squeezing the glans penis and the scrotal skin, pulling on the crines pubis, as well as anal/rectal manipulation may be effective.[21]

Suprapubic tapping must be stopped in most patients when micturition starts, permitting the fast-reacting striated sphincter to relax, whereas the slowly reacting detrusor may still remain in contraction. As soon as micturition stops, tapping has to be applied again.

Drugs or surgery may be necessary to decrease outflow resistance and to improve reflex incontinence. Videourodynamics are strongly advised to find out if the urodynamic situation is safe. Triggered voiding is contraindicated in cases of:

· inadequate detrusor contraction
· unbalanced voiding
· vesico-uretero-renal reflux
· reflux in the seminal vesicles or in the vas
· uncontrollable AD
· persistence of recurrent urinary tract infections.

Bladder expression comprises various maneuvers aimed at increasing intravesical pressure in order to enable/facilitate bladder emptying. The most commonly used are the Valsalva (abdominal straining) and the Credé (manual compression of the lower abdomen) maneuvers. Bladder expression has been recommended for a long time for patients with so-called lower motor neuron lesions, resulting in a combination of an underactive detrusor with an underactive sphincter or with an incompetent urethral closure mechanism of other origin. Clinical experience has shown that by using Valsalva or Credé maneuvers many patients are able to empty their bladders, albeit mostly incompletely. Urodynamics/videourodynamics have demonstrated that, despite high intravesical pressures during straining, the urinary flow may be very poor due to an inability to open the bladder neck, or to a mechanical obstruction at the level of the striated external sphincter by bending and compression of the urethra. Moreover, Clarke and Thomas[22] showed in flaccid male paraplegics that the major component of urethral resistance is a constant, adrenergically innervated muscular resistance in the external sphincter region.

With increasing time, more than 40% of the patients on straining show influx into the prostate and the seminal vesicles, and complications due to the high pressures such as reflux to the upper urinary tract. Measures to facilitate bladder expression can be the use of α-blockers, but they usually cause or increase urinary stress incontinence.

Contraindications are:

· sphincter hyperreflexia and detrusor-sphincter dyssynergia
· vesico-uretero-renal reflux
· reflux into the male adnexa
· hernias
· hemorrhoids
· urethral pathology
· symptomatic urinary tract infections.

Some patients use the anal sphincter stretch described by Low and Donovan[23] with success.

Intermittent catheterization and intermittent self-catheterization

Intermittent catheterization (IC) and intermittent self-catheterization (ISC) have become widely used in the last 40 years. Many studies show good results and limited complications, leading to a better prognosis and a better quality of life in many patients with neurologic bladder[24–26] (Table 13.1).

IC and ISC are nowadays considered as the methods of choice for the management of neurologic bladder dysfunction.[18]

Results depend on the techniques used, which involves the types of catheters and lubricants, the catheter manipulation and introduction, and the rules needed for a short-term and long-term successful application.

Many types of catheters are used, made of different material. Some are packed in a sheet/bag, others are reusable.[27] Some have a urethral introducer that permits bypassing the colonized 1.5 cm of the distal urethra and which resulted in a significant lower infection rate in hospitalized men with spinal cord injury.[28] Studies comparing materials in a randomized controlled way are scarce. Lundgren et al[29] found, in the rabbit, that a high osmolality is important in hydrophilic catheters with regards to removing friction and urethral trauma. Waller et al[30] had the same experience in men. Wyndaele et al[31] evaluated the use of a hydrophilic catheter in 39 male patients with neurogenic bladder using conventional catheters over a long period. The hydrophilic catheter proved as easy to use but was better tolerated. Satisfaction was better, especially in patients who experienced problems with conventional catheters. Some patients were unsatisfied for reasons of practical use or for economical reasons.

Most catheters require the use of some kind of lubricant, especially in men. Lubricants are applied on the catheter or are instilled into the urethra.[32] In some countries patients use oil or merely water as a lubricant. For patients with preserved urethral sensation, a local anesthetic jelly may be needed. Catheters with a hydrophilic and self-lubricated surface need activation with tap water or sterile water.

For adults, size 10–14 F for males and size 14–16 F for females are mostly used, but a bigger size/lumen may be necessary for those with bladder augmentation or cloudy urine that results from another origin. No studies on IC compared sizes in a randomized way.

Two main techniques have been adopted: a sterile (SIC) and a clean IC (CIC). The sterile non-touch technique advocated by Guttmann and Frankel implicates the use of

Table 13.1 *Outcome of continence study*

Authors	Number of patients	Follow-up	Adjunctive treatment	Result of continence
Iwatsubo et al[118]	60 spinal cord lesions		Overdistention during shock phase	100% continent
Kornhuber and Schultz[120]	197 multiple sclerosis			Continence improved with elimination of residual urine
Kuhn et al[121]	22 spinal cord lesions	5 years	No	Continence did not change
Lindehall et al[122]	26 meningomyeloceles	7.5–12 years		24/26 better
Madersbacher and Weissteiner[116]	12 f	2–4 years		50% dry; other 50% some grade of incontinence
McGuire and Savastano[119]	22 f	2–11 years	Surgery 27%	Continent 73%
Vaidyanathan et al[124]	7 spinal cord lesions	14–30 months	Bladder relaxant drugs intravesically	84% dry, 3 dampness at awakening
Waller et al[123]	30 spinal cord lesions	5–9 years	6 anticholinergics	22 dry, 8 incontinent
Wyndaele et al[117]	30 (18 m, 12 f)	3–30 months	6 anticholinergic, 1 colocystoplasty	73% continent + 13% improvement
Wyndaele and Maes[84]	75 (69 neurogenic)	1.5–12 years	38 anticholinergics	47 dry, 22 seldom wet, 6 wet at least once a day

f = female; m = male.

sterile materials handled with sterile gloves and forceps. In an intensive care unit, some advocate wearing a mask and a sterile gown as well. In some centers, during a bladder training program SIC used to be performed only by a catheter team, which has proven to obtain a very low infection rate.[33] Nowadays, the sterile technique is mostly used only during a restricted period of time and in a hospital setting. In the majority of cases a clean technique is used.

Self-catheterization is done in many different positions: supine, sitting, or standing. Female patients may use a mirror or a specially designed catheter to visualize the meatus. After a while, most women do not need these aids anymore.

The basic principles of urinary catheter introduction are well known: the catheter must be introduced in a noninfecting and atraumatic way. Noninfecting means cleaning hands, using a noninfected catheter and lubricant, and cleaning the meatal region before catheter introduction. Atraumatic requires a proper catheter size, sufficient lubrication, and gentle introduction through the urethra, sphincter area, and bladder neck.[34,35] The catheter has to be introduced until urine flows out. Urine can be drained

directly in the toilet, in a urinal, plastic bag, or other reservoir. The catheter should be kept in place until urine flow stops. Then it should be pulled out slowly, while gentle Valsalva or bladder expression is done in order to completely empty residual urine. When properly done, the residual urine should be maximum 6 ml.[36] However, Jensen et al measured residual urine repeatedly with ultrasonography and found residual urine in 70% of the catheterizations in their group of 12 patients with spinal cord lesion. The residual urine could exceed 50 ml and even 100 ml.[37]

Finally, the end of the catheter should be blocked to prevent backflow of the urine or air into the bladder. Hydrophilic catheters can be left in place for a short time only to prevent suction by the urethral mucosa, which may make removal difficult.

During the rehabilitation phase, clean intermittent self-catheterization (CISC) can be taught very early to patients with good hand function.[38]

When resources are limited, catheters are reused for weeks and months: some are resterilized or cleaned by soaking in an antiseptic solution or boiling water. Microwaving to resterilize rubber catheters has also been described. Reused supplies do not seem to be related to an increased likelihood of urinary tract infection.[39,40]

The frequency of catheterization needed can depend on many factors, such as bladder volume, fluid intake, post-void residual, and urodynamic parameters (bladder compliance, detrusor pressure). Usually it is recommended to catheterize 4–6 times a day during the acute phase after spinal cord lesion. Some patients will need to keep this frequency if IC is the only way of bladder emptying. Other patients will catheterize 1–3 times a day to check and evacuate residual urine after voiding or on a weekly basis during bladder retraining.[41] Use of a portable ultrasound device in IC has been evaluated.[42,43]

Adjunctive therapy to overcome high detrusor pressure is often needed. Anticholinergic drugs or bladder relaxants are often indicated in patients with bladder overactivity. For patients who develop a low-compliance bladder, upper tract deterioration or severe incontinence injection of botulinum toxin in the bladder wall or surgery as bladder augmentation may be necessary.[44,45] Where a too high diuresis is noted during the night due to diurnal variation of anti-diuretic hormone, DDAVP (desmopressin) can be safely and effectively used.[46,47] In cases of catheterization difficulty at the striated sphincter, botulinum toxin injection in the sphincter can help.[48] In individuals with tetraplegia, reconstructive hand surgery can be indicated.[49] For those with poor hand function or difficulty in reaching the meatus, assistive devices might be needed.[50]

Education is very important. Teaching programs have been successful in non-literate persons in developing countries and in quadriplegic patients.[51,52]

It is clear that IC can improve incontinence or can make patients with neurogenic bladder continent. To achieve this, bladder capacity should be sufficient, bladder pressure kept low, urethral resistance high enough, and care taken to balance between fluid intake, residual urine, and frequency of catheterization.

Not all patients starting with IC continue this treatment and several reasons can exist for this (Table 13.2). A main reason to stop is continuing incontinence. Main reasons to continue are continence and autonomy of the patients.[53] Bakke and Malt found that, among those who practiced IC independently, 25.8% were sometimes and 6% were always averse, especially young patients and females. Aversion seemed to be related above all to nonacceptance of their chronic disability.[54] A recent retrospective analysis in spinal cord injury patients showed that, of patients on CIC at discharge, 52% discontinued the method and reverted to an indwelling catheter because of dependence on caregivers, spasticity interfering with catheterization, incontinence despite anticholinergic agents, and lack of availability of external collective devices for female patients.[55]

The introduction of a catheter several times a day can give rise to complications. One of the most frequent complications is infection of the urinary tract (UTI). Prevalence of UTI varies widely in the literature. This is due to the various methods used for evaluation, the different techniques of IC, different frequencies of urine analysis, different criteria for infection and the administration or not of prophylaxis to the group of patients studied, and much more. Some publications give the percentage of sterile urine at between 12 and 88%.[24,56–61] Eleven percent prevalence for asymptomatic UTI and 53% for symptomatic bacteriuria are given in different series.[62,63] Bakke found that in 407 patients, 252 with neurogenic bladder, during an observation period of 1 year, 24.5% of patients had nonclinical UTI, 58.6% had minor symptoms, 14.3% had more

Table 13.2 *Reasons for stopping intermittent self-catheterization*

Authors	Catheter-free	Incontinence	Inconvenience	Infection	Physical status	Choice of patient
Bakke[131]	10%		5%	4%	3%	
Diokno et al[125]	17%	2%	2%		7%	
Hunt et al[132]	10%					
Maynard and Glass[126]	12%					6%
Sutton et al[130]		6%	6%	3%	3%	3%
Timoney and Shaw[129]		36%				
Whitelaw et al[127]	5%		5%		5%	5%
Webb et al[128]	9%		3%		2%	2%

comprehensive or frequent symptoms, while 2.6% claimed major symptoms.[64]

In the acute stage of spinal cord injury (SCI), with proper management, urine can be kept sterile for 15–20 days without antibiotic prophylaxis and for 16–55 days if prophylaxis is given.[65–67] Prieto-Fingerhut et al[68] determined the effect of sterile and nonsterile IC on the incidence of urinary tract infection in 29 patients after SCI in a randomized controlled trial. With urine analysis on a weekly basis they found a 28.6% UTI incidence in the group on sterile IC, whereas a 42.4% incidence was found in the nonsterile catheterization group. The cost of antibiotics for the sterile IC group was only 43% of the cost for those on nonsterile IC. However, the cost of the sterile IC kits was 371% of the cost of the kits used by the nonsterile IC group, bringing the total cost of the sterile program to 277% of the other program. Rhame and Perkash[65] found that in 70 SCI patients in the initial rehabilitation hospitalization treated with sterile catheterization and a neomycin–polymyxin irrigant, 54% of patients developed an infection, at an overall rate of 10.3 infections per 1000 patient-days on IC. Bakke and Volset[69] found that factors that may predict the occurrence of clinical UTI in patients using clean IC were low age and high mean catheterization volume in women, low age, neurogenic bladder dysfunction, and nonself-catheterization in men, in addition to urine leakage in patients with neurogenic dysfunction and the presence of bacteriuria. If antibacterial prophylaxis was used, fewer episodes of bacteriuria were noticed, but significantly more clinical UTIs were seen. Shekelle et al reviewed the risk factors for UTI in adults with spinal cord dysfunction[70] and found increased bladder residual volume to be a risk factor. Patients on IC had fewer infections than those with indwelling catheters.

In order to diagnose UTI, it should be recommended that the urine be obtained by catheterization.[71] The frequency of examining urine samples differs greatly between studies: daily use of a dipslide technique during the acute phase after SCI, once a week during the subacute phase, and monthly or a few times a year in long-term care.[72–74]

If a urine culture reveals more than 10^4 cfu/ml, this indicates significant bacteriuria. Pyuria alone is not considered reliable in patients with neurogenic bladder.[75,76] The bacteria found are mostly *Escherichia coli*, *Proteus*, *Citrobacter*, *Pseudomonas*, *Klebsiella*, *Staphylococcus aureus*, and *Streptococcus faecalis* in short-term cases, while the same bacteria plus *Acinetobacter* are found in the long-term IC patients.[77,78] *E. coli* is considered the dominant species.[64] The detection of *E. coli* on the periurethra corresponds, at a much higher percentage, with bacteriuria than if other bacteria are found.[79] *E. coli* isolates from patients who develop symptomatic UTI may be distinguished from bacteria recovered from patients who remain asymptomatic and possibly from normal fecal *E. coli*.[80]

Urinary sepsis is fortunately rare.[81,82] Previous treatment with an indwelling catheter represents a special risk to develop sepsis.[83] In his thesis Wyndaele[34] found the period of 24 hours to 3 days after changing from indwelling to IC drainage when UTI was present to be dangerous for the development of sepsis.

Wyndaele and Maes[84] found several relationships between IC and UTI. If catheterization is begun by patients with recurrent or chronic UTI and urinary retention, the incidence of infection decreases and patients may become totally free of infection. If symptomatic infections occur, improper practice of IC or misuse can often be found. Chronic infection persists after IC has been started, if the cause of the chronicity remains.

To prevent UTI, a noninfecting technique is needed. But also some additional factors can play a role in infection prevention. Nursing education is important and educational intervention by a clinic nurse is a simple, cost-effective means of decreasing the risk of UTIs in individuals with SCI on IC who are identified as at risk.[85] Anderson[67] found a fivefold incidence when IC was performed 3 times a day compared with 6 times a day. Also, prevention of bladder overdistention is important.[57,70] Crossinfection is less if IC during hospitalization is performed by a catheter team or by the patients themselves. As residual urine plays a role in infection, attention must be made to empty the bladder completely.

Treatment of UTI is necessary if the infection is symptomatic. Waites et al[86] treated men with SCI on IC and saw susceptible organisms disappear from urine in all and significantly reduced in the perineum and urethra. However, they were replaced shortly after by resistant Gram-positive cocci. This shows the importance of reserving antibiotics for symptomatic patients only and of taking into account the data from the antibiogram. The value of nontreatment for chronic nonsymptomatic bacteriuria throughout a hospitalization has been demonstrated.[87]

With antibacterial prophylaxis, several studies have shown a lowered infection rate.[88–94] Cranberry juice has been evaluated recently, but results are unclear.[94] Several studies have considered the risk of developing dangerous resistance against antibiotics when prophylaxis is given either orally or by instillation.[95–97] Galloway et al[98] state that the threat of emergence of resistant organisms, the risk to patients of side-effects of the antibiotics, the expense, and the risk to other patients from crossinfection with resistant organisms are strong arguments against prophylactic antibacterials. Therefore, it would seem logical to use antibacterial prophylaxis only for a short time, such as during the initial stage of IC. It does seem to be less indicated for long-term use, although it can help specific patients to lower the rate of symptomatic infections for which no well-defined cause is found.

Urethritis and epididymo-orchitis have been reported in several case series (Table 13.3). With a long-term

Table 13.3 *Literature data on genitourinary complications in patients on intermittent catheterization*

Author	Total no. of patients	Urethritis	Meatal stricture	Epididymitis	Urethral stricture
Bakke[131]	407 (206 m)	1%		1%	
Hellstrom et al[140]	41 (26 m)			3	
Kuhn et al[121]	22 (11 m)		1		1
Labat et al[138]	68 (48 m)	9 m		3	
Lapides et al[133]	100 (34 m)	2 m	–	–	–
Lapides et al[134]	218 (90 m)	2 m	–	2	
Maynard and Diokno[137]	28 (m?)			4 (1 with infected penile prosthesis)	
Maynard and Glass[139]	34 (m?)			3	2
Orikasa et al[135]	26 (13 m)			1	
Perkash and Giroux[142]	50 m			5	
Perrouin-Verbe et al[53]	159 (113 m)			10% short term, 28% long term	5.3%
Thirumavalan and Ransley[141]				12%	
Waller et al[123]	30 SCI (26 m)			2	4
Webb et al[128]				2%	
Wyndaele et al[136]	30 (18 m)	2 m		2	
Wyndaele and Maes[84]	75 (33 m)		3	6	7

m = male, SCI, spinal cord injury.

indwelling catheter, a larger prevalence is seen.[34] Genital infections can lower fertility in SCI patients.[99] If IC is used to empty the neurogenic bladder, better sperm quality and better pregnancy rates have been found than with indwelling catheterization.[100,101]

Prostatitis can be a cause of recurrent UTI: either acute or chronic, it is difficult to diagnose in patients with neurogenic bladder, and special tests have been developed for this.[102,103] The overall incidence was previously thought to be around 5–18%[71] but 33% may be a more realistic figure.[104]

Urethral bleeding is frequently seen in new patients and occurs regularly in one-third on a long-term basis.[105] Trauma of the urethra, especially in men, can cause false passages, meatal stenosis but the incidence is rare (see Table 13.3). The incidence of urethral strictures increases with a longer follow-up, with most events occurring after 5 years of IC.[53,84] Former treatment with an indwelling catheter causes more complications. Urethral changes were also documented in SCI men on IC for an average of 5 years, using one single reusable silicone catheter for an average of 3 years.[106] IC technique and catheter type

are claimed to be important factors.[30,107,108] Urethral trauma with false passages in neurogenic patients on CIC can be treated successfully with 5 days of antibiotics and 6 weeks of indwelling catheter. The false passage will also disappear on cystoscopy and IC can be safely restarted.[109]

Other complications such as hydronephrosis, vesico-ureteral reflux, and bladder cancer seem to relate rather to infection, bladder trabeculation, detrusor pressure, or neuropathy than to IC itself.[110]

Bladder calculi caused by the introduction of pubic hair,[111,112] loss of the catheter in the bladder,[113] bladder perforation, and bladder necrosis[114] have been case reports on rare complications of IC.

And what if IC or ISC is not possible? There can be several reasons for this: bad hand function and no relative to perform the catheterization, unwillingness of the patient, cost, lack of knowledge from carers, persistent incontinence, general bad condition, or difficulty to reach the meatus. In many cases these problems may be overcome with proper treatment. However, in some cases an indwelling catheter will be used.

Transurethral and suprapubic catheters

Transurethral and suprapubic catheters have been used for a long time. The dangers of the techniques have been well documented and the complications are well known. If they are used, it is very important to stick to good rules of management:

- Catheter size 12–14.
- Place the catheter properly with the balloon in the bladder. It is important to be especially careful in the presence of a spastic sphincter.
- Control the outflow regularly to avoid overdistention.
- Change the catheter regularly several times a week in an acute situation, every 10 days if possible, and every 4–6 weeks in a chronic patient who has few complications.
- Anticholinergic drugs may be important in patients with bladder hyperreflexia.
- Antibacterial drugs should not be used to prevent or to treat an asymptomatic infection of the urine. With an indwelling catheter, the prevalence of infection is 100% if the catheter is used for more than a couple of weeks. In the case of symptomatic infection, treatment is necessary.
- There is no general agreement on clamping of the catheter. In cases of severe incontinence unsuccessfully treated with drugs, a continuous outflow is not the only conservative possibility.
- Complications are frequent. The transurethral catheter can cause acute septic episodes, urethral trauma and bleeding, false passages, strictures, diverticuli and fistuli of the urethra, bladder stones, squamous cell bladder carcinoma, epididymo-orchitis, and prostatitis. With application of good treatment rules, many of these conditions can be largely avoided.
- The presence of an indwelling catheter should be known to all who take care of the patient: OT, PT, and of course the nursing staff.

Appliances (condom catheters, penile clamps)

Their use aims at collecting leaking urine into a device, thus preventing urinary spilling and giving better hygienic control, better control of unpleasant odor and a better quality of life. A condom catheter is indicated in all male patients with urinary incontinence provided that there is no skin/penile lesion, and intravesical pressures during storage and voiding phase are urodynamically proven to be safe.

No absolute contraindications for such appliances seem to exist.

Condom catheters are not invasive and permit us to avoid most of the complications related to indwelling catheters. Old versions were reusable external collecting devices that fitted rather loosely around the penis. They are still preferred by a few paralysed patients who have been accustomed to them for a long time, especially those with a retractile penis.

The actual types are thin conical-shaped sheaths made of different sorts of material. They fit over the shaft of the penis, fixed with some type of glue or occlusive strip. The tips are open and connected with the tube of a urinary collecting device. In recent years special condoms and special devices allowing urethral catheterization without removing the condom have been manufactured.

While the advantages of condom catheters over indwelling catheters and incontinence pads are evident, they are not without problems and complications, sometimes severe:

- Fixation to the skin can be difficult with a smaller and/or retractile penis and/or abundant pubic fat. The problem can be partly overcome by using the proper size and proper fixation glue/strip. A penile prosthesis can be a solution in the case of a retractile small penis.
- Obstruction of urine flow is a rather common problem, due to twisting or kinking of the tip of the condom or the collecting tube. To prevent this, most of the currently available condom catheters are reinforced at the tip.
- Lesions of the penis can be secondary to mechanical damage to the skin from an excessively tight condom worn for a prolonged time. One way of prevention is to discontinue the use of the condom during part of the day or night. Another source of skin lesion is allergy to the material of the condom, usually to latex. Such an allergy is not uncommon, i.e. in myelomeningocele patients. The use a latex-free condom is the solution.
- Urinary tract infection.

Newman and Price[115] found bacteriuria in more than 50% of patients using a condom catheter. One of the few factors correlated with increased risk for UTI was less than daily change of the condom.

Penile clamps are not recommended for patients with neuropathic voiding dysfunction, because of the danger of skin and urethral lesions.[18]

References

1. Wyndaele JJ. Les techniques comportementales. In: Corcos J, Schick E, eds. Les vessies neurogènes de l'adulte. Paris: Masson, 1996: 197–202.

2. Hadley EC. Bladder training and related therapies for urinary incontinence in older people. JAMA 1986; 256:372–379.

3. Dowd T, Kolcaba K, Steiner R. Using cognitive strategies to enhance bladder control and comfort. Holist Nurs Pract 2000; 14:91–103.

4. Mahoney DT, Laferte RO, Blais DJ. Integral storage and voiding reflexes; a neurophysiologic concept of continence and micturition. Urology 1980; 9:95–106.

5. Shafik A. Study of the response of the urinary bladder to stimulation of the cervix uteri and clitoris – "The genitovesical Reflex": an experimental study. Int Urogynecol J 1995; 6:41–46.

6. Laycock J. What can the specialist physiotherapist do? In: Wyndaele JJ, Laycock J, eds. Multidisciplinary conservative treatment for the neurogenic bladder. Wokingham: Incare, 2002:14–18.

7. Hoebeke P, De Paepe H, Renson C, et al. Transcutaneous neuromodulation in non-neuropathic bladder sphincter dysfunction in children: preliminary results. Neurourol Urodyn 1999; 18(4):263–264.

8. Walsh IK, Keane PF, Johnston SR, et al. Non-invasive antidromic sacral neurostimulation to enhance bladder storage. Neurourol Urodyn 1999; 18(4):380.

9. Lindstrom S, Fall M, Carlsson C-A, et al. The neurophysiological basis of bladder inhibition in response to intravaginal electrical stimulation. J Urol 1983; 129:405–410.

10. Fossberg E, Sorensen S, Ruutu M, et al. Maximal electrical stimulation in the treatment of unstable detrusor and urge incontinence. Eur Urol 1990; 18:120–123.

11. Eriksen BC, Bergmann S, Eik-Ness SH. Maximal electrostimulation of the pelvic floor in female idiopathic detrusor instability and urge incontinence. Neurourol Urodyn 1989; 8:219–230.

12. Okada N, Igawa A, Ogawa A, Nishizawa O. Transcutaneous electrical stimulation of thigh muscles in the treatment of detrusor overactivity. Br J Urol 1998; 81:560–564.

13. Plevnik S, Homan G, Vrtacnik P. Short-term maximal electrical stimulation for urinary retention. Urol 1984; 24:521–523.

14. Katona F. Stages of vegetative afferentation in reorganization of bladder control during intravesical electrotherapy. Urol Int 1975; 30:192–203.

15. De Wachter S, Wyndaele JJ. Quest for standardization of electrical sensory testing in the lower urinary tract: the influence of technique related factors on bladder electrical thresholds. Neurourol Urodyn 2002; 21:1–6.

16. Wyndaele JJ, Hoekx L, Vermandel A. Bladder biofeedback for the treatment of refractory sensory urgency in adults. Eur Urol 1997; 32:429–432.

17. Andersen JT, Blaivas JG, Cardozo L, Thuroff J. Lower urinary tract rehabilitation techniques: seventh report on the standardisation of terminology of lower urinary tract function. Neurourol Urodyn 11:593–603.

18. Madersbacher H, Wyndaele JJ, Igawa Y, et al. Conservative management in the neuropathic patient. In: Abrams P, Khoury S, Wein A, eds. Incontinence. Health Publication, 1999:775–812.

19. Stover SL, Lloyd LK, Waites KB, Jackson AB. Neurogenic urinary infection. Neurolog Clin 1991; 9:741–755.

20. Lloyd LK, Kuhlemeier KV, Stover SL. Initial bladder management in spinal cord injury: does it make a difference? J Urol 1986; 135:523–526.

21. Rossier A, Bors E. Detrusor response to perineal and rectal stimulation in patients with spinal cord injuries. Urol Int 1964; 10:181–190.

22. Clarke SJ, Thomas DG. Characteristics of the urethral pressure profile in flaccid male paraplegics. Br J Urol 1981; 53:157–161.

23. Low AI, Donovan WD. The use and mechanism of anal sphincter stretch in the reflex bladder. Br J Urol 1981; 53:430–432.

24. Guttmann L, Frankel H. The value of intermittent catheterization in the early management of traumatic paraplegia and tetraplegia. Paraplegia 1966; 4:63–83.

25. Lapides J, Diokno A, Silber S, Lowe B. Clean intermittent self-catheterization in the treatment of urinary tract disease. J Urol 1972; 107:458–461.

26. Maynard FM, Diokno A. Clean intermittent catheterization for spinal cord injured patients. J Urol 1982; 128:477–480.

27. Wu Y, Hamilton BB, Boyink MA, Nanninga JB. Re-usable catheter for longterm intermittent catheterization. Arch Phys Med Rehab 1981; 62:39–42.

28. Bennett CJ, Young MN, Razi SS, et al. The effect of urethral introducer tip catheters on the incidence of urinary tract infection outcomes in spinal cord injured patients. J Urol 1997; 158:519–521.

29. Lundgren J, Bengtsson O, Israelsson A, et al. The importance of osmolality for intermittent catheterization of the urethra. Spinal Cord 2000; 38:45–50.

30. Waller L, Telander M, Sullivan L. The importance of osmolality in hydrophilic urethral catheters a crossover study. Spinal Cord 1998; 36:368–369.

131. Wyndaele JJ, De Ridder D, Everaert K, et al. Evaluation of the use of Urocath-Gel catheters for intermittent self-catheterization by male patients using conventional catheters for a long time. Spinal Cord 2000; 38:97–99.

32. Hedlund H, Hjelmas K, Jonsson O, et al. Hydrophilic versus non-coated catheters for intermittent catheterization. Scand J Urol Nephrol 2001; 35:49–53.

33. Lindan R, Bellomy V. The use of intermittent catheterization in a bladder training program, preliminary report. J Chron Dis 1971; 24:727–735.

34. Wyndaele JJ. Early urological treatment of patients with an acute spinal cord injury. Thesis Doctor in Biomedical Science, State University of Ghent, 1983.

35. Corcos J. Traitements non médicamenteux des vessies neurogènes. In: Corcos J, Schick E, eds. Les vessies neurogènes de l'adulte. Paris: Masson, 1996:173–187.

36. Stribrna J, Fabian F. The problem of residual urine after catheterization. Acta Univ Carol Med 1961; 7:931–943.

37. Jensen AE, Hjeltnes N, Berstad J, Stanghelle JK. Residual urine following intermittent catheterisation in patients with spinal cord injuries. Paraplegia 1995; 33:693–696.

38. Wyndaele JJ, De Taeye N. Early intermittent selfcatheterization after spinal cord injury. Paraplegia 1990; 28:76–80.

39. Champion VL. Clean technique for intermittent self-catheterization. Nurs Res 1976; 25:13–18.

40. Silbar E, Cicmanec J, Burke B, Bracken RB. Microwave sterilization. Method for home sterilization of urinary catheter. J Urol 1980; 141:88–90.

41. Opitz JL. Bladder retraining: an organized program. Mayo Clin Proc 1976; 51:367–372.

42. Anton HA, Chambers K, Clifton J, Tasaka J. Clinical utility of a portable ultrasound device in intermittent catheterization. Arch Phys Med Rehab 1998; 79:172–175.

43. De Ridder D, Van Poppel H, Baert L, Binard J. From time dependent intermittent selfcatheterisation to volume dependent selfcatheterisation in multiple sclerosis using the PCI 5000 Bladdermanager. Spinal Cord 1997; 35:613–616.

44. Schurch B, Stöhrer M, Kramer G, et al. Botulinum-A toxin for treating detrusor hyperreflexia in spinal cord injured patients: a new alternative to anticholinergic drugs? Preliminary results. J Urol 2000; 164:692–697.

45. Mast P, Hoebeke P, Wyndaele JJ, et al. Experience with augmentation cystoplasty. A review. Paraplegia 1995; 33:560–564.

46. Kilinc S, Akman MN, Levendoglu F, Ozker R. Diurnal variation of antidiuretic hormone and urinary output in spinal cord injury. Spinal Cord 1999; 37:332–335.

47. Chancellor MB, Rivas DA, Staas WE Jr. DDAVP in the urological management of the difficult neurogenic bladder in spinal cord injury: preliminary report. J Am Paraplegia Soc 1994; 17:165–167.

48. Wheeler JS Jr, Walter JS, Chintam RS, Rao S. Botulinum toxin injections for voiding dysfunction following SCI. J Spinal Cord Med 1998; 21:227–229.

49. Kiyono Y, Hashizume C, Ohtsuka K, Igawa Y. Improvement of urological-management abilities in individuals with tetraplegia by reconstructive hand surgery. Spinal Cord 2000; 38:541–545.

50. Bakke A, Vollset SE. Risk factors for bacteriuria and clinical urinary tract infection in patients treated with clean intermittent catheterization. J Urol 1993; 149:527–531.

51. Parmar S, Baltej S, Vaidyanathan S. Teaching the procedure of clean intermittent catheterization. Paraplegia 1993; 31:298–302.

52. Sutton G, Shah S, Hill V. Clean intermittent self-catheterization for quadriplegic patients – a five year follow up. Paraplegia 1991; 29:542–549.

53. Perrouin-Verbe B, Labat JJ, Richard I, et al. Clean intermittent catheterization from the acute period in spinal cord injury patients. Longterm evaluation of urethral and genital tolerance. Paraplegia 1995; 33:619–624.

54. Bakke A, Malt UF. Psychological predictors of symptoms of urinary tract infection and bacteriuria in patients treated with clean intermittent catheterization: a prospective 7 year study. Eur Urol 1998; 34:30–36.

55. Yavuzer G, Gok H, Tuncer S, et al. Compliance with bladder management in spinal cord injury patients. Spinal Cord 2000; 38:762–765.

56. Pearman JW. Prevention of urinary tract infection following spinal cord injury. Paraplegia 1971; 9:95–104.

57. Lapides J, Diokno AC, Lowe BS, Kalish MD. Follow-up on unsterile intermittent self-catheterization. J Urol 1974; 111:184–187.

58. Donovan W, Stolov W, Clowers D, Clowers M. Bacteriuria during intermittent catheterization following spinal cord injury. Arch Phys Med Rehab 1978; 59:351–357.

59. Maynard F, Diokno A. Urinary infection and complications during clean intermittent catheterization following spinal cord injury. J Urol 1984; 132:943–946.

60. Murray K, Lewis P, Blannin J, Shepherd A. Clean intermittent self-catheterization in the management of adult lower urinary tract dysfunction. Br J Urol 1984; 56:379–380.

61. Wyndaele JJ. Clean intermittent self-catheterization in the prevention of lower urinary tract infections. In: Van Kerrebroeck PH, Debruyne F, eds. Dysfunction of the lower urinary tract: present achievements and future perspectives. Bussum: Medicom, 1990:187–195.

62. Sutton G, Shah S, Hill V. Clean intermittent self-catheterization for quadriplegic patients – a five year follow up. Paraplegia 1991; 29:542–549.

63. Whitelaw S, Hamonds J, Tregallas R. Clean intermittent self-catheterization in the elderly. Br J Urol 1987; 60:125–127.

64. Bakke A. Clean intermittent catheterization – physical and psychological complications. Scand J Urol Nephrol Suppl 1993; 150:1–69.

65. Rhame FS, Perkash I. Urinary tract infections occurring in recent spinal cord injury patients on intermittent catheterization. J Urol 1979; 122:669–673.

66. Ott R, Rosier AB. The importance of intermittent catheterization in bladder re-education of acute spinal cord lesions. In: Proc Eighteenth Vet Admin Spinal Cord Injury Conf 1971; 18:139–148.

67. Anderson RU. Prophylaxis of bacteriuria during intermittent catheterization of the acute neurogenic bladder. J Urol 1980; 123:364–366.

68. Prieto-Fingerhut T, Banovac K, Lynne CM. A study comparing sterile and nonsterile urethral catheterization in patients with spinal cord injury. Rehab Nurs 1997; 22:299–302.

69. Bakke A, Vollset SE. Risk factors for bacteriuria and clinical urinary tract infection in patients treated with clean intermittent catheterization. J Urol 1993; 149:527–531.

70. Shekelle PG, Morton SC, Clark KA, et al. Systematic review of risk factors for urinary tract infection in adults, with spinal cord dysfunction. J Spinal Cord Med 1999; 22:258–272.

71. Barnes D, Timoney A, Moulas G, et al. Correlation of bacteriological flora of the urethra, glans and perineum with organisms causing urinary tract infection in the spinal injuries male patient. Paraplegia 1992; 30:851–854.

72. King RB, Carlson CE, Mervine J, et al. Clean and sterile intermittent catheterization methods in hospitalized patients with spinal cord injury. Arch Phys Med Rehab 1992; 73(9):798–802.

73. Darouiche R, Cadle R, Zenon G 3rd, et al. Progression from asymptomatic to symptomatic urinary tract infection in patients with SCI: a preliminary study. J Am Parapleg Soc 1993; 16:219–224.

74. National Institute on Disability and Rehabilitation Research Consensus Statement Jan 27–29, 1992. The prevention and management of urinary tract infections among people with spinal cord injuries. J Am Parapleg Soc 1992; 15:194–204.

75. Gribble MJ, Puterman ML, McCallum NM. Pyuria: its relationship to bacteriuria in spinal cord injured patients on intermittent catheterization. Arch Phys Med Rehab 1989; 70:376–379.

76. Menon EB, Tan ES. Pyuria: index of infection in patients with spinal cord injuries. Br J Urol 1992; 69:141–146.

77. Noll F, Russe O, Kling E, Botel U, Schreiter F. Intermittent catheterisation versus percutaneous suprapubic cystostomy in the early management of traumatic spinal cord lesions. Paraplegia 1988; 26:4–9.

78. Yadav A, Vaidyanathan S, Panigraphi D. Clean intermittent catheterization for the neuropathic bladder. Paraplegia 1993; 31:380.

79. Schlager TA, Hendley JO, Wilson RA, et al. Correlation of periurethral bacterial flora with bacteriuria and urinary tract infection in children with neurogenic bladder receiving intermittent catheterization. Clin Infect Dis 1999; 28:346–350.

80. Hull RA, Rudy DC, Wieser IE, Donovan WH. Virulence factors of *Escherichia coli* isolates from patients with symptomatic and asymptomatic bacteriuria and neuropathic bladders due to spinal cord and brain injuries. J Clin Microbiol 1998; 36:115–117.

81. McGuire EJ, Diddel G, Wagner F Jr. Balanced bladder function in spinal cord injury patients. J Urol 1977; 118:626–628.

82. Sperling KB. Intermittent catheterization to obtain catheter-free bladder in spinal cord injury. Arch Phys Med Rehab 1978; 59:4–8.

83. Barkin M, Dolfin D, Herschorn S, et al. The urological care of the spinal cord injury patient. J Urol 1983; 129:335–339.

84. Wyndaele JJ, Maes D. Clean intermittent self-catheterization: a 12 year follow up. J Urol 1990; 143:906–908.

85. Barber DB, Woodard FL, Rogers SJ, Able AC. The efficacy of nursing education as an intervention in the treatment of recurrent urinary tract infections in individuals with spinal cord injury. SCI Nurs 1999; 16:54–56.

86. Waites KB, Canupp KC, Brookings ES, DeVivo MJ. Effect of oral ciprofloxacin on bacterial flora of perineum, urethra, and lower urinary tract in men with spinal cord injury. J Spinal Cord Med 1999; 22:192–198.

87. Lewis RI, Carrion HM, Lockhart JL, Politano VA. Significance of symptomatic bacteriuria in neurogenic bladder disease. Urology 1984; 23:343–347.

88. Pearman JW. The value of kanamycin-colistin bladder instillations in reducing bacteriuria during intermittent catheterization of patients with acute spinal cord injury. Br J Urol 1979; 51:367–374.

89. Haldorson AM, Keys TF, Maker MD, Opitz JL. Nonvalue of neomycin instillation after intermittent urinary catheterization. Antimicrob Agents Chemother 1978; 14:368–370.

90. Murphy FJ, Zelman S, Mau W. Ascorbic acid as urinary acidifying agent. II: Its adjunctive role in chronic urinary infection. J Urol 1965; 94:300–303.

91. Stover SL, Fleming WC. Recurrent bacteriuria in complete spinal cord injury patients on external condom drainage. Arch Phys Med Rehab 1980; 61:178–181.

92. Johnson HW, Anderson JD, Chambers GK, Arnold WJ, Irwin BJ, Brinton JR. A short-term study of nitrofurantoin prophylaxis in children managed with clean intermittent catheterization. Pediatrics 1994; 93:752–755.

93. Kevorkian CG, Merritt JL, Ilstrup DM. Methenamine mandelate with acidification: an effective urinary antiseptic in patients with neurogenic bladder. Mayo Clin Proc 1984; 59:523–529.

94. Jepson RG, Mihaljevic L, Craig J. Cranberries for preventing urinary tract infections. Cochrane Database Syst Rev 2000; (2):CD001321.

95. Dollfus P, Molé P. The treatment of the paralysed bladder after spinal cord injury in the accident unit of Colmar. Paraplegia 1969; 7:204–205.

96. Vivian JM, Bors E. Experience with intermittent catheterization in the southwest regional system for treatment of spinal injury. Paraplegia 1974; 12:158–166.

97. Pearman JW, Bailey M, Riley LP. Bladder instillations of trisdine compared with catheter introducer for reduction of bacteriuria during intermittent catheterization of patients with acute spinal cord trauma. Br J Urol 1991; 67:483–490.

98. Galloway A, Green HT, Windsor JJ, et al. Serial concentrations of C-reactive protein as an indicator of urinary tract infection in patients with spinal injury. J Clin Pathol 1986; 39:851–855.

99. Allas T, Colleu D, Le Lannon D. Fonction génitale chez l'homme paraplégique. Aspects immunologiques. Presse Med 1986; 29:2119.

100. Ohl DA, Denil J, Fitzgerald-Shelton K, et al. Fertility of spinal cord injured males: effect of genitourinary infection and bladder management on results of electroejaculation. J Am Parapleg Soc 1992; 15:53–59.

101. Rutkowski SB, Middleton JW, Truman G, et al. The influence of bladder management on fertility in spinal cord injured males. Paraplegia 1995; 33:263–266.

102. Kuhlemeier KV, Lloyd LK, Stover SL. Localization of upper and lower urinary tract infections in patients with neurogenic bladders. SCI Dig 1982:336–342.

103. Wyndaele JJ. Chronic prostatitis in spinal cord injury patients. Paraplegia 1985; 23:164–169.

104. Cukier J, Maury M, Vacant J, Mlle Lucet. L'infection de l'appareil urinaire chez le paraplégique adulte. Nouv Presse Med 1976; 24:1531–1532.

105. Webb R, Lawson A, Neal D. Clean intermittent self-catheterization in 172 adults. Br J Urol 1990; 65:20–23.

106. Kovindha A, Na W, Madersbacher H. Radiological abnormalities in spinal cord injured men using clean intermittent catheterization with a re-usable silicone catheter in developing country. Poster 86 presented during the Annual Scientific Meeting of IMSOP, Sydney, 2000:112 [Abstract].

107. Mandal AK, Vaidaynathan S. Management of urethral stricture in patients practising clean intermittent catheterization. Int Urol Nephrol 1993; 25:395–399.

108. Vaidyanathan S, Soni BM, Dundas S, Krishnan KR. Urethral cytology in spinal cord injury patient performing intermittent catheterisation. Paraplegia 1994; 32:493–500.

109. Michielsen D, Wyndaele JJ. Management of false passages in patients practising clean intermittent self catheterisation. Spinal Cord 1999; 37:201–203.

110. Damanski M. Vesico-ureteric reflux in paraplegics. Br J Surg 1965; 52:168–177.

111. Solomon MH, Foff SA, Diokno AC. Bladder calculi complicating intermittent catheterization. J Urol 1980; 124:140–141.

112. Amendola MA, Sonda LP, Diokno AC, Vidyasagar M. Bladder calculi complicating intermittent clean catheterization. Am J Roentgenol 1983; 141:751–753.

113. Morgan JDT, Weston PMT. The disappearing catheter – a complication of intermittent self-catheterization. Br J Urol 1990; 65:113–114.

114. Reisman EM, Preminger GM. Bladder perforation secondary to clean intermittent catheterization. J Urol 1989; 142:1316–1317.

115. Newman E, Price M. External catheters: hazards and benefits of their use by men with spinal cord lesions. Arch Phys Med Rehab 1985; 66:310–313.

116. Madersbacher H, Weissteiner G. Intermittent self-catheterization, an alternative in the treatment of neurogenic urinary incontinence in women. Eur Urol 1977; 3:82–84.

117. Wyndaele JJ, Oosterlinck W, De Sy W. Clean intermittent self-catheterization in the chronical management of the neurogenic bladder. Eur Urol 1980; 6:107–110.

118. Iwatsubo E, Komine S, Yamashita H, et al. Over-distension therapy of the bladder in paraplegic patients using self-catheterisation: a preliminary study. Paraplegia 1984; 22:201–215.

119. McGuire EJ, Savastano J. Comparative urological outcome in women with spinal cord injury. J Urol 1986; 135:730–731.

120. Kornhuber HH, Schutz A. Efficient treatment of neurogenic bladder disorders in multiple sclerosis with initial intermittent catheterization and ultrasound-controlled training. Eur Neurol 1990; 30:260–267.

121. Kuhn W, Rist M, Zach GA. Intermittent urethral self-catheterisation: long term results (bacteriological evolution, continence, acceptance, complications). Paraplegia 1991; 29:222–232.

122. Lindehall B, Moller A, Hjalmas K, Jodal U. Long-term intermittent catheterization: the experience of teenagers and young adults with myelomeningcele. J Urol 1994; 152:187–189.

123. Waller L, Jonsson O, Norlén L, Sullivan L. Clean intermittent catheterization in spinal cord injury patients: long-term followup of a hydrophilic low friction technique. J Urol 1995; 153:345–348.

124. Vaidyanathan S, Soni BM, Brown E, et al. Effect of intermittent urethral catheterization and oxybutynen bladder instillation on urinary continence status and quality of life in a selected group of spinal cord injury patients with neuropathic bladder dysfunction. Spinal Cord 1998; 36:409–414.

125. Diokno AC, Sonda LP, Hollander JB, Lapides J. Fate of patients started on clean intermittent self-catheterization 10 years ago. J Urol 1983; 129:1120–1122.

126. Maynard FM, Glass J. Management of the neuropathic bladder by clean intermittent catheterization: 5 year outcomes. Paraplegia 1987; 25:106–110.

127. Whitelaw S, Hamonds J, Tregallas R. Clean intermittent self-catheterization in the elderly. Br J Urol 1987; 60:125–127.

128. Webb R, Lawson A, Neal D. Clean intermittent self-catheterization in 172 adults. Br J Urol 1990; 65:20–23.

129. Timoney AG, Shaw PJ. Urological outcome in female patients with spinal cord injury: the effectiveness of intermittent catheterization. Paraplegia 1990; 28:556–563.

130. Sutton G, Shah S, Hill V. Clean intermittent self-catheterization for quadriplegic patients – a five year follow up. Paraplegia 1991; 29:542–549.

131. Bakke A. Clean intermittent catheterization – physical and psychological complications. Scand J Urol Nephrol suppl 1993; 150:1–69.

132. Hunt GM, Oakeshott P, Whitacker RH. Intermittent catheterization: simple, safe and effective but underused. BMJ 1996; 312:103–107. [References]

133. Lapides J, Diokno AC, Lowe BS, Kalish MD. Follow-up on unsterile intermittent self-catheterization. J Urol 1974; 111:184–187.

134. Lapides J, Diokno AC, Gould FR, Lowe BS. Further observations on self-catheterization. J Urol 1976; 116:169–172.

135. Orikasa S, Koyanagi T, Motomura M, et al. Experience with non-sterile intermittent selfcatheterization. J Urol 1976; 115:141–142.

136. Wyndaele JJ, Oosterlinck W, De Sy W. Clean intermittent self-catheterization in the chronical management of the neurogenic bladder. Eur Urol 1980; 6:107–110.

137. Maynard FM, Diokno A. Clean intermittent catheterization for spinal cord injured patients. J Urol 1982; 128:477–480.

138. Labat JJ, Perrouin-Verbe B, Lanoiselée JM, et al. L'autosondage intermittent propre dans la rééducation des blesses medullaires et de la queue de cheval II. Ann Réadapt Méd Phys 1985; 28:125–136.

139. Maynard FM, Glass J. Management of the neuropathic bladder by clean intermittent catheterization: 5 year outcomes. Paraplegia 1987; 25:106–110.

140. Hellstrom P, Tammela T, Lukkarinen O, Kontturi M. Efficacy and safety of clean intermittent catheterization in adults. Eur Urol 1991; 20:117–121.

141. Thirumavalan VS, Ransley PG. Epididymitis in children and adolescents on clean intermittent catheterization. Eur Urol 1992; 22:53–56.

142. Perkash I, Giroux J. Clean intermittent catheterization in spinal cord injury patients: a followup study. J Urol 1993; 149:1068–1071.

14

Systemic and intrathecal pharmacological treatment

Shing-Hwa Lu and Michael B Chancellor

Introduction

The principal causes of urinary incontinence in patients with neurogenic bladder are detrusor hyperreflexia (DH) and/or incompetence of urethral closing function. Thus, to improve urinary incontinence the treatment should aim at decreasing detrusor activity, increasing bladder capacity, and/or increasing bladder outlet resistance. Pharmacological therapy has been particularly helpful in patients with relatively mild degrees of neurogenic bladder dysfunction. Patients with more profound neurogenic bladder disturbances may require pharmacological treatment to augment other forms of management such as intermittent catheterization. The two most commonly used classes of agents are anticholinergics and α-adrenergic blockers (Table 14.1). Intravesical pharmacological therapy is discussed in Chapter 15.

Table 14.1 *Systemic drugs for incontinence due to detrusor hyperreflexia and/or low compliant detrusor*

Bladder relaxant drugs:
  Propantheline
  Oxybutynin
  Tolterodine
  Propiverine
  Trospium
  Flavoxate
  Tricyclic antidepressants

Drugs for incontinence due to neurogenic sphincter deficiency:
  Alpha-adrenergic agonists
  Estrogens
  Tricyclic antidepressants

Drugs for facilitating bladder emptying:
  Alpha-adrenergic blockers
  Cholinergics

Drugs for incontinence due to detrusor hyperreflexia and/or low-compliant detrusor

Bladder relaxant drugs

Anticholinergic agents are the commonly used pharmacological agents in the management of neurogenic bladder. Anticholinergic agents are employed to suppress DH. Although there is an abundance of drugs available for the treatment of DH, for many of them, efficacy is estimated based on preliminary open studies rather than on controlled clinical trials.[1] However, drug effects in individual patients may be practically important. In developing countries, most of the bladder relaxant drugs listed below are not available, mainly due to economical reasons, which makes the pharmacological treatment of DH in these countries difficult.

General indications of pharmacological treatment in DH are:

1. to improve or eliminate reflex incontinence
2. to eliminate or prevent a high intravesical pressure situation
3. to enhance the efficacy of intermittent catheterization (IC), triggered voiding, and indwelling catheters.

Spinal DH is mostly associated with a functional outflow obstruction due to detrusor-sphincter dyssynergia (DSD). For the most part, pharmacotherapy is used to suppress reflex detrusor activity completely and facilitate IC. Bladder relaxant drugs decrease detrusor contractility also during voiding. With this situation, residual urine increases and must then be assisted or accomplished by IC.

Propantheline

Propantheline bromide was the classically described oral antimuscarinic drug. Despite its success in uncontrolled case series, no adequate controlled study of this drug for DH is available.[1,2] The usual adult oral dosage is 7.5–30 mg three to four times daily, although higher doses are often necessary.[3]

Oxybutynin

Oxybutynin hydrochloride is a moderately potent antimuscarinic agent with a pronounced muscle relaxant activity and local anesthetic activity as well.[1,3–5]

Several double-blind controlled studies have shown its efficacy for DH.[6–11] The overall rate of good results (more than 50% symptomatic improvement) was 61–86% with 5 mg three times per day. Side-effects were noted in all studies and severity increased with dosage. The overall incidence of possible side-effects was 12.5–68%. Most of them are related to antimuscarinic action, with dry mouth as the most common complaint.

A once-a-day controlled-release formulation of oxybutynin, oxybutynin XL (Ditropan XL®), was recently developed. Parallel-group, randomized, controlled clinical trials comparing the efficacy and safety of controlled-release oxybutynin, oxybutynin XL, with conventional, immediate-release oxybutynin in patients with overactive bladder demonstrated that the urge urinary incontinence episodes declined log-linearly, and no significant difference was observed between the two formulations.[12–14] However, there was a trend toward higher efficacy with oxybutynin XL than with immediate-release oxybutynin at the same dose in one study. Dose–dry mouth analysis showed that the probability of dry mouth with an increasing dose was significantly lower with oxybutynin XL than with immediate-release oxybutynin.[15]

Recent experience with oxybutynin in neurogenic bladder patients

O'Leary et al evaluated the effects and tolerability of extended-release oxybutynin chloride on the voiding and catheterization frequency of a population of multiple sclerosis (MS) patients with neurogenic bladder.[16] This was a 12-week prospective dose titration study of extended-release oxybutynin (oxybutynin XL). Multiple sclerosis patients were recruited for this study from the MS clinic within the university. Entry criteria included a post-void residual (PVR) of <200 ml (in the noncatheterized subjects). Exclusions included those with urine results indicating pyuria in the presence of a positive urine culture. These tests were repeated at 6 and 12 weeks. After a 7-day washout period, patients recorded episodes of voiding or catheterization and incontinence for three consecutive days. Patients received initial doses of 10 mg oxybutynin XL in the first week. Doses were escalated to weekly or biweekly intervals to a maximum of 30 mg/day. Tolerability information was collected at each follow-up visit.

Twenty patients completed the study: the mean age was 46.3 years (range 24–61), and 75% of the patients were women. Subjects reported clinical improvement with decreased urinary frequency and incontinence episodes after dosing was escalated to 30 mg. Seventeen patients chose a final effective dose greater than 10 mg, with 13 patients taking at least 20 mg/day at the end of the study. There were no serious adverse events during the course of the study.

The authors concluded that controlled-release oxybutynin is safe and effective in MS patients with neurogenic bladder. The onset of clinical efficacy occurs within 1 week and daily doses up to 30 mg may be indicated and are well tolerated.

In a similar study, but performed in spinal cord injured (SCI) patients, O'Leary et al evaluated the urodynamic changes with extended-release oxybutynin chloride in SCI patients with defined DH.[17]

This was a 12-week prospective dose titration study of extended-release oxybutynin (oxybutynin XL). SCI subjects with urodynamically defined DH were recruited for this study. After a 7-day washout period, patients were evaluated by videourodynamic study and then treatment at a dose of 10 mg was initiated. Doses were increased in weekly intervals to a maximum of 30 mg/day. Micturition frequency diaries and urodynamics were completed at baseline and repeated at week 12. Tolerability information was collected at each follow-up visit.

Ten patients (mean age 49 years) with complete or incomplete SCI were enrolled. Subjects reported clinical improvement, with decreased urinary frequency and incontinence episodes after dosing was escalated to 30 mg. All patients chose a final effective dose greater than 10 mg with 4 patients taking 30 mg/day. Mean cystometric bladder capacity increased 274 ml to 380 ml ($p = 0.008$). No patient had serious adverse events during the course of the 12-week study.

The authors concluded that oxybutynin XL is safe and effective in SCI patients with detrusor hyperreflexia. The onset of clinical efficacy occurs within 1 week and daily doses up to 30 mg, if indicated, are well tolerated.

Tolterodine

Tolterodine is a new competitive muscarinic receptor antagonist.[18,19] Recently, several randomized, and double-blind controlled studies in patients with overactive bladder have demonstrated its beneficial effect.[20–28] Jonas et al reported on a randomized, double-blind, placebo-controlled study of tolterodine including urodynamic analysis in a total of 242 patients:[20] 2 mg twice daily was significantly more effective than placebo in increasing maximum cystometric bladder capacity and volume at first contraction after 4 weeks' treatment. However, there are no published reports on the specific effect on DH.

The better tolerability profile of tolterodine compared with oxybutynin has been confirmed in another randomized study on detrusor overactivity.[23] Tolterodine (2 mg twice daily) appears to be as effective as oxybutynin (5 mg three times daily), but is much better tolerated, especially in regards to dry mouth. In a meta-analysis of a four-multicenter prospective trial of 1120 patients, moderate to severe dry mouth was reported in 6% of patients receiving the placebo, 4% of patients receiving 1 mg twice daily tolterodine, 17% of patients receiving 2 mg twice daily tolterodine, and 60% of those patients receiving conventional 5 mg three times daily oxybutynin.[21] The other randomized controlled trial of tolterodine by Malone-Lee et al demonstrated superior tolerability than and comparable efficacy to oxybutynin in individuals 50 years old or older with overactive bladder.[26]

Van Kerrebroeck et al reported a comparative study of the efficacy and safety of tolterodine extended release (ER; 4 mg once daily), tolterodine immediate release (IR; 2 mg twice daily), as well as placebo in 1529 adult patients with overactive bladder.[27] The primary efficacy variable was the change in mean number of incontinence episodes per week, which decreased 53% from baseline in the tolterodine ER group, 45% with tolterodine IR, and 28% in the placebo group. Tolterodine ER and IR provided a similar significant reduction in incontinence episodes vs placebo. Post-hoc analysis of the data using median values, based on rational of skewed data distribution, demonstrated improved efficacy of tolterodine ER vs IR. Dry mouth was significantly lower with tolterodine ER than tolterodine IR (23% tolterodine ER, 31% tolterodine IR, and 8% placebo). The incidence of other side-effects was similar to placebo in the tolterodine ER and tolterodine IR groups.

A comparative study between controlled-release oxybutynin (oxybutynin XL) and immediate-release tolterodine (tolterodine IR) was recently published:[28] 378 patients were randomized to receive either oxybutynin XL 10 mg ($n = 185$) or tolterodine IR 4 mg (2 mg twice daily) ($n = 193$). The populations were evenly matched with respect to demographics. Oxybutynin XL reduced the number of weekly episodes of urge incontinence from 25.6 to 6.1 instances. Tolterodine IR decreased the number of weekly episodes from 24.1 to 7.8 instances. Oxybutynin XL demonstrated better efficacy ($p = 0.03$) compared with tolterodine IR. Dry mouth and central nervous system side-effects were similar between oxybutynin XL and tolterodine IR.

Although tolterodine has a documented effect on overactive bladder, further studies on the effect of the drug on DH in the neuropathic population are necessary. Comparative studies of tolterodine ER with propiverine, trospium, or oxybutynin XL, especially with regard to tolerability, could be useful to evaluate its position among other bladder relaxant drugs besides conventional oxybutynin or tolterodine.

Propiverine

Propiverine hydrochloride is a benzylic acid derivative with musculotropic (calcium antagonistic) activity and moderate antimuscarinic effects.[29] Several randomized double-blind, controlled clinical studies of this drug in patients with DH have been reported.[30–32] In a placebo-controlled, double-blind, randomized, prospective, multicenter trial, Stöhrer et al evaluated the efficacy and tolerability of propiverine (15 mg three times daily for 14 days) as compared to placebo in 113 patients suffering from DH caused by spinal cord injury.[30] The majority of patients practiced IC for bladder emptying. The maximum cystometric bladder capacity increased significantly in the propiverine group, on average by 104 ml. Sixty-three percent of the patients expressed a subjective improvement of their symptoms under propiverine in comparison to only 23% of the placebo group.

Takayasu et al conducted a double-blind, placebo-controlled multicenter study in 70 neurogenic patients.[31] During a treatment period of 14 days, 20 mg propiverine once daily or placebo were administered. An increase of maximum bladder capacity, a decrease of maximum detrusor pressure, and an increase of residual urine were also obtained in this Japanese study, all of which were statistically significant compared with placebo. Madersbacher et al, in a placebo-controlled, multicenter study, demonstrated that propiverine is a safe and effective drug in the treatment of DH; it is as effective as oxybutynin, but the incidence of dry mouth and its severity is less with propiverine (15 mg, three times daily) than with oxybutynin (5 mg twice daily).[32]

Trospium

Trospium is a quaternary ammonium derivative with mainly antimuscarinic actions. In a placebo-controlled, double-blind study in 61 patients with spinal DH, significant improvements in maximum cystometric capacity and maximum detrusor pressure were demonstrated with 20 mg of trospium twice daily for 3 weeks compared with placebo.[33] Few side-effects were noted, compared with placebo. Madersbacher et al compared the clinical efficacy and tolerance of trospium (20 mg twice daily) and oxybutynin (5 mg three times daily) in a randomized, double-blind, urodynamically controlled, multicenter trial in 95 patients with spinal cord injuries and DH.[34] They found that the two drugs are equal in their effects on DH (increase of the cystometric bladder capacity by 30% and decrease of the maximum detrusor pressure by 30%), but trospium has fewer severe side-effects (incidence of severe dry mouth 5% with trospium vs 25% with oxybutynin).[34]

Flavoxate

Flavoxate hydrochloride has a direct inhibitory action on detrusor smooth muscle *in vitro*. Early clinical trials with flavoxate have shown favorable effects in patients with DH.[35,36] Several randomized controlled studies have shown that the drug has essentially no effects on detrusor overactivity.[10,37,38]

Tricyclic antidepressants

Many clinicians have found tricyclic antidepressants, particularly imipramine hydrochloride, to be useful agents for facilitating urine storage, both by decreasing bladder contractility and by increasing outlet resistance.[3,39] However, no sufficiently controlled trials of tricyclic antidepressants in terms of DH in neuropathics have been reported. Nevertheless, in some developing countries tricyclic antidepressants are the only bladder relaxant substances that people can afford. The down side with tricyclic antidepressants is the narrow safety profile and side-effects. The potential hazard of serious cardiovascular toxic effect should be taken into consideration.[1] Combination therapy using antimuscarinics and imipramine may have synergistic benefits [*Level 5*].

Drugs for incontinence due to neurogenic sphincter deficiency

Several drugs, including alpha-adrenergic agonists,[40–45] estrogens,[46] beta-adrenergic agonists,[47] and tricyclic antidepressants,[48] have been used to increase outlet resistance [*Level 4*]. No adequately designed controlled studies of any of these drugs for treating neuropathic sphincter deficiency have been published. In certain selected cases of mild to moderate stress incontinence, a beneficial effect may be obtained [*Grade D*].[1]

Drugs for facilitating bladder emptying
Alpha-adrenergic blockers

Alpha adrenoceptors have been reported to be predominantly present in the bladder base, posterior urethra, and prostate. Alpha-blockers have been reported to be useful in neurogenic bladder by decreasing urethral resistance during voiding. Recently, a multicenter placebo-controlled, double-blind trials of urapidil – an alpha-blocker on neurogenic bladder dysfunction – by means of a pressure–flow study, demonstrated significant improvement of straining and of the sum of urinary symptom scores, which was associated with significant improvement of urodynamic parameters (decreases in the pressure at maximum flow rate and the minimum urethral resistance) over the placebo [*Level 1*].[49,50]

Alpha-adrenergic blockade also helps to prevent excess sweating secondary to spinal cord autonomic dysreflexia. Sweat glands, primarily responsible for thermoregulatory factors, are innervated by postganglionic cholinergic neurons of the sympathetic system. Alpha-receptor blockade inhibits this postsynaptic neuronal uptake of norepinephrine (noradrenaline) and reduces neurologic sweating.[51]

Cholinergics

In general, bethanechol chloride seems to be of limited benefit for detrusor areflexia and for elevated residual urine volume. Elevated residual volume is often due to sphincter dyssynergia. It would be inappropriate to potentially increase detrusor pressure when there is concurrent DSD.[52]

Therapy for sphincter dyssynergia

In patients with sufficient manual dexterity, the most reasonable treatment option is to abolish the involuntary detrusor contractions (to insure continence) and then to institute intermittent self-catheterization (in order to empty the bladder).[53,54] Treatment options include catheterization (either intermittent or continuous) external sphincterotomy, pharmacological therapy, urinary diversion, biofeedback, functional electrical stimulation, and several new minimally invasive alternatives to external sphincterotomy (Table 14.2).

Unfortunately, there is no class of pharmacological agents that will selectively relax the striated musculature of the pelvic floor. Several different drugs have been used to treat detrusor-external sphincter dyssynergia (DESD), including

Table 14.2 *Therapy of detrusor-external sphincter dyssynergia*

Conventional surgery:
  External sphincterotomy

Pharmacological:
  Baclofen (oral or intrathecal)
  Dantrolene
  Benzodiazepine
  Possibly alpha-adrenergic blockade
  Possibly clonidine

Minimally invasive techniques:
  Sphincter stent
  Balloon sphincter dilatation
  Laser sphincterotomy
  Botulinum toxin injection

Circumventing the problem:
  Intermittent catheterization
  Indwelling catheterization (urethral or suprapubic)
  Urinary diversion

the benzodiazepines, dantrolene, baclofen, and alpha-adrenergic blocking agents.[55–58] Baclofen and diazepam exert their actions predominantly within the central nervous system, whereas dantrolene acts directly on skeletal muscle. Although these drugs are capable of providing variable relief of muscle spasticity, their efficacy is far from complete, and troublesome muscle weakness, adverse effects on gait, and a variety of other side-effects minimize their overall usefulness.[55]

Alpha-adrenergic antagonists have been extensively used for DESD. The rationale for their use is their proven efficacy on internal urinary sphincter (bladder neck and prostate) smooth muscle obstruction. Unfortunately, there is no good clinical study to support the use of alpha blockade for DESD.

In addition, there is a report of preliminary success using oral clonidine in 4 of 5 patients with DESD.[59] Continuous intrathecal baclofen infusion has been shown to be effective in diminishing DESD in up to 40% of patients with DESD.[60]

Alpha-adrenergic blockade

Although most researchers would agree that alpha blockers exert their favorable effects on voiding dysfunction primarily by affecting the smooth muscle of the bladder neck and proximal urethra, there are suggestions that they may affect striated sphincter tone as well.[61] Other data suggest that they may exert some effects on the symptoms of voiding dysfunction by decreasing bladder contractility. Alpha antagonists have been shown to be clinically effective in relieving internal sphincter obstruction by their effect on

the bladder neck and prostate.[62,63] Whether the striated external urinary sphincter receives sympathetic innervation remains controversial. Most of the research has been carried out only in laboratory animals, where both the presence and absence of alpha receptors have been reported at the external sphincter level.[64–66] Clinical correlation of the effects of alpha antagonists on the striated external urinary sphincter during micturition is lacking. Most clinical studies have based their conclusions on effects on the passive urethral pressure profile (UPP).[67,68]

The SCI male, with both neurogenic vesical dysfunction and DESD, offers an ideal opportunity to study the interrelationship between the function of the bladder and both the internal and external urinary sphincters.[69] The effect of alpha-adrenergic innervation and its clinical significance on the two sphincters is more readily apparent in such patients.

Mobley treated 37 patients with neurogenic bladder with phenoxybenzamine and noted 78% success.[70] Unfortunately, no objective data – including urodynamic parameters, length of follow-up, or indications of improvement – were specified. Whitfield et al found a significant decrease in the UPP with alpha blockade in 25 patients with neurogenic vesical dysfunction.[71] However, actual voiding pressure was not reported.

Using intravenous phentolamine, Awad et al noted a significant decrease in pressure along the entire length of the urethra in both sexes, including the peak pressure zone.[72] Olsson et al proposed that a constant state of sympathetic tonus to the internal sphincter exists, and that inhibition of this tonus during micturition results in bladder neck opening.[73]

Research providing evidence against a clinically significant effect of a sympathetic antagonist on the external sphincter includes a report by McGuire et al.[74] They reported on 9 patients with neurogenic bladders and severe autonomic dysreflexia who demonstrated dramatic improvement with phenoxybenzamine. The urethral resistance was unassociated with spasticity of the striated muscle and was abolished by administration of phenoxybenzamine. This documents abnormal urethral smooth muscle activity in SCI patients but fails to demonstrate a sympathetic effect on the external sphincter musculature.

Rossier et al used a pudendal block plus phentolamine to study the effect on the external sphincter.[75] The authors concluded that there was no significant sympathetic innervations of striated muscle in humans. Pudendal nerve blocks have demonstrated sphincter dyssynergia to be mediated through the pudendal nerves via spinal reflex arcs. Phentolamine affects on bladder activity suggest that blockade of alpha-adrenergic receptors inhibits primarily the transmission in vesical and/or pelvic parasympathetic ganglia, and acts only secondarily through direct depression of the vesical smooth muscle. Their neuropharmacological results raise strong doubts as to the existence

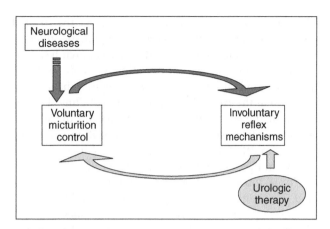

Figure 14.1
Involuntary reflex micturitional mechanisms were developed in the patients with neurological disorders. The aim of urologic therapy including neuropharmacological therapy is to convert the involuntary reflex micturition into more natural voluntary micturition control such as improving detrusor hyperreflexia (DH), and/or disorders of urethral closing function by decreasing detrusor activity, increasing bladder capacity, and/or modulating bladder outlet resistance.

of clinically significant sympathetic innervation of the striated urethral muscle in humans.

Terazosin, a selective alpha$_1$-blocker, was examined in 15 normotensive (SCI) patients.[52] DESD without obstruction of the bladder neck or prostate was documented using videourodynamic evaluation in all patients. Urodynamic testing was performed both before and after treatment was initiated with terazosin (5 mg nightly). Voiding pressure before and during terazosin therapy averaged 92 ± 17 and 88 ± 27 cmH$_2$O, respectively ($p = 0.48$). After subsequent external sphincterotomy or sphincter stent placement, the voiding pressure was reduced to 38 ± 15 cmH$_2$O ($p < 0.001$).

Nine other patients suffered from persistent voiding symptoms after previous sphincterotomy. Each was subsequently treated with oral terazosin. Of 5 patients who improved with this treatment, urodynamic parameters demonstrated obstruction only at the bladder neck, with no evidence of obstruction at the level of the external sphincter. The 4 patients who failed to improve were documented to have an open bladder neck but obstruction at the level of the external sphincter.

This study supports that even though alpha$_1$-sympathetic blockade does not significantly relieve functional obstruction caused by DESD. Also noted was that terazosin is helpful in diagnosing and treating internal sphincter (bladder neck and prostate) obstruction, especially in patients who have persistent voiding symptoms after external sphincterotomy. Other selective alpha$_1$-adrenergic blockade should yield results similar to terazosin.

Patients demonstrating clinical improvement with terazosin therapy, despite no urodynamic verification of improvement in DESD, may be responding to treatment of autonomic dysreflexia symptoms.[76,77] The patients may feel better because of diminished autonomic dysreflexia activity, despite ongoing DESD.[78] Another reason for clinical improvement without resolution of DESD may be an undiagnosed functional obstruction at the level of the urethral smooth musculature, which should improve with alpha$_1$ blockade, rather than true DESD. This is supported by studies by Yalla et al.[79]

Baclofen

Baclofen depresses monosynaptic and polysynaptic excitation of motor neurons and interneurons in the spinal cord and possibly functions as a glycine and gamma-aminobutyric acid (GABA) agonist.[55,56] GABA has been identified as the major inhibitory transmitter in the spinal cord.[80]

Baclofen has been found useful in the treatment of skeletal spasticity attributable to a variety of causes, especially multiple sclerosis and traumatic spinal cord lesions.[55] Hacken and Krucker found intravenous, but not oral, baclofen effective for patients with detrusor-sphincter dyssynergia, with the side-effects of weakness and dizziness common.[58]

Leyson et al studied high-dose oral baclofen in 25 SCI patients.[81] They concluded that baclofen was helpful in decreasing the resting urethral pressure at the level of the sphincter. Residual urine decreased in 73% of their cases. However, only 20% of the patients demonstrated a reduction in intravesical pressure at high doses of between 140 and 160 mg daily. The safety of long-term oral baclofen is also of significant concern. This study verified the very limited role, if any, that baclofen may have in the treatment of DESD.

Florante et al reported that 73% of their patients with voiding dysfunction caused by acute and chronic spinal cord injury had lower striated sphincter responses and decreased residual urine volumes after oral baclofen treatment.[82] However, a very high daily dose of 120 mg was used. The potential side-effects of baclofen include drowsiness, insomnia, rash, pruritus, dizziness, and weakness. The drug may impair the ability to walk or stand, and is not recommended for the management of spasticity resulting from cerebral lesions or disease. Sudden withdrawal has been shown to provoke hallucinations, anxiety, and tachycardia; hallucinations during treatment, which have been responsive to reductions in dosage, have also been reported.[83,84]

Benzodiazepines

Few references are available that provide valuable data on the use of any of the diazepines in the treatment of DESD.

The benzodiazepines potentiate the action of GABA at both presynaptic and postsynaptic sites in the brain and spinal cord.[85,86] We have not found the recommended oral doses of diazepam to be effective in controlling DESD. Anecdotal improvement may simply be attributable to the antianxiety effect of the drug.

Beta-adrenergic agonists

Beta-adrenergic agonists, especially those with prominent beta characteristics, are able to produce relaxation of slow-twitch skeletal muscles.[73] Gosling et al have reported that a portion of the external urethral sphincter comprising the outermost urethral wall consists exclusively of slow-twitch fibers, whereas the striated muscle fibers of the levator ani contain both fast- and slow-twitch fibers.[87] This type of action may account, at least in part, for the decrease in urethral profile parameters seen with terbutaline. There is no clinical evidence of successful treatment of DESD with beta-adrenergic agonists.

Dantrolene

Dantrolene sodium exerts its effects by a direct peripheral relaxation action on skeletal muscle.[55,85] Dantrolene has been shown to dissociate excitation–contraction coupling in the sarcoplasmic reticulum of muscle.[56] Hackler et al reported improvement in voiding function in approximately half of their patients with DESD treated with dantrolene.[57]

However, dosages significantly above the recommended daily maximum were required, whereas significant side-effects, especially weakness, were common. Harris and Benson reported that the generalized weakness which dantrolene may induce is often significant enough to compromise its therapeutic effects.[88] Other potential side-effects include euphoria, dizziness, diarrhea, and hepatotoxicity. Fatal hepatitis has been reported in approximately 0.1–0.2% of patients treated with the drug for 60 days or longer, whereas symptomatic hepatitis may occur in 0.5% of patients treated for more than 60 days; chemical abnormalities of liver function are noted in approximately 1%.[89]

Drugs to increase bladder pressure

Modalities that have been tried to increase intravesical pressure to achieve bladder emptying such as suprapubic percussion, Credé's maneuver, and use of bethanechol chloride are not effective and may potentially be detrimental.[68]

Increasing the detrusor pressure without simultaneously relaxing the outlet is associated with upper urinary tract morbidity and can aggravate autonomic dysreflexia.[90]

Intrathecal baclofen pump

The use of an intrathecal baclofen pump has also received some attention in the treatment of DESD.[60] These pumps were implanted for severe spasticity and some of the patients experienced improvement in bladder and sphincter functions. Nanninga et al reported their experience in 7 patients for relief of severe spasticity.[91] Six patients demonstrated an increase in bladder capacity and 4 were able to perform IC and remain dry. A slight decrease in maximum intravesical pressure was seen in all the patients. Talalla et al noted an inconsistent effect of intrathecal baclofen on urethral pressure in 6 SCI patients.[92] Two patients had significant reduction in maximum urethral and maximum detrusor pressures. Side-effects included half of the patients noticing that reflex erections were reduced or abolished for at least 24 hours following intrathecal baclofen. The authors reported that this side-effect has deterred other patients from considering this treatment modality.

There is also a case report of improvement in DESD with intrathecal baclofen in one patient with hereditary spastic paraplegia and voiding dysfunction.[93] However, it is not known if intrathecal baclofen merely reduced pelvic floor spasticity, eliminated lower extremity artifacts, or truly abolished DESD.[94]

At the present time intrathecal baclofen pump implantation for the primary diagnosis of DESD does not seem warranted because of the invasive spinal surgery, cost, and viable alternatives. It may be helpful for DESD in patients who also have lower severe extremities spasticity uncontrolled by oral pharmacological therapy. The intrathecal baclofen pump may also be promising for patients with refractory detrusor hyperreflexia.

Neurogenic bladder drug development

During the past few years, research in neuro-urology has stimulated the development of new therapeutic approaches for incontinence, including the intravesical administration of afferent neurotoxins such as capsaicin and resiniferatoxin. What are the research priorities for the future? It will be important to focus on the development of neuropharmacological agents that can suppress the unique components of abnormal bladder reflex mechanisms and thereby act selectively to decrease symptoms without altering normal voiding function. To end this chapter, we would like to speculate on a few areas of research which we feel may pay off within the next 5 years with new and better treatment of neuropathic urinary incontinence.

Bladder-specific K$^+$ channel openers. Can truly bladder smooth muscle or afferent neuron-specific potassium channel openers be developed. This treatment may alleviate the overactive and sensitive bladder without any dry mouth.

Intravesical vanilloid treatment. Can the clinical utility of intravesical resiniferatoxin be perfected so that the preferred therapy for neurogenic bladder is a simple outpatient 30 min instillation of 30 ml resiniferatoxin that will last 3 months without systemic side-effects?

Anticholinergic drugs. Can the pharmaceutical companies develop a truly bladder-specific and effective anticholinergic drug with no dry mouth?

Tachykinin antagonists. These substances are appealing in that they may be effective without increasing residual urine volumes. Can clinically useful and safe NK antagonists be developed?

Stress incontinence drugs. Urethral smooth and/or skeletal muscle specific alpha agonist or 5-HT reuptake inhibitor that may treat stress urinary incontinence. We need an effective drug for stress incontinence.

Advances in neuro-urology. Beyond the horizon of near-term advancement, we predict a brave new paradigm in neuro-urology. What has already started is the evolution of unstoppable forces of change in medicine that include pharmacogenomics, tissue engineering, and gene therapy. These will change how we practice urology and gynecology.

Pharmacogenomics. Medicine will be tailored to the genetic make-up of each individual. Through microarray gene chip technology, we will know how a patient metabolizes medications and the patient's receptor(s) profile and allergy risk. These factors can be screened against a list of medications prior to therapy. A physician will then be able to always prescribe the best drug for each patient without the risk of allergic reaction.

Tissue engineering. Rapid advances are being made feasible in tissue and organ reconstruction using autologous tissue and stem cells. We envisage a day, in the not too distant future, when stress incontinence is cured not with a cadaver ligament and metal screws into the bones but rather a minimally invasive injection of stem cells that will not only bulk up the deficient sphincter but also actually improve the sphincter's contractility and function.

Gene therapy. Diabetic neurogenic bladder and visceral pain may be cured with one or more injections of a gene vector that the physician will inject into the bladder or urethra. Injection of a nerve growth factor via a herpes virus vector into the bladder of a diabetic bladder may restore bladder sensation and innervation. Can the introduction of a virus that expresses the production of endorphin that is site- and nerve-specific help alleviate pelvic visceral pain, regardless of the cause?

References

1. Andersson K-E. Current concepts in treatment of disorders of micturition. Drugs 1988; 35:477.

2. Blaivas JG, Labib KB, Michalik J, Zayed AAH. Cystometric response to propantheline in detrusor hyperreflexia: therapeutic implications. J Urol 1980; 124:259.

3. Wein AJ. Neuromuscular dysfunction of the lower urinary tract and its treatment. In: Walsh, Retik, Vaughan, and Wein AJ, eds. Campbell's urology, 7th edn. 1997:953–1006.

4. Anderson GF, Fredericks CM. Characterization of the oxybutynin antagonism of drug-induced spasms in detrusor. Pharmacology 1972; 15:31.

5. Yarker YE, Goa KL, Fitton A. Oxybutynin. A review of its pharmacodynamic and pharmacokinetic properties, and its therapeutic use in detrusor instability. Drugs Aging 1995; 6(3):243.

6. Thompson IM, Lauvetz R. Oxybutynin in bladder spasm, neurogenic bladder, and enuresis. Urology 1976; 8:452.

7. Hehir M, Fitzpatrick JM. Oxybutynin and prevention of urinary incontinence in spinal bifida. Eur Urol 1985; 11(4):254.

8. Gajewski JB, Awad SA. Oxybutynin versus propantheline in patients with multiple sclerosis and detrusor hyperreflexia. J Urol 1986; 135(5):966.

9. Koyanagi T, Maru A, et al. Clinical evaluation of oxybutynin hydrochloride (KL007 tablets) for the treatment of neurogenic bladder and unstable bladder: a parallel double-blind controlled study with placebo. Nishi Nihon Hinyouki 1986; 48:1050. [in Japanese]

10. Zeegers AGM, Kiesswetter H, Kramer AEJ, Jonas U. Conservative therapy of frequency, urgency and urge incontinence: a double blind clinical trial of flavoxate hydrochloride, oxybutynin chloride, emepronium bromide and placebo. World J Urol 1987; 5:57.

11. Thüroff JW, Bunke B, Ebner A, et al. Ramdomized, double-blind, multicenter trial on treatment of frequency, urgency and urge incontinence related to detrusor hyperactivity: oxybutynin versus propantheline versus placebo. J Urol 1991; 145:813.

12. Anderson RU, Mobley D, Blank B, et al. Once a day controlled versus immediate release oxybutynin chloride for urge incontinence. J Urol 1999; 161:1809.

13. Birns J, Lukkari E, Malone-Lee JG. A randomized controlled trial comparing the efficacy of controlled-release oxybutynin tablets (10 mg once daily) with conventional oxybutynin tablets (5 mg twice daily) in patients whose symptoms were stabilized on 5 mg twice daily of oxybutynin. BJU Int 2000; 85(7):793–798.

14. Versi E, Appell R, Mobley D, et al. Dry mouth with conventional and controlled-release oxybutynin in urinary incontinence. The Ditropan XL Study Group. Obstet Gynecol 2000; 95:718.

15. Gupta SK, Sathyan G, Lindemulder EA, et al. Quantitative characterization of therapeutic index: application of mixed-effects modeling to evaluate oxybutynin dose-efficacy and dose-side effect relationships. Clin Pharmacol Ther 1999; 65:672.

16. O'Leary M, Erickson JR, Smith CP, McDermott C, Horton J, Chancellor MB. Effect of controlled release oxybutynin on neurogenic bladder function in spinal cord injury. J Spinal Cord Med 2003; 26(2):159–162.

17. O'Leary M, Erickson JR, Smith CP, et al. Bladder function in spinal cord injured patients changes in voiding patterns in multiple sclerosis patients with controlled release oxybutynin. Int MS J 2002;

18. Nilvebrant L, Andersson K-E, Gillberg P-G, et al. Tolterodine – a new bladder selective antimuscarinic agent. Eur J Pharmacol 1997; 327:195.

19. Nilvebrant L, Hallen B, Larsson G. Tolterodine – a new bladder selective muscarinic receptor antagonist: preclinical pharmacological and clinical data. Life Sci 1997; 60:1129.

20. Jonas U, Hofner K, Madersbacher H, Holmdahl TH. Efficacy and safety of two doses of tolterodine versus placebo in patients with detrusor overactivity and symptoms of frequency, urge incontinence, and urgency: urodynamic evaluation. The International Study Group. World J Urol 1997; 15:144.

21. Appell RA. Clinical efficacy and safety of tolterodine in the treatment of overactive bladder: a pooled analysis. Urology 1997; 50:90–96.

22. Rentzhog L, Stanton SL, Cardozo L, et al. Efficacy and safety of tolterodine in patients with detrusor instability: a dose-ranging study. Br J Urol 1998; 81:42.

23. Abrams P, Freeman R, Anderstrom C, Mattiasson A. Tolterodine, a new antimuscarinic agent: as effective but better tolerated than oxybutynin in patients with an overactive bladder. Br J Urol 1998; 81:801.

24. Van Kerrebroeck PE, Amarenco G, Thuroff JW, et al. Dose-ranging study of tolterodine in patients with detrusor hyperreflexia. Neurourol Urodyn 1998; 17:499.

25. Goessl C, Sauter T, Michael T, et al. Efficacy and tolerability of tolterodine in children with detrusor hyperreflexia. Urology 2000; 55:414.

26. Malone-Lee J, Shaffu B, Anand C, Powell C. Tolterodine: superior tolerability than and comparable efficacy to oxybutynin in individuals 50 years old or older with overactive bladder: a randomized controlled trial. J Urol 2001; 165:1452.

27. Van Kerrebroeck P, Kreder K, Jonas U, et al. Tolterodine once-daily: superior efficacy and tolerability in the treatment of the overactive bladder. Urology 2001; 57:414.

28. Appell RA, Sand P, Dmochowski R, et al. Prospective randomized controlled trial of extended-release oxybutynin chloride and tolterodine tartrate in the treatment of overactive bladder: results of the OBJECT Study. Mayo Clin Proc 2001; 76:358.

29. Tokuno H, Chowdhury JU, Tomita T. Inhibitory effects of propiverine on rat and guinea-pig urinary bladder muscle. Naunyn-Schmiedeberg's Arch Pharmacol 1993; 348:659.

30. Stöhrer M, Madersbacher H, Richter R, et al. Efficacy and safety of propiverine in SCI-patients suffering from detrusor hyperreflexia – a double-blind, placebo-controlled clinical trial. Spinal Cord 1999; 37:196.

31. Takayasu H, Ueno A, Tuchida S, et al. Clinical effects of propiverine hydrochloride in the treatment of urinary frequency and incontinence associated with detrusor overactivity: a double-blind, parallel, placebo-controlled, multicenter study. Igaku no Ayumi 1990; 153:459. [in Japanese]

32. Madersbacher H, Halaska M, Voigt R, et al. A placebo-controlled, multicentre study comparing the tolerability and efficacy of propiverine and oxybutynin in patients with urgency and urge incontinence. BJU Int 1999; 84:646.

33. Stöhrer M, Bauer P, Giannetti BM, et al. Effects of trospium chloride on urodynamic parameters in patients with detrusor hyperreflexia due to spinal cord injuries. A multicentre placebo-controlled double-blind trial. Urol Int 1991; 47:138.

34. Madersbacher H, Stöhrer M, Richter R, et al. Trospium chloride versus oxybutynin: a randomized, double-blind, multicentre trial in the treatment of detrusor hyperreflexia. Br J Urol 1995; 75:452.

35. Kohler FP, Morales PA. Cystometric evaluation of flavoxate hydrochloride in normal and neurogenic bladder. J Urol 1968; 100:729.

36. Pedersen E, Bjarnason EV, Hansen P-H. The effect of flavoxate on neurogenic bladder dysfunction. Acta Neurol Scand 1972; 48:487.

37. Robinson JM, Brocklehurst JC. Emepronium bromide and flavoxate hydrochloride in the treatment of urinary incontinence associated with detrusor instability in elderly women. Br J Urol 1983; 55:371.

38. Chapple CR, Parkhouse H, Gardener C, Milroy EJ. Double blind, placebo-controlled, crossover study of flavoxate in the treatment of idiopathic detrusor instability. Br J Urol 1990; 66:491.

39. Barrett D, Wein AJ. Voiding dysfunction diagnosis, classification and management. In: Gillenwater JY, Grayhack JT, Howards SS, Duckett JW, eds. Adult and pediatric urology, 2nd edn. St Louis: Mosby-Year Book, 1991:1001–1099.

40. Diokno AC, Taub M. Ephedrine in treatment of urinary incontinence. Urology 1975; 5:624.

41. Raezer DM, Benson GS, Wein AJ, Duckett JW Jr. The functional approach to the management of the pediatric neuropathic bladder: a clinical study. J Urol 1977; 177:649.

42. Awad SA, Downie JW, Kiriluta HG. Alpha-adrenergic agents in urinary disorders of the proximal urethra, part I: sphincteric incontinence. Br J Urol 1978; 50:332.

43. Ek A, Andersson K-E, Gullberg B, Ulmsten K. The effects of long-term treatment with norephedrine on stress incontinence and urethral closure pressure profile. Scand J Urol Nephrol 1978; 12:105.

44. Stewart BH, Banowski LHW, Montague DK. Stress incontinence: conservative therapy with sympathomimetic drugs. J Urol 1976; 115:558.

45. Bauer S. An approach to neurogenic bladder: an overview: Probl Urol 1994; 8:441.

46. Beisland HO, Fossberg E, Sander S. On incompetent urethral closure mechanism: treatment with estriol and phenylpropanolamine. Scand J Urol Nephrol 1981; 60(Suppl): 67.

47. Gleason D, Reilly R, Bottaccini M, Pierce MJ. The urethral continence zone and its relation to stress incontinence. J Urol 1974; 112:81.

48. Gilja I, Radej M, Kovacic M, Parazajders J. Conservative treatment of female stress incontinence with imipramine. J Urol 1984; 132:909–911.

49. Yasuda K, Yamanishi T, Homma Y, et al. The effect of urapidil on neurogenic bladder: a placebo controlled double-blind study. J Urol 1996; 156:1125.

50. Yamanishi T, Yasuda K, Kawabe K, et al. A multicenter placebo-controlled, double-blind trial of urapidil, an α-blocker, on neurogenic bladder dysfunction. Eur Urol 1999; 35: 45.

51. Chancellor MB, Erhard MJ, Hirsch IH, Staas WE. Prospective evaluation of terazosin for the treatment of autonomic dysreflexia. J Urol 1994; 151:111–113.

52. Chancellor MB, Erhard MJ, Rivas DA. Clinical effect of alpha-1 antagonism by terazosin on external and internal urinary sphincter. J Am Parapleg Soc 1993; 16:207–214.

53. Lapides J, Diokno AC, Silber SJ, Lowe BS. Clean intermittent self-catheterization in the treatment of urinary tract disease. J Urol 1972; 107:7458–7461.

54. Maynard FM, Diokno AC. Clean intermittent catheterization for spinal cord injury patients. J Urol 1982; 128:477–480.

55. Cedarbaum JM, Schleifer LS. Drugs for Parkinson's disease, spasticity, and acute muscle spasms. In: Gilman AG, Rail TW, Nies AS, Taylor P, eds. Goodman and Gilman's the pharmacological basis of therapeutics, 8th edn. New York: Pergamon, 1990:463–484.

56. Bianchine J. Drugs for Parkinson's disease: centrally acting muscle relaxants. In: Gilman AG, Goodman LS, Gilman A, eds. The pharmacological basis of therapeutics, New York: MacMillian, 1980;475–495.

57. Hackler RH, Broecker BH, Klein FA, Brady SM. A clinical experience with dantrolene sodium for external urinary sphincter hypertonicity in spinal cord injured patients. J Urol 1980; 124:78–81.

58. Hacken HJ, Krucker V. Clinical and laboratory assessment of the efficacy of baclofen on urethral sphincter spasticity in patients with traumatic paraplegia. Eur Urol 1977; 3:237–240.

59. Herman RM, Wainberg MC. Clonidine inhibits vesico-sphincter reflexes in patients with spinal cord lesions. Arch Phys Med Rehab 1991; 72:539–545.

60. Steers WD, Meythaler JM, Haworth C, et al. Effects of acuter bolus and chronic continuous intrathecal baclofen on genitourinary dysfunction due to spinal cord pathology. J Urol 1992; 148:1849–1855.

61. Hacken HJ. Clinical and urodynamic assessment of alpha adrenolytic therapy in patients with neurogenic bladder function. Paraplegia 1980; 18:229.

62. Caine M. The present role of alpha-adrenergic blockers in the treatment of benign prostatic hypertrophy. J Urol 1986; 136:1.

63. Lepor J, Gup DI, Baumann M, Shapiro E. Laboratory assessment of terazosin and alpha-1 blockade in prostatic hyperplasia. Urology 1988; [Suppl] 32:21.

64. Elbadawi A, Schenk EA. A new theory of the innervation of bladder musculature. Part 4: Innervation of the vesicourethral junction and external urethral sphincter. J Urol 1974; 111:613.

65. Awad SA, Downie JW. Sympathetic dyssynergia in the region of the external sphincter. A possible source of lower urinary tract obstruction. J Urol 1977; 118:636–640.

66. Dixon JS, Gosling JA. Light and electron microscopic observation on noradrenergic nerves and striated muscle cells of the guinea pig urethra. Am J Anat 1977; 149:121.

67. Awad SA, Downie JW. Relative contributions of smooth and striated muscles to canine urethral pressure profile. Br J Urol 1976; 48:347–354.

68. Yalla SV, Rossier AB, Fam B. Dyssynergic vesicourethral responses during bladder rehabilitation in spinal cord injury patients: effects of spurapubic percussion, crede method and bethanechol chloride. J Urol 1976; 115:575.

69. Kaplan SA, Chancellor MB, Blaivas JG. Bladder and sphincter behavior in patients with spinal cord lesions. J Urol 1991; 46:113–117.

70. Mobley DF. Phenoxybenzamine in the management of neurogenic vesical dysfunction. J Urol 1976; 116:737–738.

71. Whitfield HN, Doyle PT, Mayo ME, Poopalasingham N. The effect of adrenergic blocking drugs on outflow resistance. Br J Urol 1976; 47: 823–827.

72. Awad SA, Downie JW, Lywood DW, et al. Sympathetic activity in the proximal urethra in patients with urinary obstruction. J Urol 1976; 115:545–547.

73. Olsson AT, Swanberg E, Svedinger L. Effects of beta adrenoceptor agonists on airway smooth muscle and on slow contracting skeletal muscle: In vitro and in vivo results compared. Acta Pharmacol Toxicol 1979; 44:272.

74. McGuire EJ, Wagner F, Weiss RM. Treatment of autonomic dysreflexia with phenoxybenzamine. J Urol 1976; 115:53–55.

75. Rossier AB, Fam BA, Lee IY, et al. Role of striated and smooth muscle components in the urethral pressure profile in the traumatic neurogenic bladder: a neuropharmacological and urodynamic study. Preliminary report. J Urol 1982; 128:529–535.

76. Sizemore GW, Winternitz WW. Autonomic hyper-reflexia-suppression with alpha-adrenergic blocking agents. N Engl J Med 1970; 282:795.

77. Scott MB, Morrow JW. Phenoxybenzamine in neurogenic bladder dysfunction after spinal cord injury. II. Autonomic dysreflexia. J Urol 1978; 119:483–484.

78. Chancellor MB, Karasick S, Erhard MJ, et al. Intraurethral wire mesh prosthesis placement in the external urinary sphincter of spinal cord injured men. Radiology 1993; 187:551.

79. Yalla SV, Rossier AB, Fam BA, et al. Functional contribution of autonomic innervation to urethral striated sphincter: studies with parasympathomimetic, parasympatholytic and alpha adrenergic blocking agents in spinal cord injury and control male subjects. J Urol 1977; 117:494–499.

80. Bloom FE. Neurohumoral transmission and the central nervous system. In: Gilman AG, Rail TW, Nies AS, Taylor P, eds. Goodman and Gilman's the pharmacological basis of therapeutics, 8th edn. New York: Pergamon, 1990:244–268.

81. Leyson JFJ, Martin BF, Sporer A. Baclofen in the treatment of detrusor-sphincter dyssynergia in spinal cord injury patients. J Urol 1980; 124:82–84.

82. Florante J, Leyson J, Martin F, Sporer A. Baclofen in the treatment of detrusor-sphincter dyssynergia in spinal cord injury patients. J Urol 1980; 124:82–84.

83. Roy CW, Wakefield IR. Baclofen pseudopsychosis: case report. Paraplegia 1986; 24:318.

84. Rivas DA, Chancellor MB, Hill K, Friedman M. Neurologic manifestations of baclofen withdrawal. J Urol 1993; 150:1903–1905.

85. Davidoff RA. Antispasticity drugs: mechanisms of action. Ann Neurol 1985; 17:107.

86. Lader M. Clinical pharmacology of benzodiazepines. Ann Rev Med 1987; 38:19.

87. Gosling JA, Dixon JS, Critchley HOD, et al. A comparative study of the human external sphincter and periurethral levator ani muscles. Br J Urol 1981; 153:35.

88. Harris JD, Benson GS. Effect of dantrolene on canine bladder contractility. Urology 1980; 16:229.

89. Ward A, Chaffman MO, Sorkin EM. Dantrolene. A review of its pharmacodynamic and pharmacokinetic properties and therapeutic use in malignant hyperthermia, the neuroleptic syndrome and an update of its use in muscle spasticity. Drugs 1986; 32:130.

90. McGuire EJ, Woodside JR, Borden TA, Weiss RM. The prognostic significance of urodynamic testing in myelodysplastic patients. J Urol 1981; 126:205–209.

91. Nanninga JB, Frost F, Penn R. Effect of intrathecal baclofen on bladder and sphincter function. J Urol 1989; 142:101–105.

92. Talalla A, Grundy D, Macdonell R. The effect of intrathecal baclofen on the lower urinary tract in paraplegia. Paraplegia 1990; 8:420–427.

93. Bushman W, Steers WD, Meythaler JM. Voiding dysfunction in patients with spastic paraplegia: urodynamic evaluation and response to continuous intrathecal baclofen. Neurourol Urodynam 1993; 12:163–170.

94. Kums JJ, Delhaas EM. Intrathecal baclofen infusion in patients with spasticity and neurogenic bladder disease. World J Urol 1991; 9:153–156.

15

Intravesical pharmacological treatment

Carlos Silva and Francisco Cruz

Introduction

The increasing interest around intravesical pharmacological therapy for neurogenic bladder overactivity is essentially due to the fact that it circumvents systemic administration of active compounds. This offers two potential advantages. First, intravesical therapy is an easy way to provide high concentrations of pharmacological agents in the bladder tissue without causing unsuitable levels in other organs. Secondly, the action of effective drugs inappropriate for systemic administration can be restricted to the bladder. Although extremely attractive, it must, however, be kept in mind that intravesical pharmacological therapy should be introduced as a second-line treatment in patients refractory to conventional oral anticholinergic therapy or patients who do not tolerate its systemic side-effects.

Drugs susceptible to decreasing or abolishing detrusor contractions by the intravesical route block either the sensory input or the parasympathetic outflow to the detrusor muscle. Drugs that block the sensory input include capsaicin and resiniferatoxin, two compounds of the vanilloid family. Drugs that block the parasympathetic outflow include botulinum A toxin and anticholinergic compounds.

Vanilloid substances

Common vanilloids, VR1 receptor, and desensitization

Capsaicin, which is extracted from hot chilli peppers, and resiniferatoxin (RTX), which is extracted from *Euphorbia resinifera*, a cactus-like plant abundant in northern Africa, are the most well-studied compounds of this family. The name vanilloid derived from the presence of a homovanillyl ring in capsaicin and RTX molecules (Figure 15.1). However, such a designation became a misnomer, as new compounds with properties similar to those of capsaicin or

RTX were identified which do not possess a homovanillyl ring in their structure. Examples of such compounds include polygodial, scutigeral, and olvanil.[1]

Vanilloid substances bind to a receptor – named vanilloid receptor type 1 or VR1 – that occurs in the membrane of type C, unmyelinated sensory fibers.[2,3] VR1 is a nonselective ion channel that belongs to the transient resting potential family of ion channels, being for that reason also denominated TRPV1 in more recent publications.[4] Once activated, VR1 allows a massive Ca^{2+} and Na^+ inflow into the neuron. This causes a brief excitation, followed by a prolonged desensitization, during which the neuron is

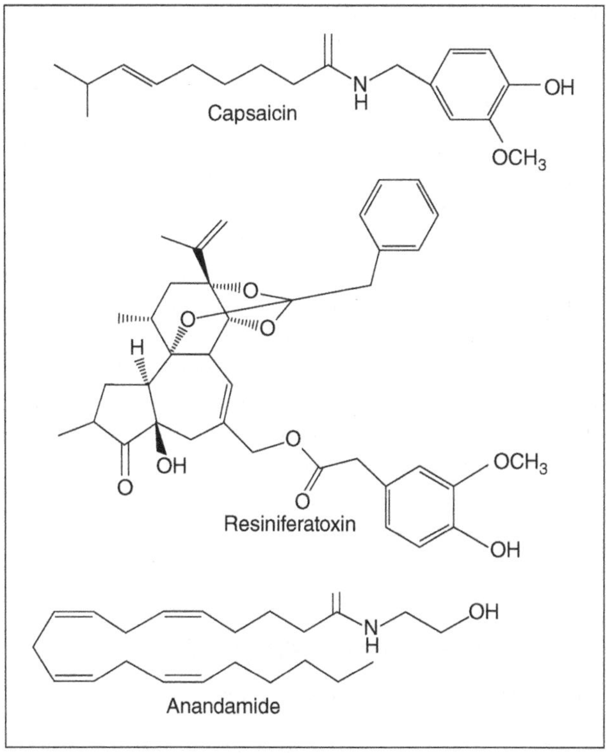

Figure 15.1
Molecular structures of capsaicin, resiniferatoxin, and anandamide.

unresponsive to natural stimuli.[1] Only desensitization has therapeutic implications. It is, however, a poorly understood phenomenon. It depends on Ca^{2+} inflow, since desensitization does not occur in sensory neurons kept in culture mediums lacking the calcium ion. It is believed that high intracellular Ca^{2+} levels arrest the voltage-sensitive Ca^{2+} conductance, disrupt metabolic critical pathways, and release neuropeptides such as substance P (SP) or calcitonin gene-related peptide (CGRP).[1] In addition, desensitization may also induce prolonged neuromessenger modifications in sensory fibers, such as a down-regulation of SP[5] and an up-regulation of galanin synthesis.[6] The latter peptide is usually not expressed by sensory neurons.[6]

It is intriguing that an endogenous vanilloid-like substance binding to VR1 has not yet been identified. At present, the endogenous substance closest to capsaicin or RTX is anandamide, a lipid synthesized in brain tissue, vascular endothelium, and macrophages.[7] Anandamide, although lacking a homovanillyl ring, has a long chain similar to that occurring in typical vanilloids (see Figure 15.1). Interestingly, anandamide also evokes Ca^{2+} inflow through VR1 receptors.[3,8]

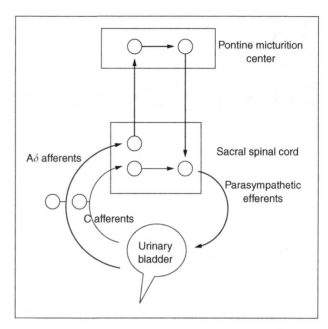

Figure 15.2
Neuronal pathways controlling micturition.

Rationale for intravesical vanilloid application

Capsaicin does not interfere with reflex detrusor contractions in intact animals but suppresses them in chronic spinal animals.[9] This finding by de Groat et al was subsequently explained by the existence of two micturition reflex pathways fed by distinct sensory input (Figure 15.2).[9] One pathway, a supraspinal loop passing through the pontine micturition center, was triggered by Aδ-fiber sensory input. The other pathway, a neuronal pathway totally lodged in the sacral spinal cord, was dependent upon C-fiber sensory input. Interestingly, the former pathway controlled micturition in intact animals, whereas the latter was active only in spinal transected animals. These experimental findings pushed Fowler et al to instill capsaicin into overactive bladders of patients with spinal cord lesions.[10] As intravesical capsaicin suppressed detrusor activity, that study indirectly confirmed the existence of a C-fiber-mediated spinal micturition reflex in man.[10]

Clinical experience with intravesical capsaicin

More than 100 patients with bladder overactivity of spinal origin received intravesical capsaicin in six non-controlled[11-16] and one controlled[17] clinical trial (Tables 15.1 and 15.2). In general, treatments followed the methodology initially suggested by Fowler et al in 1992.[10] Capsaicin was dissolved in 30% alcohol and 100–125 ml (or half of the bladder capacity if lower than that volume) of 1–2 mmol/l solutions were instilled into the bladder and left in contact with the mucosa for 30 min.

Best clinical results were found among patients with incomplete spinal cord lesions caused by multiple sclerosis, trauma, or infectious diseases who maintained some degree of bladder sensation and emptied the bladder by micturition. Success rates, defined as complete continence or satisfactory improvement, reached 70–90% (see Table 15.1).[11,15,16] In addition, capsaicin also decreased urinary frequency and attenuated urge to urinate.[11,15,16] In patients with complete spinal cord lesions the success rate was much lower. Geirsson et al[12] obtained full continence in only 20% and partial improvement in another 20% of patients with cervical cord lesions (see Table 15.1). The effect of capsaicin on micturition symptoms was long-lasting, exceeding 6 or even 9 months in some cases.[11,15,16] Upon reinstillation, capsaicin maintained the efficacy found at the first administration.[11,15,16]

Urodynamic improvement occurred in 70–90% of the patients (see Table 15.1). In particular, a 47–156% increase of bladder capacity was observed. The effect of capsaicin on maximal detrusor pressure is less clear. Although three studies have reported a 20–30 cmH$_2$O decrease in maximal detrusor pressure,[11,16,17] another study was unable to demonstrate any significant decrease.[12]

One randomized controlled study that compared capsaicin against 30% ethanol, the vehicle solution, should be mentioned (see Table 15.2).[17] Twenty cases were

Table 15.1 *Open clinical studies with intravesical capsaicin*

Study	Dose/patients	Frequency Before	Frequency After	FDC (ml) Before	FDC (ml) After	MCC (ml) Before	MCC (ml) After	DP (cmH$_2$O) Before	DP (cmH$_2$O) After	Clinical and urodynamic improvement
Fowler et al[11]	1 or 2 mmol/l 12 patients					124	274	58	40	Clinical improvement 75% Full continence 40%
Geirsson et al[12]	2 mmol/l 10 patients					195	293	82	90	Clinical improvement 40% Full continence 20% Urodynamic improvement 90%
Das et al[13]	0.1–2 mmol/l 5 patients					124	231			Clinical improvement 60%
Igawa et al[14]	1–2 mmol/l 5 patients					72	185			Clinical improvement 100%
Cruz et al[15]	1 mmol/l 10 patients	15	8	97	173	151	288			Clinical improvement 90% Full continence 80% Urodynamic improvement 70%
De Ridder et al[16]	1–2 mmol/l 49 patients					194	247	58	28	Clinical improvement 82%
Fowler (in De Ridder et al[16])	1–2 mmol/l 18 patients	12.7	6.4			169	320	68	49	Clinical improvement 78% Full continence 61%

FDC, volume to first detrusor contraction; MCC, maximum cystometric capacity; DP, maximum detrusor voiding pressure.

Table 15.2 *Comparative study between intravesical capsaicin and vehicle solution (30% ethanol)*

Study	Dose/ patients	Incontinence		Frequency		MCC (ml)		DP (cmH₂O)		Subjective improvement
		Before	After	Before	After	Before	After	Before	After	
De Séze et al[17]	1 mmol/l capsaicin 10 patients	3.9	0.6*	9.3	6.1*	169	299*	77	53*	100%
	Placebo 10 patients	5.1	4	11.1	12.2	157	182	64	69	10%

MCC, maximum cystometric capacity; DP, maximum detrusor voiding pressure; * indicates a statistically significant change.

randomized to receive capsaicin (10 cases) or 30% ethanol (10 cases). All patients that received capsaicin found significant regression of incontinence and urge sensation, whereas only one ethanol-treated patient had amelioration.

Clinical experience with intravesical resiniferatoxin

The first non-controlled trials with this vanilloid included 34 patients, most of them with incomplete spinal cord lesions (Table 15.3).[18–21] Different RTX concentrations, 10 nmol/l, 50 nmol/l, 100 nmol/l, and 10 μmol/l, were tested. RTX brought an immediate improvement or disappearance of urinary incontinence in 67–85% of the patients and a 30% decrease in their daily urinary frequency. The effect was long-lasting, up to 12 months, only in patients receiving 50 nmol/l or higher doses of RTX.[18,21] In patients treated with doses as high as 10 μmol/l, a transient urinary retention due to detrusor hypoactivity occurred.[20]

Urodynamic improvement was observed in most of the treated patients. For example, the volume to first detrusor contraction increased 40% after 50–100 nmol/l RTX. Maximal bladder capacity increased 25% after 10 nmol/l,[19] 80% after 50–100 nmol/l,[18,21] and 120% after 10 μmol/l solutions.[20] Maximal detrusor pressure was decreased only after 10 μmol/l RTX.

RTX was compared against the vehicle solution (10% ethanol in saline) in a recent randomized ongoing study (Table 15.4).[22] The discomfort was similarly low in both arms. A significant improvement of urinary frequency and incontinence was found only in the RTX arm. In addition, only patients receiving RTX had an increase of the volume to first detrusor contraction and of maximal bladder capacity, 35% and 80% above the pre-treatment values, respectively. Another three studies compared 50–100 nmol/l RTX against 1–2 mmol/l capsaicin (Table 15.5).[23–25] RTX was better tolerated and its effects on continence and urodynamic parameters were equivalent[25] or superior[24] to those induced by capsaicin.

Safety of intravesical vanilloids

The most frequent problem seen with capsaicin instillation is suprapubic burning pain felt by patients with preserved bladder sensation. It starts immediately after the beginning of the treatment and may require vigorous analgesic medication and prompt capsaicin evacuation. Preliminary bladder anesthesia with lidocaine (lignocaine) may provide partial relief.[11,15,26] In addition, a transient worsening of the urinary symptoms may occur during the first 1–2 weeks after instillation which should not be interpreted as a treatment failure.[11,15,26] Another side-effect of capsaicin needs to be stressed. In patients with high, complete spinal cord lesions, capsaicin can trigger severe episodes of autonomic dysreflexia.[12,15] In contrast, these side-effects did not occur with RTX instillation.[18,21,22]

Human contact with capsaicin and RTX was not initiated with intravesical application of these vanilloids. Capsaicin is consumed in the daily diet of millions of people and historical reports indicate that RTX has been used for medicinal purposes over many centuries, mainly as analgesic unguent.[27] Nevertheless, the contact of vanilloid compounds with the bladder mucosa represents a new challenge, the consequences of which have not yet been fully evaluated. In agreement with these concerns, bladder biopsies were obtained from patients repeatedly instilled with capsaicin[28] or RTX.[29] Examinations under the conventional and electronic microscopes were unable to detect any significant change in the transitional mucosa of those patients.

The ideal patient, the ideal vanilloid, and how to apply it

Patients with small contracted bladders or bedridden due to severe neurological disorders responded very poorly to capsaicin or RTX instillation.[11,30] In addition, in patients

Table 15.3 *Open clinical studies with intravesical resiniferatoxin*

| Study | Dose/patients | Incontinence | | Frequency | | FDC (ml) | | MCC (ml) | | DP (cmH₂O) | | Clinical improvement |
		Before	After	Before	After	Before	After	Before	After	Before	After	
Cruz et al[18]	50 or 100 nmol/l	3.6	1.5	14	10	134	184	182	330	80	70	80% at 3 months
Silva et al[21]	7 + 14 patients											
Lazzeri et al[19]	10 nmol/l							175	216	69	61	67% at 2 weeks
	6 patients											33% at 4 weeks
Lazzeri et al[20]	10 µmol/l							190	421	75	21	85% at 4 weeks
	7 patients											

FDC, volume to first detrusor contraction; MCC, maximum cystometric capacity; DP, maximum detrusor voiding pressure.

Table 15.4 *Comparative study between intravesical RTX and vehicle solution (10% ethanol)*

Study	Dose/patients	Incontinence Before	Incontinence After	Frequency Before	Frequency After	FDC (ml) Before	FDC (ml) After	MCC (ml) Before	MCC (ml) After
Cruz et al[22]	50 nmol/l RTX 12 patients	3	1.3*	9.2	7.3*	139	185*	185	326*
	Placebo 11 patients	1.8	1	10	9.6	109	110	180	189

FDC, volume to first detrusor contraction; MCC, maximum cystometric capacity; * indicates a statistically significant change.

Table 15.5 *Comparative studies between intravesical capsaicin and resiniferatoxin*

Study	Dose/patients	Incontinence Before	Incontinence After	Frequency Before	Frequency After	FDC (ml) Before	FDC (ml) After	MCC (ml) Before	MCC (ml) After	DP (cmH$_2$O) Before	DP (cmH$_2$O) After	Subjective improvement
Giannatoni et al[24]	Capasaicin 2 mmol/l 12 patients	3	2.3	5.8	5.6	165	195	183	219	76	69	33%
	RTX 100 nmol/l 12 patients	4.2	1.9*	6.6	4.8*	176	275*	196	357*	71	68	92%
de Sèze et al[25]	Capsaicin 1 mmol/l 19 patients	6	2.6*	11.1	6.4*			174	300*	75	75	67%
	RTX 50 nmol/l 21 patients	6.9	4.3	9.5	9.4			195	320*	75	71	56%
Park et al[23]	Capsaicin 2 mmol/l 7 patients							108	156*	75	60	57%
	RTX 10 nmol/l 6 patients							115	222*	58	53	83%

FDC, volume to first detrusor contraction; MCC, maximum cystometric capacity; DP, maximum detrusor voiding pressure; * indicates a statistically significant change.

with complete spinal cord transection 50–100 nmol/l RTX solutions, although increasing bladder capacity, usually do not render bladders fully arreflexic.[12] These patients might benefit from higher RTX concentrations,[20] but this aspect requires further investigation.

At present, RTX seems preferable to capsaicin, because of its reduced pungency. RTX is available only as a dry powder. A 10 μmol/l stock solution in pure ethanol (1 mg RTX dissolved in 159 ml of ethanol) must be prepared and kept at 4°C in a glass container,[18,21,22] because of RTX instability in plastic containers.[31] Solutions for instillation are then prepared immediately before treatment.[18,21,22] For example,

to prepare 100 ml of 50 nmol/l solution in 10% ethanol in saline, 0.5 ml of the stock solution should be added to 9.5 ml of pure ethanol and 90 ml of saline. Due to their low pungency, the instillation of 50–100 nmol/l RTX solutions can be carried out as an outpatient procedure without any form of preliminary bladder anesthesia.[18,21,22] A three-way urethral catheter is inserted, the urine is emptied, and the RTX solution is instilled for 30 min. Phasic detrusor contractions can occur during instillation, although they become more spaced towards the end of the treatment. Leakage of RTX solution can, however, be prevented by maintaining the urethral catheter gently pulled against the bladder neck. At the end of the treatment, the bladder is evacuated and rinsed with saline and the patients are discharged home. Urinary tract infections should be prevented by a judicious use of prophylactic antibiotics.

If capsaicin is the chosen vanilloid, 1 mmol/l solutions can be obtained by dissolving 0.3 g of capsaicin in 1000 ml of 30% ethanol in saline.[10] Instillation is carried out as described for RTX. However, in patients with some bladder sensation remaining, strong analgesic treatment is usually required to alleviate bladder pain.[11,15,16] Furthermore, patients with spinal cord transection at high levels should be carefully monitored due to their susceptibility to severe episodes of autonomic dysreflexia.[12,15] Adequate treatment must be readily accessible for immediate administration.

Botulinum A toxin

Botulinum A toxin is a neurotoxin produced by *Clostridium botulinum*, a facultative anaerobe. It causes muscular paralysis by preventing the release of acetylcholine from cholinergic nerve endings at the neuromuscular junction.[32] This property was shown to relax the external urethral sphincter and improve bladder emptying in patients with detrusor-sphincter dyssynergia.[33,34] More recently, botulinum A toxin was also shown to relax the detrusor smooth muscle and reduce bladder overactivity in spinal patients.[35] This treatment requires multiple bladder injections. Therefore, although being reviewed in this chapter, it should be realized that it implicates more than a simple bladder instillation.

Clinical experience with botulinum A toxin

Schurch et al[35] were the first to use botulinum A toxin in the treatment of bladder overactivity resistant to anticholinergic drugs. In a nonrandomized study, 17 patients with complete and 4 patients with incomplete traumatic spinal cord injuries who emptied the bladder by intermittent self-catheterization underwent botulinum A toxin detrusor injections (Table 15.6). Botulinum A toxin (Botox®) was diluted in normal saline in order to obtain a concentration of 10 units/ml. Under visual control through a cystoscope, 30 injections of 1 ml (10 units of botulinum A toxin) were performed in 30 different locations above the trigone. A flexible 6F injection needle was used to deliver the toxin in the detrusor smooth muscle. In general, detrusor paralysis started 2 weeks later. At 6 weeks, urodynamic evaluation revealed a significant increase of bladder capacity and a significant decrease in maximum

detrusor voiding pressure that was still present at 36 weeks (see Table 15.6). Seventeen patients became completely continent, 7 patients without any additional anticholinergic medication and 10 patients requiring a lower daily dose. Interestingly, in susceptible patients, episodes of autonomic dysreflexia disappeared.

The initial experience with botulinum A toxin injections was recently confirmed in a multicenter nonrandomized clinical trial conducted in Europe and involving 184 patients (see Table 15.6).[36] Detrusor relaxation and continence was achieved in all cases but two-thirds of the patients still had to maintain a daily dose of anticholinergics.[36] The long-lasting effect of the first treatment, up to 1 year, appears to be maintained in subsequent injections.

Botulinum A toxin has been recently assayed in children with myelomeningocele (see Table 15.6).[37,38] As in adults, the toxin also increased bladder capacity and decreased maximal detrusor pressure. For the moment, the success rate in terms of continence and cessation of anticholinergic medication seems inferior to that observed in adults (see Table 15.6). In children, botulinum A toxin dose (Botox®) has to be calculated according to body weight. Schulte-Baukloh et al[37] suggested a dose of 12 units/kg of weight up to a maximum dose of 300 units, whereas Corcos et al[38] used 4 units/kg. The duration of detrusor paralysis is still unknown.

Side-effects of botulinum A toxin injections in the bladder appear to be minimal: the most feared one, paralysis of the striated musculature due to circulatory leakage of the toxin, was never reported. Currently, it is not known whether the prolonged deficit of parasympathetic tonus induces detrusor muscle atrophy. Furthermore, repeated injections of botulinum A toxin may lose efficacy due to the appearance of antibodies against the toxin.

Ideal patient for botulinum A toxin treatment

Patients should understand that following botulinum A toxin injection urinary retention will occur due to detrusor paralysis. Therefore, currently, ideal patients for botulinum A toxin treatment are those performing intermittent catheterization who maintain significant incontinence or high intravesical pressures in spite of a correct anticholinergic medication.

Botulinum A toxin is available under the tradenames of Botox® and Dysport®. The two varieties have been compared in some controlled studies. Available information indicates that Botox® is roughly three times more potent than Dysport®.[39] Therefore, if the latter variety is chosen, it may be necessary to triplicate the doses indicated for Botox®. Whatever the type of botulinum A toxin used,

Table 15.6 *Experience with botulinum A toxin bladder injections*

Study	Patients	Dose/protocol	Follow-up	FDC (ml) Before	FDC (ml) After	MCC (ml) Before	MCC (ml) After	DP (cmH$_2$O) Before	DP (cmH$_2$O) After	RV (ml) Before	RV (ml) After	Compliance (ml/cmH$_2$O) Before	Compliance (ml/cmH$_2$O) After	Improvement
Schurch et al[35]	19 adults	200–300 IU 20–30 sites 10 U/ml/site Trigone spared	6 weeks	215.8	415.7	296.3	480.5	65.6	35	261.8	490.5	32.6	62.1	Urodynamic improvement 100% Full continence 89%
Reitz et al[36]	184 adults	200–300 IU 20–30 sites 10 U/ml/site Trigone spared	12 weeks			272	420	61	30	236	387	32	72	Subjective improvement 100%
			36 weeks			272	352	61	44	236	291	32	51	Subjective improvement 100%
Corcos et al[38]	16 children (8–20 years)	4 IU/kg 20–30 sites	3 months			221	307	33.7	12.3					Subjective improvement 80% Full continence 68%
Schulte-Baukloh et al[37]	17 children (mean age 10.8 years)	85–300 IU 30–40 sites	2–4 weeks	95	201	137	215	59	40			20	45	40% overall decrease in incontinence score

Open clinical trials. FDC, volume to first detrusor contraction; MCC, maximum cystometric capacity; DP, maximum detrusor voiding pressure; RV, residual urine volume.

a common drawback of this treatment is its cost. A dose of 300 units of botulinum A toxin might exceed US$1500, and to which one must add the cost of a cystoscopy. Moreover, a substantial number of patients will still require permanent anticholinergic medication.

Anticholinergic drugs

Oxybutynin is the anticholinergic drug most frequently used by the intravesical route. Intravesical oxybutynin has been offered mainly to patients in whom oral administration has no effect or evokes severe side-effects, with a 55–90% success rate.[40–45] Treatment can be maintained over long periods of time without any form of bladder toxicity.[46,47] The reason why oxybutynin is better tolerated by the intravesical rather than the oral route is still incompletely understood. As a matter of fact, plasma concentrations of oxybutynin after intravesical or oral administration were shown to be similar.[43] A plausible explanation may, therefore, rest on the level of *N*-desethyloxybutynin, an active metabolite of oxybutynin, which is in general lower after intravesical than after oral administration. However, it should be kept in mind that drug absorption through the bladder may still evoke anticholinergic systemic side-effects, leading to treatment discontinuity in a significant number of cases.[48]

At the present time, there are no oxybutynin formulations ready for intravesical application. Thus, for adult patients, a 5 mg oxybutynin tablet must be crushed and dissolved in 30 ml of distilled water or saline and instilled twice or three times daily. The solution should not be evacuated until the next voiding, since maximum effect may take 3–4 hours to occur.[49] For children, it is advisable to start with 1.25 mg (one-quarter of a 5 mg oxybutynin tablet in 5 ml of sterile water) three times daily and adjust the dose according to the response.[48] The inconvenience of crushing oxybutynin tablets before every instillation can be avoided if purified oxybutynin preparations are available, usually as 5 ml vials containing 5 mg of oxybutynin.[50]

However, the need for 2–3 daily instillations restricts intravesical oxybutynin to patients on intermittent catheterization. To obviate this inconvenience long-acting intravesical oxybutynin formulations are being investigated. Hydroxypropylcellulose that adheres to the bladder mucosa or small reservoirs that can be placed in the bladder cavity may be used in the future to induce intravesically a slow and sustained release of oxybutynin.[51,52]

Electromotive drug administration (EMDA), which uses an electrical field to enhance the migration of ionized molecules (iontophoresis) through a particular tissue, has also been suggested as an alternative to increase absorption of intravesical oxybutynin.[53,54] A Foley catheter containing a silver positive electrode is introduced and the bladder is evacuated and rinsed with distilled water to remove urinary solutes that might be dragged by the electric current. The bladder is then filled with an oxybutynin solution. Negative electrode pads are placed on the paraumbilical area.[55] Riedl et al administered, by EMDA, 15–50 mg of oxybutynin to 14 patients with detrusor hyperreflexia by applying a 15 mA electric current for 20 min. Clinical and urodynamic improvement lasting several weeks occurred in half of the patients.[55] Di Stasi et al[56] also found significant clinical and urodynamic improvement in 10 patients refractory to standard anticholinergic therapy after EMDA of 5 mg oxybutynin (5 mA electric current for 30 min). Although attractive, it is still unclear why the therapeutic effect of intravesical oxybutynin given by EMDA lasts longer than after passive instillation. Moreover, it is intriguing why oxybutynin-induced systemic side-effects are less intense after EMDA than after passive intravesical administration in spite of the fact that high doses of the drug are dragged into the bladder tissue by EMDA. Future studies are, therefore, strongly recommended before a widespread use of intravesical EMDA.

Other drugs, such as trospium chloride, verapamil, tolterodine, atropine, diltiazem, and imipramine, have been used sporadically by intravesical route to decrease bladder overactivity but their effects remain to be compared with oxybutynin.[45,57]

References

1. Szallasi A, Blumberg PM. Vanilloid (capsaicin) receptors and mechanisms. Pharmacol Rev 1999; 51:159–211.

2. Caterina MJ, Schumacher MA, Tominaga M, et al. The capsaicin receptor: a heat-activated ion channel in the pain pathway. Nature 1997; 389:816–824.

3. Hayes P, Meadows J, Gunthorpe MJ, et al. Cloning and functional expression of a human orthologue of rat vanilloid receptor-1. Pain 2000; 88:205–215.

4. Gunthorpe MJ, Benham CD, Randall A, Davies JB. The diversity in the vanilloid (TRPV) receptor family of ion channels. Trends Pharmacol Sci 2002; 23:183–191.

5. Szallasi A, Farkas-Szallasi T, Tucker JB, et al. Effects of systemic resiniferatoxin on substance P mRNA in rat dorsal root ganglia and substance P receptor mRNA in the spinal cord. Brain Res 1999; 815:177–184.

6. Avelino A, Cruz C, Cruz F. Nerve growth factor regulates galanin and *c-jun* overexpression occurring in dorsal root ganglion cells after intravesical resiniferatoxin application. Brain Res 2002; 951:264–269.

7. Di Marzo V, De Petrocellis L, Sepe N, et al. Biosynthesis of anandamide and related acylethanolamides in mouse J774 macrophages and N18 neuroblastoma cells. Biochem J 1996; 316:977–984.

8. Zygmunt PM, Peterson J, Andersson DA, et al. Vanilloid receptors on sensory nerves mediate the vasodilator action of anandamide. Nature 1999; 400:452–457.

9. de Groat WC, Kawatani M, Hisamitsu T, et al. Mechanisms underlying the recovery of urinary bladder function following spinal cord injury. J Auton Nerv Syst 1990; 30(suppl):S71–S77.

10. Fowler CJ, Jewkes D, McDonald WI, et al. Intravesical capsaicin for neurogenic bladder dysfunction. Lancet 1992; 339:1239.

11. Fowler CJ, Beck RO, Gerrard S, et al. Intravesical capsaicin for the treatment of detrusor hyperreflexia. J Neurol Neurosurg Psychiatry 1994; 57:169–173.

12. Geirsson G, Fall M, Sullivan L. Clinical and urodynamic effects of intravesical capsaicin treatment in patients with chronic traumatic spinal detrusor hyperreflexia. J Urol 1995; 154:1825–1829.

13. Das A, Chancellor MB, Watanabe T, et al. Intravesical capsaicin in neurogenic impaired patients with detrusor hyperreflexia. J Spinal Cord Med 1996; 19:190–193.

14. Igawa Y, Komiyama I, Nishizawa O, Ogawa A. Intravesical capsaicin inhibits autonomic dysreflexia in patients with spinal cord injury. Neurourol Urodyn 1996; 15:374–375. [Abstract]

15. Cruz F, Guimarães M, Silva C, et al. Desensitization of bladder sensory fibers by intravesical capsaicin has long lasting clinical and urodynamic effects in patients with hyperactive or hypersensitive bladder dysfunction. J Urol 1997; 157:585–589.

16. De Ridder D, Chandiramani V, Dasgupta P, et al. Intravesical capsaicin as a treatment for refractory detrusor hyperreflexia: a dual center study with long-term followup. J Urol 1997; 158:2087–2092.

17. de Séze M, Wiart L, Joseph PA, et al. Capsaicin and neurogenic detrusor hyperreflexia. A double blind placebo controlled study in 20 patients with spinal cord lesions. Neurourol Urodyn 1998; 17:513–523.

18. Cruz F, Guimarães M, Silva C, Reis M. Suppression of bladder hyperreflexia by intravesical resiniferatoxin. Lancet 1997; 350:640–641.

19. Lazzeri M, Beneforti P, Turini D. Urodynamic effects of intravesical resiniferatoxin in humans: preliminary results in stable and unstable detrusor. J Urol 1997; 158:2093–2096.

20. Lazzeri M, Spinelli M, Beneforti P, et al. Intravesical resiniferatoxin for the treatment of detrusor hyperreflexia refractory to capsaicin in patients with chronic spinal cord diseases. Scand J Urol Nephrol 1998; 32:331–334.

21. Silva C, Rio ME, Cruz F. Desensitization of bladder sensory fibers by intravesical resiniferatoxin, a capsaicin analog: long-term results for the treatment of detrusor hyperreflexia. Eur Urol 2000; 38:444–452.

22. Cruz F, Silva C, Ribeiro M, Avelino A. The effect of intravesical resiniferatoxin in neurogenic forms of bladder overactivity. Preliminary results of a randomised placebo controlled clinical trial. Neurourol Urodyn 2002; 21:426–427. [Abstract]

23. Park WH, Kim HG, Park BJ, et al. Comparison of the effects of intravesical capsaicin and resiniferatoxin for treatment of detrusor hyperreflexia in patients with spinal cord injury. Neurourol Urodyn 1999; 18:402. [Abstract]

24. Giannantoni A, Di Stasi SM, Stephen RL, et al. Intravesical capsaicin versus resiniferatoxin in patients with detrusor hyperreflexia: a prospective randomized study. J Urol 2002; 167:1710–1714.

25. de Sèze M, Wiart L, de Sèze M, et al. Efficacy and tolerance of intravesical instillation of capsaicin and resiniferatoxin for the treatment of detrusor hyperreflexia in spinal cord injured patients. A double-blind controlled study: preliminary results. Neurourol Urodyn 2002; 21:41–42. [Abstract]

26. Chandiramani V, Peterson T, Duthie GS, Fowler CJ. Urodynamic changes during therapeutic intravesical instillations of capsaicin. Br J Urol 1996; 77:792–797.

27. Appendino G, Szallasi A. Euphorbium: modern research on its active principle, resiniferatoxin, revives an ancient medicine. Life Sci 1997; 60:681–696.

28. Dasgupta P, Chandiramani V, Parkinson MC, et al. Treating the human bladder with capsaicin: is it safe? Eur Urol 1998; 33:28–31.

29. Silva C, Avelino A, Souto-Moura C, Cruz F. A light and electron microscope histopathological study of the human bladder mucosa after intravesical resiniferatoxin application. BJU Int 2001; 88:355–360.

30. Cruz F. Desensitization of bladder sensory fibers by intravesical capsaicin or capsaicin analogs. A new strategy for treatment of urge incontinence in patients with spinal detrusor hyperreflexia or bladder hypersensitivity disorders. Int Urogynecol J 1998; 9:214–220.

31. Szallasi A, Fowler CJ. After a decade of intravesical vanilloid therapy: still more questions than answers. Lancet Neurology 2002; 1:167–172.

32. Jankovic J, Brin MF. Botulinum toxin: historical perspective and potential new indications. Muscle Nerve 1997; 6(suppl):129–145.

33. Dykstra DD, Sidi AA. Treatment of detrusor-sphincter dyssynergia with botulinum A toxin: a double-blind study. Arch Phys Med Rehab 1990; 71:24–26.

34. Schurch B, Hauri D, Rodic B, et al. Botulinum-A toxin as a treatment of detrusor-sphincter dyssynergia: a prospective study in 24 spinal cord injury patients. J Urol 1996; 155:1023–1029.

35. Schurch B, Schmid DM, Stohrer M. Treatment of neurogenic incontinence with botulinum toxin A. N Engl J Med 2000; 342:665.

36. Reitz A, von Tobel J, Stohrer M, et al. European experience of 184 cases treated with botulinum-A toxin injections into the detrusor muscle for neurogenic incontinence. Neurourol Urodyn 2002; 21:427–428. [Abstract]

37. Schulte-Baukloh H, Michael T, Schobert J, et al. Efficacy of botulinum-A toxin in children with detrusor hyperreflexia due to myelomeningocele: preliminary results. Urology 2002; 59:325–328.

38. Corcos J, Al-Taweel W, Pippi Salle J, et al. The treatment of detrusor hyperreflexia using botulinum A toxin in myelomeningocele patients unresponsive to anticholinergic. Neurourol Urodyn 2002; 21:332–333. [Abstract]

39. Odergen T, Hjaltason H, Kaakkola, S, et al. A double blind, randomised, parallel group study to investigate the dose equivalence of Dysport® and Botox® in the treatment of cervical dystonia. J Neurol Neurosurg Psychiatry 1998; 64:6–12.

40. Brendler BCH, Radebaugh LC, Mohler JL. Topical oxybutynin chloride for relaxation of dysfunctional bladders. J Urol 1989; 141:1350–1352.

41. Madersbacher H, Jilg G. Control of detrusor hyperreflexia by the intravesical instillation of oxybutynin hydrochloride. Paraplegia 1991; 29:84–90.

42. Greenfield SP, Fera M. The use of intravesical oxybutynin chloride in children with neurogenic bladder. J Urol 1991; 146:532–534.

43. Massada CA, Kogan BA, Trigo-Rocha FE. The pharmacokinetics of intravesical and oral oxybutynin chloride. J Urol 1992; 148:595–597.

44. Weese DL, Roskamp DA, Leach GE, Zimmern PE. Intravesical oxybutynin chloride: experience with 42 patients. Urology 1993; 41:527–530.

45. Frohlich G, Burmeister S, Wiedeman A, Bulitta M. Intravesical instillation of trospium chloride, oxybutynin and verapamil for relaxation of the bladder detrusor muscle. A placebo controlled, randomized clinical test. Arzneimittelforschung 1998; 48:486–491.

46. Prasad KV, Vaidyanathan S. Intravesical oxybutynin chloride and clean intermittent catheterisation in patients with neurogenic vesical dysfunction and decreased bladder capacity. Br J Urol 1993; 72:519–522.

47. Mizunaga M, Miyata M, Kaneko S, et al. Intravesical instillation of oxybutynin hydrochloride therapy for patients with a neurogenic bladder. Paraplegia 1994; 32:25–29.

48. Palmer LS, Zebold K, Firlit CF, Kaplan WE. Complications of intravesical oxybutynin chloride therapy in the pediatric myelomeningocele population. J Urol 1997; 157:638–640.

49. Lose G, Norgaad JP. Intravesical oxybutynin for treating incontinence resulting from an overactive detrusor. BJU Int 2001; 87:767–771.

50. Buyse G, Verpoorten C, Vereecken R, Casaer P. Treatment of neurogenic bladder dysfunction in infants and children with neurospinal dysraphism with clean intermittent (self)-catheterisation and optimized intravesical oxybutynin hydrochloride therapy. Eur J Pediatr Surg 1995; 5(suppl 1):31–34.

51. Saito M, Tabuchi F, Otsubo K, Miyagawa I. Treatment of overactive bladder with modified intravesical oxybutynin chloride. Neurourol Urodyn 2000; 19:683–688.

52. Dmochowski RR A, Appell RA. Advancements in pharmacologic management of the overactive bladder. Urology 2000; 1(suppl):41–49.

53. Gurpinar T, Truong LD, Wong HY, Griffith DP. Electromotive drug administration to the urinary bladder: an animal model and preliminary results. J Urol 1996; 156:1496–1501.

54. Di Satsi SM, Giannantoni A, Massoud R, et al. Electromotive administration of oxybutynin into the human bladder wall. J Urol 1997; 158:228–233.

55. Riedl CR, Knoll M, Plas E, Pfluger H. Intravesical electromotive administration technique: preliminary results and side effects. J Urol 1998; 159:1851–1856.

56. Di Stasi SM, Giannantoni A, Vespasiani G, et al. Intravesical electromotive administration of oxybutynin in patients with detrusor hyperreflexia unresponsive to standard anticholinergics regimens. J Urol 2001; 165:491–498.

57. Mattiasson A, Ekstrom B, Andersson KE. Effects of intravesical instillation of verapamil in patients with detrusor hyperactivity. J Urol 1989; 141:174–177.

16

Transdermal oxybutynin administration

G Willy Davila

Introduction

Overactive bladder (OAB) is a chronic condition characterized by symptoms of urinary urgency, frequency, and nocturia, with or without urge incontinence, caused by involuntary contractions of the detrusor smooth muscle during bladder filling. It it estimated to affect approximately 34 million individuals in the United States, mostly women, and can have a markedly negative impact on quality of life. Long-term therapy for OAB is generally required to maintain symptomatic relief. Bladder training and other nonpharmacologic interventions may be effective in many cases, but lack of patient motivation and poor compliance restrict the long-term effectiveness of these approaches.[1,2] The mainstay of treatment for OAB is therefore pharmacologic therapy with antimuscarinic drugs. Unfortunately, they are limited in their clinical utility because of their propensity to induce dose-limiting side-effects, such as dry mouth, constipation, and sedation, thereby reducing patient compliance.

Oxybutynin, the primary antimuscarinic drug used to treat the symptoms of OAB, has been available for oral administration for more than 25 years. Although other drugs have now reached the market, oxybutynin remains a favorable treatment option.

The mechanism of action of oxybutynin, a cholinergic muscarinic receptor antagonist, is to competitively inhibit the binding of acetylcholine at postganglionic cholinergic receptor sites in the bladder smooth muscle. Oxybutynin also independently relaxes bladder smooth muscle and has local anesthetic properties.[3] Following oral administration, oxybutynin is extensively metabolized to the active compound N-desethyloxybutynin (N-DEO). N-DEO plasma levels have been associated with anticholinergic side-effects. With the development of a controlled-release oral formulation, and now with transdermal delivery, metabolism is reduced, efficacy is maintained, and side-effects are decreased. The contributions of the parent compound to efficacy and the metabolite to anticholinergic side-effects are becoming increasingly clear as more clinical experience is gained with improved delivery systems. The therapeutic effectiveness of oxybutynin is dose-related and occurs in conjunction with improvement in urodynamic parameters. Oxybutynin reduces the number of impulses reaching the detrusor muscle, thereby delaying the initial desire to void and increasing bladder capacity.[4]

As higher oral doses of oxybutynin are administered to achieve efficacy, dry mouth becomes more pronounced; therefore, alternative routes of administration have been tried. Intravesical therapy was found to alter the pharmacokinetic properties – a significantly lower concentration of the primary metabolite, N-DEO, reaches the systemic circulation, resulting in fewer anticholinergic side-effects.[5] Instillation of oxybutynin directly into the bladder is clinically effective and in most cases causes minimal or no dry mouth.[6] Because this route of administration is impractical, it is currently used only in special clinical circumstances.[7]

Recently, an oxybutynin transdermal delivery system (Oxytrol™, Watson Pharmaceuticals, Inc., Salt Lake City, Utah)[8] has been shown to provide continuous delivery of oxybutynin over 96 h, by way of a matrix-type delivery system applied to the patient's skin. This route of administration alters the pharmacokinetic profile of oxybutynin, thereby minimizing anticholinergic side-effects without compromising clinical efficacy.[9]

Transdermal drug delivery

Background

Transdermal drug administration for the pharmacologic treatment of systemic conditions has the known advantage of avoidance of presystemic gastrointestinal and hepatic 'first-pass' metabolism, which allows administration of lower doses to achieve similar plasma concentrations. Other advantages include avoidance of gastrointestinal interactions, consistent drug release over a prolonged period of time, ease of patient compliance, and utility when oral or parenteral drug administration is not ideal.

Transdermal application systems are currently in use for the treatment of angina pectoris, chronic pain syndromes, and motion sickness; to provide hormone replacement therapy and contraception; and for assistance with smoking cessation.

Transdermal systems (TDSs) vary in the technology used for delivering drugs across the stratum corneum (first layer of skin) and in their dosing frequencies. For example, the first marketed transdermal delivery system employed both a drug reservoir and rate-controlling semipermeable membrane and required daily dosing. Subsequently, hormone replacement therapy with estradiol has been administered for 3½ to 7 days using a matrix-type TDS to women with symptoms associated with menopause.

Transdermal drug therapy for the overactive bladder

The currently available oxybutynin TDS is a matrix-type system requiring twice-weekly dosing. It is composed of three layers (Figure 16.1), as follows:

- The first layer is a backing film that provides the occlusion required for drug absorption.
- The second layer is the basis of the matrix technology and contains:

  a thin film of acrylic adhesive, which enables the system to attach to the skin
  oxybutynin dissolved in an acrylic adhesive
  glycerol triacetate (triacetin, USP), a nonalcoholic permeation enhancer that improves the ability of the drug to penetrate the skin.
- The third layer is a release liner that is peeled off for application.

The design of the matrix-type delivery system allows a controlled rate of drug absorption by means of a chemical method of enhancing skin permeation. Flux enhancers, or chemical penetration enhancers, improve permeation of the drug through the dermal layer, thereby allowing for diffusion into the systemic circulation.[10]

Pharmacokinetic advantage

The oxybutynin TDS has a significant pharmacokinetic advantage over oral oxybutynin, as it avoids presystemic metabolism of the parent compound. Presystemic metabolism refers to the metabolism of the parent compound, prior to entering the systemic circulation, by the CYP450 enzyme system in the gastrointestinal tract and liver following oral administration. With transdermal oxybutynin administration, the avoidance of presystemic metabolism lowers the extent to which the primary metabolite, N-DEO, becomes available to the systemic circulation, thus resulting in fewer anticholinergic side-effects, such as dry mouth, constipation, and drowsiness.

Steady and predictable diffusion of oxybutynin across the stratum corneum has been demonstrated.[9] In studies of human subjects, it has been shown that a 39 cm^2 TDS containing 36 mg of drug will deliver an average dose of 3.9 mg/day and result in average plasma concentrations of oxybutynin of about 4 ng/ml during twice-weekly application (Figure 16.2). In human subjects, the application of oxybutynin TDS to three distinct skin sites – the buttock, hip, and abdomen – showed the same absorption profile.[11]

Bioavailability studies in human subjects showed that after the application of the first oxybutynin TDS, the parent compound becomes available to target tissues within 2 h, peaks at about 24 h, and is sustained at a steady

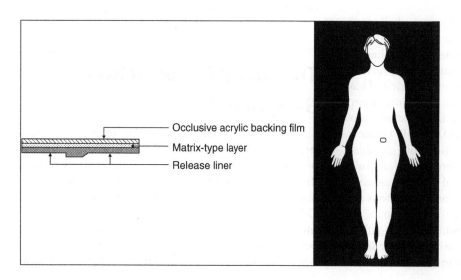

Occlusive acrylic backing film
Matrix-type layer
Release liner

Figure 16.1
A cross section of the matrix-type oxybutynin TDS (transdermal system). Placement of the oxybutynin TDS on the lower abdominal skin region.

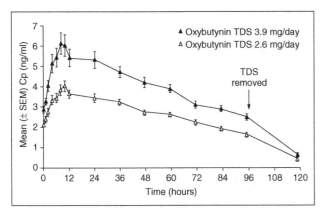

Figure 16.2
Plasma concentrations (Cp) were measured (SEM = standard error of the mean) following the subject's third application. The oxybutynin TDS (transdermal system) was removed after 96 hours.

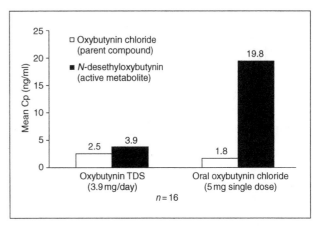

Figure 16.3
Mean plasma concentrations (Cp) were measured after a single 96-hour application of oxybutynin TDS 3.9 mg/day and a single 5 mg oral dose of oxybutynin chloride in 16 healthy subjects.

level for over 96 h. Steady-state concentrations are reached with the second application.[9]

In patients with OAB, plasma concentrations showed a linear relationship between the dose of oxybutynin TDS and plasma concentrations of both the parent compound, oxybutynin, and the active metabolite, N-DEO. This occurred from the lower (1.3 mg/day) to the upper (5.2 mg/day) dose studied.[12]

To show the alteration in first-pass hepatic and gastrointestinal metabolism of the parent oxybutynin compound during transdermal delivery, 16 human subjects participated in a study in which the plasma concentrations of the active metabolite and parent compound were measured following both oral and transdermal drug administration.[13] In the oral oxybutynin group, the average plasma concentration for N-DEO was 19.8 ng/ml and for the parent compound was 1.8 ng/ml, a ratio of approximately 10:1. In the oxybutynin TDS group, average plasma concentrations for N-DEO, the active metabolite, and the parent compound were 3.9 and 2.5 ng/ml, respectively, a ratio of approximately 1.2:1, showing the contrast of transdermally to orally administered oxybutynin in pharmacokinetic properties (Figure 16.3).

Clinical efficacy in the overactive bladder

The efficacy of oxybutynin TDS in the treatment of OAB was demonstrated in two clinical trials. The pivotal trial enrolled 520 patients and consisted of a 12-week, double-blind, placebo-controlled initial phase in which three doses of oxybutynin TDS (1.3, 2.6, and 3.9 mg/day) were compared with placebo. For patients receiving oxybutynin

TDS 3.9 mg/day, the median number of episodes of urinary incontinence decreased from 31 per week at baseline to 12 per week at end point (Figure 16.4), showing significance ($p = 0.017$) in the end-point change from baseline comparison to placebo (-19 vs -14.5, respectively). A supportive efficacy end point, the mean daily urinary frequency, decreased by 2.3 urinations per day from a baseline of 12 and was significant ($p = 0.046$) in comparison to placebo (-2.3 vs -1.7, respectively). In addition, the measured urinary voided volume increased significantly and quality of life scores improved in the group receiving oxybutynin TDS 3.9 mg/day.[14] Patients in all TDS treatment groups then entered a 12-week, open-label, dose-titration period and again experienced reductions in the number of urinary incontinence episodes per week.

In an earlier 6-week, dose-identification trial, 76 patients who had previously responded to treatment with oral oxybutynin were randomized to active treatment with either TDS or oral immediate-release oxybutynin. Dosages were titrated for each group, according to anticholinergic side-effects at weeks 2 and 4. Mean daily incontinence episodes were reduced from washout to end of treatment by approximately 5 in both groups ($p < 0.0001$), with no significant difference between transdermal and oral therapy (Figure 16.5). After 6 weeks of treatment, daily incontinence episodes were reduced to 2.4 ± 2.4 in the transdermal group and 2.6 ± 3.3 in the oral group.[12] A total of 8 patients in the TDS group and 10 patients in the oral group were continent on completion of the study.

Cystometry was performed before and at the end of treatment (Figure 16.6). Bladder volume (mean $\pm$ SD) at first detrusor contraction increased by 66 ± 126 ml for the transdermal group ($p = 0.005$) and 45 ± 163 ml in the oral group ($p = 0.1428$). Maximum bladder capacity

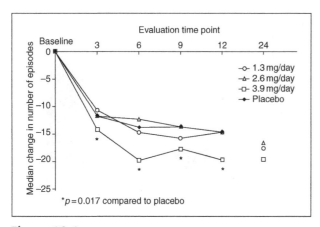

Figure 16.4
Patients taking oxybutynin TDS 3.9 mg/day had a significant decrease in the number of urinary incontinence episodes per week from baseline (BL) to end point.

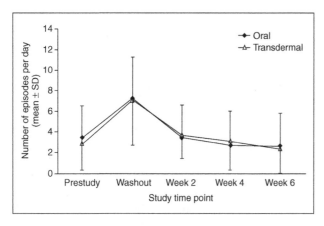

Figure 16.5
Incontinence episodes (mean ± SD) in 72 patients receiving titrated doses of both oral and transdermal oxybutynin during 6 weeks of treatment.

(mean ± SD) increased 53 ± 8 and 51 ± 138 ml in the transdermal ($p = 0.0011$) and the oral ($p = 0.0538$) groups, respectively.[12]

Side-effect profile

The improved anticholinergic side-effect profile of oxybutynin TDS over oral oxybutynin is the most important clinical consequence of this novel route of oxybutynin administration.

In the pivotal trial of 520 patients who received either TDS oxybutynin in doses of 1.3 mg/day, 2.6 mg/day, or 3.9 mg/day, or placebo, the overall frequency of dry mouth was 7.0% for the oxybutynin TDS group and 8.3% for

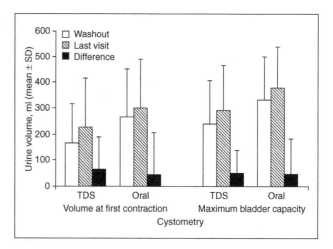

Figure 16.6
Bladder volume at first contraction and maximum bladder capacity in patients receiving TDS ($n = 33$) and oral ($n = 30$) oxybutynin in patients at washout and after 6 weeks of treatment. Patients received titrated doses of oxybutynin between time points.

placebo. Constipation, which can be especially troublesome in older patients, occurred in only 3% of subjects receiving either TDS oxybutynin or placebo. The incidence of dizziness and somnolence was similar to that of the placebo group.[14] The most common adverse event of TDS oxybutynin is a skin reaction at the application site – generally pruritus (16.8%) or erythema (5.6%). In all clinical trials for patients treated with the largest available patch, 3.9 mg/day of TDS oxybutynin ($n = 331$), application site reaction occurred in 14.8% of patients and was mostly mild or moderate in severity and completely reversible.[14]

A review of published clinical trial reports, such as the OBJECT study, shows the incidence of anticholinergic side-effects for oral oxybutynin formulations to be higher than reported in the TDS oxybutynin pivotal clinical trial (Table 16.1).

Dose escalation and occurrence of dry mouth

The first clinical trial of oxybutynin TDS ($n = 76$) was designed to determine the dose limitation in patients with OAB, based on tolerability of anticholinergic side-effects in two parallel groups taking either oral or TDS oxybutynin. Patients entered the trial based on their pre-study dose of oral oxybutynin at one of three TDS dose levels – 2.6, 3.9, or 5.2 mg/day – and had their dose increased every 2 weeks to the maximum of 5.2 mg/day, according to their tolerance of dry mouth. At the 6-week study visit, 68% of the patients receiving oxybutynin TDS had titrated to the maximal dose of 5.2 mg/day compared with 32% of

Table 16.1 *Incidence of dry mouth for orally administered anticholinergic drugs*

Published clinical trials	OXY (%)	OXY er (%)	TOL (%)	OXY TDS (%)	PLA (%)
Appell et al:[15] OXY er, 10 mg/d TOL, 2 mg bid		28.1	33.2		
Davila et al:[12] OXY TDS, 2.6–5.2 mg od OXY, 10–20 mg od	94[b]			38[b]	
Dmochowski et al:[14] OXY TDS, 3.9 mg od PLA				9.6	8.3
Tapp et al:[16] OXY, 5 mg qid PLA	29				10
Thuroff et al:[17] OXY, 5 mg tid PLA	48				12
Birns et al:[18] OXY, 5 mg bid OXY er, 10 mg od	16.7	22.6			
Versi et al:[19] OXY, 5–20 mg[a] OXY er, 5–20 mg[a]	7 (5 mg) 26 (10 mg) 39 (15 mg) 45 (20 mg)	4 (5 mg) 9 (10 mg) 19 (15 mg) 40 (20 mg)			
Anderson et al:[20] OXY, 5 mg od-qid[a] OXY er, 5–30 mg, od[a]	87	68			
Burgio et al:[21] OXY, 2.5 mg od to 5 mg tid[a]	96.9				

[a] Titrated doses.

[b] At maximum tolerated dose.

OXY, oxybutynin; TOL, tolterodine; TDS, transdermal system; PLA, placebo; er, extended-release formulation; od, daily; bid, twice daily; tid, three times daily; qid, four times daily.

patients taking oral oxybutynin.[12] No patient using the oxybutynin TDS had intolerable dry mouth; 62% did not report any dry mouth; and only 11% had moderate, tolerable dry mouth at the final visit.[12] This low incidence of dry mouth, the major anticholinergic side-effect of oxybutynin, contrasts with incidences of 9% intolerable and 59% moderate but tolerable incidence for oral oxybutynin.

Convenience and quality of life

Patients may exercise, shower, or bathe with the TDS in place. The translucent nature of the oxybutynin TDS improves aesthetic acceptability to the patient. The quality of life (QoL) Incontinence Impact Questionnaire showed a significant improvement ($p < 0.05$) compared with that of placebo (Figure 16.7).

Discussion

Transdermal delivery is a novel approach for the administration of oxybutynin to patients with OAB. Although oxybutynin has a long-established history of efficacy in reducing the number of episodes of urge incontinence, a large percentage of patients discontinue oral oxybutynin because of intolerable anticholinergic side-effects, dry mouth in particular. Because side-effects are dose-related, it has not been possible for most patients to tolerate higher,

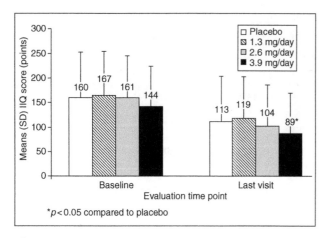

Figure 16.7
Patients with oxybutynin TDS reported improved quality of life on the Incontinence Impact Questionnaire (IIQ) during the double-blind treatment period. Numerical values are in inverse relation to quality of life.

more therapeutically effective doses. The TDS was developed to minimize anticholinergic side-effects by modifying the metabolism and plasma concentration profile of oxybutynin.

By avoiding presystemic gastrointestinal and hepatic metabolism, transdermal delivery of oxybutynin reduces the incidence of anticholinergic side-effects, specifically dry mouth, while maintaining its efficacy in controlling the symptoms of OAB. The incidence of dry mouth is dose-related and reported to be 7.0% overall for oxybutynin TDS and similar to placebo (8.3%).

In conclusion, the pharmacokinetic changes that result from transdermal administration of oxybutynin make it possible to achieve higher plasma levels of oxybutynin with much lower dosing compared to oral administration. Dosing of oxybutynin can thus be optimized without intolerable anticholinergic side-effects. The TDS offers a convenient, efficacious, and well-tolerated route of administering oxybutynin to patients with symptoms of OAB.

References

1. Frewen W. Role of bladder training in the treatment of the unstable bladder in the female. Urol Clin N Am 1979; 6:273–277.

2. Oldenburg B, Millard RJ. Predictors of long term outcome following a bladder re-training programme. J Psychosom Res 1986; 30:691–698.

3. Rovner ES, Wein AJ. Modern pharmacotherapy of urge urinary incontinence in the USA: tolterodine and oxybutynin. BJU Int 2000; 86:44–54.

4. United States Pharmacopeial Convention. Oxybutynin: systemic. In: United States Pharmacopeial Convention, ed. Drug information for the health care professional. Englewood, CO: Micromedex, 2001:2300–2302.

5. Buyse G, Waldeck K, Verpoorten C, et al. Intravesical oxybutynin for neurogenic bladder dysfunction: less systemic side effects due to reduced first pass metabolism. J Urol 1998; 160:892–896.

6. Dmochowski RR, Appell RA. Advancements in pharmacologic management of the overactive bladder. Urology 2000; 56:41–49.

7. Madersbacher H, Jilg G. Control of detrusor hyperreflexia by the intravesical instillation of oxybutynin hydrochloride. Paraplegia 1991; 29:84–90.

8. Watson Pharmaceuticals I. Data on File, Oxytrol™ NDA 21-351. 2001.

9. Zobrist RH, Thomas H, Sanders SW. Pharmacokinetics and metabolism of transdermally administered oxybutynin. Clin Pharmacol Ther 2002:P94. [Abstract]

10. Ranade VV. Drug delivery systems: 6. Transdermal drug delivery. J Clin Pharmacol 1991; 31:401–418.

11. Sanders SW, Thomas H, Zobrist RH. Population pharmacokinetics of transdermally administered oxybutynin. Clin Pharmacol Ther 2002:P34. [Abstract]

12. Davila GW, Daugherty CA, Sanders SW. A short-term, multicenter, randomized double-blind dose titration study of the efficacy and anticholinergic side effects of transdermal compared to immediate release oral oxybutynin treatment of patients with urge urinary incontinence. J Urol 2001; 166:140–145.

13. Zobrist RH, Schmid B, Feick A, et al. Pharmacokinetics of the R- and S-enantiomers of oxybutynin and N-desethyloxybutynin following oral and transdermal administration of the racemate in health volunteers. Pharm Res 2001; 18:1029–1034.

14. Dmochowski RR, Davila GW, Zinner NR, et al. Efficacy and safety of transdermal oxybutynin in patients with urge and mixed urinary incontinence. J Urol 2002; 168:580–586.

15. Appell RA, Sand P, Dmochowski R, et al. Prospective randomized controlled trial of extended-release oxybutynin chloride and tolterodine tartrate in the treatment of overactive bladder: results of the OBJECT Study. Mayo Clin Proc 2001; 76:358–363.

16. Tapp AJ, Cardozo LD, Versi E, Cooper D. The treatment of detrusor instability in post-menopausal women with oxybutynin chloride: a double blind placebo controlled study. Br J Obstet Gynaecol 1990; 97:521–526.

17. Thuroff JW, Bunke B, Ebner A, et al. Randomized, double-blind, multicenter trial on treatment of frequency, urgency and incontinence related to detrusor hyperactivity: oxybutynin versus propantheline versus placebo. J Urol 1991; 145:813–816.

18. Birns J, Lukkari E, Malone-Lee JG. A randomized controlled trial comparing the efficacy of controlled-release oxybutynin tablets (10 mg once daily) with conventional oxybutynin tablets (5 mg twice daily) in patients whose symptoms were stabilized on 5 mg twice daily of oxybutynin. BJU Int 2000; 85:793–798.

19. Versi E, Appell R, Mobley D, et al. Dry mouth with conventional and controlled-release oxybutynin in urinary incontinence. Obstet Gynecol 2000; 95:718–721.

20. Anderson RU, Mobley D, Blank B, et al. Once daily controlled versus immediate release oxybutynin chloride for urge urinary incontinence. J Urol 1999; 161:1809–1812.

21. Burgio KL, Locher JL, Goode PS, et al. Behavioral vs drug treatment for urge urinary incontinence in older women: a randomized controlled trial. JAMA 1998; 280:1995–2000.

17

Management of autonomic dysreflexia

Waleed Altaweel and Jacques Corcos

Autonomic dysreflexia (AD) is a life-threatening condition, and is considered a medical emergency. It is important for physicians dealing with spinal cord injury (SCI) patients to recognize and to be aware of the signs and symptoms of this syndrome. However, the signs and symptoms of AD might be minimal or absent, despite elevated blood pressure. SCI patients might have difficulty disclosing their symptoms when AD presents due to cognitive and verbal communication impairments. The key to successful management is prevention, through patient and family education, proper bladder, bowel, and skin care, and identification and avoidance of noxious stimuli. Health care providers should be aware of the potential causes of AD or treat it when it occurs.

Acute treatment

Normally, patients with SCI at T6 or above have normal systolic blood pressure of 90–110 mmHg. A sudden 20–40 mmHg increase of both systolic and diastolic blood pressure over baseline that is frequently associated with bradycardia may be a sign of AD.

If blood pressure is elevated, the patient needs to be placed upright in the sitting position. This maneuver pools blood in the lower limbs and might reduce the blood pressure.[1,2]

Tight clothing or any constrictive devices should be loosened to allow the blood to pool in the abdomen and lower extremities.[1,2]

SCI patients usually suffer impaired autonomic regulations. During AD, the blood pressure has the potential to fluctuate; therefore it should be monitored frequently (every 5 min) until the patient has stabilized.[1–6]

Triggering factors should be removed; the most common cause of AD is **bladder distention**:

- If an indwelling catheter is not in place, catheterize the patient.[3,7–10] Since catheterization can exacerbate AD, use intraurethral lidocaine (lignocaine) jelly and wait for 2 min to decrease sensory input and to relax the sphincter (Table 17.1).

- If the patient has a Foley catheter, check for obstruction or kinks.
- If the catheter is blocked, try to irrigate with 10–15 ml of warm saline; the use of a large volume or of a cold solution can exacerbate the autonomic dysreflexia. Avoid bladder distention and suprapubic percussion because it can worsen the condition. If this fails to decompress the bladder, change the catheter with lidocaine jelly.
- During bladder decompression, monitor the patient's blood pressure because sudden decompression will normalize it. However, hypotension might occur, especially if the patient has been given antihypertensive medication.
- If blood pressure elevation persists, then suspect **fecal impaction**. It is the second most common cause of AD.[3,7]
- Appropriate precaution should be taken before disimpaction, since additional stimulation could further aggravate AD.[11–13] Use intrarectal lidocaine jelly and wait 2 min before checking for the presence of stool.
- If present, gently disimpact it. If AD worsens, stop the manual evacuation and recheck after 20 min. However, if blood pressure is above 150 mmHg, consider **pharmacological management** before disimpaction:

1. Nifedipine or nitrates are the most commonly used medications during acute attack.[14–16] Nifedipine 10 mg, bitten and swallowed in the immediate-release form, is the preferred method of administration; treatment can be repeated in 30 min. Extreme caution should be exercised in the elderly or in patients with coronary artery disease, as it has been reported that nifedipine can cause hypotension and reflex tachycardia in individuals without SCI.[17]

2. Phenoxybenzamine, 10 mg orally, an alpha-receptor blocker, can be given to treat acute AD. It has been shown that phenoxybenzamine causes relaxation of the internal sphincter and controls the symptoms.[18,19]

3. Glyceryl trinitrate 300–600 µg S/L can be administered in appropriately monitored settings for rapid blood pressure control. It can be repeated

Table 17.1 *Practical acute management of AD*
1. If an indwelling urinary catheter is not in place, catheterize the patient
2. If an indwelling urinary catheter is already in place, check the system along its entire length for position, kinks, folds, constrictions, or obstructions
3. If the catheter appears to be blocked, gently irrigate the bladder with a small amount of fluid, such as normal saline, at body temperature. Avoid manually compressing or tapping on the bladder
4. If the catheter is draining and the blood pressure remains elevated, suspect fecal impaction; check the rectum for stool, using intrarectal lidocaine jelly as lubricant
5. If the situation is not corrected, administer an antihypertensive agent with rapid onset and short duration while the causes of AD are being investigated: • nifedipine 10 mg to be repeated every 30 min if necessary. It should be in the immediate-release form; bite-and-swallow is the preferred method, *not* sublingual treatment   • nitrates (e.g. glyceryl trinitrate). To be avoided the patient took sildenafil in the past 24 hours   • phenoxybenzamine 10 mg orally   • captopril 25 mg orally
6. Use antihypertensives with extreme caution in older persons or people with coronary artery disease
7. Monitor the individual's symptoms and blood pressure for at least 2 hours after resolution of the AD episode to ensure that blood pressure elevation does not reoccur. AD may resolve because of medication, not because of resolution of the underlying cause
8. If the response to treatment is poor and/or if the cause of the AD has not been identified, admit the patient for close monitoring, maintenance of pharmacological blood pressure control, and investigation of other possible causes

after 10 min. Sildenafil is being increasingly used to treat erectile dysfunction in SCI patients. Nitrates are contraindicated in patients taking sildenafil. The resulting blood pressure decrease may be huge and dangerous. If sildenafil is used within the last 24 h, another short-acting antihypertensive medication should be given.

4. Captopril 25 mg is an alternative for the management of hypertensive emergencies in AD. It acts within 30 min, achieves levels within 1–3 h and, has a half-life of 2–4 h. A pilot study has shown that it is safe and effective in treating patients with hypertension from AD.[20]

• Blood pressure should be monitored for symptomatic hypotension. If present, the patient should lie down and elevate his legs. If not controlled, then consider intravenous fluids and adrenergic agonist. If the precipitating cause has still not been determined, check for the least-frequent cause.

capable of preventing an AD attack if given shortly before stimulation (Table 17.2).[21] In patients with recurrent attacks, terazosin results in complete suppression of dysreflexic symptoms; a nightly dose of 5 mg reduces the severity, but does not eliminate the need for careful monitoring during provocative procedures.[22]

Anesthetic techniques for controlling AD include topical application for cystoscopy, general anesthesia, and spinal and epidural anesthesia. Lidocaine jelly decreases the sensation and relaxes the sphincter during cystoscopy, but bladder distention may trigger an AD episode despite local anesthesia. In one case report AD occurred despite general anesthesia.[23] Studies have shown that halothane anesthesia is more effective than other agents.[24–26] Spinal anesthesia has been reported to give excellent control,[9] and has been recommended to manage acute AD refractory to medical management.[27] Preoperative evaluation should include determination of the level of injury and history of dysreflexic episodes. Intraoperative and postoperative cardiac monitoring is recommended.[28–30]

Prophylactic treatment of autonomic dysreflexia and anesthetic considerations

Surgical, cystoscopic, urodynamic, and radiological procedures might precipitate acute AD. Nifedipine 10 mg is

Autonomic dysreflexia treatment during pregnancy and labor

Spinal cord injury patients should be monitored for urinary tract infections, fecal impaction, and blood

Table 17.2 *Preventive measures against autonomic dysreflexia*
• Frequent pressure relief in bed/chair
• Avoidance of sunburn/scalds
• Maintenance of regular bowel program
• A well-balanced diet and adequate fluid intake
• Compliance with medications

• For patients with an indwelling catheter:
  • keep the tubing free of kinks
  • keep the drainage bags empty
  • check daily for deposits inside the catheter

• If patients are on an intermittent catheterization program, they should catheterize themselves as often as necessary to prevent overfilling
• If patients void spontaneously, make sure that they have an adequate output
• Patients should carry an intermittent catheter kit when they are away from home
• In all cases: perform routine skin assessments
• Inform the health care staff if you tend to develop AD
• Carry Adalat (nifedipine) 10 mg; give 10 mg orally 30 min before stimulation

pressure during both gestation and labor. AD during pregnancy has the same pathophysiology and management. In addition, before vaginal examinations, urinary catheterizations, or rectal manipulation, use an anesthetic jelly to reduce stimulation. Bladder catheter drainage should be initiated and monitored frequently to avoid obstruction during labor.[31] It has also been proposed that monitoring during labor and delivery should ideally include:

1. an intra-arterial catheter for continuous blood pressure reading
2. telemetry for cardiac rhythm monitoring continuously
3. constant electronic fetal monitoring to identify fetal distress.[32]

A complete anesthesia consultation should be undertaken prior to labor. Epidural anesthesia with a combination of morphine, with bupivacaine,[33] or meperidine alone[34] has been reported in cases of successful deliveries in women with spinal cord lesions. Oral nifedipine, intravenous hydralazine, or trimethaphan has been recommended to control extremely high blood pressures in this population during labor.[33] Intravenous nitroprusside is not recommended because of elevated fetal cyanide levels.[35] Ganglionic-blocking agents with a short duration of action, such as a 0.1% solution of trimethaphan in 5% dextrose by intravenous drip, can be administered in refractory AD cases during labor that are not adequately controlled by regional anesthesia.[35]

Autonomic dysreflexia is a common complication of pregnancy SCI or patients. Prevention remains the most important factor in AD management to avoid morbidity and mortality in patients or their fetus. Patient and health worker should understand the pathophysiology, and causes and management of this syndrome to avoid serious complications.

Conclusion

Autonomic dysreflexia is an emergency often secondary to urological or gynecological problems or manipulations. Its management starts primarily with its prevention. Easy measures can avoid this highly risky event. Facing such events, physicians must be aware of simple procedures and the possible cascade of treatment that could be administered. Pregnancy and anesthesia have to be considered as precipitating factors supporting preventive and aggressive management.

References

1. Cole TM, Kotte FJ, Olsen M, et al. Alterations of cardiovascular control in high spinal myelomalacia. Arch Phys Med Rehab 1967; 48:359–368.

2. Guttman L, Frankel HL, Paeslack V. Cardiac irregularies during labor in paraplegic women. Paraplegia 1965; 66:144.

3. Colachis SC. Autonomic hyperreflexia in spinal cord injury. J Am Parapleg 1992; 15:171.

4. Erickson RP. Autonomic hyperreflexia, pathophysiology and medical management. Arch Phys Med Rehab 1980; 61:431.

5. Kewalramani LS. Autonomic dysreflexia in traumatic myelopathy. Am J Phys Med 1980; 59:1.

6. Kuric J, Hixon AK. Clinical practice guideline: autonomic dysreflexia. Jackson Height, NY: Eastern Paralyzed Veterans Association, 1996.

7. Lee BY, Karmakar MG, Herz BL, et al. Autonomic dysreflexia revisited. J Spinal Cord Med 1995; 18:75. [Review]

8. Lindun R, Joiner E, Frechafer AA, et al. Incidence and clinical features of autonomic dysreflexia in patients with spinal cord injury. Paraplegia 1980; 18:285.

9. Trop CS, Bennett CJ. Autonomic dysreflexia and its urological implications. J Urol 1992; 146:1461. [Review]

10. Wurster RD, Randall WC. Cardiovascular response to bladder distension in patients with spinal transection. Am J Physiol 1975; 228:1288.

11. O'Donnell WF. Urological management in the patient with acute spinal cord injury. Crit Care Clin 1987; 3:599.

12. Silver JR. Vascular reflexes in spinal shock. Paraplegia 1971; 8:231.

13. Muzumdar AS. The mass reflex; an emergency in the quadriplegic patient. Can Med Ass J 1982; 126:376.

14. Braddom RL, Rocco JF. Autonomic dysreflexia: a survey of current treatment. Am J Phys Med Rehab 1991; 70:234.

15. Dyskstra DD, Sidi AA, Anderson LC. The effect of nifedipine on cystoscopy induced autonomic dysreflexia in patients with high spinal cord injuries. J Urol 1987; 138:1115.

16. Thyberg M, Ertzgaard PE, Gylling M, et al. Effect of nifedipine on cystometry, induced elevation of bladder pressure in patients with reflex urinary bladder after a high level spinal cord injury. Paraplegia 1994; 32:308.

17. Grossman E, Messerli FH, Grodzicki T, Kowey P. Should a moratorium be placed on sublingual nifedipine capsules given for hypertensive emergencies and pseudo-emergencies?. JAMA 1996; 276:1328–1331.

18. Scott MB, Marrow JW. Phenoxybenzamine in neurogenic bladder dysfunction after spinal cord injury. Autonomic dysreflexia. J Urol 1978; 119:483.

19. McGuire J, Wagner FM, Weiss RM. Treatment of autonomic dysreflexia with phenoxybenzamine. J Urol 1976; 115:53.

20. Esmail Z, Shalansky K, Sunderji R, et al. Evaluation of captopril for the management of hypertension in autonomic dysreflexia. Pilot study. Arch Phys Med Rehab 2002; 38:604.

21. Lindan R, Lettler EJ, Kedia KR. A comparison of the efficacy of alpha adrenergic blocker and slow calcium channel blocker in autonomic dysreflexia. Paraplegia 1985; 23:34.

22. Viadyanathan S, Soni BM, Sett P, et al. Pathophysiology of autonomic dysreflexia: long-term treatment with terazosin in adult and pediatric spinal cord injury patients manifesting recurrent dysreflexic episodes. Spinal Cord 1998; 36:761.

23. Raeder JC, Gisvold SE. Perioperative autonomic hyperreflexia in high spinal cord lesions: a case report. Case report. Acta Anast Scand 1986; 30:672–673.

24. Ciliberti BJ, Goldfein J, Rovenstine EA. Hypertension during anesthesia in patients with spinal cord injures. Anesthesiology 1954; 15:273–279.

25. Alderson JD, Thomas DG. The use of halothane anesthesia to control autonomic hyperreflexia during transurethral surgery in spinal cord injury patient. Paraplegia 1975; 13:183.

26. Drinker AS, Helrich M. Halothane anesthesia in paraplegic patients. Anesthesiology 1963; 24:399.

27. Nieder RM, O'Higgins JW, Aldrete JA. Autonomic hyperreflexia in urologic surgery. JAMA 1970; 213:867–869.

28. Deasmon J. Paraplegia: problem confronting the anaesthesiologist. Cnad Anesth Soc J 1970; 17:435.

29. Schonwald G, Fish K, Perkash I. Cardiovascular complications during anesthesia in chronic spinal cord injured patients. Anesthesiology 1981; 55:550–558.

30. Fraser A, Edmonds-Seal J. Spinal cord injuries. A review of the problems facing the anesthetist. Anesthesia 1982; 37:1084–1098.

31. Greenspoon JS, Paul RH. Paraplegia and quadriplegia. Special consideration during pregnancy and labor and delivery. Am J Obstet Gynecol 1986; 155:738–741.

32. Gross LL, et al. Pregnancy, labour, delivery and post spinal cord injury. Paraplegia 1992; 30:890.

33. Crosby E, St. Jean B, Reid D, Elliott RD. Obstetrical anesthesia and analgesia in achronic spinal cord-injured women. Can J Anasth 1992; 36:487–494.

34. Baraka A. Epidural meperidine for control of autonomic hyperreflexia in a paraplegic paturient. Anesthesiology 1985; 62:688–690.

35. Tabsh K, Crinkman C, Reff R. Autonomic dysreflexia in pregnancy. Obstet Gynecol 1982; 60:119.

18

Peripheral electrical stimulation

Magnus Fall and Sivert Lindström

General background

Important prerequisites for continence are intactness of the vesicourethral supportive structures and of the smooth and the striated muscles of the urethra, the latter being composed of the intramural striated sphincter and the paraurethral components of the pelvic floor muscles. Most striated muscles of the body are composed of three motor unit types, one with slowly contracting muscle fibers and two with fast contraction properties.[1] The intramural urethral sphincter is special in being composed of slow fibers only, whereas the paraurethral striated muscles have varying numbers of all three types. The three motor unit types differ with respect to their maximal force development, fusion frequency – that is the activation frequency for a smooth sustained contraction – and resistance to fatigue. The slow units develop little force but are resistant to fatigue. Their fusion frequency is about 10 Hz. The fastest units can produce 10–20 times more contraction force but fatigue rapidly. Their fusion frequency is around 40–50 Hz. The intermediate fast units are somewhat weaker but considerably more fatigue-resistant. It follows that the intramural striated sphincter can generate a well-sustained but rather limited increase in urethral pressure. The main function of this muscle seems to be to accomplish urethral closure during bladder filling at rest, when there is little physical stress. In more provocative situations, when the intra-abdominal pressure suddenly increases, e.g. lifting, coughing, and running (when most women with stress urinary incontinence leak), the fast motor units of the paraurethral pelvic floor muscles provide a rapidly induced, strong closing force upon the urethra. This contraction is in fact governed by the central motor program during self-generated increases of the intra-abdominal pressure, thereby allowing these muscles to contract in advance of the pressure rise. They are also promptly reflexly engaged by pressure increases from the outside caused by a sudden push towards the abdominal wall, but in this situation the contraction lags behind the pressure increase. The pressures generated by the pelvic floor muscles upon the urethra clearly exceed the maximal detrusor or

intra-abdominal pressures in intact subjects. Thus, there is normally a reliable safety margin.

Bladder filling is detected by mechanoreceptors in the bladder wall. These receptors respond both to passive distention and to active contraction of the detrusor.[2] The afferent signals are transmitted, mainly via the pelvic nerves, to the spinal cord, and ascend bilaterally in the dorsolateral white matter. The information eventually reaches the cerebral cortex in the medial region of its somatosensory area[3,4] and gives rise to the sensation of bladder filling and urgency. The afferent signal also influences neurons in Barrington's micturition center in the upper pons.[5] When appropriately activated, descending neurons in this center drive preganglionic bladder pelvic neurons in the sacral cord, and thereby induce a micturition contraction. Once initiated, the micturition reflex is self-sustained by a positive feedback mechanism. The reflex detrusor contraction generates an increased bladder pressure and an enhanced activation of bladder mechanoreceptors. This afference, in turn, reinforces the activation of the pontine micturition center and the pelvic motor output to the bladder, resulting in a further increase in bladder pressure and mechanoreceptor afference. When urine enters the urethra, the reflex is further enhanced by activation of urethral receptors.[6] Normally, this positive feedback mechanism ascertains a complete emptying of the bladder during micturition. As long as there is any fluid left in the lumen, the intravesical pressure will be maintained above the threshold for the mechanoreceptors, which will provide a continuous drive for the detrusor.

A drawback with this arrangement is that the reflex system may easily become unstable. Any stimulus that elicits a small burst of impulses in mechanoreceptor afferents may trigger a micturition reflex. To prevent this from happening during the filling phase, the micturition reflex pathway is controlled by several inhibitory mechanisms at spinal and supraspinal levels.[7] The micturition reflex has normally an all-or-nothing character. The pelvic efferents to the bladder are silent during the filling phase but, due to the positive feedback system, they fire maximally during micturition contractions.

Activation of continence reflexes by electrical stimulation

Penile,[8] clitoris,[9] and vaginal electrical stimulation[10,11] activates the motor fibers to the pelvic floor and the intramural urethral sphincter, either directly or by reflex mechanisms, or both.[10–13] At these sites of stimulation, further reflexes are evoked with the afferent limb in the pudendal nerve and with three concomitant central actions: activation of hypogastic inhibitory fibers to the bladder; central inhibition of the pelvic outflow to the bladder; and central inhibition of the ascending afferent pathway from the bladder.[4,12,14] This reflex is silent at rest and seems to be designed to prevent bladder contractions during coitus. Anal stimulation[15,16] inhibits the bladder in a similar fashion by a reflex with its afferent limb in pelvic nerve branches to the anal region,[17] a reflex designed to inhibit the bladder during defecation. Thus, perineal methods for electrical stimulation utilize natural reflexes that are silent during normal, everyday life but capable of sustained bladder inhibition when evoked by continuous or intermittent electrical stimulation.

It is generally believed that in the normal situation, bladder inhibition follows pelvic floor contraction and that bladder inhibition elicited by electrical stimulation would result from pelvic floor activation.[14] However, in animal experimental studies it has been demonstrated that there is rather activation of specific inhibitory pudendal afferents. Lindström et al[12] showed that complete relaxation of the pelvic floor by succinylcholine did not abolish the inhibitory effect of stimulation. Subsequently, it has been demonstrated that there are separate systems for bladder and urethral sphincter activation. In patients with so-called uninhibited overactive bladder there was a dissociation of the ability to exhibit bladder inhibition and sphincter activation, respectively, in 21% of patients.[18] In experiments in cats, Blok and Holstege[19] described separate centers for micturition (M-region pontine center) and storage (L-region pontine center). The M region excites bladder muscle through projections to its motoneurons and inhibits the urethral sphincter through γ-aminobutyric acid (GABA) interneurons, which inhibits the sphincter. The L region acts independently and excites the sphincter motoneurons.

The therapeutic effects of functional electrical stimulation (FES), on the bladder as well as the sphincter mechanism, depends on artificial activation of nerves. The first requirement for an effect is that the stimulation intensity is high enough to evoke an activity in the relevant nerves. The threshold intensity varies inversely with the fiber diameter, distance between the nerves and the stimulating electrodes, and the pulse configuration. Large myelinated fibers, like efferents to the pelvic floor, have the lowest threshold. Anogenital cutaneous afferents involved in bladder inhibition and pelvic floor muscle reflexes (bulbocavernosus reflex) have intermediate values, whereas afferents responsible for pain sensation have the highest. In practice the distance between electrode and nerve fiber is more important. Thus, all external electrodes induce skin or mucosal sensations at much lower intensities than pelvic floor contractions by direct stimulation of the motor fibers. For the same reason, the difference between the detection threshold and the pain effects is quite narrow, with the maximal tolerance level reached at intensities about 1.5–2 times the detection threshold.[20] From experimental studies it is clear that the tolerance level is well below that required for maximal bladder inhibition or pelvic floor contraction. It follows that proper electrode design that permits positioning of the electrodes close to the relevant nerves is mandatory to achieve good clinical effects.

Any pulse configuration would do for nerve activation, provided the stimulators can generate high enough intensities (in mA or V). Short square-wave pulses (0.2–0.5 ms) are most effective, however, in terms of charge transfer for a given biological effect.[28,29] To minimize electrochemical reactions at the electrode–mucosa interphase, it is preferable to use biphasic or polarity alternating pulses.

Stimulation frequency is another crucial factor. Due to the contractile properties of the fast and slow motor units, a high stimulation frequency, 50–100 Hz is required for maximal urethral closure. The bladder inhibitory reflex systems operate at much lower frequencies. Maximal inhibition via the sympathetic route is obtained at about 5 Hz, and 5–10 Hz is also the best frequency for central inhibition of the pelvic outflow to the bladder. Since the lower frequency may be unpleasant, 10 Hz stimulation has been recommended as a practical compromise. In clinical experiments in women with detrusor overactivity, cystometric registrations and isobaric volume recordings were performed to document effects during intravaginal electrical stimulation.[21] With these procedures it was easy to demonstrate an abolishment of phasic detrusor contractions and an increase in bladder volume during stimulation, an effect most evident at low-frequency stimulation (10 Hz). Vereecken et al[22] and Vodusek et al[23] observed similar effects but did not see any difference in the degree of bladder inhibition at stimulation frequencies between 5 and 20 Hz. All frequencies in that range do elicit bladder inhibition and it is quite plausible that different clinical conditions, like idiopathic phasic detrusor overactivity vs detrusor overactivity in spinal cord injury, may require somewhat different technique for an optimal response. Detrusor inhibition has likewise been demonstrated by anal[16] or penile surface[8] electrodes. The frequency characteristics are similar for reflexes elicited from anal or genital stimulation. Engagement of larger pudendal nerve branches or selective stimulation of clitoris or penile nerve branches has been found to optimize the effect. It has been suggested that the effect on the bladder can be further improved if the pudendal nerve stimulation is calibrated by electrophysiological monitoring of the 'maximal motor response'.[24]

In trials without drugs, adequate urethral closure was obtained at 20–50 Hz, the lower frequency being a good compromise for patients with mixed stress and urge incontinence. Muscle fatigue is an important problem. When using FES for incontinence, intermittent trains of impulses have been found to reduce this problem.[25,26] Another factor to consider is the long-term effect of chronic stimulation on the pelvic floor muscles. As one effect, it has been proposed that chronic stimulation increases the relative number of slow-twitch fibers in the paraurethral muscles,[27] since it has previously been found for leg muscles that long-lasting slow stimulation may transform intermediate fast motor units to such with mainly slow properties.[28] Slow and intermediate motor units are also recruited first in reflex activation of the motor pool. Intermittent high-frequency stimulation would, if anything, be expected to have the opposite effect, though. To improve urethral closure at sudden increases of the intra-abdominal pressure, stronger fast-twitch fibers would be desirable, not the opposite.

A clinically most significant result of peripheral electrical stimulation is the carry-over or re-education effect: in some patients there is long-term remission of symptoms after repeated electrical stimulation,[10,29–31] sometimes lasting for years.[32] The physiological basis of this seemingly curative effect of stimulation is not yet fully explained but no doubt involves modulation of central nervous activity. A change of peripheral receptor activity after chronic stimulation has been suggested, too,[33,34] which may contribute to a normalization of micturition pattern. Recently, Jiang,[35] during anogenital electrical stimulation in the rat, demonstrated that 5 min stimulation at 10 Hz induced a prolonged increase in the micturition threshold volume, which was maintained for 40 min, presumably involving modulation of synaptic transmission in the central micturition pathway. When intravesical electrical stimulation (IVES) was used, the opposite result was achieved: i.e. prolonged enhancement of the micturition reflex. In further experiments, the specific antagonist CPPene was used to block central glutaminergic receptors of the NMDA type. The IVES-induced decrease in micturition threshold was blocked by prior administration of CPPene. This finding indicates that the IVES-induced modulation of the micturition reflex is due to an enhanced excitatory synaptic transmission in the central micturition reflex pathway.[36] Similar modulation of the inhibitory, central mechanisms during electrical stimulation at relevant sites seems quite likely. A further plausible mechanism is that continence reflexes, once upgraded by artificial electrical stimulation, will be maintained when micturition is normalized, providing the chance of daily voiding and withholding training sessions.

Table 18.1 *Requirements of a stimulator for clinical use*
Adequate electrode design
Sufficient and adjustable stimulation intensity
Short pulse width (range 0.2–0.5 ms)
Biphasic pulses
Variability of stimulation frequency (range 10–50 Hz), depending on clinical demands
Continuous or intermittent stimulation, depending on clinical demands

A further possibility is that chronic stimulation can improve the central motor programs for activation of the relevant striated muscles, in analogy with the stimulation-induced re-education in urge incontinence. Stimulation may also improve the reinervation of partly denervated muscle fibers by enhancing sprouting of surviving motor axons. Activation in animal experiments has been observed to promote the development of large motor units with many muscle fibers.[37] In line with these observations, Smith et al[38] and Fall, Hjälmås, and Lindehall (unpublished work) observed an improvement of stress incontinence in children and youngsters with myelomeningocele and partly denervated pelvic floor.

It is worth noting that electrical pelvic floor stimulation involves the coordinated bladder and urethral function. When treating bladder overactivity, an effect on the sphincter mechanism may be as significant for the patient. It is not an unusual observation that, during ongoing treatment, the patients may still experience urgency and frequency of urination but have regained control of the sphincter. They can thereby postpone voiding – an effect of utmost importance for their ability to resume normal activities of daily life.

Clinical techniques of electrical stimulation

There are two main options for clinical treatment. *Long-term stimulation* implies chronic stimulation at low intensity and requires several hours of treatment per day during several months. This modality was first used by Caldwell et al,[29] who implanted electrodes into the pelvic floor muscles and connected them to a radiolinked stimulator activated from an outside antenna. It was subsequently found that external electrodes yielded similar good results. Different shapes of vaginal and anal electrodes have been tried on a long-term basis. Advantages of long-term external stimulation are that hospital attention is not required and treatment is cheap and self-controlled by the patient.

A disadvantage is that the procedure demands patient persistence. Many patients also find the different devices uncomfortable to wear for a prolonged period of time. Most patients using this treatment prefer to use the device during sleep at night. Today, because of the slow progress of treatment, most of the devices for long-term treatment have gone out of the market.

A different approach was presented by Godec et al.[39] Using anal plug electrodes and needle electrodes inserted into the levator ani muscle, they applied a 15–20 min continuous train of pulses at high intensity, so-called *acute maximal stimulation*. The applications were repeated up to 10 times in the outpatient clinic. Plevnik and Janez[40] and Kralj[41] used a modified technique with only surface electrodes and obtained a successful result in more than 50% of patients. Acute maximal stimulation may be preferable as treatment in urge incontinence owing to an overactive bladder. High-amplitude stimulation induces a more pronounced bladder inhibition and fewer stimulation sessions are required for a curative effect.[12,24] A limiting factor for maximal stimulation by means of external electrodes is that the effective range up to the maximum tolerable level is rather narrow.[20] A stronger effect may be obtained in selected cases by direct stimulation of the pudendal nerve trunk by means of needle electrodes.[42] A combined approach of clinical and home high-intensity stimulation by means of a personal stimulator (*home maximal stimulation*) now seems to be the most popular alternative.[43]

Up to half of the patients regain permanent control (re-education) of the bladder and/or the urethral sphincters after a period of long-term or a sequence of maximal electrical stimulation.[16,32,40–45] In some patients only a temporary improvement may be achieved, and recurrence of symptoms is encountered after a few weeks or months. In these cases, repeated sessions of treatment usually restore control. However, very frequent periods of treatment or daily stimulation is demanding and not readily accepted by all patients. In such a situation, implantation of a sacral root or pudendal nerve stimulator may be a better solution (see Chapter 20).

The problem of randomized controlled trials and functional electrical stimulation

One problem with FES is the relative lack of randomized controlled studies (RCTs). In clinical practice today no treatment is fully accepted if active treatment is not superior to placebo. FES requires the sensation of stimulation to be effective. It has still not been possible to design a study with a genuine placebo equivalent, i.e. electrical stimulation producing the sensation of stimulation with no other effect in the control arm. A nonfunctioning stimulator as control is too easy for the patient to reveal and thus is not an ideal placebo. In an early trial, this method was tested, but the study was not completed because of dropouts in the group having nonfunctioning stimulation devices.[46] Recently, trials have been presented using this principle,[47,48] and a statistically significant effect on stress urinary incontinence was found during active home maximal stimulation compared to the group wearing a device without stimulation. Yamanishi et al[49] treated patients with detrusor overactivity with 15 min stimulation twice daily for 4 weeks, which is comparably a low quantity of stimulation. Still, subjective improvement in the active arm compared with inactive treatment was accomplished, as well as increase of cystometric capacity. Other reports have been contradictory, such as the one by Luber and Wolde-Tsadik[50] treating patients with genuine stress incontinence twice daily for 3 months with no difference between active and control groups.

Control studies are important to determine the 'real' efficacy of varying FES modalities for different diagnoses. They are also desirable to get acceptance of the methods by health insurance authorities. In the recent report of the International Consultation on Incontinence, electrical stimulation was claimed to have an insufficient evidence base depending on the limited number of positive RCTs. Too much emphasis on RCTs, disregarding extensive experience presented in open studies, may lead to a short-sighted abandonment of further experimentation and development of techniques and includes the risk that a useful and harmless option for treatment of stress incontinence and detrusor overactivity is disregarded. Studies of electrical stimulation also entail other risks and problems. If treatment is applied with suboptimal techique, an effect may be overlooked and researchers may be disencouraged to continue further trials.

Electrical stimulation in various neurogenic lower urinary tract dysfunctions

Established indications are **stress urinary incontinence** caused by pelvic floor insufficiency, the efficacy of FES being similar to that of pelvic floor exercises. It has been demonstrated that female stress incontinence depends not only on a defect of the urethral supporting structures but also on partial damage of the innervation to the pelvic floor muscle complex caused by delivery or other traumatic insults.[51] Up to 75% of patients referred for surgery of their stress incontinence may be sufficiently improved by FES so that an operation becomes unnecessary.[16,32,41] Some patients using pelvic floor exercises have defective perception and cannot recognize the relevant muscles, making training impossible. By means of intravaginal stimulation, muscle identification may be possible, and a combined treatment may reinforce their training. In stress incontinence, long-term stimulation at 20–50 Hz is recommended.

The standard therapy of an **overactive bladder** is anticholinergic drug treatment, however limited in usefulness because of more or less pronounced side-effects owing to general effects on the receptor systems. Functional electrical stimulation circumvents this problem by acting directly on the micturition reflex mechanism. Urge incontinence due to detrusor overactivity (DO) is an ideal indication for electrical stimulation.[40,42,44,45,52] Detrusor overactivity is a typical feature of suprasacral spinal cord lesion as well as supraspinal neuropathy. There is an ongoing debate on the etiology and pathogenesis of detrusor overactivity in patients with so-called idiopathic DO. When making a thorough examination, however, subtle neurologic signs may frequently be revealed, mainly affecting the lower extremities,[53] which indicate that we are dealing with a neurogenic bladder disorder. Another feature of DO relevant for the application of electrical stimulation, is that different functional subtypes may be identified. The **uninhibited overactive bladder** subtype[54] responds fairly well to maximal stimulation at 10 Hz, few other methods being applicable. The results are even better in subjects with **phasic detrusor instability**,[54] many of which attain the unique re-education effect, too. In mixed incontinence, an individual assessment is mandatory. If stress urinary incontinence dominates, surgery is usually preferred, but electrical stimulation at 10–20 Hz may be contemplated as an alternative. When DO dominates, electrical stimulation is the therapy of choice, either as repeated maximal stimulation or as self-administered home-maximal stimulation at 10 Hz.

Detrusor overactivity may be a severe symptomatic distress in spinal cord injury with **spinal detrusor hyperreflexia**. In cases refractory to anticholinergic drugs, penile electrical stimulation has been demonstrated to reduce hyperreflexic contractions and urinary leaks.[22,23] Recently, Shah[55] utilized penile electrical stimulation in a physiological study to modulate DO in a homogeneous series of subjects with spinal cord injury. Optimal inhibition of detrusor contraction required currents at least twice the pudendo-anal reflex, irrespective of pulse width, and was achieved with stimulation frequencies between 15 and 20 Hz. Repetitive stimulation resulted in increasing filling volumes before contraction with slow poststimulation return to the baseline volume, indicating not only acute but also prolonged modulation of detrusor inhibitory mechanisms. No doubt, this option of treatment warrants further exploration in this group of patients.

In patients refractory to noninvasive procedures, other techniques are justified, e.g. perineally inserted or implanted electrodes for direct stimulation of the pudendal main nerve trunk.[42,56] Another option is percutaneous stimulation of the sacral nerves, a successful test being followed by implantation of a stimulator for chronic use.

Acknowledgment

The authors acknowledge the support of the Swedish Medical Research Council (Project Nos. 009902-02 and 04767) and the Medical Faculty, Göteborg University.

References

1. Burke RE, Levine DN, Tsairis P, Zajac FE 3rd. Physiological types and histochemical profiles in motor units of the cat gastrocnemius. J Physiol 1973; 234(3):723–748.

2. Iggo A. Tension receptors in the stomach and the urinary bladder. J Physiol 1955; 128:593–607.

3. Badr G, Fall M, Carlsson C-A, et al. Cortical evoked potentials obtained after stimulation of the lower urinary tract. J Urol 1984; 131:306–309.

4. Jiang C-H, Lindström S, Mazières L. Segmental inhibitory control of ascending sensory information from bladder mechanoreceptors in cat. Neurourol Urodyn 1991; 10:286–288.

5. Barrington FJF. The relation of the hind-brain to micturition. Brain 1921; 44:23–53.

6. Barrington FJF. The nervous mechanism of micturition. Q J Exp Physiol 1914; 8:33–71.

7. Lindström S, Fall M, Carlsson C-A, Erlandson B-E. Rhythmic activity in pelvic afferents to the bladder: an experimental study in the cat with reference to the clinical condition "unstable bladder". Urol Int 1984; 39:272–279.

8. Nakamura M, Sakurai T. Bladder inhibition by penile electrical stimulation. Br J Urol 1984; 56:413–415.

9. Madersbacher H, Kiss G, Mair D. Transcutaneous electrostimulation of the pudendal nerve for treatment of detrusor overactivity. Neurourol Urodynam 1995; 14:501–502.

10. Alexander S, Rowan D, Millar W, Scott R. Treatment of urinary incontinence by electric pessary. A report of 18 patients. Br J Urol 1970; 42:184–190.

11. Fall M, Erlandson B-E, Carlsson C-A, Lindström S. The effect of intravaginal electrical stimulation of the feline urethra and urinary bladder. Neuronal mechanisms. Scand J Urol Nephrol 1978; Suppl 44:19.

12. Lindström S, Fall M, Carlsson C-A, Erlandson B-E. The neurophysiological basis of bladder inhibition in response to intravaginal electrical stimulation. J Urol 1983; 129:40.

13. Trontelj TV, Janko M, Godec C, et al. Electrical stimulation for urinary incontinence: a neurophysiological study. Urol Int 1974; 29:213.

14. Teague CT, Merrill DC. Electric pelvic floor stimulation. Mechanism of action. Invest Urol 1977; 15:65–69.

15. Glen E. Effective and safe control of incontinence by the intra-anal plug electrode. Br J Surg 1967; 54:802.

16. Eriksen BC, Bergmann S, Mjolnerod OK. Effect of anal electrostimulation with the 'Incontan' device in women with urinary incontinence. Br J Obstet Gynaecol 1987; 94:147–156.

17. Lindström S, Sudsuang R. Functionally specific bladder reflexes from pelvic and pudendal nerve branches: an experimental study in the cat. Neurourol Urodyn 1989; 8:392–393.

18. Geirsson G, Fall M, Lindström S. Cystometric classification of bladder overactivity: assessment of a new system in 501 patients. Int Urogyn J 1993; 4:186–193.

19. Blok BF, Holstege G. Two pontine micturition centers in the cat are not interconnected directly: implications for the central organisation of micturition. J Comp Neurol 1999; 403:209–218.

20. Ohlsson BL. Effects of some different pulse parameters on the perception of intravaginal and intraanal electrical stimulation. Med Biol Eng Comput 1988; 26:503–505.

21. Fall M, Erlandson B-E, Sundin T, Waagstein F. Intravaginal electrical stimulation. Clinical experiments on bladder inhibition. Scand J Urol Nephrol 1978; (suppl) 44:41–47.

22. Vereecken RL, Das J, Grisar P. Electrical sphincter stimulation in the treatment of detrusor hyperreflexia of paraplegics. Neurourol Urodyn 1984; 3:145–154.

23. Vodusek DB, Light JK, Libby JM. Detrusor inhibition induced by stimulation of pudendal nerve afferents. Neurourol Urodyn 1986; 5:381–389.

24. Vodusek DB, Plevnik S, Vrtacnik P, et al. Detrusor inhibition on selective pudendal nerve stimulation in the perineum. Neurourol Urodyn 1988; 6:389–393.

25. Collins CD. Intermittent electrical stimulation. Urol Int 1974; 29:221.

26. Rottembourg JL, Ghoneim MA, Fretin J, Susset JG. Study on the efficiency of electric stimulation of the pelvic floor. Invest Urol 1976; 13:354–358.

27. Bazeed MA, Thuroff JW, Schmidt RA, et al. Effect of chronic electrostimulation of the sacral roots on the striated urethral sphincter. J Urol 1982; 128:1357–1362.

28. Ridge RM, Betz WJ. The effect of selective, chronic stimulation on motor unit size in developing rat muscle. J Neurosci 1984; 4:2614–2620.

29. Caldwell KP, Cook PJ, Flack FC, James ED. Stress incontinence in females: report on 31 cases treated by electrical implant. J Obstet Gynaecol Br Commonw 1968; 75:777–780.

30. Eriksen BC, Erik-Nes SH. Long-term electrostimulation of the pelvic floor: primary therapy in female stress incontinence? Urol Int 1989; 44:90–95.

31. Fall M, Erlandson B-E, Nilson AE, Sundin T. Long-term intravaginal electrical stimulation in urge and stress incontinence. Scand J Urol Nephrol 1978; (suppl) 44:55–63.

32. Fall M. Does electrostimulation cure urinary incontinence? J Urol 1984; 131:664–667.

33. Janez J, Plevnik F, Korosec L, et al. Changes in detrusor receptor activity after electric pelvic floor stimulation. In: Proceedings of International Continence Society's XIth Meeting, Lund, Sweden; 1981:22.

34. Ishigooka M, Hashimoto T, Sasagawa I, Nakada T. Reduction in norepinephrine content of the rabbit urinary bladder by alpha-2 adrenergic antagonist after electrical pelvic floor stimulation. J Urol 1994; 151:774–775.

35. Jiang CH. Prolonged modulation of the micturition reflex by electrical stimulation. Thesis, Linköping University Medical Dissertations No. 582. Faculty of Health Sciences, Linköping University, Sweden, 1999.

36. Jiang C-H. Modulation of the micturition reflex pathway by intravesical electrical stimulation: an experimental study in the rat. Neurourol Urodyn 1998; 17:543–553.

37. Salmons S, Vrbova G. The influence of activity on some contractile characteristics of mammalian fast and slow muscles. J Physiol 1969; 201:535–549.

38. Schmidt RA, Kogan BA, Tanagho EA. Neuroprostheses in the management of incontinence in myelomeningocele patients. J Urol 1990; 143:779–782.

39. Godec C, Cass AS, Ayala GF. Bladder inhibition with functional electrical stimulation. Urology 1975; 6:663–666.

40. Plevnik S, Janez J. Maximal electrical stimulation for urinary incontinence: report of 98 cases. Urology 1979; 14:638–645.

41. Kralj B. Treatment of female urinary incontinence by stimulators of the pelvic floor muscles. Artif Org 1981; (suppl)5:609–612.

42. Ohlsson BL, Fall M, Frankenberg-Sommar S. Effects of external and direct pudendal nerve maximal electrical stimulation in the treatment of the uninhibited overactive bladder. Br J Urol 1989; 64:374–380.

43. Plevnik S, Janez J, Vrtacnik P, et al. Short-term electrical stimulation: home treatment for urinary incontinence. World J Urol 1986; 4:24–26.

44. Eriksen BC, Bergmann S, Erik-Nes SH. Maximal electrostimulation of the pelvic floor in female idiopathic detrusor instability and urge incontinence. Neurourol Urodyn 1989; 8:219.

45. Primus G, Kramer G. Maximal external electrical stimulation for treatment of neurogenic or non-neurogenic urgency and/or urge incontinence. Neurourol Urodyn 1996; 15:187–194.

46. Shepherd AM, Blannin JP, Winder A. The English experience of intravaginal electrical stimulation in urinary incontinence – a double blind trial. Proc International Continence Society's 15th Annual Meeting, London, 1985:224–225.

47. Sand PK, Richardson DA, Staskin DR, et al. Pelvic floor electrical stimulation in the treatment of genuine stress incontinence: a multicenter, placebo-controlled trial. Am J Obstet Gynecol 1995; 173:72–79.

48. Yamanishi T, Yasuda K, Hattori T, et al. Pelvic floor electrical stimulation in the treatment of stress incontinence: a placebo-controlled double-blind trial. Neurourol Urodyn 1996; 15:397.

49. Yamanishi T, Yasuda K, Sakakibara R, et al. Randomized, double-blind study of electrical stimulation for urinary incontinence due to detrusor overactivity. Urology 2000; 55:353–357.

50. Luber KM, Wolde-Tsadik G. Efficacy of functional electrical stimulation in treating genuine stress incontinence: a randomized clinical trial. Neurourol Urodyn 1997; 16:543–551.

51. Allen RE, Hosker GL, Smith AR, Warrell DW. Pelvic floor damage and childbirth: a neurophysiological study. Br J Obstet Gynaecol 1990; 97:770–779.

52. Abel I, Ottesen B, Fischer-Rasmussen W, Lose G. Maximal electrical stimulation of the pelvic floor in the treatment of urge incontinence: a placebo controlled study. Neurourol Urodyn 1996; 15:283–284.

53. Ahlberg J, Edlund C, Wikkelsö C, Rosengren L, Fall M. Neurological signs are common in patients with urodynamically verified "idiopathic" bladder overactivity. Neurourol Urodyn 2002; 21:65–70.

54. Fall M, Geirsson G, Lindström S. Toward a new classification of overactive bladders. Neurourol Urodyn 1995; 14:635–646.

55. Shah N. Thesis, University College London Medical School, London, 2002.

56. Janez J, Plevnik S, Vrtacnik P. Maximal electrical stimulation in patients with lower motor neuron lesion. Proc International Continence Society's XIIth Annual Meeting, Leiden, The Netherlands, 1982:115–118.

19

Emptying the neurogenic bladder by electrical stimulation

Graham H Creasey

Principles

Electrical stimulation has been investigated for many years for the purpose of restoring function to the neurogenic bladder, whose functions of micturition and continence may be impaired by either paralysis or hyperreflexia of the detrusor and/or sphincter mechanisms. Ideally, the functions of both emptying and storage should be restored. This would require coordinated contraction of the detrusor and relaxation of the sphincter mechanism for voiding, alternating with relaxation of the detrusor and adequate contraction of the sphincters for continence.

Electrical stimulation is usually thought of as producing muscle contraction, but there are also ways of using it to prevent contraction or produce relaxation. Reflex contraction or relaxation of muscle may be produced by stimulating sensory nerves. When stimulation is applied in this way, modifying activity in the central nervous system, it is sometimes called neuromodulation; this is discussed in other chapters in this book. When stimulation is applied directly to efferent nerves to improve function by producing contraction of muscles it is sometimes called functional neuromuscular stimulation or functional electrical stimulation. This chapter describes such stimulation of sacral efferent nerves to produce emptying of the neurogenic bladder. This process clearly requires that efferent nerves to the bladder be intact, specifically the preganglionic parasympathetic efferents from the sacral segments of the cord which run via the sacral anterior nerve roots, sacral nerves, and pelvic plexus. It is therefore applicable to patients with lesions of the spinal cord above the sacral segments, who can now derive considerable clinical benefit from electrical stimulation to produce safe and effective bladder emptying. Restoration of continence to the neurogenic bladder by electrical stimulation is still under investigation, and chemical or surgical methods are still needed in many cases.

Location of stimulation

A variety of sites of stimulation have been used in patients with suprasacral spinal cord injury or disease, with electrodes on the bladder wall, the pelvic splanchnic nerves, the conus medullaris, the sacral anterior roots, or the mixed sacral nerves. In practice only the latter two sites have reached clinical significance (Figure 19.1).

Electrodes on the bladder wall produced poor results, probably for several reasons including breakage of electrodes with bladder movement, the difficulty of recruiting enough of the detrusor muscle, and the stimulation of afferents producing unwanted reflexes.[1,2] If these problems

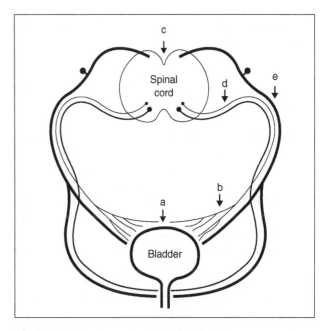

Figure 19.1
Potential sites of stimulation: (a) bladder wall; (b) pelvic nerves; (c) conus medullaris; (d) sacral anterior roots intradurally; and (e) sacral nerves extradurally.

could be solved it might be useful to stimulate postganglionic parasympathetic neurons in the bladder wall for patients whose preganglionic neurons have been damaged by injuries to the sacral segments of the spinal cord or the cauda equina; such patients do not gain bladder function from electrical stimulation at present.

The pelvic splanchnic nerves appear to be a theoretically desirable site but surgical access is difficult and it may be difficult to avoid stimulating sympathetic fibers to the bladder neck and afferent fibers. Good results were claimed in a few patients but little has been published on this route.[3,4]

Stimulation of the conus medullaris was developed by Nashold et al.[5] A laminectomy from T12 to L2 was performed and a pair of electrodes inserted into the gray matter of the conus medullaris at the spinal level giving the highest bladder pressures on electrical stimulation of the dorsal surface of the conus. Nashold reported a good result in 16 of 27 patients followed for 3–10 years; however, the technique has not gained wide acceptance, perhaps because of the difficulty of identifying a location in the cord which could produce coordinated micturition.

Stimulation of the sacral anterior roots was developed by Brindley.[6,7] This site has the advantage that these roots do not usually contain sensory neurons, so direct activation of reflexes rarely occurs. The sacral anterior roots do, however, contain efferent neurons to both detrusor and external urethral sphincter. The lower motor neurons to the sphincter have a lower threshold for electrical activation than the parasympathetic efferent neurons to the detrusor, so it is possible to activate the sphincter without the bladder but not usually the bladder without the sphincter. It used to be thought that attempts to produce voiding would therefore be ineffective and possibly dangerous, by causing co-contraction of detrusor and sphincter. However, Brindley made use of the fact that the smooth muscle of the detrusor contracts and relaxes much more slowly than the striated muscle of the external urethral sphincter. Stimulation in bursts of a few seconds, separated by longer gaps, allows a sustained pressure to be built up in the bladder while allowing the external sphincter to relax rapidly between the bursts, allowing urine to flow during these gaps.[8] Careful long-term clinical follow-up has shown that the brief co-contraction of the sphincter during the bursts does not cause bladder trabeculation or upper tract damage, and effective emptying of the bladder can be produced.

Sensory nerves in the end organs can nevertheless respond to muscle activity, and this may produce reflex contraction, or failure to relax, at the sphincter, even during the gaps between stimulation, a condition resembling detrusor-sphincter dyssynergia, which can hinder the flow of urine in some patients.[9] Sauerwein developed the addition of posterior sacral rhizotomy to this stimulation, carrying out both procedures simultaneously at the level of the cauda equina.[10] This has the great advantage of reducing not only reflex contraction of the sphincter but also reflex contraction

of the bladder, protecting the upper tracts from back pressure and abolishing reflex incontinence. It also abolishes autonomic dysreflexia triggered from contraction of the bladder or lower bowel. It does, however, have other disadvantages, which are discussed below.

If posterior sacral rhizotomy is performed, similar function can be obtained by applying bursts of stimulation to the mixed sacral nerves whose afferent connections to the cord have been divided. Electrodes and cables can thus be implanted extradurally in the sacral spinal canal. The rhizotomy is still best performed intradurally where it is easier to separate sensory from motor roots. It is easiest to separate these where they diverge to enter the conus medullaris and the sensory roots can be divided with little handling of the motor roots. The combination of extradural electrodes and intradural rhizotomy at the conus was developed by Sarrias et al. and is sometimes called the Barcelona technique.[11] However, this involves a second laminectomy at the level of the conus. If there has been a previous spinal fracture or internal fixation at the thoracolumbar junction it is probably safer not to risk destabilizing the spine at this level and to carry out the rhizotomy in the cauda equina. This can be done conveniently at the lower end of the dural sac through the same laminectomy used for implanting extradural electrodes (Figure 19.2).

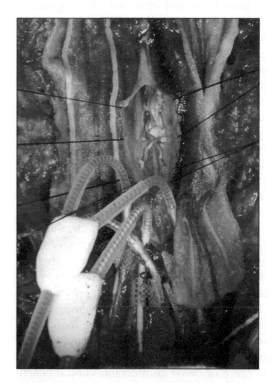

Figure 19.2
Alternative site of posterior rhizotomy with extradural electrodes. The lower end of the dural sac is shown held open with stay sutures to display the divided posterior roots; the electrodes have been attached to the sacral nerves caudal to the end of the dural sac.

Methods

Surgery

General anesthesia should be carried out without anticholinergic medication, which could reduce bladder contraction, and preferably without long-acting skeletal muscle relaxants, so that lower limb muscle responses can be used to assist in identifying nerves. Laminectomy is carried out according to the technique selected from Table 19.1. After opening the dura, sensory roots are distinguished from motor roots by intraoperative stimulation using hook electrodes while recording bladder pressure via a urethral catheter. Under general anesthesia sensory roots do not produce bladder contraction though they may produce reflex contraction of the lower limbs and reflex rises in blood pressure that can be rapid. It is therefore advisable to monitor blood pressure intra-arterially. After division of posterior roots, usually S2–5, electrodes are implanted on the nerves or roots that produce bladder pressure on stimulation, usually S3–4. Electrodes may also be implanted on S2, even if these roots do not produce bladder pressure, for the purpose of producing penile erection. The cables from the electrodes are passed subcutaneously through a cannula, usually to a temporary pocket in the flank. After repositioning the patient, they can be passed subcutaneously to the front of the body, where they are attached to a stimulator implanted in a subcutaneous pocket over the lower chest or abdomen. Detailed instructions are given in Brindley's *Notes for Surgeons and Physicians*, available from the manufacturer.[12]

Equipment

Equipment includes implanted components, external components, and equipment used during surgery. Implantable intradural and extradural electrodes are shown in Figure 19.3. Cables from the electrodes are connected via plugs and sockets to an implantable receiver (Figure 19.4). A 3-channel receiver is typically used if S2–4 are to be stimulated individually with intradural electrodes, whereas a 2-channel receiver can be used if S3 and S4 are stimulated by the same channel, as is often done with extradural electrodes.

The implantable components contain no batteries but are powered and controlled by radio transmission from an external controller programmed by the clinician and operated by the user. Analog and digital versions of the controller are available; their batteries can be charged weekly.

During surgery, hook electrodes connected to a battery-powered nerve stimulator are used for identification of nerves. Medical adhesive is used to seal the connections between plugs and sockets.

The equipment is approved by the US Food and Drug Administration (FDA) as a Humanitarian Use Device and in Europe is CE Marked under the requirements of the Active Implantable Medical Device Directive 90/385/EEC.

Preoperative investigation

It is essential to know that the parasympathetic efferent fibers from the sacral cord to the bladder are capable of producing bladder contraction. This may be tested by cystometry in which it is desirable to see a reflex bladder contraction of at least 35 cmH$_2$O in a woman and 50 cmH$_2$O in a man.[12] Anticholinergics may need to be stopped several days before this procedure, in which case it may be necessary to prepare the patient for increased incontinence and autonomic dysreflexia. The presence of other sacral reflexes such as the anocutaneous reflex, bulbocavernosus reflex, or ankle tendon reflexes and a history of reflex erection help to confirm sacral function.

It is also desirable to confirm adequate bladder capacity and exclude severe fibrosis of the bladder wall. This can usually be determined from the patient's history, particularly when using anticholinergics, but in case of doubt can be confirmed by repeating cystometry under spinal anesthesia.

It is of course desirable to document urinary tract function thoroughly, as well as penile erection and bowel

Table 19.1 *Potential sites of surgery; criteria for selecting a site are given under Discussion*			
Technique	Electrodes	Posterior rhizotomy	Laminectomies
Classical technique	Intradural	Mid cauda equina	L3–5
Barcelona technique	Extradural	Conus medullaris	S1–3 and T12–L1
Alternative technique	Extradural	Low cauda equina	S1–3

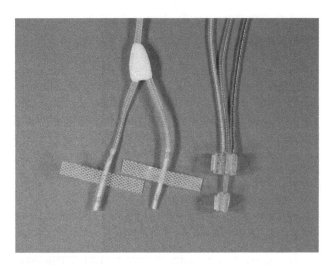

Figure 19.3
Electrodes. On the right is shown an array of intradural electrodes, with three cables corresponding to S2, S3, and S4. On the left is shown a pair of extradural electrodes, for application to left and right sacral nerves at a given segmental level, with a common lead. Three pairs of extradural electrodes may be implanted for S2–4, but more commonly the S3 and S4 nerves are stimulated together, allowing two pairs to be used.

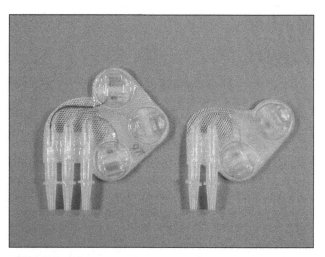

Figure 19.4
Receivers. On the left is shown a 3-channel receiver and on the right a 2-channel receiver. During implantation, cables from the electrodes are attached to the receivers using plugs and sockets located within the vertical tubular structures.

function. The appearance of the bladder neck on videocystometry probably has prognostic value for stress incontinence, as described below.[13] Bladder diverticula are not necessarily a contraindication but may result in some persistence of urinary tract infection. Ureteric reflux or hydronephrosis are not necessarily a contraindication and may be a strong indication for posterior rhizotomy. If a subject has a suprapubic catheter it is probably preferable to revert to urethral catheterization before surgery to allow adequate closure of the stoma before generating bladder pressure with the stimulator. Prior bladder augmentation, if successful, abolishes the ability of the bladder to generate pressure and therefore renders the patient unsuitable.

Imaging of the lumbosacral spine can be used to exclude structural abnormalities. Separation of the spinal roots intradurally can be complicated by adhesions due to previous subarachnoid hemorrhage (such as from a bullet or stab wound) or spinal meningitis or myelography with an oily contrast medium,[12] and magnetic resonance imaging (particularly with gadolinium enhancement) may aid in the preoperative detection of these adhesions[14] as well as confirming the position of the conus medullaris.

Postoperative management

Extradural electrodes may be tested and brought into use on the first postoperative day. Cystometry and clinical examination should show that rhizotomy is effective; on the rare occasion that bladder reflexes persist, it is easier to return to surgery and complete the rhizotomy before the wound is healed. It is wise to check residual volumes after stimulator-driven voiding for the first few days and adjust the stimulator if necessary with urodynamic monitoring of voiding pressure and flow rate. Many patients may have a high fluid output initially as a result of intravenous fluids or the habit of a high fluid intake, so it may be necessary to void frequently until this is adjusted. Overdistention of the bladder can result in poor contractility and the need to revert to catherization until the bladder recovers.

Some surgeons prefer to postpone the use of intradural electrodes for a few days after surgery to reduce the risk of leakage of cerebrospinal fluid along the cables, but the implant should be tested within 3–4 days; reduced responses at 1 week, particularly of somatic muscles, may indicate nerve damage due to handling at operation. However, the patient can be reassured that the motor responses seen in the first week are likely to return.[12]

Delay in the use of the stimulator can contribute to postoperative constipation, but thereafter regular use of the stimulator usually improves bowel function, though patients may take a few weeks to adjust to a new bowel habit. Initial follow-up by telephone is helpful and thereafter follow-up is recommended at 3 months and annually.

Results

This technique has now been used in several thousand patients, primarily in Europe, where the intradural technique has been predominant, with others in

North America, the Far East, New Zealand, and Australia. Reports have been published from many single-center studies,[10,13,15–22] as well as multi-center studies[23–26] and surveys.[27,28] The stimulator was the subject of conferences at Le Mans, France in 1989,[29] Halifax, Nova Scotia in 1992,[30] Innsbruck, Austria in 1996, and Sydney, Australia in 2000.

Micturition

The majority of subjects with the stimulator use it routinely for producing micturition at home 4–6 times per day. Of the 184 patients reported by van Kerrebroeck et al, 157 (85%) used the stimulator alone; a further four required a subsequent sphincterotomy in order to use it, and a further eight combined its use with intermittent catheterization; 7.6% did not use it for various reasons.[27] Residual volume in the bladder following implant-driven micturition was reduced in 151 patients (89% of users) to less than 30 ml, and in 95% of users to less than 60 ml. No user had a residual greater than 200 ml.

Urine infection

A substantial decrease in urinary tract infection is one of the main benefits of the technique, and has been reported by many groups following the use of the implant.[15,17,23,27,29,31] The reduction in residual volume is probably the main reason, together with greatly reduced use of intermittent or indwelling catheterization. As a result, antibiotic use is also greatly reduced.

Continence of urine

Reflex incontinence due to spinal reflexes is abolished by posterior sacral rhizotomy from S2–5. Some female patients have reported that incontinence can return temporarily if they have a urinary tract infection; this is probably a local reflex as a result of inflammation of the bladder wall, as it always improves following eradication of the infection.

Stress incontinence may persist following surgery in 10–15% of patients, particularly in those who have had previous sphincterotomy or bladder neck resection. McDonagh et al. reported that the state of the bladder neck on videourodynamics prior to sacral rhizotomy appeared to have a bearing on subsequent continence. All patients in their series with a closed bladder neck preoperatively became continent, except one patient who had had two previous sphincterotomies; another patient with previous sphincterotomy but a closed bladder neck prior to rhizotomy became continent. However, three out of four patients with an open bladder neck preoperatively had some degree of incontinence. Pre- or postoperative sphincterotomy appeared to be less of a risk to continence than bladder neck resection.[13] Of 41 early users followed up for 5–13 years, 35 reported continence day and night; of the six who were not continent, four had had previous bladder neck resections.[32] Stress incontinence may also occur *de novo* in a few patients; this is probably in those with an open bladder neck whose continence has been maintained preoperatively by hyperreflexia of the external urethral sphincter; abolition of this hyperreflexia may then result in stress incontinence.

Most paraplegic patients dispense with urine collection devices, but some tetraplegic patients wear a condom and leg bag because of their limited hand function.

Urodynamics

Bladder capacity

Posterior rhizotomy dramatically increases bladder capacity by abolishing detrusor hyperreflexia; urodynamic filling of the areflexic bladder is best limited to under 400 ml to avoid stretching of the detrusor. McDonagh et al showed that functional bladder capacity increased by at least 140 ml, and an average of 404 ml (range 140–680), in all patients who had posterior rhizotomy, an increase that was statistically significant at the level of $p < 0.00001$.[13] Van Kerrebroeck et al, who took particular care not to overdistend the bladder postoperatively, found an average increase in cystometric capacity of 332 ml ($p < 0.001$) in patients who had undergone posterior rhizotomy.[33]

Bladder compliance

Since compliance is volume-dependent, it is desirable to compare it at the same volumes pre- and postoperatively; Van Kerrebroeck used the maximal preoperative cystometric capacity of each patient as this volume, and found that patients who had undergone posterior rhizotomy had a statistically significant increase in compliance from 8 to 53 ml/cmH$_2$O. The postoperative compliance, at 500 ml, was over 50 ml/cmH$_2$O in 12 of 13 patients.[33]

Detrusor pressure

Detrusor pressure can be controlled by programming the external controller, and fluctuates with bursts of stimulation. Pressures in the bladder during electrically activated micturition have been reported by several authors. Cardozo et al reported that the maximum voiding pressure was on average 55 cmH$_2$O with a range of 22–82 cmH$_2$O.[34]

Arnold et al recorded a mean peak pressure of 88 cmH$_2$O and mean trough pressure of 40 cmH$_2$O and concluded that this did not appear to be harmful.[15] Madersbacher et al reported a mean peak pressure of 71 cmH$_2$O (range 55–90) and noted that post-stimulus voiding did not appear to induce detrusor hypertrophy.[17] In the first 50 patients to receive the implant, bladder trabeculation was reported to have decreased in 13 patients when followed up at 1–9 years, and no patient in this group showed evidence of increased trabeculation.[32] Van Kerrebroeck recorded a mean peak voiding pressure of 89 cmH$_2$O.[33] It is likely that voiding pressure is less significant for the upper tracts than storage pressure, which is usually reduced by posterior rhizotomy.

Upper tracts

The improvement in bladder capacity and compliance which follow posterior rhizotomy reduce the risk of upper tract damage and can result in improvement in pre-existing ureteric reflux or hydronephrosis.[10] In a multicenter review of 184 patients, reflux was present in nine patients before the operation: after implantation it was improved or abolished in seven of these and persisted in two. No patient in this group developed reflux with the use of the stimulator.[27] Eight of the 184 subjects showed upper tract dilatation preoperatively: of these, the dilatation improved in seven and deteriorated in one. No patient in this series developed upper tract dilatation *de novo* after implantation of the stimulator.[27]

Pain

Stimulation is never painful in patients with complete spinal cord injury and almost never in patients who undergo posterior rhizotomy. Intradural stimulation of anterior roots would usually be expected to be painless, even without rhizotomy, since these roots are usually purely motor. However, among the first 50 patients, implanted over 20 years ago, all of whom had intradural implants but not all of whom had rhizotomy, three were unable to use the implant because of pain on stimulation, and four others found use of the stimulator to some extent painful. All these patients had preserved pain sensitivity in the sacral dermatomes preoperatively.[35] It may be that current can sometimes spread from the intradural electrodes to activate nearby sensory roots, but a few patients have continued to experience pain on stimulation in spite of a thorough sacral posterior rhizotomy. This led to the belief that some anterior roots can contain sensory fibers, which has been confirmed experimentally.[36] A modified implant with a larger number of channels has been developed for use in such patients, to allow more selective stimulation of individual roots.[12] Extradural stimulation of mixed sacral nerves would be unacceptably painful if pain sensitivity was present in the sacral dermatomes and rhizotomy was not performed.

Autonomic dysreflexia

The symptoms of autonomic dysreflexia associated with contraction of the bladder or lower bowel are greatly reduced by posterior rhizotomy. Slight rises in blood pressure may occur with stimulation in rhizotomized patients, perhaps as a result of somatic muscle contraction in the sacral segments, or the presence of afferent nerves in anterior roots, but these are not sufficient to prevent use of the device.[37] If rhizotomy were not performed, extradural stimulation of mixed sacral nerves would be likely to cause significant blood pressure rises, at least in patients with cervical and upper thoracic lesions.

Nerve damage

Accidental damage to motor nerve fibers at the time of operation is less likely to occur with extradural electrodes than intradural, because of the greater surgical handling of anterior roots in the latter procedure and the lack of supporting fibrous tissue intradurally. It is dependent on surgical care and experience. It can be most sensitively detected by testing for any loss of skeletal muscle responses to the use of the stimulator during the first postoperative week, and may also become evident as a temporary loss of bladder response. It usually takes the form of neuropraxia or axonotmesis and is therefore temporary, but bladder responses may take from 2 to 6 months to return as the axons regrow, thus delaying the use of the implant for micturition.

Some patients have now been using the stimulator for 20 years or more without apparent deterioration in nerve function. The histological appearance of stimulated nerves was reported as normal in the case of two patients who died (one by suicide and one from myocardial infarction) after using the implant for 3 and 5 years, respectively.[31]

Leakage of cerebrospinal fluid

Early intradural implants sometimes had leakage of cerebrospinal fluid along the cables passing through the dura. The implant has since been modified by the addition of a grommet to seal the cables to the dura, and the incidence of this complication appears to have been greatly reduced.

It is rarely a problem with extradural electrodes, even though the dura may have been opened in the vicinity of the cables to perform rhizotomy.

Implant infection

Infection of the implants has been rare, particularly since a technique of coating them with antibiotics was introduced in 1982. Rushton et al reported in 1989 that one out of 104 coated implants had become infected, and in this case infection appeared to have been introduced at a subsequent operation to close a leak of cerebrospinal fluid.[38] Brindley reported a 1% infection rate for the first 500 implants.[28] The infection rate for a variety of similar implants has been shown to be significantly reduced by antibiotic coating, but not by systemic perioperative antibiotics.[38] Nevertheless, many surgeons use systemic perioperative antibiotic prophylaxis aimed at both Gram-positive and Gram-negative organisms.

If the receiver becomes infected, and this is detected promptly before infection has spread along the cables, it is sometimes possible to divide the cables at a sterile location in the flank and remove the receiver, leaving the electrodes in place. If the infection has spread along the cables to the electrodes, it is necessary to remove all the implanted components. In either case, vigorous treatment with antibiotics followed by a waiting period of at least 6 months is advisable before reimplanting a stimulator.

Implant reliability

The implanted components have proved to be remarkably reliable. A survey of the first 500 implants showed that faults occurred on average once every 19.2 implant-years.[39] The commonest site for faults has been in cables, which are sometimes mechanically damaged by movement. Repair or replacement of the device is usually possible, often with minor surgery, and special equipment is available from the manufacturer to facilitate repairs.[12]

Failures in the external transmitter have been more common and have primarily been due to breaks in the antenna lead, but do not require reoperation.

Penile erection

In about 60% of patients, sustained full erection sufficient for coitus can be produced by stimulation of S2, although not all of these patients use it for coitus.[23] In many of the remaining 40% of patients, a partial erection is produced and this may be useful when attaching a condom for urine drainage. Some centers have reported less success with erection when using extradural electrodes; these require higher levels of stimulation to pass equivalent current through the epineurium.

Bowel function

Stimulation, primarily of S3, produces contraction of the lower bowel as far proximal as the splenic flexure, and increases the frequency of defecation, probably by enhancing colonic motility.[40–43] By careful adjustment of the Finetech stimulator, MacDonagh et al were able to produce defecation routinely with the stimulator alone in 6 of 12 patients, and to reduce the time spent each week in bowel emptying from 2.5 h to half an hour.[44]

Costs

A prospective three-center study in the Netherlands collected the actual costs of hospital care, self-care, and travel expenses associated with bladder function of 52 patients before and after the procedure and through 2 years of follow-up. A model of the long-term costs indicated a break-even point of approximately 8 years, after which the procedure resulted in reduced costs.[25] In the USA a retrospective study of costs of bladder and bowel care using structured interviews in 12 patients indicated a break-even point of 5 years; the lower figure may be related to a shorter length of postoperative hospitalization in the North American patients.[45]

Discussion
Selection of patients

Patients with complete spinal cord injury above the conus medullaris and inefficient reflex micturition may be considered at any time after the first few months of injury, particularly if they have complications such as frequent or chronic urine infection, reflex incontinence resistant to medication, or autonomic dysreflexia triggered by bladder or bowel.

In patients with incomplete injuries:

1. it is wise to wait until 2 years after injury to allow any recovery to occur
2. it is necessary to determine whether the implant is likely to be painful
3. it is particularly important to weigh the advantages of posterior rhizotomy against any loss of function which it may cause.

Some patients with multiple sclerosis are suitable, subject to the reservations above. A few adult patients with suprasacral meningomyelocele may also be suitable, but the growth of young children might displace the electrodes if implanted in them. Betz has investigated the use of extensible leads, and has implanted stimulators in patients as young as 14 after evaluation of their skeletal maturity.[46,47] Children with spinal cord injury have a significant risk of developing scoliosis during adolescence, so it may be worth waiting until this is unlikely, or combining implantation with spinal instrumentation if that is needed.

In assigning priorities the following generalizations may be of use:

- Patients with complete spinal cord lesions are more straightforward to investigate and treat by this technique than patients with incomplete lesions.
- Women with reflex incontinence have more to gain than men, because of the lack of satisfactory urine-collecting devices for females, and have less to lose from posterior rhizotomy.
- Patients with recurrent infection have more to gain than those without. Those with persistently high reflex bladder pressures endangering renal function or with autonomic dysreflexia triggered by bladder or bowel are likely to benefit from posterior rhizotomy; this operation provides the opportunity to implant a stimulator, which may then provide them with a preferable alternative to intermittent catheterization.
- Men with poor or absent reflex erection have more to gain and less to lose than those whose reflex erections already suffice for coitus.
- Paraplegic men are more likely to benefit from continence, whereas some tetraplegic men may continue to wear a condom and leg bag at least during the day because of the difficulty in handling urine bottles and clothing.

Selection of surgical technique

Each of the techniques described above can produce excellent results in the hands of a careful surgeon who performs the operation sufficiently often to maintain skill.

The classical technique, implanting electrodes and performing the rhizotomy at the level of the cauda, has the advantage of a single laminectomy. There is a slight risk of cerebrospinal fluid leakage along the cables, and if the cables later break at the site of exit through the dura they are difficult to repair at this site; extradural electrodes can be added to restore function. If the rhizotomy at the cauda later proves to be incomplete it can be revised at the conus.

The Barcelona technique, implanting extradural electrodes and performing intradural rhizotomy at the conus,

has the advantage that it is easier to distinguish sensory from motor roots at the conus and little handling of the motor roots is necessary; in addition, the sacral nerves extradurally have a fibrous covering continuous with the dura and are more robust than the intradural anterior roots. It is therefore probably less likely that the motor neurons will be damaged by intraoperative handling, at least in the hands of a new operator. Extradural electrodes may be the only type possible if there is severe intradural arachnoiditis. If the rhizotomy at the conus proves to be incomplete, it can be revised within a few days at the same site or later at the cauda, provided that intrathecal bleeding has not led to arachnoiditis.

The alternative technique, implanting extradural electrodes and performing rhizotomy at the lower end of the cauda, combines the advantages of a single laminectomy with those of the Barcelona technique, and avoids any risk of destabilizing the spine at the thoracolumbar junction if there has been a previous fracture or internal fixation at that level. It is slightly more difficult to identify all the posterior roots in the cauda than at the conus, so there may be a slightly higher incidence of incomplete rhizotomy.

Extradural separation of sensory and motor fibers is difficult and may damage the nerves, and is rarely performed.[48]

Detrusor-sphincter dyssynergia

Many of the complications of the neurogenic bladder are due to co-contraction of the external urethral sphincter or its failure to relax, and many forms of electrical stimulation produce contraction of the sphincter in addition to the detrusor. Several approaches to reducing sphincter contraction during electrical stimulation have been investigated. Tanagho et al used a variety of surgical procedures such as pudendal neurotomy, levatorotomy, pudendal nerve stimulation, and increasingly extensive posterior rhizotomy,[49] but effective voiding was only produced in about one-third of subjects.

Brindley and Craggs suggested the use of anodal block to prevent propagation of action potentials in the large somatic axons to the external sphincter while allowing propagation in the small parasympathetic fibers to the detrusor.[50] They demonstrated the principle experimentally and early models of the Brindley stimulator included the option of a triangular waveform for this purpose. This option was later omitted when clinical follow-up showed that post-stimulus voiding was safe and effective for voiding, at least when combined with posterior rhizotomy.

In our laboratory we showed in chronically spinalized dogs that anodal block could be used to produce contraction of the bladder with little contraction of the external urethral sphincter. However, voiding was still hindered by reflex activation of urethral muscle unless posterior rhizotomy was performed.[51,52]

High-frequency stimulation can also be applied selectively to large axons to produce either fatigue or block, while allowing smaller axons and their muscles to be activated. This has been applied by implants in chronically spinalized dogs in Montreal.[53] Although voiding pressures were not significantly different with selective stimulation, the urethral pressures were much lower and voiding was produced with low residual volumes without evidence of reflux over a 6-month period in these animals.

The role of posterior rhizotomy

Division of all the posterior roots from S2 to S5 can produce substantial benefits to a patient with a neurogenic bladder; it can also have some significant disadvantages and has therefore been a subject of some debate.

During the early 1980s sacral anterior root implants, using intradural electrodes to stimulate motor nerves, were often done without deliberate rhizotomy, though posterior roots may have been damaged accidentally in some cases.[35] Most of these patients had useful function, though some may have had persisting autonomic dysreflexia and some needed subsequent sphincterotomy.

Tanagho et al reported extradural implants on 22 patients, most of whom had other procedures to reduce outlet resistance; with increasing experience, they commented that 'more extensive dorsal rhizotomy is essential to achieve good voiding'.[49]

Talalla et al placed electrodes extradurally in seven patients without posterior rhizotomy or pudendal neurectomy and, although initial results were promising,[54] Talalla and Bloom subsequently concluded that this combination was not effective.[9]

Kirkham et al recently implanted extradural electrodes without rhizotomy in five patients with spinal cord injury. Reflex bladder contraction was preserved and could be inhibited by using the electrodes to stimulate only afferent neurons in the sacral nerves, but voiding was hindered in several patients, probably by reflex contraction of the sphincter.[55]

The major advantages of posterior rhizotomy are:

1. A great increase in bladder compliance and capacity (except in the few cases where poor compliance is due to fibrosis), thereby protecting the upper tracts from ureteric reflux and hydronephrosis.
2. The abolition of uninhibited reflex bladder contractions, thereby reducing reflex incontinence and the need for anticholinergic medication and its side-effects.
3. The abolition of reflex contraction of the sphincter, thereby reducing detrusor-sphincter dyssynergia.
4. The abolition of autonomic dysreflexia triggered from the bladder or rectum.

The disadvantages of posterior rhizotomy include:

1. The loss of perineal sensation if present.
2. The loss of reflex erection and reflex ejaculation if present, although these are not always functional after spinal cord injury. Some patients are capable of a modified form of orgasm by stimulating the sacral dermatomes after spinal cord injury and this too would be abolished by sacral rhizotomy. Erection is commonly produced by the implant and even more effectively by injection of papaverine or prostaglandins into the corpora cavernosa. Seminal emission can now be produced from a high proportion of spinal cord injured men by rectal probe electrostimulation, even after rhizotomy, and the procedure does not damage the implant.
3. The loss of reflex micturition and reflex defecation. The micturition produced by the implant is usually much more effective than reflex micturition, but if the implant is not used for any reason a patient will have to resort to intermittent or indwelling catheterization. Similarly, a patient with rhizotomy who uses the implant will generally become less constipated, but will be more constipated if the implant is not used.

A decision about posterior rhizotomy should therefore be made in each case. Brindley suggests the following policy:

- In women with complete lesions – who have less to lose and much to gain from continence – complete posterior rhizotomy is usually advised.
- In men with complete lesions and without useful reflex erection or ejaculation, the same policy may be followed, but if useful reflexes or sensation are present, the advantages and disadvantages of rhizotomy should be weighed with the patient.

The advantages of the combined procedure are such that implantation of the stimulator is now rarely performed without posterior rhizotomy, and this practice is likely to continue until a suitable alternative to surgical rhizotomy is found.

References

1. Bradley W, Timm G, Chou S. A decade of experience with electronic simulation of the micturition reflex. Urol Int 1971; 26:283–303.

2. Halverstadt D, Parry W. Electronic stimulation of the human bladder: nine years later. J Urol 1975; 113:341–344.

3. Burghele T. Electrostimulation of the neurogenic urinary bladder. In: Lutzmeyer Wea, ed. Urodynamics. Upper and lower urinary tract. Berlin: Springer-Verlag, 1973:319–322.

4. Kaeckenbeeck B. [Electrostimulation of the bladder in paraplegia. Method of Burghele–Ichim–Demetrescu.] Acta Urol Belg 1979; 47:139–140.

5. Nashold BS Jr, Friedman H, Grimes J. Electrical stimulation of the conus medullaris to control the bladder in the paraplegic patient. A 10-year review. Appl Neurophysiol 1981; 44:225–232.

6. Brindley GS. An implant to empty the bladder or close the urethra. J Neurol Neurosurg Psychiatry 1977; 40:358–369.

7. Brindley GS, Polkey CE, Rushton DN. Sacral anterior root stimulators for bladder control in paraplegia. Paraplegia 1982; 20:365–381.

8. Brindley GS. Emptying the bladder by stimulating sacral ventral roots. J Physiol 1974; 237:15P–16P.

9. Talalla A, Bloom J. Sacral electrical stimulation for bladder control. In: Illis LS, ed. Functional stimulation (spinal cord dysfunction, III). Oxford: Oxford University Press, 1992:206–218.

10. Sauerwein D. [Surgical treatment of spastic bladder paralysis in paraplegic patients. Sacral deafferentation with implantation of a sacral anterior root stimulator.] Urologe A 1990; 29:196–203.

11. Sarrias M, Sarrias F, Borau A. The "Barcelona" technique. Neurourol Urodyn 1993; 12:495–496.

12. Brindley G. The Finetech–Brindley Bladder Controller: Notes for surgeons and physicians. Welwyn Garden City, Herts, England: Finetech Medical Ltd., 1998.

13. MacDonagh RP, Forster DMC, Thomas DG. Urinary continence in spinal injury patients following complete sacral posterior rhizotomy. Br J Urol 1990; 66:618–622.

14. Delamarter RB, Ross JS, Masaryk TJ, et al. Diagnosis of lumbar arachnoiditis by magnetic resonance imaging. Spine 1990; 15:304–310.

15. Arnold E, Gowland S, MacFarlane M, et al. Sacral anterior root stimulation of the bladder in paraplegics. Aust NZ J Surg 1986; 56:319–324.

16. Herlant M, Colombel P. Electrostimulation intra-durale des racines sacrees anterieures chez les paraplegiques. Historique, reultats, indications. Annales de Réadaptation et de Médecine physique 1986; 29:405–411.

17. Madersbacher H, Fischer J, Ebner A. Anterior sacral root stimulator (Brindley): experiences especially in women with neurogenic urinary incontinence. Neurourol Urodyn 1988; 7:593–601.

18. Robinson L, Grant A, Weston P, et al. Experience with the Brindley anterior sacral root stimulator. Br J Urol 1988; 62:553–557.

19. Nordling J, Hald T, Kristensen JK, et al. [An implantable radiocontrolled sacral nerve root stimulator for control of urination.] Ugeskr Laeger 1988; 150:978–980.

20. Borau A, Vidal J, Sarrias F, et al. Electro-estimulación de las raices sacras anteriores para el control esfinteriano en el lesionado medular. Médula Espinal 1995; 1:128–133.

21. Schurch B, Rodic B, Jeanmonod D. Posterior sacral rhizotomy and intradural anterior sacral root stimulation for treatment of the spastic bladder in spinal cord injured patients. J Urol 1997; 157:610–614.

22. van der Aa HE, Alleman E, Nene A, Snoek G. Sacral anterior root stimulation for bladder control: clinical results. Arch Physiol Biochem 1999; 107:248–256.

23. Egon G, Barat M, Colombel P, et al. Implantation of anterior sacral root stimulators combined with posterior sacral rhizotomy in spinal injury patients. World J Urol 1998; 16:342–349.

24. Van Kerrebroeck PEV, van der Aa HE, Bosch JLHR, et al. Sacral rhizotomies and electrical bladder stimulation in spinal cord injury: clinical and urodynamic analysis. Eur Urol 1997; 31:263–271.

25. Wielink G, Essink-Bot ML, Van Kerrebroeck PEV, Rutten FFH. Sacral rhizotomies and electrical bladder stimulation in spinal cord injury: cost-effectiveness and quality of life analysis. Eur Urol 1997; 31:441–446.

26. Creasey G, Grill J, Korsten M, et al. An implantable neuroprosthesis for restoring bladder and bowel control to patients with spinal cord injuries: a multi-center trial. Arch Phys Med Rehab 2001; 82:1512–1519.

27. Van Kerrebroeck P, Koldewijn E, Debruyne F. Worldwide experience with the Finetech-Brindley sacral anterior root stimulator. Neurourol Urodyn 1993; 12:497–503.

28. Brindley GS. The first 500 patients with sacral anterior root stimulator implants: general description. Paraplegia 1994; 32:795–805.

29. Colombel P, Egon G. [Electrostimulation of the anterior sacral nerve roots. An International Congress – Le Mans – 24–25 November 1989.] Ann Urol Paris 1991; 25:48–52.

30. Brindley GS. History of the sacral anterior root stimulator, 1969–1982. Neurourol Urodyn 1993; 12:481–483.

31. Brindley GS, Rushton DN. Long-term follow-up of patients with sacral anterior root stimulator implants. Paraplegia 1990; 28:469–475.

32. Brindley GS. Sacral anterior root stimulators for bladder control in paraplegia: the first 50 cases. J Neurol Neurosurg Psychiatry 1986; 49:1104–1114.

33. Van Kerrebroeck P, Koldewijn E, Wijkstra H, Debruyne F. Urodynamic evaluation before and after intradural posterior rhizotomies and implantation of the Finetech-Brindley anterior sacral root stimulator. Urodinamica 1992; 1:7–16.

34. Cardozo L, Krishnan KR, Polkey CE, et al. Urodynamic observations on patients with sacral anterior root stimulators. Paraplegia 1984; 22:201–209.

35. Brindley G, Polkey C, Rushton D, Cardozo L. Sacral anterior root stimulators for bladder control in paraplegia: the first 50 cases. J Neurol Neurosurg Psychiatry 1986; 49:1104–1114.

36. Schalow G. Efferent and afferent fibres in human sacral ventral nerve roots: basic research and clinical implications. Electromyogr Clin Neurophysiol 1989; 29:33–53.

37. Schurch B, Knapp PA, Jeanmonod D, et al. Does sacral posterior rhizotomy suppress autonomic hyper-reflexia in patients with spinal cord injury? Br J Urol 1998; 81:73–82.

38. Rushton DN, Brindley GS, Polkey CE, Browning GV. Implant infections and antibiotic-impregnated silicone rubber coating. J Neurol Neurosurg Psychiatry 1989; 52:223–229.

39. Brindley GS. The first 500 sacral anterior root stimulators: implant failures and their repair. Paraplegia 1995; 33:5–9.

40. Varma JS, Binnie N, Smith AN, et al. Differential effects of sacral anterior root stimulation on anal sphincter and colorectal motility in spinally injured man. Br J Surg 1986; 73:478–482.

41. Binnie N, Smith A, Creasey G, Edmond P. Motility effects of electrical anterior sacral nerve root stimulation of the parasympathetic supply of the left colon and anorectum in paraplegic subjects. J Gastrointest Mot 1990; 2:12–17.

42. Binnie N, Smith A, Creasey G, Edmond P. The effects of electrical anterior sacral nerve root stimulation on pelvic floor function in paraplegic subjects. J Gastrointest Mot 1991; 3:39–45.

43. Binnie NR, Smith AN, Creasey GH, Edmond P. Constipation associated with chronic spinal cord injury: the effect of pelvic parasympathetic stimulation by the Brindley stimulator. Paraplegia 1991; 29:463–469.

44. MacDonagh RP, Sun WM, Smallwood R, et al. Control of defecation in patients with spinal injuries by stimulation of sacral anterior nerve roots. Br Med J 1990; 300:1494–1497.

45. Creasey GH, Dahlberg JE. Economic consequences of an implanted neuralprosthesis for bladder and bowel management. Arch Phys Med Rehab 2001; 82:1520–1525.

46. Akers JM, Smith BT, Betz RR. Implantable electrode lead in a growing limb. IEEE Trans Rehab Eng 1999; 7:35–45.

47. Merenda LA, Spoltore TA, Betz RR. Progressive treatment options for children with spinal cord injury. SCI Nurs 2000; 17:102–109.

48. Sauerwein D, Ingunza W, Fischer J, et al. Extradural implantation of sacral anterior root stimulators. J Neurol Neurosurg Psychiatry 1990; 50:681–684.

49. Tanagho EA, Schmidt RA, Orvis BR. Neural stimulation for control of voiding dysfunction: a preliminary report in 22 patients with serious neuropathic voiding disorders. J Urol 1989; 142:340–345.

50. Brindley GS, Craggs MD. A technique for anodally blocking large nerve fibres through chronically implanted electrodes. J Neurol Neurosurg Psychiatry 1980; 43:1083–1090.

51. Grunewald V, Bhadra N, Creasey GH, Mortimer JT. Functional conditions of micturition induced by selective sacral anterior root stimulation: experimental results in a canine animal model. World J Urol 1998; 16:329–336.

52. Bhadra N, Grunewald V, Creasey G, Mortimer JT. Selective suppression of sphincter activation during sacral anterior nerve root stimulation. Neurourol Urodyn 2002; 21:55–64.

53. Abdel-Gawad M, Boyer S, Sawan M, Elhilali MM. Reduction of bladder outlet resistance by selective stimulation of the ventral sacral root using high frequency blockade: a chronic study in spinal cord transected dogs. J Urol 2001; 166:728–733.

54. Talalla A, Bloom JW, Nguyen Q. Successful intraspinal extradural sacral nerve stimulation for bladder emptying in a victim of traumatic spinal cord transection. Neurosurgery 1986; 19:955–961.

55. Kirkham AP, Knight SL, Craggs MD, et al. Neuromodulation through sacral nerve roots 2 to 4 with a Finetech-Brindley sacral posterior and anterior root stimulator. Spinal Cord 2002; 40:272–281.

20

Central neuromodulation

Philip EV Van Kerrebroeck

Introduction

A multitude of neurological disorders can affect the bladder and although the incidence of lower urinary tract dysfunction is different among the various neurological entities, an important percentage of patients develop voiding dysfunction.[1] Incontinence and poor evacuation of urine with residual urine and recurrent urinary tract infections can cause important morbidity. In patients with spinal cord injury the lack of ability to control the storing and evacuation function of the bladder is one of the most prominent aspects of their handicap.

Besides these bladder problems with a proven neurological basis, a vast group of patients suffers from lower urinary tract dysfunction without an evident neurological cause. These are patients with different forms of so-called idiopathic dysfunctional voiding.

Therapeutic modalities are pharmacological treatment, eventually in combination with clean intermittent catheterization. Lifelong continuation of this therapy, however, is a major issue mainly because of side-effects. Furthermore, in most patients, especially in females, incontinence remains a problem even with maximal pharmacological treatment. The failure of pharmacological manipulation has led to the development of surgical approaches such as augmentation cystoplasty, sphincteric incisions, and artificial sphincter implantation. However, a considerable number of patients with neurogenic bladder dysfunction continue to have significant urological problems although maximal classical therapy is applied. Therefore the use of electrical stimulation to control storage and evacuation of urine has become an important tool in the urological treatment of voiding dysfunction.

The aim of electrical stimulation for voiding dysfunction is to treat incontinence due to a lack of activity in the striated muscles of the urethral closure mechanism by improvement of the contraction of the sphincter mechanism or to overcome incontinence due to detrusor hyperactivity by reduction of detrusor contractions. Furthermore, electrical stimulation can be used to permit evacuation of a paraplegic bladder by provocation of detrusor contractions or to control micturition in the hyperreflex bladder by a combination of dampening of spontaneous reflex excitability and controlled activation of the detrusor.

These aims can be fulfilled by stimulation of the efferent nerves to the lower urinary tract or by modulation of reflex activity as a consequence of stimulation of afferent nerves. Different modalities to apply electrical current to the lower urinary tract are available. Surface electrodes can be used as nonimplantable devices.[2] Insertable plugs in the anal canal or the vagina are applied to treat incontinence.[3–5] Intravesical electrostimulation is performed in children with meningomyelocele.[6–8] Implantable prostheses are available to induce bladder contraction in order to evacuate urine in paraplegic bladders or to control detrusor contraction in hyperreflexic bladders.[9–11] Another type of prosthesis permits the modulation of symptomatic voiding dysfunction such as urge incontinence, urgency/frequency syndrome, and retention.[12,13]

Electrical stimulation for chronic lower urinary tract dysfunction

Chronic lower urinary tract dysfunction, such as urge incontinence, urgency/frequency syndrome, and bladder evacuation problems, presents a challenge. Most patients are initially treated conservatively with bladder retraining, pelvic floor exercises, and biofeedback. In the majority, this regimen will be supplemented with drugs. However, about 40% of patients with these forms of lower urinary tract dysfunction do not achieve an acceptable condition with these forms of treatment and remain a therapeutic problem. Alternative procedures with variable success rates such as bladder transection, transvesical phenol injection of the pelvic plexus, augmentation cystoplasty, and even urinary diversion are being advocated.

During recent decades, functional electrical stimulation has gained interest in the treatment of this type of lower urinary tract dysfunction. Different stimulation sites, such as the vagina or the anus, have been reported to be successful. Since the 1960s, transcutaneous neurostimulation applied to the third or fourth sacral foramen has been tried as a method of controlling functional lower urinary tract disorders.[14] Unilateral sacral segmental stimulation with a permanent electrode at the level of the sacral foramen S3 or S4 (sacral neuromodulation) can offer an alternative nondestructive mode of treatment for patients presenting with voiding dysfunction and chronic pelvic pain refractory to conservative measures. Since 1981 a clinical trial has been underway to evaluate the effectiveness of this method. Since that time, experience has been gathered in the evaluation, surgery, and follow-up of patients presenting with voiding dysfunction and pelvic pain who have been treated with sacral foramen electrode implants.[15] The goal of such treatment is to relieve the symptoms by rebalancing micturition control.

The mode of action of this so-called sacral neuromodulation is still unclear but it has been hypothesized that the electrical current modulates reflex pathways involved in the filling and evacuation phase of the micturition cycle.[16] Stimulation of Aδ myelinated fibers of the sacral roots S3 and S4 decreases the spastic behavior of the pelvic floor and enhances the tone of the urethral sphincter. The threshold for the somatic component of the spinal nerve that innervates the pelvic floor is lower than that for the autonomic component to the bladder. Therefore, simultaneous bladder contraction is avoided during stimulation. In many subjects the primary voiding dysfunction appears to begin with unstable urethral activity, which activates the voiding reflexes, leading to detrusor instability and the associated urgency, frequency, and incontinence. The inhibitory effect of the enhanced urethral sphincter tone suppresses detrusor instability and stabilizes detrusor activity.

Ideal candidates for neuromodulation are patients presenting with urge incontinence, urinary urgency/frequency, and evacuation problems. Patients who have failed numerous other therapies should not be excluded from neuromodulation as they often show an excellent response to this technique.

Sacral neuromodulation is planned as a long-term treatment, but patients are first tested by means of a temporary trial stimulation for 3–7 days. This trial stimulation consists of two steps. The first phase is the acute testing, followed by the so-called subchronic phase. During an outpatient procedure and under local anesthesia, one of the sacral foramina, preferably the third one, is punctured with a 20-gauge hollow needle. The proximal and distal tip of the needle is not isolated and allows electrical stimulation.

Typical responses to stimulation of each nerve level are seen at both the local (perineum) and distant (foot and toe) sites. S3 stimulation produces a contraction of the levator muscles (bellows-like contraction) as well as detrusor and urethral sphincter contraction. Signs of S3 stimulation in the lower extremities include plantar flexion of the great toe. Subjectively, patients report a pulling sensation in the rectum during S3 stimulation, with variable sensations being perceived in the scrotum and the tip of the penis by men or the labia and vagina in women. S4 stimulation results in a contraction of the levator ani muscle (bellows-like contraction), with no activity being noted in the foot or leg. The sacral root at either site with the best clinical (subjective) or urodynamic response is selected and the intensity of the current adapted to the sensation of stimulation.

Through the needle a temporary electrode is placed and the needle is removed. This electrode remains in the vicinity of the sacral root selected and passes through the sacral foramen, subcutaneous tissue, and the skin. When the acute motoric responses with stimulation are confirmed, the electrode is connected to an external stimulator. Then starts the subchronic phase of the trial stimulation. Patients will check the effect for 3–7 days based on voiding diaries. Urodynamic examination is a possible other control of the effect.

Patients with a good clinical and preferably urodynamic result can be candidates for a permanent implant. This implant consists of a surgically implanted electrode with four contact points (Pisces quad lead Model 3886, Medtronic Inc., Minneapolis, Minnesota, USA) connected to a pacemaker (Interstim stimulator, Medtronic Interstim, Tolchenau, Switzerland).

Implantation is performed under general anesthesia. After a midline incision over the sacrum, the fascia overlying the foramina at one side of the sacrum is opened, giving access to the foramen selected. Acute stimulation with a needle will be repeated in order to confirm the motoric responses. The permanent electrode is positioned in the foramen with the four contact points in the neighborhood of the sacral nerve. The electrode is fixed to the posterior wall of the sacral with nonresorbable sutures and passed subcutaneously to an incision in one of the flanks. After closure of the wounds, the patient is placed in a lateral position. A subcutaneous pocket is created lateral of the umbilicus. The flank wound is opened and the electrode is connected with the pulse generator using a connection cable that is passed subcutaneously to an abdominal pocket. The pacemaker is fixed to the rectus fascia. Recently an alternative technique has been presented in which a gluteal pocket is created to receive the pulse generator. This method has the advantage that the surgery can be performed in one position. Furthermore, morbidity, especially pain at the implant side, seems to be reduced.

Generally, low amplitudes (1.5 to 5.5 V, 210 μs pulse duration at 10 to 15 cycles/s) are sufficient for stimulation of the somatic nerve fibers. With these parameters, no dyssynergia of the bladder and striated urethral musculature is induced even when voiding is initiated with the stimulator on.

Previous reports indicate an overall success rate of 60–75% at initial trial stimulation.[15] Of the patients selected after subchronic trial stimulation who underwent permanent implantation, up to 83% have derived major benefit from the definitive procedure.[17] This effect appears to be durable, as evidenced by the late results. However, about 20% of patients who respond well on trial stimulation fail to reproduce the same result after chronic stimulation. Based on clinical parameters it appears that patients with detrusor overactivity and urethral instability have the best result.[18]

Recently, the results of a multinational, multicenter clinical trial of this method were presented.[19] In a group of 155 patients with therapy-resistant urge incontinence, 98 (63%) reacted sufficiently on the temporary trial stimulation. Of these, 38 were followed for 1 year with a successful outcome in 30 (79%).

Similar multicenter, multinational studies in patients with urgency/frequency and chronic voiding problems have been published with similar results.[20,21] Also, with long-term follow-up, results seem to be persistent over time.[22] However after permanent implantation about 20% of patients with initially favorable PNE test results fail to respond for yet unknown reasons. Further research to indicate additional parameters that may be used as reliable predictors of success is necessary.

Neuromodulation seems to be an effective treatment modality in patients with various forms of lower urinary tract dysfunction. This technique is a valuable addition to our treatment options when conservative measures fail.

References

1. Wein AJ, Raezer DM, Benson GS. Management of neurogenic bladder dysfunction in the adult. Urology 1976; 8:432–443.

2. Bradley WE, Timm GW, Chou SN. A decade of experience with electronic stimulation of the micturition reflex. Urol Int 1971; 26:283–302.

3. Godec C, Cass AS, Ayala GF. Electrical stimulation for incontinence. Technique, selection and results. Urology 1976; 7:388–397.

4. Merrill DC. The treatment of detrusor incontinence by electrical stimulation. J Urol 1979; 122:515–517.

5. Fall M. Does electrostimulation cure urinary incontinence? J Urol 1984; 131:664–667.

6. Katona F. Stages of vegetative afferentiation in reorganization of bladder control during intravesical electrotherapy. Urol Int 1975; 30:192–203.

7. Seiferth J, Heising J, Larkamp H. Experiences and critical comments on the temporary intravesical electrostimulation of neurogenic bladder in spina bifida children. Urol Int 1978; 33:279–284.

8. Madersbacher H, Pauer W, Reiner E. Rehabilitation of micturition by transurethral electrostimulation of the bladder in patients with incomplete spinal cord lesions. Paraplegia 1982; 20:191–195.

9. Caldwell KP, Flack FC, Broad AF. Urinary incontinence following spinal injury treated by electronic implant. Lancet 1965; 39:846–847.

10. Brindley GS, Polkey CE, Rushton DN, Cardozo L. Sacral anterior root stimulators for bladder control in paraplegia: the first 50 cases. J Neurol Neurosurg Psychiatry 1986; 49:1104–1114.

11. Tanagho EA, Schmidt RA, Orvis BR. Neural stimulation for control of voiding dysfunction: a preliminary report in 22 patients with serious neuropathic voiding disorders. J Urol 1989; 142:340–345.

12. Markland C, Merrill D, Chou S, Bradley W. Sacral nerve root stimulation: a clinical test of detrusor innervation. J Urol 1972; 107:772–776.

13. Schmidt RA. Advances in genitourinary neurostimulation. Neurosurgery 1986; 18:1041–1044.

14. Habib HN. Experiences and recent contributions in sacral nerve stimulation for both human and animal. Br J Urol 1967; 39:73–83.

15. Schmidt RA. Applications of neurostimulation in urology. Neurourol Urodyn 1988; 7:585.

16. Thon WF, Baskin LS, Jonas U, et al. Neuromodulation of voiding dysfunction and pelvic pain. World J Urol 1991; 9:38.

17. Bosch JLHR, Groen J. Sacral (S_3) segmental nerve stimulation as a treatment for urge incontinence in patients with detrusor instability: results of chronic electrical stimulation using an implantable neural prosthesis. J Urol 1995; 154:504–507.

18. Koldewijn EL, Rosier PF, Meuleman EJ, Koster AM, Debruyne FM, Van Kerrebroeck PE et al. Predictors of success with neuromodulation in lower urinary tract dysfunction: results of trial stimulation in 100 patients. J Urol 1994; 152:2071–2075.

19. Janknegt RA, Van Kerrebroeck PhEV, Lycklama à Nijeholt AA, et al. Sacral nervemodulation for urge incontinence: a multinational, multicenter randomized study. J Urol 1997; 157, 4:1237.

20. Hassouna MM, Siegel SW, Nyeholt AA, et al. Sacral neuromodulation in the treatment of urgency-frequency symptoms: a multicenter study on efficacy and safety. J Urol 2000; 163(6):1849–1854.

21. Jonas U, Fowler CJ, Chancellor MB, et al. Efficacy of sacral nerve stimulation for urinary retention: results 18 months after implantation. J Urol 2001; 165:15–19.

22. Bosch JL, Groen J. Sacral nerve neuromodulation in the treatment of patients with refractory motor urge incontinence: long-term results of a prospective longitudinal study. J Urol 2000; 163(4):1219–1222.

21

Intravesical electrical stimulation of the bladder

Helmut G Madersbacher

Background

Already in 1887 the Danish surgeon Saxtorph[1] described intravesical electrical stimulation (IVES) for the 'atonic bladder' by inserting a transurethral catheter with a metal stylet in it and with a neutral electrode on the lower abdomen. In 1899 two Viennese surgeons, Frankl-Hochwart and Zuckerkandl,[2] stated that intravesical electrotherapy was more effective in inducing detrusor contractions than external faradization. In 1975 Katona[3] introduced this method for the treatment of neurogenic bladder dysfunction. Ebner et al[4] demonstrated in cat experiments that intravesical electrostimulation activates the mechanoreceptors within the bladder wall.

Further basic research was undertaken by Jiang et al,[5] who demonstrated that IVES at low frequencies (≥ 20 Hz) had a better modulatory effect than at higher frequencies. Jiang[6] proved in the animal experiment that IVES induced modulation of the micturition reflex due to an enhanced excitatory synaptic transmission in the central micturition reflex pathway. The observed modulation may account for the clinical benefit of IVES treatment.

The afferent stimuli induced by IVES travel along afferent pathways from the lower urinary tract to the corresponding cerebral structures. This 'vegetative afferention'[3] results in the sensation of bladder filling/urge to void, with subsequent enhancement of active contractions and possibly also voluntary control over the detrusor (Figure 21.1).

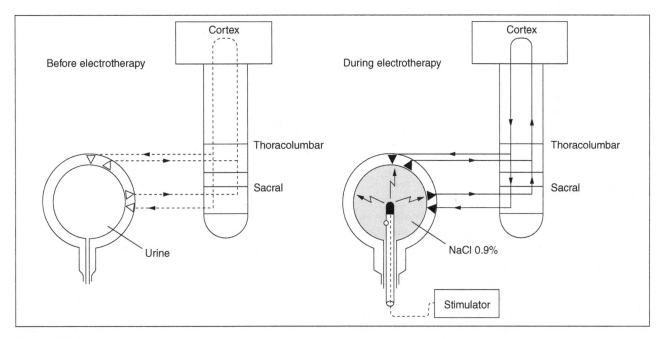

Figure 21.1
Intravesical electrostimulation activates the mechanoreceptors within the bladder wall, thus increasing the efferent input from the bladder and consequently the efferent output to the bladder. (Reproduced with permission from Ebner et al.[4])

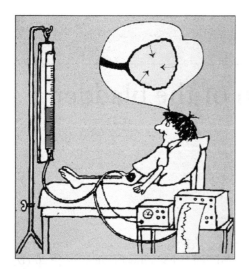

Figure 21.2
With intravesical electrostimulation a feedback training is
mediated by enabling the patient to observe the change of
the detrusor pressure on a water manometer: the patient is
able to realize when a detrusor contraction takes place.

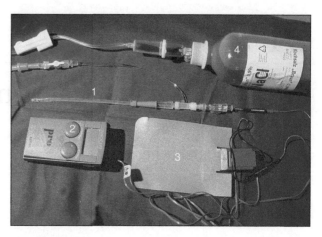

Figure 21.3
IVES armamentarium: 1, Disposable catheter with the
electrode in it; 2, battery-operated stimulator; 3, neutral
electrode; 4, saline (0.9%).

Colombo et al[7] demonstrated that intravesical electrostimulation also induces electrical changes on higher micturition centers, measured by electroencephalography
(EEG). The evaluation of viscerosensory cortical evoked
potentials after transurethral electrical stimulation has
been proved to be useful in determining whether a patient
is suitable for IVES or not.[8]

A feedback training is mediated by enabling the patient
to observe the change of the detrusor pressure on a water
manometer; thus the patient is able to realize when a
detrusor contraction takes place. This also facilitates voluntary control (Figure 21.2).

Various synonyms were used in the literature for intravesical electrical stimulation, such as bladder stimulation,
intravesical bladder stimulation, transurethral electrostimulation of the bladder, and intravesical, transurethral
bladder stimulation.

Technique

The technique involves a catheter, with a stimulation electrode (cathode) in it, being introduced into the bladder
and connected to a stimulator. Saline (0.9%) is used as the
current leading medium within the bladder. The anode
(neutral) electrode (14 × 9 cm) is attached to the skin in
an area with preserved sensation, usually in the lower
abdomen (Figure 21.3). According to Ebner et al[4] the following stimulation parameters have proved to be most
effective in the animal experiment: pulse width, 2 ms; frequency, 20 Hz; and current, 1–10 mA. Some researchers
use square unipolar pulses for continuous stimulation,[9]

whereas others use intermittent stimulation with bursts
and gaps that can be varied (1–10 s) along with the rise
time and the time of the plateau within the burst. With
intermittent electrostimulation, each therapy session takes
60–90 min, with continuous stimulation 20 min, on a daily
basis, 5 days a week, until the maximum response is
reached. For patients who have never experienced the urge
to void – e.g. children with myelomeningocele or children
who have lost this ability – IVES is combined with a
biofeedback training: on a water manometer attached to
the system the patient is able to observe the change in the
detrusor pressure. This way he is able to realize that the
sensation experienced is caused by a bladder contraction.
This external feedback also facilitates achievement of
voluntary control.

Results

The results presented are based on 31 studies: 6 are basic
research papers (animal experiments and clinical research),
one is a randomized controlled trial, there are 2 reviews
within an editorial, one pro and one contra IVES, and the
others are case series.

Intravesical electrical stimulation of the bladder is still a
controversial therapy for patients with neurogenic detrusor dysfunction, although basic research during the last
decade has evidenced the mechanism of its action and its
efficacy.[4,6] At least, in animal experiments, optimal parameters have been determined.[4,10]

The controversy about the value of IVES for detrusor
(re-)habilitation is also reflected in an editorial recently
published, in which Kaplan[11] reported favorable results in
288 children who received at least one series (20 outpatient

sessions, 90 min long): 87% of patients have control and void or catheterize with sensation or have improved bladder compliance. Eighteen percent have gained full control, they void synergistically and are continent, whereas before they were either voiding poorly and incontinent or used clean intermittent catherization and were more or less dry. Forty-four percent void with sensation and are in biofeedback to try and gain control. Finally, in 13% the treatment failed, but the patients maintained their condition. Moreover, the results seen in an 'early' group were followed up 10 years later. As long as no intervening neurosurgical insult occurred, less than 3% of cases needed to return for a tune-up to maintain their 'healthy bladder'. The average number of daily sessions to achieve these results was 47.

In contrast, the results reported by Decter[12] were less favorable. In 25 patients during a 5-year period with, all together, 938 sessions of stimulation, bladder capacity increased greater than 20% in regards to the age-adjusted and end-filling bladder pressure and showed clinically significant decreases in 28% of patients. In response to a questionnaire, 56% of parents noted a subjective improvement in their childrens' bladder function. However, the urodynamic improvements achieved after IVES did not significantly alter the daily voiding routine in these children.[13]

The only randomized controlled prospective clinical trial[14] could not find differences between active and sham treatment; however, only 15 sessions were performed at first and another 15 sessions of IVES were applied after a 3-month hiatus. Moreover, the inclusion criteria were not defined.

Other studies are either individual case-controlled studies (*Level of evidence 3B*) or case series (*Level of evidence 4*). They cannot be compared due to different or non-defined inclusion criteria, different technique details (different time of electrostimulation, varying follow-ups), and some with only a small number of patients included.[15–31] Recently, Gladh[9] presented the results of 44 children (mean age 10.5 years), 20 of them with neurogenic bladder dysfunction: with a mean follow-up of 2.5 years, 64% had their bladder emptying normalized, 11 of 15 children on clean intermittent catheterization (CIC) have terminated catheterization, 8 of them with neurogenic bladder dysfunction; 7 children had no remaining benefit of the treatment.

Prerequisites for successful intravesical electrical stimulation

None of the research really focused on the inclusion criteria. According to the basic research, only those with some intact afferent fibers from the bladder to the cortex and those with spinal cord lesions with the presence of pain sensation in the sacral dermatomes S3 and S4 can benefit from IVES. According to Nathan and Smith,[32] the pathways of the bladder proprioception and for pain lie close together. The value of viscerosensoric cortical evoked potentials from the bladder neck was demonstrated by Kiss et al.[8] A precise indication seems to be one prerequisite for a good result. Regarding children with myelomeningocele, one must also take into account that myelomeningocele bladders at birth may have a threefold increase in connective tissue compared to normal controls.[33] According to clinical experience, significant decrease of receptors tempers the enthusiasm for intravesical electrical stimulation in this particular group of patients.

Implications for practice

Basically, intravesical electrotherapy is able to improve neurogenic bladder dysfunction, primarily by stimulating Aδ mechanoafferents inducing bladder sensation and the urge to void and consequently increasing the efferent output with improvement of micturition and conscious control. Therefore, IVES is the only available option to induce/improve bladder sensation and to enhance the micturition reflex in incomplete central or peripheral nerve damage. However, proper indication is crucial and this type of therapy should only be applied in those with intact afferent fibers between the bladder and the cortex if possible, proved by the evaluation of viscerosensoric cortical evoked potentials. *If these premises are respected, IVES is effective.*

Intravesical electrical stimulation is *safe*; no side-effects have been reported, beyond an occasional urinary infection. The question of cost-effectiveness was raised by Kaplan,[11] who stated that the most commonly used alternative for these patients is bladder augmentation, which is 'miles apart in terms of cost, discomfort and short- and long-term complications'.

One benefit of IVES was noted by most of the authors: improved sensation documents satisfactory long-term results. The patients with successful IVES get great satisfaction from knowing when their bladder is full and when it is time to catheterize or to void. Moreover, even without direct bowel stimulation, patients noted significant improvement in the warning of bowel fullness and gained greater control for their bowel movements.

IVES can only be effective with certain prerequisites, the most important being that at least some afferent fibers between the bladder and the CNS are intact and the detrusor is able to contract. The method is safe, and no real complications have been reported.

Conclusions

- Basic research during the last decade has proved the underlying working concept.
- The results reported in the literature are controversial, mainly because of different inclusion and exclusion criteria.
- In the only sham-controlled study the treatment period is too short and the inclusion and exclusion criteria are not really defined.
- The alternative may be either life long intermittent catheterization or bladder augmentation. In this regards, IVES is *cost-effective*.
- It is worthwhile to apply intravesical electrostimulation, bearing in mind inclusion and exclusion criteria, especially when trying to verify functioning afferent fibers between the bladder and the cortex.

Recommendations

- Intravesical electrotherapy is able to improve neurogenic bladder dysfunction, primarily by stimulating Aδ mechanoreceptor afferents inducing bladder sensation and the urge to void and consequently increasing the efferent output with improvement of micturition and conscious control.
- IVES is the only available option to induce/improve bladder sensation and to enhance the micturition reflex in patients with incomplete central or peripheral nerve damage.
- Indication is crucial and IVES should only be applied if afferent fibers between the bladder and the cortex are still intact and if the detrusor muscle is still able to contract.
- *If these premises are respected, IVES is effective.*
- The ideal indication is the neuropathic underactive – hyposensitive and hypocontracile – detrusor.

Further research

There is definitely a need for placebo-(sham-)controlled prospective studies with clear inclusion and exclusion criteria and clear definitions of the aims. Recently De Wachter and Wyndaele[34] demonstrated in animal experiments and models that the position of the stimulating electrode, as well as the amount of saline within the bladder, may be crucial for the effect. Additional research is needed to clarify these aspects of IVES.

References

1. Saxtorph MH. Stricture urethrae – fistula perinee – retentio urinae. Clinisk Chirurgi. Copenhagen: Gyldendalske Fortlag 1878:265–280.

2. Frankel vL, Zuckerkandl O. In: Hrsg. H Senator, Die erkrankungen der blase. Wien: Alfred Höbler Verlag, 1899:101.

3. Katona F. Stages of vegetative afferentiation in reorganization of bladder control during electrotherapy. Urol Int 1975; 30:192–203.

4. Ebner A, Jiang CH, Lindström S. Intravesical electrical stimulation – an experimental analysis of the mechanism of action. J Urol 1992; 148:920–924.

5. Jiang CH, Lindström S, Mazières L. Segmental inhibitory control of ascending sensory information from bladder mechanoreceptors in cat. Neurourol Urodyn 1991; 10:286–288.

6. Jiang CH. Modulation of the micturition reflex pathway by intravesical electrical stimulation: an experimental study in the rat. Neurourol Urodyn 1998; 17(5):543–553.

7. Colombo T, Wieselmann G, Pichler-Zalaudek K, et al. Central nervous system control of micturition in patients with bladder dysfunctions in comparison with healthy control probands. An electrophysiological study. Urologe A 2000; 39(2):160–165.

8. Kiss G, Madersbacher H, Poewe W. Cortical evoked potentials of the vesicourethral junction – a predictor for the outcome of intravesical electrostimulation in patients with sensory and motor detrusor dysfunction. World J Urol 1998; 16(5):308–312.

9. Gladh G. Intravesical electrical stimulation in children with micturition dysfunction. Proc ICS 2002, Heidelberg, 2002: 22. [Abstract]

10. Buyle S, Wyndaele JJ, D'Hauwers K, et al. Optimal parameters for transurethral intravesical electrostimulation determined in an experiment in the rat. Eur Urol 1998; 33(5):507–510.

11. Kaplan WE. Intravesical electrical stimulation of the bladder: Pro. Editorial. Urology 2000; 56(1):2–4.

12. Decter RM. Intravesical electrical stimulation of the bladder: Contra. Editorial. Urology 2000; 56(1):2–4.

13. Decter RM, Snyder P, Laudermilch C. Transurethral electrical bladder stimulation: a follow-up report. J Urol 1994; 152:812–814.

14. Boone TB, Roehrborn CG, Hurt G. Transurethral intravesical electrotherapy for neurogenic bladder dysfunction in children with myelodysplasia: a prospective, randomized clinical trial. J Urol 1992; 148:550–554.

15. Eckstein HG, Katona F. Treatment of neuropathic bladder by transurethral electrical stimulation. Lancet 1974; 1:780–781.

16. Nicholas JL, Eckstein HB. Endovesical electrotherapy in treatment of urinary incontinence in spina bifida patients. Lancet 1975; 2:1276–1277.

17. Denes J, Leb J. Electrostimulation of the neuropathic bladder. J Pediatr Surg 1975; 10(2):245–247.

18. Janneck C. Electric stimulation of the bladder and the anal sphincter – a new way to treat the neurogenic bladder. Prog Pediatr Surg 1976; 9:119–139.

19. Seiferth J, Heising J, Larkamp H. Intravesical electrostimulation of the neurogenic bladder in spina bifida children. Urol Int 1978; 33(5):279–284.

20. Seiferth J, Larkamp H, Heising J. Experiences with temporary intravesical electro-stimulation of the neurogenic bladder in spina bifida children. Urologe A 1978; 17(5):353–354.

21. Schwock G, Tischer W. The influence of intravesical electrostimulation on the urinary bladder in animals. Z Kinderchir 1981; 32(2): 161–166.

22. Madersbacher H, Pauer W, Reiner E, et al. Rehabilitation of micturition in patients with incomplete spinal cord lesions by transurethral electrostimulation of the bladder. Eur Urol 1982; 8:111–116.

23. Kaplan WE, Richards I. Intravesical bladder stimulation in myelodysplasia. J Urol 1988; 140:1282–1284.

24. Madersbacher H. Intravesical electrical stimulation for the rehabilitation of the neuropathic bladder. Paraplegia 1990; 28:349–352.

25. Lyne CJ, Bellinger MF. Early experience with transurethral electrical bladder stimulation. J Urol 1993; 150:697–699.

26. Kölle D, Madersbacher H, Kiss G, Mair D. Intravesical electrostimulation for treatment of bladder dysfunction. Initial experience after gynecological operations. Gynakol Geburtshilfliche Rundsch 1995; 35(4):221–225.

27. Cheng EY, Richards I, Kaplan WE. Use of bladder stimulation in high risk patients. J Urol 1996; 156:479–752.

28. Cheng EY, Richards I, Balcom A, et al. Bladder stimulation therapy improves bladder compliance: results from a multi-institutional trial. J Urol 1996; 156:761–764.

29. Primus G, Trummer H. Intravesical electrostimulation in detrusor hypocontractility. Wien Klin Wochensch 1993; 105(19):556–557.

30. Kroll P, Jankowski A, Martynski M. Electrostimulation in treatment of neurogenic and non-neurogenic voiding dysfunction. Wiad Lek 1998; 51(Suppl 3):92–97.

31. Pugach JL, Salvin L, Steinhardt GF. Intravesical electrostimulation in pediatric patients with spinal cord defects. J Urol 2000; 164:965–968.

32. Nathan PW, Smith MC. The centripetal pathway from the bladder and urethra within the spinal cord. J Neurol Neurosurg Psychiatry 1951; 14:262–280.

33. Shapiro E, Becich MJ, Perlman E, Lepor H. Bladder wall abnormalities in myelodysplastic bladders: a computer assisted morphometric analysis. J Urol 1991; 145(5):1024–1029.

34. De Wachter S, Wyndaele JJ. Personal Communication, 2001.

22

Surgery to improve reservoir function

Manfred Stöhrer

Introduction

Compensated bladder storage is a function that is decisive for the quality of life and life expectancy of patients with neurogenic lower urinary tract dysfunction. It is characterized by low-pressure storage with physiological storage pressure as the maximum value. Storage pressure does not increase significantly before filling volume reaches 300 ml. The volume at which this pressure increase occurs is defined as the reflex volume.[1] Continence is better and the pressure load on the upper urinary tract is lower when the reflex volume is higher. When this condition cannot be achieved by medical treatment, a number of surgical interventions are available. Electrical stimulation and intestinal replacement are described elsewhere. The surgical procedures outlined here are effective for the majority of patients and are minimally invasive.

Two prerequisites are fundamental: intact detrusor musculature (no fibrosis) and satisfactory management of bladder emptying, preferably by intermittent catheterization. Should detrusor elasticity be impaired by morphologic conditions, (partial) bladder replacement is the only option. These changes, caused by tissue scarring, are the result of 'mismanagement' over several years. When the patient is treated correctly, this pathology will seldom occur.

In principle, to normalize the detrusor muscle its nervous supply can be altered by chemical receptor blockers, such as botulinum A toxin, which is the simplest and most promising method of ensuring compensated storage.[2,3]

For non-responders or when the effect is unsatisfactory, detrusor myectomy (partial auto-augmentation) is a possible alternative.[4,5] Some authors have expanded this simple intervention, with the use of omentum or gastrointestinal components to cover the mucosa at the site of the muscular defect after surgery.[6–9]

Should these procedures fail, clam cystoplasty offers a compromise before embarking on extensive enterocystoplasty.[10] All three methods can help patients with both complete or incomplete lesions.

Available for high and complete lesions, deafferentation by transection of the S2–S4 vertebral roots is an additional procedure to completely block detrusor overactivity.[11] In these cases, alternative emptying (preferably by intermittent catheterization) is necessary too, unless sacral root electrostimulation is applied.[12,13]

Table 22.1 presents an overview of the surgical options that could improve storage function in patients with neurogenic detrusor overactivity.

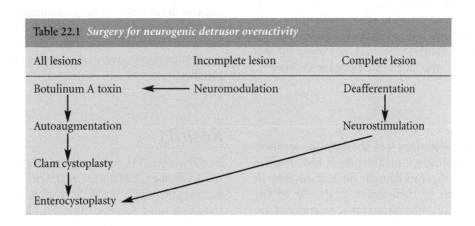

Table 22.1 *Surgery for neurogenic detrusor overactivity*

All lesions	Incomplete lesion	Complete lesion
Botulinum A toxin ← Neuromodulation		Deafferentation
↓		↓
Autoaugmentation		Neurostimulation
↓		
Clam cystoplasty		
↓		
Enterocystoplasty		

Botulinum A toxin injections in the detrusor

Botulinum A toxin has been known for many years to be not only one of the most potent venoms but also a very effective drug for the suppression of chronic muscular spasticity. It has been applied since 1980 to spastic striated muscles in many neurologic and orthopedic domains.[14,15] Aesthetic plastic surgeons use it much more extensively.[16] In urology, it was injected initially in the external sphincter to treat detrusor-sphincter dyssynergia.[17] In 1998, detrusor injections were given to patients with neurogenic lower urinary tract dysfunction in Germany and Switzerland. The first results were published in 1999.[2,3]

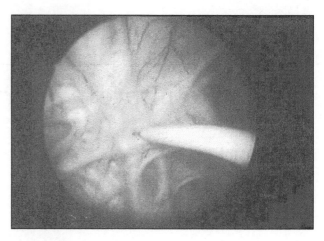

Figure 22.1
Botulinum A toxin injection in detrusor trabecule.

Mode of action

Botulinum toxin has several subtypes. Subtype A is the most effective, and the only one that is available commercially: a product of *Clostridium botulinum*, it is a strong natural venom. The molecule is composed of light and heavy nucleic acid chains connected by a disulfide ring. It blocks presynaptic nerve endings at the cholinergic neuron and prevents acetylcholine secretion, leading to temporary chemical denervation and loss of nerve activity in the target organ. The process is reversible by nerve regeneration, as new nerve endings will sprout from the neuron and reconstitute connections to the target organ. The time course of this process is dependent on the target organ type and is individually variable; it takes roughly between 3 and 4 months in the urethral sphincter, and 6–14 months in the detrusor. The average efficacy period in patients studied after detrusor injection is 10–12 months. Maximal efficacy is observed after about 2 weeks, remains pronounced until about 3 months after the injection, and then subsides slowly and continually.

Two varieties of botulinum A toxin are available: Botox® and Dysport®. The efficacy ratio between these two products is about 1:3. Dysport demonstrates greater dispersion. It thus appears rational to use a lower dilution to avoid its dispersion into the circulation. This mechanism may explain the isolated cases of generalized muscle weakness described in the literature.[18] We have not observed this effect in our patients who have been treated with Botox®.

Indication

Botulinum A toxin injections into the detrusor are indicated when anticholinergic medication is not effective or not tolerated. As this procedure is the least invasive of all available options in these cases, it should be the method of first choice when conservative treatment fails.

Its fundamental prerequisite is an effective bladder emptying after the treatment. Our experience shows that aseptic intermittent catheterization is preferred. When the detrusor overactivity is enhanced by acute urinary tract infection, the action of the toxin is insufficient to suppress it, and episodes of reflex incontinence may occur.

Method of application

Botox 300 IU (or Dysport 750–1000 IU) are given for the treatment of neurogenic detrusor overactivity. The agent is dissolved in 15 ml saline and injected in 0.5 ml aliquots through a standard endoscopic needle (30 injection sites) over the entire muscle. For children, the dosage is reduced in relation to body weight. The injections are administered preferably in visible muscular structures (trabecules) (Figure 22.1). The trigone and ureteric orifices are spared to prevent possible reflux. Thus, 10 IU Botox are injected at each site. An indwelling catheter is placed for 24 h. Antibiotic prophylaxis is started preoperatively and continued for 1 week. After removal of the indwelling catheter the patient practices intermittent catheterization – most patients adopt this routine before treatment. Peroperative anticholinergic treatment is continued during the first postoperative week and then discontinued completely.

Results

In our center, 141 patients were treated from early 1998 until October 2002: 222 treatment sessions were performed, including multiple treatments. The underlying condition was traumatic spinal cord lesion in the majority of patients, with small groups suffering from multiple sclerosis or myelomeningocele. Patients with low bladder compliance caused by structural changes in the detrusor wall (fibrosis) secondary to neurological disease were excluded from this treatment. Patients at risk from autonomic dysreflexia or who preserved their bladder sensation were treated under local or general anesthesia.

The condition of these patients and of those who were evaluated in cooperation with the center in Zurich was checked by videourodynamics preoperatively and at 12 and 36 weeks postoperatively. The parameters studied were reflex volume, maximal voiding detrusor pressure, cystometric bladder capacity, detrusor compliance, and continence status (Figures 22.2–22.5). Patient satisfaction and the post-treatment dosage of anticholinergics were also recorded. Significant improvement of all parameters was achieved in nearly all patients (95%). Reflex volume and cystometric capacity showed considerable amelioration after 6 weeks and most responders (>90%) were continent, unless urinary tract infection was present. Spontaneous voiding was eliminated, and thus the residual

was equal to the capacity. Treatment was successful, even in children. The condition of many patients with pre-existing autonomic dysreflexia improved significantly. It was not known why 5% of patients did not respond to botulinum A toxin injections, although immunity caused against the toxin by the presence of antibodies after earlier contact with it might be one reason.

Blocked nerve endings regenerate slowly – after 36 weeks, the condition of patients had deteriorated in comparison to that at 6 weeks, but was still significantly better than preoperatively. The mean efficacy period in our patients was 10–12 months. These results have been confirmed in a European multicenter study comprising over 200 patients.

Repeated botulinum A treatment sessions did not result in any loss of efficacy. In our patients, 51 had two injection sessions, 21 had three, 6 had four, and 3 had five, and increased toxin tolerance was not found.

Botox or Dysport application led to essentially similar outcomes, but generalized muscle weakness was observed in three patients after Dysport application. As discussed above, dispersion and dilution could have been determining

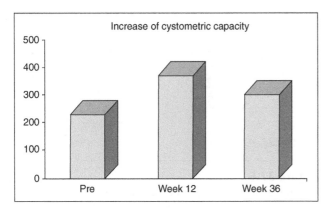

Figure 22.2
Increase of cystometric capacity at 12 and 36 weeks after botulinum treatment.

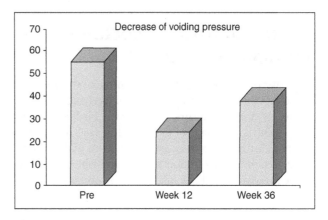

Figure 22.4
Decrease of voiding pressure at 12 and 36 weeks after botulinum treatment.

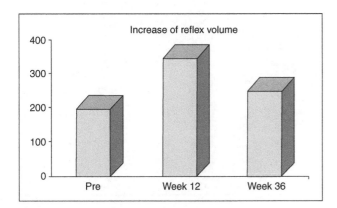

Figure 22.3
Increase of reflex volume at 12 and 36 weeks after botulinum treatment.

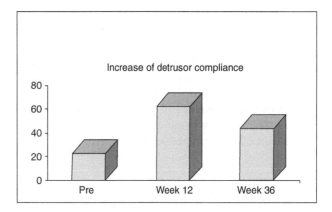

Figure 22.5
Increase of detrusor compliance at 12 and 36 weeks after botulinum treatment.

factors here; thus, we decided to reduce the dilution volume to 7.5 ml when using Dysport. Whether this will diminish or prevent the occurrence of these generalized adverse effects is still an open question.

In summary, detrusor injections of botulinum A toxin represent an effective treatment for neurogenic detrusor overactivity. Because this therapy has not been approved by the medical authorities in most countries, its use should be considered only with the appropriate precautions and documentation.

Recent literature

This procedure[2,3] has raised much interest since its introduction, but, apart from conference reports, the number of publications in the literature is still sparse. Its mechanism of action has been studied in rats[19] and preliminary trials have confirmed its efficacy also in myelomeningocele children.[20]

Partial detrusor myectomy (autoaugmentation)

The basis of this therapy is partial removal of the overactive detrusor without compromising the underlying mucosa. It decreases storage pressure and increases bladder capacity. The essential advantage of the procedure is its low invasivity and abstinence from covering the defect with intestinal tissue sections. This option remains available when later, more invasive procedures might become necessary.

Indication

Aggressive detrusor overactivity that is refractory to conservative treatment and that also does not respond to botulinum A toxin can be corrected by autoaugmentation. After this treatment, intermittent catheterization is compulsory. The functional transformation caused by the procedure needs time to be expressed. This period is at least 1 year, and the procedure is contraindicated if enough time is not available due to the patient's condition. Degenerative changes in the detrusor musculature, causing a reduction of anesthetic bladder capacity, are also a contraindication.

Method

The bladder anterior wall and dome are approached, and the peritoneum is freed from the bladder until about halfway down the bladder posterior wall. The bladder is filled to about 200 ml, and a circular section of the detrusor muscle with a radius of about 4 cm around the urachus is resected. The mucosa is left intact (Figures 22.6 and 22.7). The diverticulum created in this way will reduce storage pressure and improve bladder capacity after a period of 1–2 years. An indwelling catheter is left for 2 days when the mucosa has not been perforated during the procedure. When mucosal perforation has occurred, the indwelling catheter is placed for a maximum of 2 weeks and is clamped intermittently for 3–4 days, putting a low-grade load on the diverticulum.[5,21] In a few patients, ancillary injection with botulinum A toxin to accelerate the process of functional transformation has recently shown partial success.

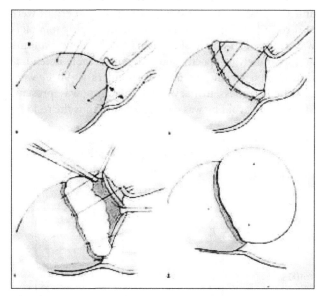

Figure 22.6
The autoaugmentation procedure (side view).

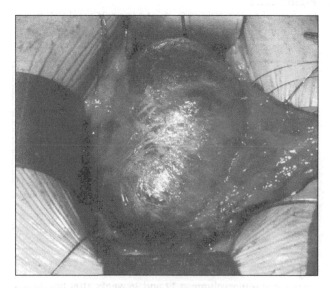

Figure 22.7
Surgical view during autoaugmentation procedure.

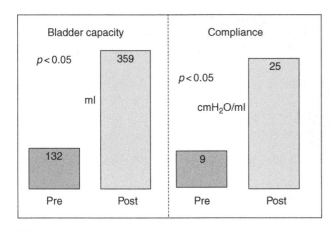

Figure 22.8
Bladder capacity and detrusor compliance after autoaugmentation.

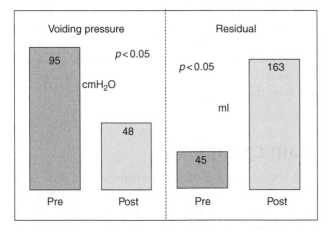

Figure 22.9
Voiding pressure and residual after autoaugmentation.

In 1989, Cartwright and Snow published a paper on a similar procedure in dogs and in a child.[4] Also in 1989, we performed this for the first time in a man with an incomplete spinal cord lesion. Cartwright and Snow attached the bladder to the iliopsoas, whereas we only do the simple resection. This simpler approach produces good results. The peritoneum remains closed, and covering of the defect is unnecessary.[5,21]

Results

From 1989 to October 2002 we treated 93 patients by this method. After the introduction of botulinum A toxin injections for the same indication, the number of autoaugmentations declined considerably, but nonresponders to botulinum A toxin are good candidates for autoaugmentation. The efficacy of this procedure has been documented by videourodynamics, preoperatively, 6–12 weeks and 1 year postoperatively, and at 1–2 year intervals thereafter. Its outcome parameters are improvement of incontinence, bladder compliance, maximum detrusor pressure during voiding, cystometric capacity, residual urine, reduced use of anticholinergics, and patient satisfaction. All parameters are significantly ameliorated after a mean follow-up period of over $6\frac{1}{2}$ years in about two-thirds of patients (Figures 22.8 and 22.9). Patients who have been lost to follow-up are rated as nonresponders. The patient population consists mainly of complete and incomplete spinal cord lesions, plus multiple sclerosis and myelomeningocele. The interval between surgery and a satisfactorily improved functional condition was 3 months to 2 years (Figures 22.10 and 22.11). One woman who

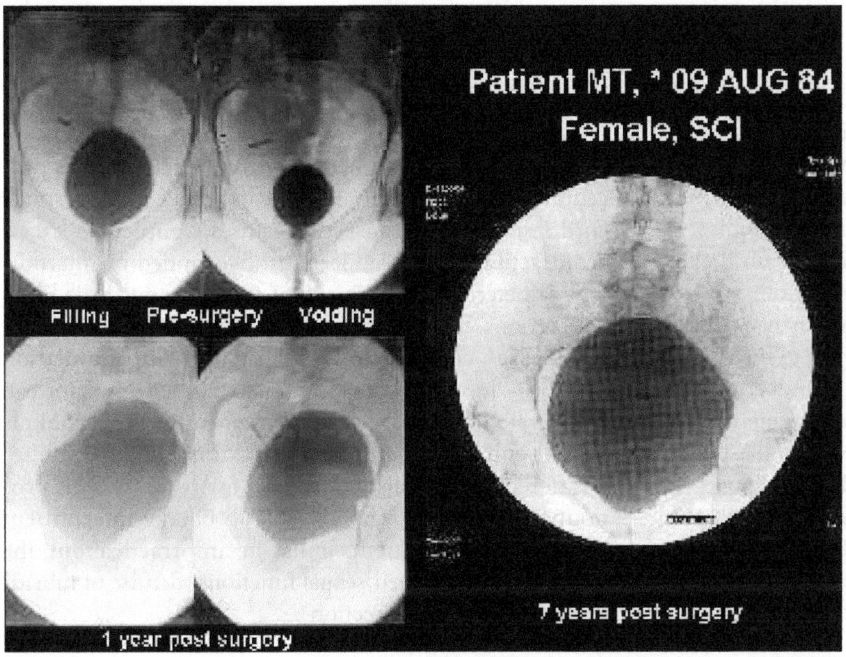

Figure 22.10
X-ray views of female patient pre, and 1 and 7 years post autoaugmentation.

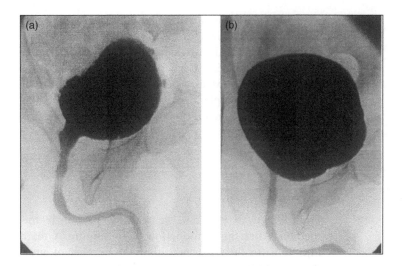

Figure 22.11
X-ray views of male patient pre (a) and 5 months after (b) autoaugmentation.

received an artificial sphincter after autoaugmentation and thus lost the opportunity for overflow incontinence suffered a bladder rupture at 600 ml capacity. Her condition was resolved by surgery without any sequelae. Four patients submitted to further procedures with intestinal replacement.

It is of the utmost importance to realize that functional improvement does not occur immediately after treatment, but may take a long time. One of our patients had already elected for intestinal augmentation but after 2 years a positive result was obtained. Published modifications of the method, including covering the defect with omentum or intestinal sections, have not produced better outcomes. One major advantage of this uncomplicated procedure is that the peritoneum is not opened. Based on my 13 years of experience, I thus see no need to change it.

Recent literature

In a review comparing enterocystoplasty and detrusor myectomy,[22] it is stated that: 'For most clinical indications detrusor myectomy has offered comparable success or significant improvement in bladder function without incurring the significant complication rate of enterocystoplasty.' Another review[23] attests that: 'The principle of urothelial preservation, introduced by autoaugmentation, is very promising in the effort to create a compliant urinary reservoir without metabolic disturbance and without the risk of cancer.' In a review comparing Ingelman–Sundberg bladder denervation, detrusor myectomy, and augmentation cystoplasty,[24] it is argued that augmentation cystoplasty has the highest success rate but a 'much higher likelihood of early and late post-operative complications' and, thus, the less invasive methods should be favored if feasible. Two long-term follow-up studies on children[25,26] underscore the contraindication of hypertonic/poorly compliant bladders.

In this author's view, the use of backing tissue to cover the detrusor defect[26–28] does not contribute to improvement of the clinical result. The procedure, as presented in this chapter, offers fast repair of – nearly inevitable – mucosal perforations. This is probably the reason why a laparoscopic access for this surgery has not become established.[29,30]

Clam cystoplasty

This relatively simple bladder augmentation with only slight per-operative risks inserts an intestinal segment in the bladder defect that is made by incision of the posterior bladder wall.[10] The results so far are good,[31,32] but the procedure is far more invasive than autoaugmentation and might induce late complications from bowel use.

S2–S4 Deafferentation

Another option to achieve a low-pressure bladder without intestinal patches is the transection of the S2–S4 roots on both sides. Unlike the methods described above, this procedure is indicated only in patients with complete spinal cord lesions. The transection causes complete detrusor acontractility – the bladder must be emptied by intermittent catheterization. As many of these patients have high-level lesions, the required dexterity is often unavailable. In those cases, combination with sacral electrostimulation (e.g. Brindley stimulator) is feasible, as the stimulator can be operated quite easily.[12] Improvement of the technique might enhance the quality of stimulated voiding.[33] Deafferentation is also an option for patients with pronounced spasticity who are able to handle intermittent catheterization. Patients must be informed about the adverse effects on their sexual functions (demise of lubrification, loss of reflex erection).

Conclusion

The procedures described in this chapter are sufficient to achieve compensated storage in the vast majority of patients. More complicated interventions, necessary for nonresponders, are described in other chapters of this book.

References

1. Stöhrer M, Goepel M, Kondo A, et al. The standardization of terminology in neurogenic lower urinary tract dysfunction with suggestions for diagnostic procedures. Neurourol Urodyn 1999; 18:139–158.

2. Stöhrer M, Schurch B, Kramer G, et al. Botulinum-A toxin in the treatment of detrusor hyperreflexia in spinal cord injury: a new alternative to medical and surgical procedures? Neurourol Urodyn 1999; 18:401–402.

3. Schurch B, Stöhrer M, Kramer G, et al. Botulinum A-toxin for treating detrusor hyperreflexia in spinal cord injured patients: a new alternative to anticholinergic drugs? Preliminary results. J Urol 2000; 164:692–697.

4. Cartwright PC, Snow BW. Bladder auto-augmentation: early clinical experience. J Urol 1989; 142:505–508.

5. Stöhrer M, Kramer G, Goepel M, et al. Bladder autoaugmentation in adult patients with neurogenic voiding dysfunction. Spinal Cord 1997; 35:456–462.

6. Dewan PA, Stefanek W. Autoaugmentation gastrocystoplasty: early clinical results. Br J Urol 1994, 74:460–464.

7. Nguyen DH, Mitchell ME, Horowitz M, et al. Demucosalized augmentation gastrocystoplasty with bladder autoaugmentation in pediatric patients. J Urol 1996; 156:206–209.

8. Carr MC, Docimo SG, Mitchell ME. Bladder augmentation with urothelial preservation. J Urol 1999; 162:1133–1136.

9. Perovic SV, Djordjevic ML, Kekic ZK, Vukadinovic VM. Bladder autoaugmentation with rectus muscle backing. J Urol 2002; 168:1877–1880.

10. Mast P, Hoebeke P, Wyndaele JJ, et al. Experience with augmentation cystoplasty. A review. Paraplegia 1995; 33:560–564.

11. Diokno AC, Vinson RK, McGillicuddy J. Treatment of the severe uninhibited neurogenic bladder by selective sacral rhizotomy. J Urol 1977; 118:299–301.

12. Sauerwein HD. The use of nerve deafferentation and stimulation in the paraplegic female patient. In: Raz S, ed. Female urology. Philadelphia: WB Saunders, 1996: 656–664.

13. Van Kerrebroeck PE, Koldewijn EL, Debruyne FM. Worldwide experience with the Finetech–Brindley sacral anterior root stimulator. Neurourol Urodyn 1993; 12:497–503.

14. National Institutes of Health. Clinical use of botulinum toxin. National Institutes of Health Consensus Development Conference Statement, Nov. 12–14, 1990. Arch Neurol 1991; 48:1294–1298.

15. Jankovic J, Schwartz KS. Longitudinal experience with botulinum toxin injections for treatment of blepharospasm and cervical dystonia. Neurology 1993; 43:834–836.

16. Bulstrode NW, Grobbelaar AO. Long-term prospective follow-up of botulinum toxin treatment for facial rhytides. Aesthetic Plast Surg 2002; 26:356–359.

17. Schurch B, Hauri D, Rodic B, et al. Botulinum-A toxin as a treatment of detrusor-sphincter dyssynergia: a prospective study in 24 spinal cord injury patients. J Urol 1996; 155:1023–1029.

18. Wyndaele JJ, Van Dromme SA. Muscular weakness as side effect of botulinum toxin injection for neurogenic detrusor overactivity. Spinal Cord 2002; 40:599–600.

19. Smith CP, Somogyi GT, Chancellor AM. Emerging role of botulinum toxin in the treatment of neurogenic and non-neurogenic voiding dysfunction. Curr Urol Rep 2002; 3:382–387.

20. Schulte-Baukloh H, Michael T, Schobert J, et al. Efficacy of botulinum-A toxin in children with detrusor hyperreflexia due to myelomeningocele: preliminary results. Urology 2002; 59: 325–327.

21. Stöhrer M, Kramer A, Goepel M, et al. Bladder auto-augmentation – an alternative for enterocystoplasty: preliminary results. Neurourol Urodyn 1995; 14:11–23.

22. Leng WW, Blalock HJ, Fredriksson WH, et al. Enterocystoplasty or detrusor myectomy? Comparison of indications and outcomes for bladder augmentation. J Urol 1999; 161:758–763.

23. Cranidis A, Nestoridis G. Bladder augmentation. Int Urogynecol J Pelvic Floor Dysfunct 2000; 11:33–40.

24. Westney OL, McGuire EJ. Surgical procedures for the treatment of urge incontinence. Tech Urol 2001; 7:126–132.

25. Marte A, Di Meglio D, Cotrufo AM, et al. A long-term follow-up of autoaugmentation in myelodysplastic children. BJU Int 2002; 89:928–931.

26. Carr MC, Docimo SG, Mitchell ME. Bladder augmentation with urothelial preservation. J Urol 1999; 162:1133–1136.

27. Oge O, Tekgul S, Ergen A, Kendi S. Urothelium-preserving augmentation cystoplasty covered with a peritoneal flap. BJU Int 2000; 85:802–805.

28. Perovic SV, Djordjevic ML, Kekic ZK, Vukadinovic VM. Bladder autoaugmentation with rectus muscle backing. J Urol 2002; 168:1877–1880.

29. McDougall EM, Clayman RV, Figenshau RS, Pearle MS. Laparoscopic retropubic auto-augmentation of the bladder. J Urol 1995; 153:123–126.

30. Siracusano S, Trombetta C, Liguori G, et al. Laparoscopic bladder auto-augmentation in an incomplete traumatic spinal cord injury. Spinal Cord 2000; 38:59–61.

31. Chartier-Kastler EJ, Mongiat-Artus P, Bitker MO, et al. Long-term results of augmentation cystoplasty in spinal cord injured patients. Spinal Cord 2000; 38:490–494.

32. Arikan N, Turkolmez K, Budak M, Gogus O. Outcome of augmentation sigmoidoplasty in children with neurogenic bladder. Urol Int 2000; 64:82–85.

33. Schumacher S, Bross S, Scheepe JR, et al. Restoration of bladder function in spastic neuropathic bladder using sacral deafferentation and different techniques of neurostimulation. Adv Exp Med Biol 1999; 462:303–309.

23

Surgery to improve bladder outlet function

Gina Defreitas and Philippe Zimmern

Introduction

The bladder outlet in patients with neurogenic voiding dysfunction is subject to two main abnormalities: outlet underactivity, leading to urine leakage with increased intra-abdominal pressure; nonrelaxing urethral sphincter obstruction, resulting in reduced urine flow at the time of bladder emptying.[1] This chapter is therefore divided into two sections: surgical treatment of the underactive or incompetent bladder outlet and surgical treatment of the nonrelaxing or hyperactive bladder outlet (detrusor-sphincter dyssynergia or DSD). Procedures currently used to alleviate sphincteric deficiency in the neurogenic bladder population are injection of urethral bulking agents, slings, artificial urethral sphincters, bladder neck reconstruction procedures, and bladder neck closure. The surgical options currently available for the treatment of intractable DSD are sphincterotomy, insertion of a temporary or permanent urethral stent, balloon dilatation of the external sphincter, and use of a chronic indwelling catheter. The choice of surgical treatment depends on a number of factors, the most important of which are sex of the patient, the patient's comorbidities and functional status, the severity of urine leakage, whether or not the patient has had previous anti-incontinence procedures, patient and caregiver preferences, and, last but not least, the experience and expertise of the surgeon.

This chapter will focus on indications, surgical techniques, results, and complications of the various treatment options currently employed to treat bladder outlet pathology in the neurogenic bladder population. Literature dealing with the use of these surgical procedures in patients with non-neurogenic voiding dysfunction will not be discussed. Definitions and urodynamic terminology will conform to the recommendations published in the most recent report of the standardization sub-committee of the International Continence Society.[1]

Surgical management of the incompetent bladder outlet

Urethral bulking agents

Introduction

The first use of an injectable substance to treat urinary incontinence dates back to 1938 when Murless instilled sodium murrhate into the anterior vaginal wall.[1] Since then, a number of advancements have been made in agent composition, patient selection, and injection technique. Agents that have been employed for urethral injection include autologous fat, polytetrafluoroethylene (polytef, Teflon), bovine collagen (Contigen), and pyrolytic carbon-coated zirconium oxide beads (Durasphere). In 1984, Lewis et al performed periurethral Teflon injections in female patients with neurogenic bladder on intermittent catheterization and noted a favorable result on continence.[2] Subsequently, several investigators have published data on the use of urethral bulking agents to treat urinary incontinence in patients with neurogenic voiding dysfunction. Although the bulk of the literature deals with children, adults with neuropathic bladder have been addressed in a few case series. Since the majority of experience has been accrued with glutaraldehyde cross-linked bovine collagen, and it is currently the most widely used bulking agent for the treatment of urinary incontinence, this section will focus on the results obtained with this substance. The Food and Drug Administration (FDA), secondary to problems with granuloma formation and particle migration, has not approved Teflon for the treatment of urinary incontinence.[3] To date there have not been any studies published dealing with the use of autologous fat or Durasphere in patients with neurogenic bladder dysfunction.

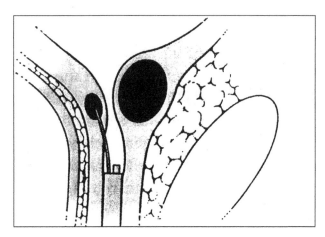

Figure 23.1
Correct placement of periurethral collagen. Injection should be at the proximal urethra in the submucosal plane. (Reproduced with permission from Functional reconstruction of the urinary tract and gynaeco-urology, 1st edn, 2002, Fig. 9.79 c and d.)

The use of bulking agents to treat incontinence has several advantages. Delivery is minimally invasive, relatively easy to learn, and entails low morbidity. Furthermore, treatment with injectable substances does not jeopardize the performance and efficacy of other anti-incontinence procedures later on. The liabilities of this technology stem from a lack of durability and poorer effectiveness when compared to other, albeit more invasive, treatment modalities. This disadvantage often leads to repeat injections, which can elevate the cost of a procedure already known to be expensive.[4]

Collagen biocompatibility, durability, and allergenicity

The collagen used for urethral injection is harvested from bovine corium, which is treated to decrease its antigenicity, and then cross-linked with glutaraldehyde to improve its durability and resistance to degradation by host collagenase.[5] Comprised of 95% type I collagen and 5% type III collagen, it is marketed under the trade names Contigen, Zyderm, and Zyplast (Bard Corp., Atlanta, GA and Collagen Corp., Palo Alto, CA). Bovine collagen has weak antigenicity in humans with 1–3% of patients having a positive skin test.[5] Concerns over developing an autoimmune response to human collagen after injection with bovine collagen appear to be unfounded, since no direct relation between collagen injection and autoimmune disease has been demonstrated in clinical practice.[6] The product is not latex-free, and for this reason, the manufacturer package insert states that a positive skin test may be more prevalent in myelomeningocele patients; however, no literature or experimental data exist to substantiate this finding.

Bovine collagen was approved by the FDA for treatment of intrinsic sphincter deficiency in 1993. Since then, no reports of local or distant migration in animals or humans have surfaced. The host inflammatory response is mild and little granuloma formation occurs. The substance is supposed to undergo gradual degradation over the course of 3–19 months and becomes a matrix for host collagen deposition and neovascularization.[7] Three-dimensional ultrasonographic imaging of the urethra, however, has found persistence of bovine collagen in the tissues up to 4 years post-injection,[8] indicating that resorption of this substance may be slower and more variable than was previously proposed.

Mechanism of action

In the neuropathic urethra, sphincteric deficiency is caused by denervation of the musculature of the bladder neck, proximal urethra, external sphincter, and pelvic floor.[9]

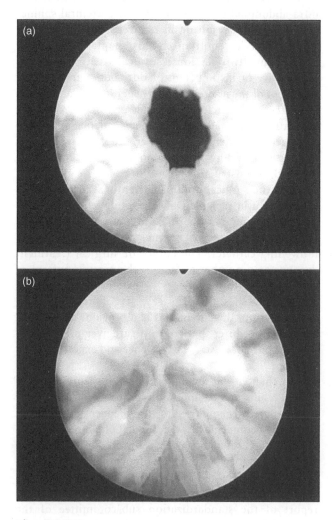

Figure 23.2
(a) Intraoperative cystoscopic view of open proximal urethra before collagen injection. (b) Intraoperative cystoscopic view of properly coapted proximal urethra after collagen injection.

Collagen and other injectable agents theoretically work by increasing the length of bladder neck and proximal urethral mucosa apposition, thereby improving the efficiency of compression of the sphincter mechanism in response to increases in intra-abdominal pressure.[9,10] McGuire et al have determined that injectable agents exert their mechanism of action by increasing the Valsalva leak point pressure (VLPP) but not the detrusor leak point pressure (DLPP) or voiding pressure.[11] This finding has been substantiated by several other authors including Bomalaski et al, who found that in neurogenic bladder patients who experience clinical improvement with collagen injections, the VLPP increased an average of 26 cmH_2O, compared with an increase of only 8 cmH_2O in patients who were not helped by the treatment.[4]

Urethral bulking agents are not thought to increase bladder outlet resistance and, therefore, the pressure at which the bladder empties. For this reason, they are postulated to have an advantage in the treatment of neurogenic incontinence over slings and artificial sphincters, which may cause elevated detrusor pressures and upper tract deterioration.[12,13] So far, there have been no reports of renal compromise related to the use of injectable agents. Chernoff et al, however, have reported significant postoperative urodynamic changes in 3 children with neurogenic bladder who were treated with transurethral collagen injections with decreased compliance and appearance of a DLPP where none had previously existed. These investigators warn of possible bladder decompensation in patients with small-capacity, low-compliance bladders who undergo injection of urethral bulking agents.[14]

Delivery methods

There are three methods for the injection of bulking agents in the treatment of stress urinary incontinence: periurethral, transurethral, and antegrade.[15] Before the use of collagen, 0.1 ml of skin test collagen must be injected subcutaneously into the volar surface of the forearm and observed for 4 weeks to rule out sensitivity. If the test is negative, then collagen injections can proceed. The skin test must be readministered prior to any repeat collagen treatments. Prior to injection, all patients should have a negative urine culture and receive perioperative antibiotics to prevent urosepsis post-procedure. This is especially important for the neurogenic bladder population, in whom urinary tract infections (UTIs) and bacteriuria are common. Children require a general anesthetic, but most adults, especially if they are insensate below the waist secondary to neurologic pathology, can tolerate the injection under local anesthetic or intravenous sedation. Some urologists prefer to inject all patients under general anesthetic in order to have better control over placement of the submucosal blebs. The patient is placed in the dorsal lithotomy position no matter which method of injection is used.

Periurethral technique. This method is often used in women. The urethra is injected with 2% lidocaine (lignocaine) jelly, and 1% lidocaine is injected periurethrally at 3 and 9 o'clock. A 20-gauge spinal needle is inserted at the 3 o'clock position and advanced under cystoscopic vision within the submucosal space toward the urethral lumen just distal to the bladder neck and proximal urethra. The bulking agent is slowly injected with the needle bevel facing the lumen until a mucosal bleb is raised. This process is repeated on the opposite side at 9 o'clock until the cystoscopic appearance of the lumen resembles that of lateral prostatic lobes meeting in the midline.

Transurethral technique. Although preferred for males, this method is often used in females as well. It requires a 21–24F cystoscope that can accommodate a 5F working element. A zero, 12, or 30 degree lens can be used.[16] The cystoscope is placed in the urethral lumen just proximal to the external sphincter and a needle delivery system (often 20-gauge) is placed through the working port of the cystoscope. The submucosal space is entered at 3 or 9 o'clock with the needle bevel pointing towards the urethral lumen. The bulking material is slowly injected until a sufficient bleb is raised. The process is repeated on the opposite side or anywhere else necessary to achieve good coaptation. Care should be taken to avoid more than one puncture at any single injection site in order to minimize extrusion. As with the periurethral technique, the cystoscope should not be advanced past the injection sites, because this can result in compression or extrusion of material and loss of the mucosal bleb.

Antegrade technique. This approach was developed in an attempt to achieve better closure of the bladder neck in males with scarred, noncompliant urethras postprostatectomy. It can also be used in children or adults with previous bladder neck reconstruction in whom the urethral passage may not be wide enough or compliant enough to accommodate a cystoscope of the caliber needed to employ the needle delivery system. It can be done under general anesthetic, intravenous sedation, or spinal anesthesia. The bladder is distended with irrigation fluid and a suprapubic cystotomy is performed under cystoscopic guidance, then dilated to allow placement of a sheath large enough to accommodate the cystoscope. Antegrade cystoscopy is performed and the material is injected submucosally around the bladder neck until coaptation occurs. A suprapubic tube is left in postoperatively for 24–72 hours.

Postoperative care

Patients are discharged once they are able to void. If they go into retention, they can be taught intermittent catheterization with a small-caliber catheter. Some investigators place narrow-lumen urethral catheters for 24–72 hours post-procedure.[17] If the patient was performing intermittent catheterization preoperatively, he can usually resume catheterization with an 8–12F tube the same day of the procedure with little fear of significant molding of the material.[9,12]

Indications and patient selection

The role of injectable agents for the treatment of urinary incontinence in the neurogenic bladder population remains hard to define. Perhaps this is because there are no randomized controlled trials comparing one treatment modality with another in this subset of patients, and the literature mainly consists of case series comprised of small numbers and short follow-up. In examining these data, however, a few patterns emerge.

It is often said that the ideal candidate for urethral collagen injection has a stable, compliant, good capacity bladder with low VLPP.[12,14] Many investigators believe that detrusor overactivity or decreased compliance should be treated with anticholinergics and/or augmentation cystoplasty before attempting to treat an incompetent outlet with bulking agents.[12,18] Perez et al, however, in their series of 32 patients with neurogenic bladder, found that the presence of detrusor overactivity and decreased compliance did not adversely affect the clinical outcome.[19]

In addition to its role in leakage prevention, injection of collagen into the bladder neck and proximal urethra has also been used to provide outlet resistance in order to increase the bladder capacity of children with exstrophy-epispadias complex prior to bladder neck reconstruction.[20] Although this technique has been successful in a small number of patients, not every author has found this to be the case.[14]

Many investigators regard urethral bulking agents as adjuncts to other forms of treatment, but do not believe them capable of providing a durable cure for incontinence in the majority of patients with neurogenic voiding dysfunction when used as the sole source of intervention.[13,17,21] This is particularly true in the subset of children with exstrophy-epispadias complex who have undergone bladder neck reconstruction yet remain incontinent. Many of these patients were rendered dry or experienced substantial improvement after collagen injection.[12,17,19,20] Bomalaski et al, in their study of 40 children with neurogenic bladder, found statistically greater improvement in continence and postoperative satisfaction in the exstrophy-epispadias group than in the myelomeningocele group.[4]

Groups of investigators in Canada have determined that preoperative urodynamic data could not predict the clinical result of collagen injection.[12,18] Chernoff et al, however, in their series of 11 children, found that a preoperative VLLP of greater than 45 cmH$_2$O was predictive of injection failure.[14] A patulous bladder neck was thought to be

a positive predictor of success by Kim et al, whose series of patients undergoing collagen injection contained 8 children with neurogenic bladder, 4 of whom had this finding on examination and were dry post-injection. These authors speculated that this cystoscopic feature, although indicative of a severely incompetent bladder outlet, may be a sign of more pliable, less-scarred tissue which would allow for optimal injection and, therefore, improved long-term treatment success.[22]

Contraindications to the use of injectable collagen for the treatment of urinary incontinence are known collagen sensitivity (a positive skin test), untreated detrusor overactivity, and untreated urinary tract infection. Scarring secondary to previous surgery or radiation treatment may decrease retention of collagen in tissue, thus contributing to its relatively poor efficacy.[9,17]

Results

Analysis of the studies published in the last 10 years on treatment of urinary incontinence with collagen injection reveals that the benefits derived from this agent by patients with neuropathic voiding dysfunction are comparable to those seen in the non-neurogenic incontinence population (Table 23.1). The proportion of patients rendered dry ranges from 20 to 50% in the majority of studies, although cure rates as low as 5% have been reported. The improvement rate, which is often the only outcome stated, ranges anywhere from 15 to 76%. The data are difficult to interpret and compare, since there is no standard definition of cure and improvement, and these terms are not always clearly delineated within the methodology of each study.

Most patients received between 1 and 4 injections, with the majority of responders having had only 1 or 2 treatments before assessment of clinical efficacy was made. The total volume of collagen injected ranged from 0.4 to 55 ml, with a total of less than 10 ml typically administered by most authors. In our experience, continence is rarely attained if a trial of 1 or 2 injections fails to achieve any improvement. We have recently begun to employ three-dimensional ultrasound of the urethra as an objective outcome measure to aid in the decision as to whether or not to offer repeat collagen injection to patients who have failed to experience clinical improvement.[8] The administration of further collagen may be costly and delay more effective treatment, particularly if postoperative three-dimensional ultrasound imaging demonstrates either poor or good retention of collagen, and the patient's incontinence persists.

Although most studies reported moderate treatment efficacy with follow-up of 1–6.3 years, some investigators found collagen to be disappointing in terms of treatment outcome. In 20 children with neurogenic stress incontinence, Sundaram et al reported only 30% improvement in leakage status post-collagen injection, while the rest

Table 23.1 *Results of glutaraldehyde cross-linked collagen in patients with neurogenic incontinence*

Investigator	Year and patient population	Number of patients	Mean follow-up (months)	Mean amount collagen (ml)	Results	Complications	Comments
Capozza et al[20]	1995 pediatric	25 – 9 NB, 16 EE	Range 9–36; no mean given	3 range 2.1–4.5	76% improved 9/9 NB, 10/16 EE	None	EEC patients had prior NB reconstruction
Bennett et al[9]	1995 adult	11 – 5 MMC, 5 SCI, 1 SC tumor	24 range 12–32	Females – 55 Males – 56	28% cured 36% improved	1 transient difficulty catheterizing	Series contained 9 men, 2 women
Ben-Chaim et al[17]	1995 3 adults, 16 children	19 – all EE	26 range 9–84	4 range 0.4–12	53% improved	1 UTI/epididymo-orchitis, 1 bladder perforation	15 patients had prior NB reconstruction
Perez et al[14]	1996 pediatric	32 – 24 MMC, 7 EE, 1 sacral teratoma	10 range 3–19	10 MMC, 7.5 EE range 3.5–17	MMC – 20% dry, 28% improved EEC – 43% dry, 14% improved	1 urosepsis, 2 transient worsening of incontinence	3/7 EEC patients had undergone previous NB reconstruction
Bomalaski et al[4]	1996 pediatric	40 – 25 MMC, 12 EE, rest non-neurogenic	25.2 range 3–75.6	10.2 range 2.5–22.5	22% cure, 54% improved Statistically significant decrease in pad use, dry interval, incontinence grade	None	8 patients followed for 4.5 years had overall cure/improvement of 86% Greater success with EE than with MMC
Leonard et al[12]	1996 pediatric	18 – 10 MMC, 6 EE	15 range 5–21	5 range 2.4–13	MMC – 3/6 cured, 2 improved EE – 2 cured, 2 improved	None	4 patients had ileocysto-plasty, 7 had NB reconstruction, 4 had epispadias repair
Chernoff et al[14]	1997 pediatric	11 – 7 MMC, 1 SCI, 2 EE, 1 uro-genital sinus defect	14.4 range 4–20	Maximum injected 15 ml	36% dry, 18% improved	None	4 patients had previous ileocystoplasty, 3 had NB reconstruction
Sundaram et al[21]	1997 pediatric	20 – 12 MMC, 4 EE, 4 other neurogenic bladder causes	15.2 range 9–23	7.3 range 3–18	5% dry, 25% improved, 10 had transient improvement	None	2 patients had prior NB reconstruction
Kassouf et al[18]	2001 pediatric	20 – all MMC	50.4	6.3 range 2–13	10% dry, 15% improved, 14 had transient improvement	None	80% on CIC, all had stable bladder preoperation

CIC, clean intermittent catheterization; EEC, MMC, myelomeningocele; EE, exstrophy-epispadias complex; SCI, spinal cord injury; NB, neurogenic bladder.

experienced transient improvement lasting an average of 52 days.[21] In children with myelomeningocele on intermittent catheterization, Kassouf et al found that only one-quarter of patients had a durable treatment response, with the rest failing at 3 months.[18] Suboptimal outcomes have been attributed in part to disruption of the collagen blebs by catheterization shortly after injection, but Sundaram et al did not find any difference in the outcome between patients on intermittent catheterization and those who voided spontaneously.[21]

Complications have been few and minor, consisting of UTI, urosepsis, epididymo-orchitis, transient difficulty with catheterization, and temporary worsening of urinary incontinence.[9,17,19] One patient sustained a bladder perforation requiring laparotomy and operative repair 3 days after injection which was felt by the investigators to be secondary to overfilling at the time of the procedure and subsequent difficulty emptying the bladder completely.[17]

Conclusion

In summary, treatment of stress urinary incontinence with glutaraldehyde cross-linked bovine collagen in the neurogenic bladder population has been demonstrated to be safe and variably successful, with follow-up extending past 5 years. Almost all the literature, however, deals with children, and very little data exist for adults with spinal cord injury or other acquired forms of neuropathic voiding dysfunction. Children with exstrophy-epispadias who have had previous bladder neck reconstruction have been found to be suitable candidates for collagen injection, as have patients with myelomeningocele. The relative efficacy of

injectable agents, coupled with their minimally invasive nature and ease of administration, has continued to fuel the search for novel substances. Animal and human studies examining the feasibility of submucosal injection of autologous ear chondrocytes and autologous muscle-derived cells are currently underway in an attempt to find more durable, more biocompatible, and less allergenic alternatives to bovine collagen.[23,24] The ideal injectable agent has not yet been devised.

Bladder neck slings and wraps

Introduction

The fascial sling and the artificial urethral sphincter (AUS) are the two most commonly employed surgical treatments for patients with urinary incontinence secondary to neurogenic outlet incompetence. The pros and cons of bladder neck sling and artificial urethral sphincter are listed in Table 23.2. The issue of how much tension to place on the fascial sling is not as problematic in the neurogenic bladder population as it is in patients with stress urinary incontinence (SUI), since retention in a patient with neurogenic bladder who already performs intermittent catheterization (IC) is usually a treatment goal rather than a complication. Furthermore, the incidence of tension-induced erosion is low when autologous fascia is utilized as the sling material. Unfortunately, long-term experience with the bladder neck sling in the neurogenic bladder population is seldom reported, with most case series documenting mean follow-up times of less than 4 years. It is thus unknown whether

Table 23.2 *Advantages and disadvantages of fascial bladder neck sling and artificial urethral sphincter (AUS)*

Surgical option	Advantages	Disadvantages
Bladder neck sling	1. No foreign body insertion 2. 'Pop-off' valve – allows leakage to occur at high intravesical pressure, protecting upper tracts 3. No concern with contamination of surgical field and infection seeding when performing a concomitant bladder augment	1. Majority of patients must catheterize to empty bladder 2. Less efficacious in males than females
AUS	1. Highly effective even for severe outlet incompetence 2. No 'pop-off' valve – may lead to upper tract deterioration in patients with poor preoperative compliance and high intravesical pressures 3. Allows some patients to void spontaneously without need for catheterization	1. Risk of revision for mechanical failure 2. Risk of infection and erosion

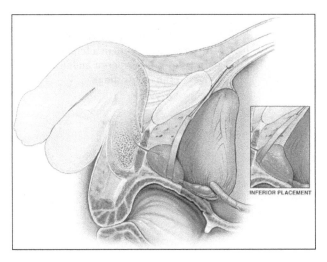

INFERIOR PLACEMENT

Figure 23.3
Placement of rectus fascia sling in a male patient. Sling is placed at the bladder neck posterior to the seminal vesicles.

or not the fascial sling in young women with myelomeningocele may be disrupted by pregnancy and childbirth.[25]

Indications and patient selection

The ideal candidate for this procedure is a female patient with bladder outlet incompetence, preserved urethral length, and a well-managed bladder on IC.

Whether or not to perform enterocystoplasty in addition to a procedure to occlude the bladder outlet is a complex decision based on preoperative urodynamic and radiographic assessment. Bladder augmentation alone may be sufficient to cure incontinence in some neurogenic bladder patients despite low outlet resistance,[26] particularly in male children who have the potential for increased outlet competence with pubertal prostate growth. Conversely, supporting the bladder neck with a sling may be enough to abolish leakage if the preoperative urodynamic assessment, performed with some form of bladder outlet occlusion, shows a stable bladder with sufficient capacity and normal compliance.[27] Whether or not to perform both procedures together, or to do one before the other, is somewhat controversial. In general, a cystogram showing a wide open bladder neck and a VLPP less than 30 cmH$_2$O are indications of intrinsic sphincter deficiency, in which case a procedure to improve bladder outlet competence is recommended. Adherence to these guidelines, however, cannot always predict the patient's postoperative status. As Kreder and Webster demonstrated, a bladder neck sling may cause de-novo detrusor overactivity (DO) or decreased bladder capacity and compliance if performed without enterocystoplasty, despite a preoperative urodynamic work-up documenting normal detrusor parameters.[27] To avoid

subjecting the patient to a second operation, some investigators have advocated the routine performance of concomitant enterocystoplasty and rectus fascial sling in all patients with neurogenic incontinence.[28,29] One such proponent of this practice, Decter, found that the rate of postoperative leakage was higher in patients who did not undergo bladder augmentation along with bladder neck sling compared with patients who had both procedures.[29] The downside of this systematic approach, however, is that even though it saves some patients the morbidity of a second surgery, it may needlessly subject some others to the risks of enterocystoplasty.

Surgical techniques

Prior to undergoing a bladder neck sling, patients must have a negative urine culture. Perioperative broad-spectrum antibiotics are administered and, if a bladder augmentation is performed, they are continued postoperatively for a few days.

A bowel preparation should be considered in all patients undergoing concomitant enterocystoplasty. When performing both a sling and a bladder augment, the fascial harvest and bladder neck dissection are usually performed prior to the augmentation. Once the augment is completed, the fascial sling is positioned and secured in place.

A midline incision provides the best exposure if an enterocystoplasty is also to be done, but a Pfannenstiel incision can be employed, staying extraperitoneal, if only a sling is required.[30] The bladder neck dissection is often done via the abdominal incision, but a transvaginal or combined transabdominal–transvaginal approach can be employed in adult women, and has even been accomplished in adolescent girls with the help of a mediolateral episiotomy.[31] In the transabdominal dissection, the endopelvic fascia is incised bilaterally, the bladder neck and proximal urethra are freed circumferentially, and a Penrose drain is placed around the bladder neck. A finger in the vagina, or the rectum in males, can aid in the posterior dissection.[30] Some surgeons prefer just to clear a tunnel beneath the bladder neck rather than mobilizing around it completely.[28] In males, the dissection is identical to that performed for AUS bladder neck cuff placement, in that a plane is entered posterior to the bladder neck but anterior to the seminal vesicles.[32] The transvaginal dissection, if employed, is approached via a vertical midline or inverted U incision in the anterior vaginal wall. The incision should extend from 1.5 cm proximal to the urethral meatus to 1 cm proximal to the bladder neck, which is identified with the aid of the balloon of a urethral Foley catheter. The vaginal mucosa is dissected off the underlying periurethral fascia to expose the urethrovesical junction. After perforating the endopelvic fascia, the retropubic space is entered on either side of the bladder neck using a combination of sharp and

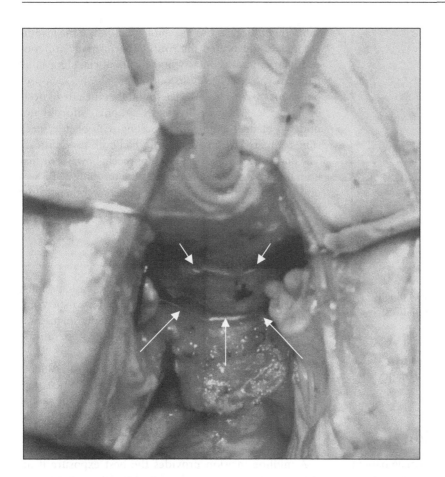

Figure 23.4
Correct placement of rectus fascia sling at the proximal urethra in a female patient (arrows indicate superior and inferior edges of the rectus sling).

blunt dissection. This dissection allows a ligature carrier to be passed safely from the suprapubic region to the vaginal area under fingertip guidance.

A strip of autologous rectus fascia 1.5–2 cm in width and 6–10 cm in length is usually employed, although fascia lata may also be used. Marlex slings have also been placed, but the likelihood of infection and erosion is increased compared to autologous fascia.[32] The rectus fascia can be harvested transversely or longitudinally as a free graft, or one end of the fascial strip may be left attached to the anterior abdominal wall as a pedicle and secured to the opposite rectus sheath. In males, the sling is usually placed around the bladder neck and superior aspect of the prostate, although some surgeons place it around the distal prostatic urethra, where coaptation may be easier to achieve.[33] In females, the fascial strip is positioned around the bladder neck and proximal urethra. The sling is often sutured to the lateral edges of the bladder neck with absorbable suture to prevent rolling and displacement that may cause excessive urethral angulation or compression. If employing a free fascial graft, a zero or number one polypropylene stitch is passed through each end of the graft before the sling is positioned around the bladder neck. When the operation is done transvaginally, the sutures are brought out through the lower anterior abdominal wall using a ligature carrier

passed through the retropubic space into the vaginal incision under fingertip guidance. The sutures are then tied down suprapubically at the end of the procedure. Some investigators have used Gortex bolsters or pledgets to prevent suture pull-through,[25,31] but this is not essential. Alternatively, the edges of fascia can be secured to Cooper's ligament[4] or the symphysis pubis.[29]

Several techniques have been recommended to optimize sling tension. In patients with neurogenic bladder on IC there is little concern with causing retention, but one should avoid tying the sutures too tightly to prevent urethral erosion and atrophy.[34] Elder describes filling the bladder with saline via a suprapubic tube and increasing tension on the sling until urethral leakage no longer occurs with manual bladder compression.[25] Other authors have tied the sutures so that no further movement of a Foley balloon at the bladder neck occurs, or so that 1 or 2 fingers can be placed between the knots and the fascia.[31] The sling sutures can also be tightened under cystoscopic control until the bladder neck appears closed.[29,30] Decter has suggested that because of the prostate bulk, more tension needs to be applied to the sutures in males than in females to achieve adequate urethral elevation and compression.[29] The surgeon should ensure that catheterization can be performed before finalizing sling tension.[28]

Some surgeons leave a suprapubic tube and urethral Foley catheter in postoperatively, remove the Foley catheter within 1–2 weeks, and then the suprapubic tube once catheterization can be performed with no difficulties. Others leave just a suprapubic tube, which is removed after 1–3 weeks, depending on whether or not an enterocystoplasty was also performed.

Wrap procedures in which a pedicle of bladder detrusor, a strip of rectus fascia, or a distally based rectus/pyramidalis myofascial flap is used to encircle the bladder neck completely, have been employed by various authors in order to provide circumferential compression, tapering, and suspension of the bladder outlet.[33,35,36] In some cases, one end of the wrap is secured to the anterior abdominal wall fascia in order to elevate the bladder neck.[35] It has been theorized that catheterization may be easier with the bladder neck wrap than with the sling, since the suspending force is evenly distributed around the bladder neck, thereby avoiding urethral kinking.[33,36]

Some investigators, in addition to placing a sling support beneath the bladder neck, have tapered it to improve urethral coaptation and reduce sling tension, in an attempt to decrease the likelihood of erosion.[32] Techniques which have been described include excising a full-thickness diamond of tissue along the anterior aspect of the bladder neck and reapproximating the edges of mucosa and detrusor muscle with absorbable sutures, or, alternatively, excising full-thickness wedges of anterior bladder neck and prostate from the edges of a vertical midline incision extending to the level of the verumontanum, and tapering it over a 16F catheter.[30,32]

Results and complications

The literature on bladder neck slings to treat neurogenic urinary incontinence consists largely of case series, made up of pediatric or a mixture of pediatric and adult patients (Table 23.3). Mean follow-up ranges from 9 months to 4.5 years. Published success rates depend on the definition of dryness used by the author. Continence has been described as no leakage occurring in between intermittent catheterization intervals of 3–4 hours or more, wearing less than 1 pad per day, or dry during the daytime only, with no consideration given to nocturnal incontinence. Most investigators report overall continence rates greater than 70%, with women faring better (85%) than men (69%) in some studies.[28,29,31–33] Kurzrock et al suggest that this discrepancy in sling effectiveness between the sexes may be because the prostate makes it more difficult to close and elevate the proximal urethra.[33] Fascial bladder neck wraps have not been found to be any more effective at preventing urinary leakage than slings.[33,35,36]

Complications specific to the rectus fascia sling are relatively rare and include sling breakdown resulting in postoperative leakage as a result of fascial breakage or suture pullout and urethral erosion.[29,30] The urethra may become angulated, resulting in difficulty with catheterization or retraction of the meatus into the vaginal introitus.[30] Care needs to be taken when passing a cystoscope via the urethra post-sling insertion. Elder[25] and Barthold et al[35] have described cases in which patients who were initially dry after surgery became incontinent after the performance of transurethral instrumentation. Bladder perforation may occur in patients with augmented bladders and bladder neck slings who are not compliant with IC, or in whom catheterization has become difficult.[28,35,37] Other reported complications are incisional hernia, de-novo DO, retroperitoneal hematoma, and bladder neck contracture when the outlet is tapered along with sling insertion.[30,32]

Conclusion

The rectus fascia bladder neck sling has been shown to be a versatile and valuable addition to the armamentarium of the reconstructive surgeon. Despite its lower rate of success in males with neurogenic incontinence, the lack of requirement for foreign materials and relative ease of implantation make it an attractive option for treatment of the incompetent reservoir outlet in a wide variety of patients. The long-term durability of the bladder neck sling, however, is still unknown. This is an important consideration, particularly for children, in whom the procedure may have to last decades. Many authors speculate that with growth the sling should maintain its functional obstruction of the bladder outlet, but longer follow-up is required.

Artificial urinary sphincters

Introduction

Ever since the first published clinical report in 1973 by Scott, the AUS has been used extensively to treat sphincteric incontinence.[38] High rates of efficacy and patient satisfaction, but also substantial revision rates secondary to mechanical failure as well as problems with infection and erosion resulting in sphincter removal have been reported. The high initial cost of the device, compounded with the cost of replacing components when they malfunction or wear out, makes it an expensive treatment option. Despite its availability since the 1970s, concerns have also been raised regarding silicone shedding, particularly in children, since the long-term sequelae of silicone migration is unknown.[39] There have been relatively few large series of AUS use in neurogenic patients, and there are no controlled trials comparing its efficacy to that of fascial slings or bladder neck reconstruction.

Table 23.3 *Results of fascial slings and wraps in patients with neurogenic bladder outlet incompetence*

Study	Year and patient population	Number and type of patients	Mean follow-up (months)	Surgical technique	Results	Other surgical procedures
Elder[25]	1990 adult and pediatric M and F	14: 10 F, 4 M all MMC	12 range 7–27	Periurethral or peri-prostatic RF sling, tied on abdominal wall	85.7% dry 1 nocturnal enuresis only	12 concomitant bladder augmentation
Herschorn and Radomski[32]	1992 adult M	13: 10 MMC, 3 SCI	34.3 range 5.5–49	2 Marlex, 11 RF pedicle sutured to opposite rectus sheath, BN tapering	69.2% dry	All had concomitant augmentation
Decter[29]	1993 adult and pediatric M and F	10: 6 F, 4 M 8 MMC, 2 SA	26.4	RF sling in 5, fascia lata in 5, symphyseal fixation	67% with augment dry, 25% without augment dry	6 concomitant bladder augmentations
Chancellor et al[113]	1993 adult F	14: neurogenic, patulous urethras	24 range 6–60	RF pedicle sling sutured to opposite abdominal wall	100% dry	5 concomitant augmentations, 5 cutaneous urostomy
Gormley et al[31]	1994 F adolescents	15: 8 MMC, 2 SA, 1 imperforate anus, 3 BN trauma	54 range 6–102	RF sling, combined abdominal and vaginal dissection, tied over abdominal wall	84.6% dry (2 redos using larger piece of RF) 1 using 1 pad/day	2 concomitant augmentations, 5 prior bladder outlet procedures
Walker et al[30]	1995 adult and pediatric M and F	17: 9 F, 8 M 10 MMC, 3 sacral lipoma, 4 other	16.2	RF sling, some with bladder neck tapering	94.1% dry 1 has some SUI	11 concomitant augmentations, 9 prior BN procedures
Kakizaki et al[34]	1995 adult and pediatric mostly M	13: 10 M, 3 F 8 MMC, 2 pelvic surgery, 1 SCI, 2 non-neurogenic patients	36 range 4–63	Sling of RF in 8, fascia lata in 5; BN placement in 11, bulbous urethra in 2; tied over abdominal wall	69.2% dry 23% improved	9 concomitant bladder augmentations

Reference	Year/population	Patients	Follow-up (months)	Procedure	Results	Comments
Kurzrock et al[33]	1996 pediatric M and F	24: 9 F, 15 M all MMC	Range 9–14	Bladder wall pedicle wrap suspended to pubic symphysis	100% F dry 66.7% M dry	6 prior augmentations, 1 prior RF sling
Fontaine et al[28]	1997 adult F	21: 9 MMC, 8 SCI, 3 SA, 1 sacral lipoma	28.6 range 6–60	RF sling done transabdominally, sutured to Cooper's	85.7% dry day and night 95.2% dry day only	All had concomitant bladder augmentation
Barthold et al[35]	1999 pediatric mostly F	27: 20 F, 7 M 21 MMC, 2 SA, 4 other	Wrap 43.2 sling 25.2	10 RF slings, 18 RF wraps, both secured to anterior abdominal wall	Wrap 28% dry, sling 50% dry ($p > 0.05$) 14.3% M dry, 50% F dry ($p = 0.02$)	19 concomitant, 1 prior, 2 subsequent augmentations, 17 Mitrofanoffs
Austin et al[37]	2001 pediatric M and F	18: 10 M, 8 F 16 MMC, 2 SCI	21.2 range 6–57	RF sling tied over anterior abdominal wall	78% dry; 2 dry with repeat sling	4 concomitant, 2 prior augmentations
Mingin et al[36]	2002 pediatric and adult M and F	37: 14 M, 23F 36 neurogenic, 1 traumatic	48 range 6–120	Distally based rectus/pyramidalis myofascial flap wrapped around BN and sewn to contralateral RF	92% (34) dry 2 M failures, 1 F failure	33 concomitant augmentations, 9 Mitrofanoff stomas, 5 reimplantations

MMC, myelomeningocele; SCI, spinal cord injury; SA, sacral agenesis; M, male; F, female; RF, rectus fascia; BN, bladder neck; SUI, stress urinary incontinence.

History and design evolution

The AUS 800 represents the culmination of a number of design modifications which have occurred since 1975 when the patent for the original device, the AMS 721, was issued to American Medical Systems (Minnetonka, Minnesota). This early model operated on the hydraulic principle still employed by the modern AUS, but there was no way to control the occlusive force applied to the urethra and the large number of components made it difficult to implant.[40] In 1980, the AMS 721 was altered to overcome these problems by streamlining the design and incorporating a pressure-regulating balloon reservoir, which was then marketed as the AMS 761. The AMS 742, 791, and 792 represented further design simplifications and introduced the concept of delayed activation in order to allow for tissue healing. With these devices, a second surgical procedure was needed to activate the pump.[40]

In 1982, the AMS 800 was introduced and is the only AUS currently available on the market.[41] Like its predecessors, it consists of three components: a cuff which fits around the urethra or bladder neck; a balloon fluid reservoir which is implanted in the abdomen; and a pump which is implanted in the scrotum or labia to control activation. The cuff is composed of an outer layer of Dacron (polyethylene terephthalate) monofilament backing an inner silicone shell, and is available in sizes ranging from 4 to 11 cm with 0.5 cm increments. Three different balloon reservoirs are available with plateau pressures of 51–60 cmH_2O, 61–70 cmH_2O and 71–80 cmH_2O. The pump and reservoir are also made of silicone and are connected to each other and the pump by kink-resistant color-coded tubing. The sphincter is implanted fully primed with isotonic radiopaque fluid or normal saline in its deactivated state.

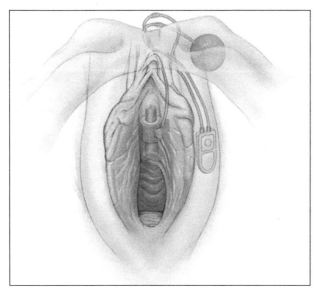

Figure 23.5
Placement of the AMS-800 in a female patient. (Reproduced with permission from The urinary sphincter, Chapter 34, Fig. 5.)

The device is activated a few weeks later by sharply squeezing the bulb of the pump. This maneuver allows fluid to exit the reservoir and enter the hollow cuff, thereby occluding the urethra or bladder neck lumen. When the patient wishes to void, he pumps the bulb to direct fluid out of the cuff and back into the reservoir. Fluid moves back into the cuff, closing it automatically within 3–5 min. Should urethral or bladder instrumentation be necessary, the unit can be locked or deactivated by pressing a button on the pump.

In 1988, a cuff with Dacron backing that was narrower than the silicone surface facing the urethra (narrow-backed cuff) was incorporated into the AMS 800 design along with alterations in the manufacturing process used to make the reservoir. These modifications improved durability and decreased urethral pressure atrophy.[42] There have been no further changes to the AMS 800 design.

Indications and patient selection

All patients in whom an AUS is being considered should undergo preoperative urodynamic testing to document the severity and mechanism of incontinence and to assess bladder function. Determination of detrusor parameters may require bladder neck occlusion with a Foley catheter balloon during the filling phase.[43] As for the fascial sling, the ideal candidate for an AUS should have a stable bladder with good compliance and capacity as well as a good emptying. Elevated detrusor pressures can lead to upper tract deterioration once the outlet is occluded by the sphincter cuff. De Badiola et al compared the preoperative and postoperative urodynamic parameters of 23 pediatric patients who received an AUS for neurogenic sphincteric incompetence. Patients with filling pressures of less than 50 cmH_2O with preoperative bladder capacities greater than or equal to 60% of that expected for age and/or a preoperative compliance greater than 2 ml/cmH_2O, were less likely to require subsequent augmentation for persistent incontinence and upper tract changes.[44] The average time to cystoplasty in patients who developed high intravesical pressures after AUS implantation was 14 months.[44]

Many authors advocate an AUS as primary treatment for patients who can void spontaneously.[45] Patients, however, should be informed that IC may have to be performed in the future, particularly if they receive a bladder augment or, in men, if prostatic growth later in life produces outlet obstruction. The AUS has also been employed as secondary treatment for patients who have failed other forms of bladder outlet surgery. Aliabadi and Gonzalez described 15 patients who had failed multiple urethral and bladder neck surgeries and were salvaged with an AUS, resulting in an overall continence rate of 73%.[46]

The optimal timing for US insertion in the pediatric population with neurogenic incontinence is controversial.

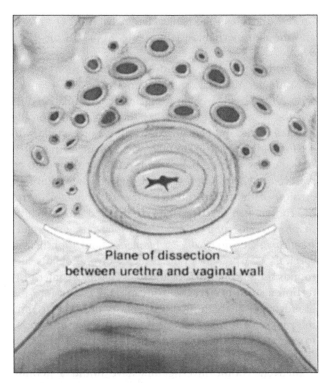

Figure 23.6
Transvaginal view of urethra and anterior vaginal wall to show dissection plane between the vagina and urethra/bladder neck.

Kryger et al found no difference in the number of AUS removals, continence rate, revision rate, augmentation rate, or number of complications in patients who received an AUS before age 11 compared to those placed later in life. AUS insertion, in fact, may be easier in prepubertal patients secondary to the shallower pelvis and lesser degree of periurethral venous plexus engorgement. Revisions for retraction of the pump in the scrotum were uncommon, occurring only in 1 of their 25 patients.[45] Levesque et al also found no increase in the rate of AUS revision post-puberty, with a follow-up of 12.1 years.[47]

Although Fulford et al[41] have reported a cuff erosion rate of 44% in females, and Levesque et al[47] found a higher rate of erosion in girls who had previous bladder neck surgery, other investigators have not. Salisz et al described successful AUS insertion in women despite intraoperative injuries to the vagina, bladder, or urethra. Their technique involved closing the injury primarily, placing the cuff within a different plane of dissection around the bladder neck, and delaying sphincter activation for a minimum of 6 weeks.[48]

Surgical technique

AUS insertion can be performed under general or spinal anesthesia. The cuff is usually placed around the bladder neck in women and children and around the bulbar urethra in males. The dorsal lithotomy position is favored in order to access the perineum for bulbar urethral placement, or to place a finger in the vagina to aid in transabdominal dissection of the bladder neck. The urine should be sterile before surgery and the skin should be free of dermatitis or candidiasis. Broad-spectrum perioperative intravenous antibiotics are administered. Strict sterile precautions are followed in the operating room and many surgeons prepare the patient with a 10–15 min antiseptic soap scrub before painting the abdomen and perineum with an antiseptic solution. Once the patient has been draped, a Foley catheter is inserted into the bladder.

Dissection of the bladder neck proceeds in much the same fashion as for placement of a fascial sling (see earlier). A 2-cm wide window behind the bladder neck is adequate for cuff placement, and a right-angled clamp is used to pass the measuring device around the bladder neck. Bladder neck cuff sizes range from 6 to 11 cm in diameter. Limited injuries to the bladder or vagina can be repaired primarily, but rectal injuries require abortion of the procedure. Once the appropriate-sized cuff is placed around the bladder neck, the cuff tubing is brought out through the rectus fascia via a separate stab incision superior to the pubis. The reservoir is placed in the retropubic space with its tubing penetrating the rectus fascia near the cuff tubing. A 71–80 cmH$_2$O balloon is often used for bladder neck occlusion. The reservoir can also be inserted into the peritoneal cavity, a location preferred by some to permit better balloon expansion.[40]

The anterior rectus sheath is closed and the balloon reservoir is filled with 22 ml of normal saline or an iso-osmotic contrast solution for postoperative X-ray imaging of the AUS. The pump mechanism is placed subcutaneously in the most dependent part of the scrotum or the labia. This space is created by passing a long curved Kelly clamp or sponge forceps from the lower edge of the suprapubic incision into the hemiscrotum or labium. The site of pump placement depends on whether the patient is left- or right-handed. A Babcock clamp can be placed around the pump tubing to prevent it from riding up while the components are being assembled. All tubing must be cleared of bubbles and blood clots before being connected. Straight or right-angled connectors can be used and secured with the quick-connect system or hand-tied with 2–0 or 3–0 polypropylene sutures in revision cases. The device should be cycled intraoperatively to make sure the cuff inflates and deflates properly. Some surgeons perform this maneuver while visualizing the cuff directly with flexible cystoscopy. Others perform perfusion sphincterometry to confirm proper sphincter function, to exclude unsuspected urethral injury, and to determine the refill time of the device.[49] All AUS components and incisions are irrigated copiously with antibiotic solution throughout the procedure. Before closing the incision, the AUS is deactivated by squeezing the button on the pump before it refills completely.

Placement of the cuff around the bulbar urethra begins by making a vertical incision in the perineum with its midpoint at the lower edge of the ischeal tuberosities. A Lonestar or Turner–Warwick retractor is recommended for better exposure. After incising the bulbocavernosus muscle along its midline, the bulbar urethra is mobilized circumferentially for a distance of 2–3 cm. If the urethra is injured, then the procedure should be terminated and the Foley catheter left indwelling after the injury is repaired with fine absorbable suture. A measuring device is passed around the urethra and the appropriate-sized cuff is placed. Most adult male patients will be fitted a 4.5 cm cuff, but sizes of 4 and 5 cm are also available. The cuff tubing and tab are withoriented laterally so that neither one abuts the base of the penis, which can be uncomfortable postoperatively. The reservoir is placed in the retropubic space through a separate abdominal incision. The operation proceeds as described above.

To circumvent retention secondary to edema, a catheter is usually left in the bladder overnight and removed the next morning. Patients are discharged on oral antibiotics for 10–14 days after completing 24–48 hours of intravenous therapy. Patients should avoid heavy lifting, straining, and intercourse for 4–6 weeks. The AUS is activated in the clinic 4–6 weeks after its insertion and the patient is instructed in its use. Patients should inform medical personnel that they have an AUS when entering the hospital for surgery or any other procedure that may involve bladder catheterization, since the cuff should be deactivated beforehand to avoid damage to the device and the urethra. Patients should also carry the AUS information card provided by the manufacturer and obtain a Medicalert bracelet in case of accident or injury.

Results and complications

In patients with neurogenic sphincteric incontinence, the AUS has been reported to result in continence rates from 59–92%, revision rates of 27–57%, and removal rates of 19–41% (Table 23.4).[45,47,50–55] Perioperative and immediate postoperative complications include bladder neck, urethral and rectal perforations, UTIs, wound infections, and scrotal hematomas.[50,51] In the long term, mechanical problems are the most common reason for revision surgery and include tubing kinks, fluid loss secondary to pump, reservoir or cuff leaks, pump migration, pump dysfunction, and connector separation.[42,52,53,55] Non-mechanical complications consist of urethral atrophy, infection, erosion, and elevated bladder storage pressures which can result in reflux, hydronephrosis, and renal insufficiency.[42,47,50] In the Mayo Clinic series of 323 AUS patients, 26 of whom had myelomeningocele, both types of complications were shown to decrease after 1988 with incorporation of the narrow-backed cuff and improved manufacturing

process: the rate of mechanical failure fell from 21 to 7.5% and the non-mechanical failure rate dropped from 17 to 9%.[42]

Infection, one of the most dreaded complications, results in sphincter removal, and accounts for 4–5% of most series.[40] Proposed mechanisms include contamination during the procedure, exposure of the AUS to chronically infected urine, and hematogenous spread of bacteria with seeding of the device.[56] The presence of an infection is often indicated by skin erythema, induration at the pump or reservoir site, erosion of the cuff through the urethra, or erosion of the pump through the scrotal or labial skin. Microorganisms recovered from infected AUS include *Staphylococcus epidermidis*, β-streptococcus, *Bacteroides fragilis*, *Escherichia coli*, *Pseudomonas*, and diphtheroid species.[56–58] A pseudocapsule made of myofibroblasts surrounds the silicone parts of the AUS and may confer protection against bacteria, which can be liberated into the bloodstream at the time of cystoplasty or with systemic infections.[57] The infection rate does not appear to increase in patients who catheterize compared to those who void spontaneously or who empty their bladders using the Credé maneuver.[57] Some investigators have found a definite increase in the occurrence of infection when cystoplasty is performed concomitantly with AUS insertion.[47,51] Holmes et al found an increased incidence of infection to be associated with prior bladder neck surgery in the neurogenic bladder population and recommended performing the AUS insertion before doing the augmentation in patients who have this risk factor.[56] Miller et al performed simultaneous bladder augmentation and AUS insertion using a variety of different bowel segments and found a 6.9% infection rate (2/29 patients). They suggested performing gastrocystoplasty along with AUS insertion since there were no infections associated with the use of stomach in their series.[58]

Erosion rates range from 6 to 31% in contemporary neurogenic bladder series and are the major cause of sphincter removal. Erosion can occur secondary to infection, ischemia from high cuff pressures, devascularization from prior surgery or radiation, and traumatic catheterization.[41,50,56] Factors which increase the likelihood of erosion include prior bladder neck surgery, placement of the cuff around the bulbar urethra in children, and placement of the cuff around the bowel used to form a neobladder.[41,50,55] Guralnick et al recently described AUS cuff placement through a dissection plane deep to the tunica albuginea of the corporal bodies in 31 men who experienced erosion or atrophy at the original cuff site. They were able to salvage continence in 84% of cases, but there was the potential for postoperative deterioration of erectile function.[59]

Patients who receive an AUS must undergo long-term urologic follow-up with urodynamic bladder monitoring and serial upper tract imaging to detect the onset of upper tract deterioration. High intravesical pressure requires the institution of anticholinergic medications, or, if this fails,

Table 23.4 *Results of artificial urinary sphincter insertion for the treatment of incontinence in patients with neurogenic bladder*

Study	Year	Patient population	Type and location of sphincter	Mean follow up time	Results	Complications
Bellioli et al[53]	1992	Adolescents 37: 35 male, 2 female 33 MMC, 3 SA, 1 pelvic surgery	2 AMS 792, 35 AMS 800 33 BN, 4 BU	4.5 years range 1–8.5	59% dry day and night 90% dry day only	2 upper tract deteriorations 38% reoperation rate for mechanical problems 1 infection, 1 BN perforation, 1 scrotal hematoma
Gonzalez et al[52]	1995	Pediatric 19 males all neurogenic	11 AMS 800 8 AMS 721 or 792 all BN placement	8 years	84.2% continent 73.8% catheterizing	36.8% postoperative augmentation rate 1 renal loss 10% new hydro
Levesque et al[47]	1996	Adult and pediatric Most with MMC 36: 22 male, 14 female before 1985 18 children	Before 1985: 6 AMS 792, 18 AMS 292, 12 AMS 800 After 1985: all AMS 800 All BN placement	13.7 years	Mean survival time 12.1 years 82% dry 64% catheterizing 59% continent	6 developed renal failure 42% required postoperative augmentation
Singh and Thomas[51]	1996	Mostly adult 90: 75 male, 15 female 65 MMC, 19 SCI, 5 SA, 1 sacral angioma	82 AMS 800 8 AMS 792 BU and BN	4 years range 1–10	92% continent 79% with detrusor overactivity required augmentation 78% catheterizing	28% reoperation rate 6 infections, 7 erosions, 8 system failures, 2 pump failures, 1 cut tube, 1 rectal perforation, 1 bladder perforation
Simeoni et al[50]	1996	Pediatric 107: 74 male, 33 female 92 MMC	AMS 800 98 BN, 9 BU	61 months minimum of 12	41% continent with no revisions 21% augmentation rate	Immediate: 4 UTI, 2 wound infection, 3 scrotal hematoma, 3 urinary fistula, 2 retention 25% removal rate 59% revision rate 13% erosion rate

Table 23.4 Continued

Table 23.4 *Continued*

Study	Year	Patient population	Type and location of sphincter	Mean follow up time	Results	Complications
Fulford et al[41]	1997	Adult and pediatric 61: 43 male, 18 female 34 neurogenic, 15 post-radiation prostatectomy, 12 other	Combination of AMS 791, 792, and 800 BU and BN placement	10–15 years	75% functioning	49 with 1 or more revision 13% continent with original AUS *in situ* 31% erosion rate, 2/3 in 1st year after placement
Elliot and Barrett[42]	1998	Adult 323: 313 male, 10 female 70 neurogenic	All AMS 800 139 without narrow cuff backing 184 with narrow cuff backing 272 BU, 51 BN	68.8 months range 18–153	Males 27% reoperation rate, females: 60% reoperation rate 90.4% functioning at 5 years, 72% no reoperation at 5 years	Mechanical failure: 21% pre-cuff, 7.6% post-cuff Non-mechanical failure: 17% pre-cuff, 9% post-cuff
Kryger et al[45]	2001	Pediatric 32: 25 male, 7 female Group 1 – insertion before age 11 (21) Group 2 – insertion after age 11 (11)	AMS 800 – 21 Pre-AMS 800 – 11	1 year 15.4 years	Group 1 – 54% intact, all dry Group 2 – 64% intact, 86% dry No statistical significant difference between groups	56% revision rate Group 1 – 43% removed: 4 infection, 5 erosion Group 2 – 36% removed: 1 infection, 3 erosions
Castera et al[55]	2001	Pediatric 49: 39 male, 10 female 38 MMC, 7 exstrophy, 4 trauma	All AMS 800 29 BN 20 BU	7.5 years range 2–11	67% dry: 86% dry with no prior surgery, 37.5% dry with prior BN surgery	20% erosion, 4% infection, 12% mechanical failure
Spiess et al[54]	2002	Pediatric 30 males with MMC	All AMS 800	6.5 years	63% dry, 20% slightly wet	Only 8.3% lasted >100 months, mean lifetime 4.9 years

MMC, myelomeningocele; SA, sacral agenesis; SCI, spinal cord injury; BN, bladder neck; BU, bulbar urethra; UTI, urinary tract infection.

augmentation. Hydronephrosis or reflux is usually refractory to medical management and indicates a need for cystoplasty. The proportion of AUS recipients with neurogenic bladder who ultimately require augmentation cystoplasty ranges from 4 to 42%.[46,50,52,55] Patients who are noncompliant with surveillance protocols may develop upper tract damage. A number of authors have described the occurrence of chronic renal failure in patients with incontinence of neurologic etiology who received an AUS and were then lost to follow-up for long periods of time.[42,46,53]

Conclusions

When it was first marketed in the early 1970s, the AUS represented a major advancement in the treatment of patients with severe incontinence secondary to sphincteric deficiency. The device has undergone many design modifications since its first inception, all of which have served to increase its efficacy and lower its complication rate. Erosion and infection rates are low in well-selected patients. The possibility of requiring repeat surgery for mechanical failure is high, as is the cost of these revisions, but the AUS will, no doubt, continue to be utilized in the treatment of urinary incontinence.

Bladder neck reconstruction

Introduction

In 1908, Young described a technique for increasing bladder outlet resistance by narrowing the urethra and bladder neck lumen to the size of a silver probe.[60] Since this first description of bladder neck reconstruction was published, there have been many modifications to the surgical procedure. At first, reconfiguring the bladder outlet to increase its resistance was thought to be contraindicated in the neurogenic bladder population because of the subsequent necessity for IC.[61] Many investigators, however, have found this technique to be a viable alternative to bladder neck sling, AUS, or urinary diversion in patients with neurologic lesions who require treatment for severe sphincteric incompetence provided that the patient and/or caregiver is capable of performing IC and is compliant with this routine. These procedures are technically challenging and a successful outcome is highly dependent on the operative experience of the surgeon.

The main types of bladder neck reconstruction that have been utilized in the neurogenic bladder population are the Kropp anterior bladder wall flap valve and the Salle anterior bladder wall flip-flap. The Young–Dees–Leadbetter posterior bladder wall flap is primarily used for the treatment of bladder exstrophy, but has been reported in patients with neurogenic sphincteric deficiency. The Tanagho and Smith bladder neck reconstruction, which is mostly of historic interest, has been described in patients with post-prostatectomy incontinence and will not be covered in this section.[61,62] The majority of the literature deals with the pediatric population, since it is in this age group that urologic intervention is first sought. The Kropp and Salle procedures work on the flap valve principle popularized by Mitrofanoff. As the bladder fills with urine, increases in intravesical pressure are transmitted to the valve constructed from anterior bladder wall, thereby increasing leak point threshold and preventing incontinence.[63] The Young–Dees–Leadbetter reconstruction prevents urine leakage by increasing bladder neck and urethral length and decreasing their caliber, two maneuvers which result in an increase in outlet resistance.[60]

Young–Dees–Leadbetter procedure

The Young–Dees–Leadbetter bladder neck reconstruction, as it was first described by Leadbetter in 1964, involves lengthening the urethra and creating a new bladder neck using a flap of posterior bladder wall which incorporates the trigone. The ureters are reimplanted 3–4 cm superiorly so that the trigonal muscle can be utilized. The posterior bladder wall is not mobilized in order to keep the blood and nervous supply intact, thereby helping to prevent slough and denervation of the bladder wall flap. The vertical midline cystotomy which was made to reimplant the ureters is carried into the urethra, and longitudinal lateral incisions are made on either side of the urethra and bladder neck. These incisions begin at the apex of the midline urethral incision and extend along the bladder base through the old ureteric orifice sites and 1–2 cm beyond them on the posterior bladder wall.

The resulting lateral bladder flaps are denuded of mucosa to leave a posterior strip of bladder 1.5 cm wide and 3 cm long.[64] These flaps are then folded over on each other using an 8–10F urethral catheter as a guide to caliber and closed in two layers. The mucosal layer is closed with interrupted fine absorbable suture and the muscle layer is opposed in an overlapping fashion using a fine running suture of absorbable material. The bladder neck closure is completed in layers: mucosa, muscle, and serosa. The end result is a urethra which is lengthened by 4–5 cm. The dog ears of bladder that remain are incorporated into the bladder wall closure, since resection of these segments can result in a substantial decrease in bladder capacity.[60] A urethral catheter and suprapubic tube are often placed, although some surgeons prefer to forgo urethral stenting. If employed, the urethral Foley catheter is removed within 3–4 weeks and the suprapubic tube is discontinued once the patient is able to empty the bladder by voiding or intermittent catheterization.

Placement of a silicone sheath around the bladder neck reconstruction to facilitate the insertion of an artificial urethral sphincter cuff later on if required was advocated by Mitchell et al in 1985. These authors, however, later abandoned this practice upon experiencing a 67% erosion rate at a mean of 4 years after operation.[65] Ransley's group, however, has reported a lower erosion rate of 14% after decreasing the thickness of the silicone sheath and interposing omentum between the sheath and the bladder neck.[65,66]

Kropp bladder neck reconstruction

The Kropp procedure was first described by Kropp and Aangwafo in 1986. It lengthens the urethra by attaching it to a tube of bladder muscle which is implanted into the posterior bladder wall through a submucosal tunnel to create a one-way flap valve that allows a catheter to be passed but prevents urine from leaking out. A rectangular flap 5–7 cm × 2–2.5 cm is outlined on the anterior bladder wall with stay sutures. This flap is left attached to the bladder neck and the bladder is separated completely from the bladder neck. The anterior wall flap is rolled into a tube over a 10–12F Foley catheter and sutured together with 4–0 chromic catgut. A submucosal tunnel is developed between the ureteric orifices, and the tube is pulled through this tunnel. The bladder is drawn back down to the bladder neck and sutured with absorbable sutures. The ostia of the new urethra is sutured to the posterior bladder wall. This method can also be accomplished using a posterior strip of bladder, which is tunneled into the anterior bladder wall.[67]

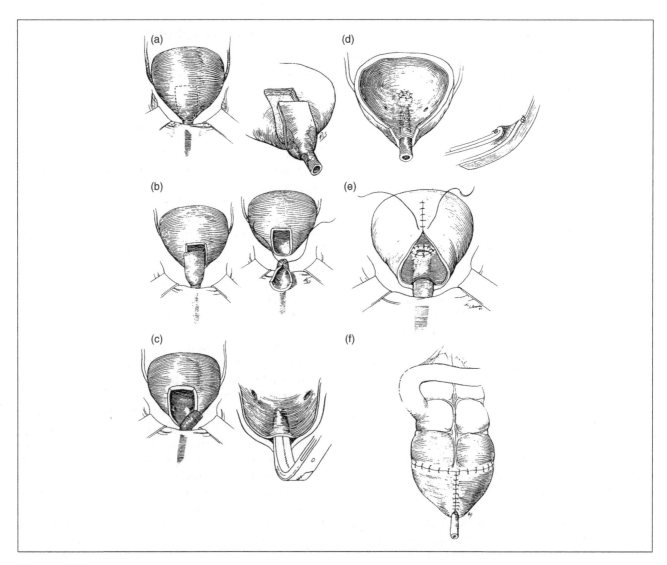

Figure 23.7
Kropp anterior flap-valve bladder neck reconstruction. (Reproduced with permission from Kropp and Angwolfo, J Urol 1986; 135:533–536.)

Two modifications to the Kropp bladder neck reconstruction were described by Belman and Kaplan and subsequently adopted widely by other surgeons, including the originator of the Kropp procedure.[68] These alterations involve leaving the bladder neck attached to the bladder and making a groove in the posterior bladder wall into which the tube is laid, then suturing the epithelium over the tube rather than creating a submucosal tunnel.[69] Mollard et al demuscularized the bladder tube, leaving only mucosa to tunnel in some cases, and reimplanted one of the ureters cephalad to make more room to tunnel the tube in the posterior bladder wall.[63]

Pippi Salle bladder neck reconstruction

In 1994, Pippi Salle described his own version of the anterior wall flap valve in 15 dogs and 6 children with myelomeningocele. The Salle bladder neck reconstruction is a modification of the Kropp design in which the urethra is lengthened with an anterior bladder wall flap 4–5 cm × 1–1.7 cm, which is sutured to the posterior wall in an onlay fashion. In the original description, the ureters are reimplanted superiorly using the Cohen cross-trigonal technique. A border of mucosa 0.1 cm wide is removed from the flap to obtain separate non-overlapping suture lines. The edges of the posterior bladder wall are then sewn over the lengthened urethra to create a flap valve. A urethral catheter is left in for 2–3 weeks.[70] In 1997 Salle and colleagues described a number of modifications to the original technique. The first involved making two longitudinal incisions in the trigonal mucosa to better expose the muscle for suturing to the exposed muscle edges of the anterior wall flap, then suturing the lateral edges of posterior wall mucosa over the flap to help prevent leakage of urine and fistula formation. The second modification was to widen the base of the flap to improve its blood supply but to leave the distal tip narrow to attain the correct lumen size when fashioning the neourethra. In some cases, a superior extension of mucosa was taken with the anterior wall flap and folded back over the intravesical urethra to cover it and prevent fistula formation. Lastly, the authors described the creation of a lateral anterior wall flap in 4 patients who had a midline scar in the anterior bladder wall from previous surgery. Ureteric reimplantations were not performed routinely in this later series.[71]

Indications and patient selection

All patients being considered for bladder neck reconstruction should undergo urodynamic assessment and

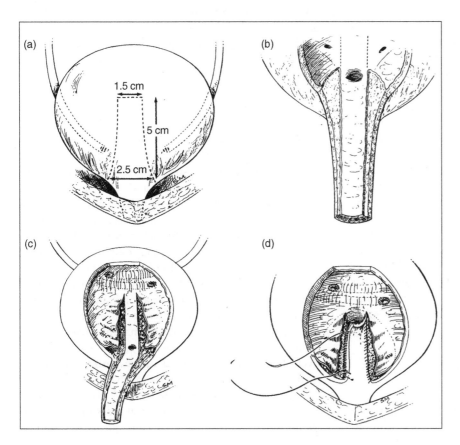

Figure 23.8
Pippi Salle flip-flap bladder reconstruction. (Reproduced with permission from Pippi-Salle, J Urol 1994; 152:803–806.)

voiding cystourethrogram to document the mechanism of incontinence and the degree of urethral incompetence. The filling phase should be carried out with a Foley balloon occluding the bladder outlet to determine bladder capacity, stability, and compliance.[43] Cystoscopy may aid in assessing the characteristics of the bladder wall and outlet before surgery. The urodynamic prerequisites for bladder neck reconstruction are similar to those for the AUS or bladder neck sling: a stable, adequate capacity bladder (see above). The majority of authors recommend the concomitant performance of bladder augmentation, since increasing outlet resistance will often lead to elevated storage pressures and the use of bladder wall to reconstruct the outlet can significantly decrease bladder capacity.[72,73]

Although bladder neck reconstruction can be performed as a salvage procedure for patients who have failed bladder neck sling or AUS insertion,[74] many authors advocate considering it as a primary option in patients who have total incontinence secondary to a patulous, wide-open bladder neck, since compromised blood supply from previous surgery will decrease the success of the operation.[69] Bladder neck reconstruction in general is not suitable for the correction of mild stress urinary incontinence, since it has a significant complication rate.

The Young–Dees–Leadbetter bladder neck reconstruction is mainly employed in the treatment of anatomic bladder outlet defects encountered in the exstrophy-epispadias complex; there have been few reports of its use in patients with neurogenic bladder. Continence rates are not as high in patients with neuropathic outlet incompetence as they are in the exstrophy population, and some investigators have documented better results in females than in males.[75]

The Kropp procedure was specifically designed for the treatment of neurogenic incontinence and functions on the assumption that all patients will need to catheterize to empty the bladder. It is often performed as a last resort to achieve continence before AUS insertion. Mollard et al[63] and Snodgrass[73] prefer to use the Kropp procedure as first-line bladder outlet management in females and reserve the AUS for males, with the rationale that lengthening the urethra in boys may make it more difficult for them to perform IC. Waters et al, however, in a review of catheterization problems in patients who had had Kropp reconstruction, found that the problem was experienced by equal numbers of boys and girls.[68] The Salle technique has been employed with equal success in patients with incontinence secondary to neurogenic bladder and exstrophy-epispadias complex.[70,71,76,77]

Results and complications

The Young–Dees–Leadbetter procedure and its numerous modifications have produced continence rates up to 60–80% when performed in the exstrophy population.[78,79] Published series employing this technique in neurogenic bladder patients are small, but success has been reported to be lower, with continence rates of 50–60% over a follow-up period of greater than 5 years.[75,80,81] Complications have included UTIs, de-novo vesicoureteral reflux (VUR), urethral and bladder neck fistulas, SUI, difficulty catheterizing, and bladder neck strictures, particularly in patients who have had previous bladder neck surgery.[75,79]

The Kropp bladder neck reconstruction has enjoyed continence rates of 80–94%, but this has been tempered by difficult catheterization rates of 10–44% (Table 23.5).[63,67–69,72,73] This problem is thought to occur secondary to the tube being compressed as it passes through the submucosal tunnel, or the suture line running along the back wall of the tube causing formation of an elevated scar.[67,70] An overdistended bladder resulting from delay in catheterization can also compress the valve, making it difficult to pass a drainage tube.[72] In later series, investigators have noted a decrease in the occurrence of catheterization problems when the urethral catheter was left in 4–5 weeks after bladder neck reconstruction.[69] In most cases, this situation is alleviated by passing a catheter under cystoscopic guidance and leaving it in for a few weeks, then having the patient resume catheterization.[68] Other patients who have trouble passing a catheter require bladder neck dilatation or endoscopic resection of the roof of the neourethra. Occasionally, open revision of the flap valve is required.[67,72] Snodgrass has described the performance of an appendicovesicostomy concomitant to the Kropp procedure as a means of providing an alternative route of bladder drainage should the patient be unable to catheterize via the reconstructed bladder outlet.[73]

Other complications encountered with the Kropp technique include pyelonephritis, peritonitis secondary to bladder perforation, de-novo VUR, and fistula formation between the valve and the bladder resulting in incontinence. The Kropp procedure is highly effective at increasing bladder neck resistance and can result in the attainment of a VLPP of greater than 60 cmH$_2$O in many patients.[69] This high level of continence, coupled with the possibility of difficult catheterization in a patient who may also have an enterocystoplasty, can result in perforation of the augmented portion of the bladder, with subsequent peritonitis, cases of which have culminated in death.[72] New-onset VUR is thought to be a consequence of elevated intravesical pressures as a result of increased outlet resistance, disruption of the trigonal musculature when tunneling the tube, or VUR which was present preoperatively but was not observed on cystourethrogram.[71,73] A small proportion of patients who develop de-novo VUR fail to resolve it spontaneously and require ureteric reimplantation. Fistulas can occur at areas of devascularization along suture lines or as a consequence of traumatic

Table 23.5 *Results of Kropp bladder neck reconstruction in patients with neurogenic incontinence*

Procedure	Study	Year	Patients	Follow-up time	Concomitant surgeries	Results	Complications
Kropp	Kropp and Angwafo[67]	1986	Pediatric 7 male, 6 female 13 MMC	8–36 months	6 augments, 2 reimplants, 2 undiversions	92% dry	4/6 IC problems 4 de-novo VUR
Kropp	Belman and Kaplan[69]	1989	Pediatric 18: 16 MMC, 2 SA, 10 male	Not stated	14 augments	78% dry, 4 hours	44% IC problems 4 de-novo VUR, 1 pyelonephritis
Kropp	Nill et al[72]	1990	Pediatric and adult 24: MMC and MS 14 female	1.5–7 years	19 reoperations to perform bladder augmentation	83% dry	46% IC problems 1 vesicocutaneous fistula, 5 reoperations on valve, 9 peritonitis, 8 bladder stones, 10 de-novo VUR
Kropp	Mollard et al[63]	1990	Pediatric 16 girls 15 MMC, 1 other	Not stated	6 augments, 7 reimplants	81% dry	12.5% IC problems 2 valve failures
Kropp (Belman and Kaplan modifications)	Snodgrass[73]	1997	Pediatric 23: 13 male all MMC	Mean 27 months range 3–72	20 augments	91% dry	17% IC problems all in males, 2 valve fistulas, 50% de-novo VUR

MMC, myelomeningocele; SA, sacral agenesis; IC, intermittent catheterization; VUR, vesicoureteric reflux.

Table 23.6 *Results of Salle and Young–Dees–Leadbetter bladder neck reconstruction in patients with neurogenic incontinence*

Procedure	Study	Year	Patients	Follow-up time	Concomitant surgery	Results	Complications
Salle	Pippi Salle et al[70]	1994	Pediatric 6: 3 males All with MMC	Mean 16.8 months range 7–24	Not stated	4/6 (67%) dry	1 flap fistula, 1 re-operation to narrow flap, 1 de-novo VUR, 1 pyelo
Salle	Rink et al[77]	1994	Pediatric 3 MMC females	12–15 months	Cohen reimplants 2 augments	2/3 dry, 1 nocturnal leakage	None
Salle	Mouriquard et al[76]	1995	Pediatric 8 girls: 7 MMC, 1 other	Mean 6.7 months range 2–18	6 augments	38% dry day and night 88% dry during day	1 flap fistula, 1 bladder calculi
Salle	Pippi Salle et al[71]	1997	Pediatric 17: 13 neurogenic, 4 EE	Mean 25.6 months range 9–49	Not stated	70% dry 9/13 neurogenic dry, 3/4 EE dry	2 flap fistulas, 2 IC problems (all in EEC), 12% de-novo VUR
Young–Dees–Leadbetter vs AUS	Sidi et al[80]	1987	Pediatric 11 BN reconstruction: 9 female 16 AUS: all male 17 MMC, 6 SA, 4 other	BNR Mean 3.2 years range 1–5 AUS Mean 5.7 years range 1–12	BNR: 64% dry AUS: 69% dry	BNR reoperation rate 0.8/patient AUS reoperation rate 1.5/patient	BNR: 9 augments AUS: 2 augments
Young–Dees–Leadbetter	Donnahoo et al[75]	1999	Pediatric 38: 25 female 32 MMC, 3 SA, 13 other	Mean 9 years range 1–17	8 silicone sheath placements, 36 reimplants, 22 augments	50% dry 12.5% partially dry 63% girls vs 25% boys dry with primary bladder neck reconstruction	10.5% IC problems 62.5% silicone sheath erosion, 14% perforation of augmented bladder

MMC, myelomeningocele; SA, sacral agenesis; EE, exstrophy-epispadias; IC, intermittent catheterization; VUR, vesicoureteric reflux; AUS, artificial urethral sphincter; BNR, bladder neck reconstruction instrumentation or catheterization and usually require open revision of the flap valve in order to achieve continence.

The Salle anterior bladder wall flap has continence rates which are slightly lower than the Kropp procedure, but does not have the high incidence of catheterization difficulty which has plagued the other technique. The occurrence of fistulas between the flap valve and bladder is a problem particularly noted with the Salle procedure and catheterization problems were experienced by some of the exstrophy patients in the later series published by Pippi Salle et al (Table 23.6).[70,71]

Conclusion

In summary, bladder neck reconstruction is one of the earliest surgical treatments devised for treating urinary incontinence secondary to an incompetent bladder neck and proximal urethra. All these procedures, while they have the advantage of utilizing the patient's own tissue, are technically challenging and are associated with a number of complications, some of which may require numerous surgical revisions. Bladder neck reconstruction should not be performed in patients who have mild degrees of urinary incontinence that may be cured by urethral collagen injections or a fascial sling. Bladder neck reconstruction should be reserved for patients with severe outlet incompetence and should only be performed by an experienced surgeon. Despite the availability of the AUS and popularity of the fascial sling, bladder neck reconstruction in its many forms continues to have a role in the treatment of patients with neurogenic bladder and exstrophy-epispadias complex who suffer from total urinary incontinence.

Bladder neck closure

Introduction

Bladder neck closure is considered a last-resort procedure.[82] It is indicated in patients with outlet incompetence who have failed multiple anti-incontinence procedures, patients who are poor surgical candidates and cannot tolerate lengthy, complex reconstructive procedures, and in patients with destroyed urethras which cannot be rebuilt.[83] Closure of the bladder neck can be combined with a catheterizable cutaneous stoma or a chronic indwelling suprapubic tube depending on the constitutional and functional status of the patient.

In female spinal cord injury patients who have been managed with a chronic indwelling Foley catheter, bladder neck closure and suprapubic tube insertion can improve quality of

life by eliminating leakage of urine alongside the tube, which can cause chronic skin breakdown, and facilitate return to sexual activity by eliminating the urethral catheter.[84,85]

The disadvantages of bladder neck closure are its irreversibility; its abolishment of the pop-off valve, which necessitates long-term monitoring of the upper tracts to prevent occult renal deterioration;[86] and unpredictable effects on potency and ejaculation when performed in young males.[82] Patients who are managed with bladder neck closure and a chronic suprapubic tube must undergo surveillance cystoscopy in order to monitor for the formation of bladder calculi and squamous neoplasia.[83] There is also a persistent risk of infection secondary to the indwelling catheter.[84]

Transposition of the female urethra to the suprapubic area to form a continent catheterizable stoma has been described, but it is not suitable for obese patients or patients with a significant amount of periurethral scarring secondary to previous surgical procedures or years of chronic indwelling urethral Foley management.[83,84,86] Reconstruction using vaginal wall or bowel has also been attempted in females with destroyed urethras but the success rate with these procedures is low.[87] Alternatively, a tight fascial sling can be used to achieve a functional bladder neck closure, provided that the patient has a urethral length of at least 1.5–2 cm.[88]

Surgical technique

Bladder neck closure can be performed via the transabdominal or transvaginal route. In the transabdominal approach, a transverse suprapubic incision or vertical midline incision is made and the bladder neck is mobilized. In males, the bladder is transected just cranial to the prostate after ligating the superficial dorsal venous complex and dissecting the neurovascular bundles away. The prostate is usually left intact in order to preserve fertility and antegrade ejaculation. In cases of urethral stricture or prostatorectal fistula which compromise drainage of prostatic secretions and act as a nidus of infection, the prostate is removed to avoid abscess formation. In females the bladder is transected at the vesicourethral junction once the deep dorsal vein has been ligated. Intravenous indigo carmine or ureteric catheters are used to help identify the ureteric orifices. The bladder is mobilized posteriorly to the level of the ureteric orifices. A sponge stick in the vagina can aid in identifying the correct plane of dissection.

Once the posterior and inferior aspects of the bladder have been mobilized out of its dependent position in the pelvis, the bladder neck opening is closed ventrally in two layers: mucosa and muscle with serosa. A suprapubic tube is placed and brought out through a separate stab incision before closing the bladder neck completely, and if the bladder closure is to be combined with a continent catheterizable stoma it is constructed and attached to the bladder at this stage. The urethral stump is closed dorsally in two layers and an omental flap is mobilized and placed between the closed urethral stump and the bladder neck closure to prevent fistula formation.[82,84] A drain is usually left in the space of Retzius. Postoperatively, anticholinergics are administered to prevent bladder spasms. Reid et al have described a different technique of bladder neck closure which involved denuding the bladder neck mucosa through a midline cystotomy, excising a cuff of bladder neck, then closing the denuded muscle with a purse string suture.[89]

The transvaginal approach is typically employed in females with urethral destruction secondary to chronic

indwelling Foley catheter drainage who are to be managed with bladder neck closure and suprapubic tube placement. The patient is placed in the dorsal lithotomy position and a suprapubic tube is placed using a Lowsley retractor. This technique is employed to circumvent the difficulty inherent in distending a small contracted bladder with an incompetent outlet.

The patient is placed in the Trendelenburg position to displace the bowels cephalad and the curved Lowsley retractor is inserted into the urethra and pointed towards the anterior abdominal wall 1–2 cm above the pubic symphysis. A small fascial incision is made over the tip of the retractor, which is pushed out through the skin incision.

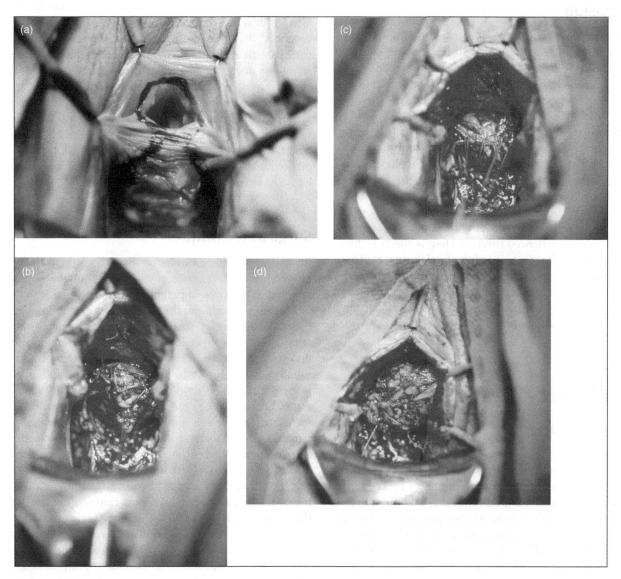

Figure 23.9
Transvaginal bladder neck closure. (a) Creation of anterior vaginal wall flap. Destroyed urethra is circumscribed. (b) Bladder neck is mobilized and urethral reminant excised. First tension-free layer of bladder neck closure. (c) Transversal second layer closure to protect against a secondary vesicovaginal fistula. (d) Placement of Martius flap tunneled beneath labia minora. (Reproduced with permission from Glenn's Urologic Surgery, 5th edn, 1998, Chapter 49, Figs 49.1–49.4.)

The tip of a large-bore Foley catheter is grasped in its jaws and pulled back into the bladder. Intravesical placement of the catheter can be confirmed by irrigation of the tube or cystoscopic inspection.[90]

An incision circumscribing the urethral opening is extended into an inverted U incision on the anterior vaginal wall. The endopelvic fascia is pierced on either side of the bladder neck in order to free it up completely from the pubic bone and the pubourethral ligaments are transected. Intravenous indigo carmine is given to visualize the ureteric orifices. The scarred urethra, if present, is excised and the bladder neck closed in two layers: first in the vertical, and then in the horizontal direction. The second suture line should contain tissue from the bladder neck to the anterior wall located behind the symphysis to transfer the closed bladder neck to the retropubic space and remove it from a dependent position. The integrity of the closure is checked by filling the bladder through the suprapubic tube. A Martius flap is interposed between the bladder neck and anterior vaginal wall to help prevent vesicovaginal fistula formation and the vaginal wall flap is closed over the Martius flap as a third layer. A vaginal pack containing antibiotic solution is left in for 24 hours,[83] and anticholinergics are administered to prevent bladder spasms.

Bladder neck closure is highly effective at treating incontinence secondary to an incompetent bladder outlet. Continence rates of 75–100% have been reported in the literature, with mean follow-up times ranging from 1.5 to 3 years.[82–87,91,92] The main technical complication is bladder neck fistulization with continued leakage of urine, which has been reported to occur in 6–25% of cases.[84,89–92] The rate of fistulization is low in series which adhere to the following surgical principles: mobilization of the bladder from its dependent position in the pelvis, closure of the bladder neck and urethral stump in multiple layers without tension, and interposition of well-vascularized tissue such as omentum or a labial fat pad between the urethra and bladder neck. No adverse effect on potency or ejaculation was noted by Hoebeke et al, who performed the procedure in nine young males.

Surgical treatment of the hyperactive bladder outlet

Introduction

For several years it has been recognized that detrusor-external sphincter dyssynergia (DESD), a common condition in patients with suprasacral spinal cord lesions, is associated with elevated intravesical pressure, which can result in substantial morbidity and mortality. DESD is defined as a detrusor contraction concurrent with an involuntary contraction of the urethral and/or peri-urethral striated muscle during voiding.[93] During urodynamic assessment, DESD is denoted by an increase in electromyographic activity of the sphincter or pelvic muscles associated with an involuntary detrusor contraction. On voiding cystourethrogram or videourodynamic assessment, dilation of the bladder neck due to a contracted external sphincter is observed during bladder emptying.[94] The condition leads to a complication rate in excess of 50%, resulting in urosepsis, hydronephrosis, nephrolithiasis, and vesicoureteric reflux, all of which can terminate in renal insufficiency and, eventually, dialysis.[95,96] DESD is also associated with autonomic dysreflexia, particularly in patients with injuries above the T5 spinal cord level. Since its description by Emmett et al in 1948, sphincterotomy has been recommended to treat DESD in a subset of spinal cord injured males who are at risk for renal damage.[97] By incising the external sphincter to render it incompetent, one can transform intermittent incontinence into continous incontinence, which can be managed with a condom catheter drainage device.[98] Sphincterotomy is irreversible and has been associated with intraoperative bleeding and erectile dysfunction. A reduction in long-term efficacy has also been observed which may require repeat external sphincter or bladder neck incision.[99] Long-term use of a condom catheter can lead to skin ulceration, urethrocutaneous fistula, and penile retraction.[98] Despite these drawbacks, sphicterotomy is still considered the gold standard to which other treatments for DESD are compared.

A urethral stent was first used by Milroy et al in 1988 to treat stricture disease.[100] Subsequently, it has been employed in benign prostatic hyperplasia (BPH) therapy and as an alternative to sphincterotomy in patients with DESD. Most of the experience with external sphincter stenting has been with the Urolume prosthesis (American Medical Systems, Minnetonka, Minnesota), a nonmagnetic superalloy woven into a mesh cylinder which is inserted endoscopically across the external sphincter to hold it open. The geometry and elasticity of the stent material exerts a radial force which maintains its position within the urethral lumen until epithelialization occurs.[101] Other urethral stents which have been used to circumvent DESD include the Ultraflex (Boston Scientific Corp., Boston, MA), which is made of a single elastalloy wire, and the Memokath (Engineers and Doctors A/S, Homback, Denmark), a coil made of thermosensitive titanium/nickel alloy. Sphincteric stenting has several advantages over sphincterotomy. It is an easier and quicker procedure that is associated with shorter hospital stay and cost.[101] Unlike sphincterotomy, stent insertion is potentially reversible, a characteristic which appeals to spinal cord injured patients still hoping for a cure.[94] Furthermore, sphincteric stents are

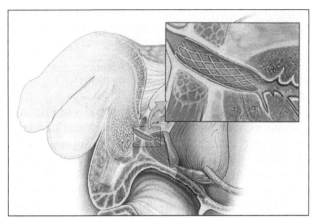

Figure 23.10
Sagittal view of male pelvis to show placement of urethral stent across external sphincter.

not associated with diminished erectile ability or significant blood loss.[94] Despite these advantages, insertion of a stent across the external sphincter raises some legitimate concerns. The stent is a foreign body which is placed in contact with urine, resulting in encrustation.[94] Difficult removal of the Urolume stent occasionally resulting in urethral injury has also been reported.[102,103]

Another minimally invasive treatment for the dyssynergic external sphincter, balloon dilatation, has also recently been described.[104] More experience is needed to determine its long-term merit.

Indications and patient selection

Both sphincterotomy and urethral stents are employed in the treatment of DESD in male spinal cord injured patients with DO refractory to anticholinergics and IC, or in those unable or unwilling to carry out this conservative treatment.[99] Sphincteric stents have been used not only as primary treatment for DESD but also for patients who have failed previous sphincterotomy.[94,105] Relative contraindications to stenting include patients who are known to be recurrent stone formers, patients who have had previous bladder neck (BN) incisions or TURP (transurethral rejection of the prostate), and patients who have an artificial urinary sphincter.[94,105,106] Chancellor et al, in the North American Multicenter Urolume Trial, found that a wide-open bladder neck secondary to previous bladder neck or prostatic surgery predisposed patients to stent migration.[94] McInerney and colleagues placed stents in 3 men with spinal cord injuries and DESD who had artificial urinary sphincters.[105] The voiding parameters of these men were not improved, and, due

to perineal discomfort, one stent was eventually removed with great difficulty.

The Memokath stent has been found to be easier to remove than the Urolume device and has been advocated as a short-term treatment option for DESD. This stent may be used as an alternative to an indwelling catheter in recent spinal cord injured patients who are likely to regain enough upper extremity function to be able to perform self-catheterization, or for patients who would like to try condom catheter drainage before committing themselves to Urolume or sphincterotomy.[107] Men who are undergoing electroejaculation may also benefit from the Memokath, since the device can be easily removed and replaced later on.[107]

Sphincterotomy or sphincteric stenting with condom catheter drainage is preferable to a chronic indwelling Foley catheter, which is still often used as the management of last resort in quadriplegic patients who do not have the manual dexterity or caregiver support to perform IC or change a condom catheter. Chronic indwelling catheters are associated with recurrent urosepsis, bladder calculi, and squamous cell carcinoma in this patient population.[108]

Sphincterotomy techniques

Before proceeding with incision of the external sphincter, the patient should have a negative urine culture. The patient is placed in the dorsal lithotomy position and perioperative intravenous antibiotic prophylaxis is administered. The type of anesthesia required depends on the amount of sensation and severity of autonomic dysreflexia experienced by the individual. Intravenous sedation with or without calcium channel or alpha-antagonist prophylaxis for hypertensive crisis may be all that is needed.

Sphincterotomy is usually performed under endoscopic video control with a 24F resectoscope and Collins knife or loop electrocautery attachment. A cut is made anteriorly at the 12 o'clock or 11 o'clock position away from the neurovascular bundles to minimize the risk of bleeding and erectile dysfunction. The incision is taken from the prostatic urethra just proximal to the verumontanum to the proximal bulbar urethra. The cut must extend through the muscle fibers of the sphincter to the level of the corpus spongiosum tissue of the proximal bulb.[109] Hemostasis is attained with the electrocautery, and a 22F three-way Foley catheter is placed in the bladder. Continuous bladder irrigation is run for 24–48 hours to prevent clot retention and the patient is discharged once the urine is clear. The catheter is removed 4–7 days after the procedure and a condom catheter is applied to the penis for bladder drainage.

Sphincterotomy performed with the Nd:YAG contact laser has been described as an alternative to electrocautery.[110,111] A chisel or round-tip probe is deployed through the instrument port of a 21 or 23F cystoscope with a 30 degree lens. The sphincterotomy is performed anteriorly, as with electrocautery, with the probe tip in contact with the tissue to be vaporized. Repeated passes are made over the area until the required depth is attained. Cutting tissue requires settings of 25–50 W and hemostasis is achieved with lower energy settings of 15–25 W. Laser sphincterotomy may take a longer time than conventional electrocautery, especially if there is a large amount of scarring from previous surgery.[111]

Whether or not to perform bladder neck incision concomitant with sphincterotomy to optimize bladder emptying is somewhat controversial. Some investigators state that the bladder neck should not be incised immediately, as there is often delayed relaxation of the bladder outlet after sphincterotomy, and performing a bladder neck incision will result in complete incontinence with continuous urine leakage.[99] Other surgeons cut the bladder neck in addition to the external sphincter when preoperative urodynamics demonstrate bladder neck obstruction.[109,110] In their series of laser sphincterotomies, Perkash[110] performed concomitant laser bladder neck incisions at 3 and 9 o'clock, whereas Rivas et al[111] cut the bladder neck in the midline at 6 o'clock.

Results and complications of sphincterotomy

The results of some contemporary series of spinal cord patients treated with sphincterotomy are listed in Table 23.7. Incising the external sphincter results in statistically significant decreases in maximum detrusor pressure, post-void residual, and the occurrence of autonomic dysreflexia. Bladder capacity is usually maintained. Complications include bleeding, clot retention, urosepsis, erectile dysfunction, and sphincterotomy failure secondary to urethral scarring. Making the incision anteriorly at 12 or 11 o'clock, rather than posterolaterally, has lowered the likelihood of damage to the urethral blood supply and cavernous body innervation, resulting in decreased rates of clot retention and erectile dysfunction compared with older series.[109,111] The need for repeat sphincterotomy secondary to scarring and stenosis of the external sphincter is usually evident within 12 months of having the procedure, but can occur years later.[99] Repeat sphincterotomy rates range from 9%, when the laser is employed, to 31%, with the use of conventional electrocautery.[109,110] Other complications said to be decreased with laser sphincterotomy compared to electrocautery are severe bleeding and erectile dysfunction. In the absence of a prospective randomized trial, there is no conclusive

proof of the superiority of laser to electrocautery. The post-void residual often persists after incising the external sphincter, but many authors do not consider this finding an indication of treatment failure unless the patient continues to have recurrent UTIs due to urinary stasis.[98,109] Treatment failure despite a technically perfect sphincterotomy occurs in 10–50% of men treated for DESD. Reasons for failure include problems fitting the condom catheter as well as detrusor areflexia, which can result in poor bladder emptying despite an incompetent bladder outlet.[98,109,112]

Sphincteric stenting techniques

As with sphincterotomy, the patient is placed in the dorsal lithotomy position and is given perioperative antibiotic coverage. The Urolume device is packaged in a preloaded 24F cystoscopic insertion tool that accommodates a zero degree urethroscope. The Urolume comes in lengths of 2, 2.5, and 3 cm. The Ultraflex device comes in 2–5 cm lengths with 0.5 cm increments. The 3 cm length is usually adequate for two-thirds of patients being treated for DESD,[113] and, with the 5 cm Ultraflex prosthesis, only 10% of patients were found to need placement of a second stent.[114] If required, however, more than one device can be placed in order to span the entire external sphincter. Temporary suprapubic drainage is established intraoperatively to ensure good visibility and postoperative bladder drainage. Under direct vision, the insertion tool is introduced into the urethra and advanced to the level of the verumontanum, then released. The stent usually retracts 1–2 mm after deployment, and this should be accounted for when deciding on the position to release the device.[110,111] The stent should cover the caudal half of the verumontanum, leaving the ejaculatory ducts unblocked. The distal end should extend at least 5 mm into the bulbar urethra, well beyond the distal aspect of the external sphincter. If placement is incorrect, the Urolume can be moved or removed with endoscopic forceps. The Ultraflex can be pulled back using a suture located on its distal end which is removed after confirmation of proper placement.[114] When needed, a second stent should be placed overlapping the first by approximately 5 mm to completely bridge the sphincteric area.[115]

The Memokath stent is also inserted under direct vision mounted on a flexible or rigid cystoscope. Intraoperative fluoroscopy is used after filling the bladder with 200 ml of dilute contrast to monitor for distal movement that may occur with removal of the scope after stent deployment.[112] Once the stent is positioned correctly within the urethral lumen, saline warmed to 50°C is instilled into the device to cause expansion. Irrigation of the stent with cold saline (<10°C) renders it soft for easy removal with alligator forceps.[116]

Table 23.7 *Contemporary results of sphincterotomy in the treatment of detrusor-external sphincter dyssynergia*

Study	Year	Number and type of patients	Type of sphincterotomy	Mean follow-up (months)	Previous surgery	Results	Complications
Rivas et al[111]	1994	22 SCI males 14 quads 8 paras	Nd:YAG contact laser (round probe)	14 range 3–20	7% previous electrocautery sphincterotomy	18 successful Decreased voiding pressure and PVR ($p < 0.01$)	13.6% repeat sphincterotomy 1 skin ulceration, 1 urethrocutaneous fistula
Vapneck et al[109]	1994	16 SCI males 13 quads 3 paras	14 electrocautery 1 open 1 cold knife	39 range 3–96		50% success 8/16 still used condom drainage	5 repeat sphincterotomy, 1 spinal headache, 1 urosepsis/ADR Long term: 3 recurrent UTIs, 2 penile skin problems, 2 ADR, 1 combo of above
Perkash[110]	1996	76 SCI males 32% – bladder neck stenosis or BPH 32% bulbar strictures 54% quads 46% paras	Nd:YAG contact laser (chisel tip probe) Sphincterotomy ± bladder neck/prostatic incisions	27 range 16–41	56% previous electrocautery sphincterotomy	Decreased voiding pressure ($p < 0.0003$), decreased ADR	Overall 11.8% 7 repeat sphincterotomy 2 blood loss >100 ml
Fontaine et al[98]	1996	92 SCI males 47 quads 45 paras	Electrocautery	20.6		Objective improvement in 83.7% Subjectively improved in 73%, ADR resolution in 93.2%, decreased PVR ($p < 0.001$)	Overall 10.6% 8.1% repeat sphincterotomy 4 hematurias 1 transfusion 4 de-novo ADR 2 bacteremia

SCI, spinal cord injury; ADR, autonomic dysreflexia; PVR, post-void residual; quad, quadraplegic; para, paraplegic; BPH, benign prostatic hyperplasia.

Postoperative oral antibiotics are usually continued for 10–14 days.[94,111] A condom catheter is used to drain the bladder postoperatively. The patient can be discharged within 24 hours. A pelvic X-ray is recommended to confirm proper position of the prosthesis before discharge. The suprapubic tube can be removed a few days later once adequate bladder emptying via the condom catheter is documented. Urethral catheterization should be avoided for at least 3 months to avoid displacement of the stent before epithelialization occurs.

Stent removal can be accomplished under intravenous sedation or general anesthesia. The resectoscope on low cutting current is used to remove all epithelium overlying the stent. The prosthesis is then grasped with alligator forceps and pulled through the scope or pushed into the bladder and removed through the scope obturator.[103,113] The stent may unravel into individual wires and may need to be removed piece-by-piece. When the stent begins to separate, more than one procedure may be required in order to remove the prosthesis completely.[115] Fluoroscopy or a pelvic X-ray should be obtained to ensure complete stent removal.

Results and complications of sphincteric stenting

Several series examining the performance of urethral stents in the treatment of DESD have found statistically significant decreases in voiding pressure, post-void residual, and autonomic dysreflexia with no change in bladder capacity (see Table 23.8).[94,102,114] In a prospective nonrandomized trial comparing sphincterotomy to the Urolume stent, Rivas et al found no statistically significant differences in treatment outcomes between these two modalities.[101] The stent, however, was associated with a significantly shorter operative time, decreased length of hospital stay, and less blood loss when compared to sphincterotomy. Long-term complications that have been found to occur with the Urolume include epithelial hyperplasia, stent encrustation, stent migration, urethral obstruction, secondary bladder neck obstruction, and difficult stent removal.[94,100,103,106] The Memokath device is associated with a high rate of migration, recurrent UTIs, and calcification, making it more suitable for the short-term treatment of DESD.[102,112]

Urothelial hyperplasia first occurs during growth of urethral mucosa over the stent, and usually resolves by the time the stent is completely covered, a process which can take anywhere from 3 months to 1 year.[94] Incorporation of the device into the urethral wall lowers the likelihood of stone formation, infection, and migration.[100,114] Epithelial hyperplasia can lead to stent obstruction in 5% of cases, which can be remedied with endoscopic resection.[94] Calcific encrustation may occur at the ends of the

Urolume device, which are the last areas to become epithelialized.[102]

Stent migration is the most common reason for stent removal and can usually be diagnosed by cystoscopy or a pelvic X-ray. The most recent report of the North American Multicenter Urolume Trial found a 28.7% rate of stent migration, with approximately 40% of cases occurring within the first 3 months after insertion.[94] Reasons for stent migration include previous bladder neck or prostatic surgery, previous sphincterotomy, urethral catheterization before epithelialization took place, and dislodgement during stool disimpaction or patient transfers.[94,103] Wilson et al, in a recent review of stent failures, discovered urethral obstruction in one patient who had had tandem stents placed, secondary to one stent telescoping on the other more proximal stent.[103] The long-term rate of secondary bladder neck obstruction is 26.3% with the Urolume endoprosthesis,[94] and is thought to be a result of bladder neck dyssynergia masked by the presence of DESD.[106] If conservative management with alpha-blockade fails, then bladder neck incision or resection can be performed.

Despite several large series detailing the ease with which the Urolume can be removed even when completely epithelialized, many investigators have reported cases of stent explantation which were difficult and tedious.[102,103] Despite following the manufacturer's directions for prosthesis removal, the stent has been known to disintegrate and unravel, requiring piecemeal removal of each individual wire in a time-consuming process. Wilson et al described two cases of challenging stent removal, one of which required making a perineal incision, and the other resulting in avulsion of the urethral mucosa.[103]

Balloon dilatation of the external urethral sphincter

The concept of dilating the urethra with a balloon in order to treat high intravesical pressure was first described by Bloom et al, who employed this technique to lower the leak point pressures of 18 children with myelomeningocele.[117] Since then, Chancellor et al have compared the short-term results of balloon dilatation of the external sphincter to sphincterotomy and stent insertion in the treatment of spinal cord injured men with DESD. All three modalities were found to be equivalent in terms of decreasing voiding pressure, post-void residual, and autonomic dysreflexia at a mean follow-up time of 15 months. Complications occurring in 20 cases of balloon dilatation were blood transfusion (1), recurrent sphincteric obstruction (3), and bulbar urethral stricture (1).[104]

Table 23.8 *Results of urethral stents for the treatment of detrusor-external sphincter dyssynergia*

Study	Year	Number and type of patients	Type of stent	Mean follow-up (months)	Previous surgery	Results	Complications
Rivas et al[101]	1994	26 had stent, 20 sphincterotomy	Urolume vs sphincterotomy Patients selected treatment	Range 6–20		Shorter OR time, hospitalization time, lower blood loss, no difference in decrease in PVR, voiding pressure, or capacity	Stents – 15.4% migration, 2 BNO Sphincterotomy – 2 transfusions, 2 repeat ORs, 1 erectile dysfunction
Sauerwein et al[115]	1995	51 SCI males	Urolume (see above)	Range 12–36	All had sphincterotomy, 22 BNI, 18 TURBN	All had lowered ADR and voiding pressures, increased compliance	25.5% initial ADR, 9.8% migration, 5.9% explantation, 1 poor emptying
McFarlane et al[106]	1996	11 SCI males	Wallstent (American Medical Systems, UK) now Urolume	69.6 range 36–89		36.4% success – decreased PVR, maximum detrusor pressure	1 urosepsis at insertion, 5 BNO, 2 explantations, 1 recurrent UTI, 1 encrustation
Shaw et al[107]	1997	14 SCI males	Memokath (see above)	Maximum 24		50% success – decreased PVR, hydro, ADR	42.9% migration 1 mucosal hyperplasia, 1 recurrent UTI
Low and McRae[112]	1998	24 SCI males	Memokath (Engineers and Doctors A/S, Hornback, Denmark)	16 range 2–24	13 had 1 or more sphincterotomies 4 TURP, 4 other	29.1% success – decreased PVR, ADR, and UTIs	20.8% migration 25% recurrent UTIs, 12.5% de-novo ADR, 16.7% poor emptying, 4.1% encrustation
Chancellor et al[116]	1999	160 males 100 SCIs, 8 MS, 1 spinal vascular accident, 1 SC tumor	Urolume (American Medical Systems, Minnetonka, Minnesota)	60	46 had 1 or more sphincterotomies 11 TURP, 11 TURBN, 4 BNI	Significantly decreased voiding pressure, PVR, ADR, hydro, UTIs	15% explanted 28.7% migration 33% hematuria 26.3% BNO 2 urosepsis
Chartier-Kestler et al[114]	2000	40 males 30 SCI, 6 MS, 4 other	Ultraflex (Boston Scientific Corp., Boston, MA)	16.9	5 – 1 or more sphincterotomies 4 TUIP, 2 TURP, 3 VIU	Decreased PVR, decreased ADR in 63.1%	1 explantation for UTIs, 2 BNOs\ transient hematuria

SCI, spinal cord injury; PVR, post-void residual; ADR, autonomic dysreflexia; BNO, bladder neck obstruction; UTI, urinary tract infection; BPH, benign prostatic hyperplasia; TURP transurethral resection of the prostate; BNI, bladder neck incision; TURBN, transurethral resection of bladder neck contracture.

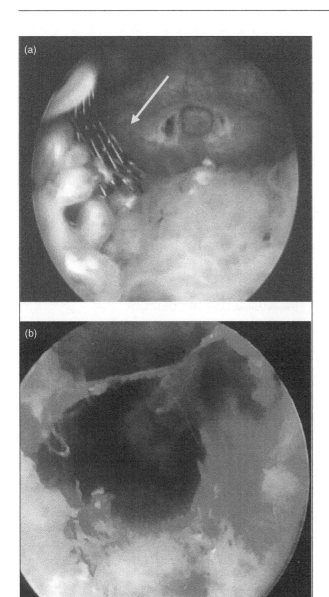

Figure 23.11
Urethral avulsion (a) stent exposed on right side (arrow); (b) after stent removal.

Conclusion

In summary, treatment of the male neurogenic bladder patient with refractory DESD continues to be challenging. Sphincterotomy and urethral stents will undoubtedly continue to be used in the management of these difficult cases. While there are now several different surgical options to choose from in addition to sphincterotomy, none of these treatment modalities has been shown to be superior to another with respect to efficacy, and each is fraught with its own unique liabilities and complications. Hopefully, future technical advances in the construction and composition of urethral stents will decrease their rate of migration and improve the ease of explantation. The results of balloon

dilatation are still too preliminary to speculate as to whether this technique will become a viable option for the treatment of DESD.

Conclusions

The surgeon endeavoring to treat a patient with urinary incontinence secondary to neuropathic bladder outlet incompetence has a number of surgical options at his disposal. Injectable agents are often employed in female patients with mild degrees of incontinence, patients who leak small amounts post-bladder neck sling or reconstruction, and patients who are not operative candidates or who are reluctant to undergo open surgery. The sling and AUS are commonly used when a more durable, long-term solution for incontinence is required. Because slings may be more successful in females than in males, some surgeons prefer to use slings as their first-line treatment in females and AUS as their primary treatment in males with neurogenic sphincteric incompetence. Reluctance to utilize the AUS in females stems from concerns of cuff erosion. The fascial sling may be preferable to the AUS in patients who do not wish to have a foreign body implanted or who, because of their comorbidities or surgical history, are at high risk for cuff erosion or infection of the device. Bladder neck reconstruction techniques are still performed at some specialized centers with experience in treating myelomeningocele and exstrophy-epispadias patients, but their popularity is waning secondary to high complication rates, especially in patients who have already undergone bladder neck surgery. Bladder neck closure is a suitable option for select patients who have failed multiple surgical attempts to increase outlet resistance or who have poor functional and constitutional status.

Sphincterotomy and urethral stents have both been shown to be effective at treating DESD. As some recent reports have illustrated, however, the currently available urethral stents many not be as easily removed or as complication-free as was once thought. Choice of treatment option is often guided by what the patient perceives as the irreversibility of sphincterotomy compared to urethral stenting.

References

1. Murless BC. The injection treatment of stress incontinence. J Obstet Gynaecol 1938; 45:67–73.

2. Lewis RI, Lockhart JL, Politano VA. Periurethral polytetrafluroethylene injections in incontinent female subjects. J Urol 1984; 131:459–462.

3. Malizia AA Jr, Reiman HM, Myers RP, et al. Migration and granulomatous reaction after periurethral injection of Polytef (Teflon). JAMA 1984; 251:3277–3281.

4. Bomalaski MD, Bloom DA, McGuire EJ, Panzi A. Glutaraldehyde cross-linked collagen in the treatment of urinary incontinence in children. J Urol 1996; 155:699–702.

5. Kryger JV, Gonzalez R, Barthold JS. Surgical management of urinary incontinence in children with neurogenic sphincteric incompetence. J Urol 2000; 163:256–263.

6. Cooperman L, Micheli D. The immunogenicity of injectable collagen II. A retrospective review of 72 tested and treated patients. J Am Acad Dermatol 1984; 10:647–651.

7. Leonard MP, Carring DA, Epstein JI. Local tissue reaction to the suburereral injection of glutaraldehyde cross-linked bovine collagen in humans. J Urol 1990; 143:1209.

8. Defreitas GA, Wilson TS, Zimmern PE, Forte TB. Three dimensional ultrasonography: an objective outcome tool to assess collagen distribution in women with stress urinary incontinence. Urology 2003; 62(2):232–236.

9. Bennett JK, Green BG, Foote JE, Gray M. Collagen injections for intrinsic sphincter deficiency in the neuropathic urethra. Paraplegia 1995; 33:697–700.

10. Wan J, McGuire EJ, Bloom DA, Ritchey ML. The treatment of urinary incontinence in children using glutaraldehyde cross-linked collagen. J Urol 1992; 148:127–130.

11. McGuire EJ, Fitzpatrick CC, Wan J, et al. Clinical assessment of urethral sphincteric function. J Urol 1993; 150:1452–1454.

12. Leonard MP, Decter A, Mix LW, et al. Treatment of urinary incontinence in children by endoscopically directed bladder neck injection of collagen. J Urol 1996; 156:637–641.

13. McGuire EJ, Apell RA. Transurethral collagen injection for urinary incontinence. Urology 1994; 43:413–415.

14. Chernoff A, Horowitz M, Combs A, et al. Periurethral collagen injection for the treatment of urinary incontinence in children. J Urol 1997; 157:2303–2305.

15. Kershen RT, Atala A. New advances in injectable therapies for the treatment of incontinence and vesicoureteral reflux. Urol Clin N Am 1999; 26:81–94.

16. Nataluk EA, Assimos DG, Kroov RL. Collagen injections for treatment of urinary incontinence secondary to intrinsic sphincter deficiency. J Endourol 1995; 9:403–406.

17. Ben-Chaim J, Jeffs RD, Peppas DS, Gearhart JP. Submucosal bladder neck injections of glutaraldehyde cross-linked bovine collagen for the treatment of urinary incontinence in patients with the exstrophy/epispadias complex. J Urol 1995; 154:862–864.

18. Kasouff W, Capolicchio G, Berardinucci G, Corcos J. Collagen injection for treatment of urinary incontinence in children. J Urol 2001; 165:1666–1668.

19. Perez LM, Smith EA, Parrot TS, et al. Submucosal bladder neck injection of bovine dermal collagen for stress urinary incontinence in the pediatric population. J Urol 1996; 156:633–636.

20. Capozza N, Caione P, De Gennaro M, et al. Endoscopic treatment of vesico-ureteric reflux and urinary incontinence: technical problems in the pediatric patient. Br J Urol 1995; 75:538–542.

21. Sundaram CP, Reinberg Y, Aliabadi HA. Failure to obtain durable results with collagen implantation in children with urinary incontinence. J Urol 1997; 157:2306–2307.

22. Kim YH, Kattan MW, Boone TB. Correlation of urodynamic results and urethral coaptation with success after transurethral collagen injection. Urology 1997; 50:941–948.

23. Bent AE, Tutrone RT, McLennan MT, et al. Treatment of intrinsic sphincter deficiency using autologous ear chondrocytes as a bulking agent. Neurourol Urodyn 2001; 20:157–165.

24. Yokoyama T, Yoshimura N, Dhir R, et al. Persistence and survival of autologous muscle derived cells versus bovine collagen as potential treatment of stress urinary incontinence. J Urol 2001; 165:271–276.

25. Elder JS. Periurethral and puboprostatic sling repair for incontinence in patients with myelodysplasia. J Urol 1990; 144:434–437.

26. Raz S, McGuire EJ, Ehrlich RM, et al. Fascial sling to correct male neurogenic sphincter incompetence: the McGuire/Raz approach. J Urol 1988; 139:528–531.

27. Kreder KJ, Webster G. Management of the bladder outlet in patients requiring enterocystoplasty. J Urol 1992; 147:38–41.

28. Fontaine E, Bendaya S, Desert JF, et al. Combined modified rectus fascial sling and augmentation ileocystoplasty for neurogenic incontinence in women. J Urol 1997; 157:109–112.

29. Decter RM. Use of the fascial sling for neurogenic incontinence: lessons learned. J Urol 1993; 150:683–686.

30. Walker RD, Flack CE, Hawkins-Lee B, et al. Rectus fascial wrap: early results of a modification of the rectus fascial sling. J Urol 1995; 154:771–774.

31. Gormley EA, Bloom DA, McGuire EJ, Ritchey ML. Pubovaginal slings for the management of urinary incontinence in female adolescents. J Urol 1994; 152:822–825.

32. Herschorn S, Radomski SB. Fascial slings and bladder neck tapering in the treatment of male neurogenic incontinence. J Urol 1992; 147:1073–1075.

33. Kurzrock EA, Lowe P, Hardy BE. Bladder wall pedicle wraparound sling for neurogenic urinary incontinence in children. J Urol 1996; 155:305–308.

34. Kakizaki H, Shibata T, Shinno Y, et al. Fascial sling for the management of urinary incontinence due to sphincter incompetence. J Urol 1995; 153:644–647.

35. Barthold JS, Rodriguez E, Freedman AL, et al. Results of the rectus fascial sling and wrap procedures for the treatment of neurogenic sphincteric incontinence. J Urol 1999; 161:272–274.

36. Mingin GC, Youngren K, Stock JA, Hanna MK. The rectus myofascial wrap in the management of urethral sphincter incompetence. BJU Int 2002; 90:550–553.

37. Austin PF, Westney L, Leng WW, et al. Advantages of rectus fascial slings for urinary incontinence in children with neuropathic bladders. J Urol 2001; 165:2369–2372.

38. Scott FB, Bradley WE, Timm GW. Treatment of urinary incontinence by an implantable prosthetic device. Urology 1973; 1:252–259.

39. Reinberg Y, Manivel JC, Gonzalez R. Silicone shedding from artificial urinary sphincter in children. J Urol 1993; 150:694–696.

40. Hajivassiliou CA. The development and evolution of artificial urethral sphincters. J Med Eng Technol 1998; 22:154–159.

41. Fulford SCV, Sutton C, Bales G, et al. The fate of the 'modern' artificial urinary sphincter with a follow-up of more than 10 years. Br J Urol 1997; 79:713–716.

42. Elliot DS, Barrett DM. Mayo Clinic long-term analysis of the functional durability of the AMS 800 artificial sphincter: a review of 323 cases. J Urol 1998; 159:1206–1208.

43. Woodside JR, McGuire EJ. Technique for detection of detrusor hypertonia in the presence of urethral sphincteric incompetence. J Urol 1982; 127:740–743.

44. De Badiola FIP, Castro-Diaz D, Hart-Austin C, Gonzalez R. Influence of preoperative bladder capacity and compliance on the outcome of artificial sphincter implantation in patients with neurogenic sphincter incompetence. J Urol 1992; 148: 1483–1495.

45. Kryger JV, Lerverson G, Gonzalez R. Long-term results of artificial urinary sphincters in children are independent of age at implantation. J Urol 2001; 165:2377–2379.

46. Aliabadi H, Gonzalez R. Success of the artificial sphincter after failed surgery for incontinence. J Urol 1990; 143:987–990.

47. Levesque PE, Bauer SB, Atala A, et al. Ten year experience with the artificial urinary sphincter in children. J Urol 1996; 156:625–628.

48. Salisz JA, Diokno AC. The management of injuries to the urethra, bladder or vagina encountered during the difficult placement of the artificial urinary sphincter in the female patient. J Urol 1992; 148:1528–1530.

49. Leach GE, Raz S. Perfusion sphincterometry. Method of intraoperative evaluation of artificial urethral sphincter function. Urology 1983; 21:312–314.

50. Simeoni J, Guys JM, Mollard P, et al. Artificial urinary sphincter implantation for neurogenic bladder: a multi-institutional study in 107 children. Br J Urol 1996; 78:287–293.

51. Singh G, Thomas DG. Artificial urinary sphincter in patients with neurogenic bladder dysfunction. Br J Urol 1996; 77:252–255.

52. Gonzalez R, Merino FG, Vaughn M. Long-term results of the artificial urinary sphincter in male patients with neurogenic bladder. J Urol 1995; 154:769–770.

53. Bellioli G, Campobasso P, Mercurella A. Neuropathic urinary incontinence in pediatric patients: management with artificial sphincter. J Ped Surg 1992; 27:1461–1464.

54. Spiess PE, Capolicchio JP, Kiruluta G, et al. Is an artificial sphincter the best choice for incontinent boys with spina bifida? Review of our long term experience with the AS-800 artificial sphincter. Can J Urol 2002; 9:1486–1491.

55. Castera R, Podesta ML, Ruarte A, et al. 10-year experience with artificial urinary sphincter in children and adolescents. J Urol 2001; 165:2373–2376.

56. Holmes NM, Kogan BA, Baskin LS. Placement of artificial urinary sphincter in children and simultaneous gastrocystoplasty. J Urol 2001; 165:2366–2368.

57. Light K, Lapin S, Vohra S. Combined use of bowel and the artificial urinary sphincter in reconstruction of the lower urinary tract: infectious complications. J Urol 1995; 153:331–333.

58. Miller EA, Mayo M, Kwan D, Mitchell M. Simultaneous augmentation cystoplasty and artificial urinary sphincter placement: infection rates and voiding mechanisms. J Urol 1998; 160:750–753.

59. Guralnick ML, Miller E, Toh KL, Webster GD. Transcorporal artificial urinary sphincter cuff placement in cases requiring revision for erosion and urethral atrophy. J Urol 2002; 167:2075–2079.

60. Leadbetter GW. Surgical correction of total urinary incontinence. J Urol 1964; 91:261–266.

61. Tanagho EA. Bladder neck reconstruction for total urinary incontinence: 10 years experience. J Urol 1981; 125:321–326.

62. Tanagho EA, Smith DA, Meyers FH, Fisher R. Mechanism of urinary continence II. Technique for surgical correction of incontinence. J Urol 1969; 101:305–313.

63. Mollard P, Mouriquand P, Joubert P. Urethral lengthening for neurogenic urinary incontinence (Kropp's procedure): results of 16 cases. J Urol 1990; 143:95–97.

64. Ferrer FA, Tadros YE, Gearhart J. Modified Young–Dees–Leadbetter bladder neck reconstruction: new concepts about old ideas. Urology 2001; 58:791–796.

65. Kropp BP, Rink RC, Adams MC, et al. Bladder outlet reconstruction: fate of the silicone sheath. J Urol 1993; 150:703–706.

66. Hollowell JG, Ransley PG. Surgical management of incontinence in bladder extrophy. Br J Urol 1991; 68:543–548.

67. Kropp KA, Angwafo FF. Urethral lengthening and reimplantation for neurogenic incontinence in children. J Urol 1986; 135:533–536.

68. Waters PR, Chehade NC, Kropp KA. Urethral lengthening and reimplantation: incidence and management of catheterization problems. J Urol 1997; 158:1053–1056.

69. Belman AB, Kaplan GW. Experience with the Kropp anti-incontinence procedure. J Urol 1989; 141:1160–1162.

70. Pippi Salle JL, Fraga JCS, Amarante A, et al. Urethral lengthening with anterior bladder wall flap for urinary incontinence: a new approach. J Urol 1994; 152:803–806.

71. Pippi Salle JL, McLorie GA, Bagli DJ, Khoury AE. Urethral lengthening with anterior bladder wall flap (Pippi Salle procedure): modifications and extended indications of the technique. J Urol 1997; 158:585–590.

72. Nill TG, Peller PA, Kropp KA. Management of urinary incontinence by bladder tube urethral lengthening and submucosal reimplantation. J Urol 1990; 144:559–563.

73. Snodgrass W. A simplified Kropp procedure for incontinence. J Urol 1997; 158:1049–1052.

74. Gearhart JP, Canning DA, Jeffs RD. Failed bladder neck preconstruction: options for management. J Urol 1991; 146:1082–1084.

75. Donnahoo KK, Rink RC, Cain MP, Casale AJ. The Young–Dees–Leadbetter bladder neck repair for neurogenic incontinence. J Urol 1999; 161:1946–1949.

76. Mouriquand PDE, Phillips SN, White J, et al. The Kropp-onlay procedure (Pippi Salle procedure): a simplification of the technique of urethral lengthening. Preliminary results in eight patients. Br J Urol 1995; 75:656–662.

77. Rink RC, Adams MC, Keating MA. The flip-flap technique to lengthen the urethra (Salle procedure) for treatment of neurogenic urinary incontinence. J Urol 1994; 152:799–802.

78. Lepor H, Jeffs RD. Primary bladder closure and bladder neck reconstruction in classical bladder extrophy. J Urol 1983; 130:1142–1145.

79. Leadbetter GW. Surgical reconstruction for complete urinary incontinence: a 10 to 22-year followup. J Urol 1985; 133: 205–206.

80. Sidi AM, Reinberg Y, Gonzalez R. Comparison of artificial sphincter implantation and bladder neck reconstruction in patients with neurogenic urinary incontinence. J Urol 1987; 138:1120–1122.

81. Rink RC, Mitchell M. Bladder neck reconstruction in the incontinent child: bladder neck/urethral reconstruction in the neuropathic bladder. Dial Ped Urol 1987; 10:5.

82. Hoebeke P, De Kuyper P, Goeminne H, et al. Bladder neck closure for treating pediatric incontinence. Eur Urol 2000; 38:453–456.

83. Zimmern PE, Hadley HR, Leach GE, Raz S. Transvaginal closure of the bladder neck and placement of a suprapubic catheter for destroyed urethra after long-term indwelling catheterization. J Urol 1985; 134:554–557.

84. Syme RRA. Bladder neck closure for neurogenic incontinence. Aust NZ J Surg 1981; 2:197–200.

85. Chancellor MB, Erhard MJ, Kilholma PJ, et al. Functional urethral closure with pubovaginal sling for destroyed female urethra after long-term urethral catheterization. Urology 1994; 43:499–505.

86. Das S, Amar AD. Abdominal transposition of the female urethra. J Urol 1986; 135:373–375.

87. Litweller SE, Zimmern PE. Closure of bladder neck in the male and female. In: Graham SD, Glen JF, eds. Glenn's Urologic surgery, 5th edn. Wolters Kluwer, 1998: 407–414.

88. Chancellor MB, Erhard JM, Kilholma PJ, et al. Functional urethral closure with pubovaginal sling for destroyed female urethra after long-term urethral catheterization. Urology 1994; 43:499–505.

89. Reid R, Schneider K, Fruchtman B. Closure of the bladder neck in patients undergoing continent vesicostomy for urinary incontinence. J Urol 1978; 120:40–42.

90. Zeidman EJ, Chiang H, Alarcon A, Raz S. Suprapubic cystotomy using the Lowsley retractor. Urology 1988; 32:54.

91. Hensle TW, Kirsch AJ, Kennedy WA, Reiley EA. Bladder neck closure in association with continent urinary diversion. J Urol 1995; 154:883–885.

92. Jayanathi VR, Churchill BM, McLorie GA, Khoury AE. Concomitant bladder neck closure and Mitrofanoff diversion for the management of intractable urinary incontinence. J Urol 1995; 154:886–888.

93. Abrams P, Cardozo L, Fall M, et al. The standardization of terminology of lower urinary tract function: report from the standardization sub-committee of the International Continence Society. Neurourol Urodyn 2002; 21:167–178.

94. Chancellor MB, Gajewski J, Ackman CF. Long-term followup of the North American Multicenter Urolume Trial for the treatment of external detrusor-sphincter dyssynergia. J Urol 1999; 161:1545–1550.

95. Kaplan SA, Chancellor MB, Blaivas JG. Bladder and sphincter behavior in patients with spinal cord lesions. J Urol 1991; 146:113.

96. McGuire EJ, Brady S. Detrusor-sphincter dyssynergia. J Urol 1979; 121:774.

97. Emmett J, Paut R, Dunn J. Role of the external urethral sphincter in the normal bladder and cord bladder. J Urol 1948; 59:439–454.

98. Fontaine E, Hajari M, Rhein F, et al. Reappraisal of endoscopic sphincterotomy for post-traumatic neurogenic bladder: a prospective study. J Urol 1996: 155:277–280.

99. Noll F, Sauerwein D, Stohrer M. Transurethral sphincterotomy in quadraplegic patients: long term follow up. Neurourol Urodyn 1995; 14:351–358.

100. Milroy EJG, Chapple CR, Cooper JE, et al. A new treatment for urethral strictures. Lancet 1988; 1(8600):1424–1427.

101. Rivas DA, Chancellor MB, Bagley D. Prospective comparison of external sphincter prosthesis placement and external sphincterotomy in men with spinal cord injury. J Endourol 1994; 8:89–93.

102. Shaw PJR, Milroy EJG, Timoney AG, et al. Permanent external striated sphincter stents in patients with spinal injuries. Br J Urol 1990; 66:297–302.

103. Wilson TS, Lemack GE, Dmochowski RR. Urolume stents: lessons learned. J Urol 2002; 167:2477–2480.

104. Chancellor MB, Rivas DA, Abdill CK, et al. Prospective comparison of external sphincter balloon dilatation and prosthesis placement with external sphincterotomy in spinal cord injured men. Arch Phys Med Rehab 1994; 75:297–305.

105. McInerney PD, Vanner TF, Harris SAB, Stephenson TP. Permanent urethral stents for detrusor sphincter dyssynergia. Br J Urol 1991; 67:291–294.

106. McFarlane JP, Foley SJ, Shah PJR. Long-term outcome of permanent urethral stents in the treatment of detrusor-sphincter dyssynergia. Br J Urol 1996; 78:729–732.

107. Shah NC, Foley SJ, Edhem I, Shah PJR. Use of Memokath temporary urethral stent in treatment of detrusor-sphincter dyssynergia. J Endourol 1997; 11:485–488.

108. Watanabe T, Rivas DA, Smith R, et al. The effect of urinary tract reconstruction on neurologically impaired women previously treated with an indwelling urethral catheter. J Urol 1996; 156:1926–1928.

109. Vapnek JM, Couillard DR, Stone AR. Is sphincterotomy the best management of the spinal cord injured bladder? J Urol 1994; 151:961–964.

110. Perkash I. Contact laser sphincterotomy: further experience and longer follow-up. Spinal Cord 1996; 34:227–233.

111. Rivas DA, Chancellor MB, Staas WE, Gomella LG. Contact neodymium:yttrium-aluminum-garnet laser ablation of the external sphincter in spinal cord injured men with detrusor sphincter dyssynergia. Urology 1995; 45:1028–1031.

112. Low AI, McRae PJ. Use of the Memokath for detrusor-sphincter dyssynergia after spinal cord injury – a cautionary tale. Spinal Cord 1998; 36:39–44.

113. Chancellor MB, Karusick S, Erhard MJ, et al. Placement of a wire mesh prosthesis in the external urinary sphincter of men with spinal cord injuries. Radiology 1993; 187:551–555.

114. Chartier-Kastler EJ, Bussel TB, Chancellor MB, Denys P. A urethral stent for the treatment of detrusor-striated sphincter dyssynergia. BJU Int 2000; 86:52–57.

115. Sauerwein D, Gross AJ, Kutzenberger J, Ringert RH. Wallstents in patients with detrusor-sphincter dyssynergia. J Urol 1995; 154:495–497.

116. Chancellor MB, Rivas DA, Linsenmeyer T, et al. Multicenter trial in North America of Urolume urinary sphincter prosthesis. J Urol 1994; 152:924–930.

117. Bloom DA, Knechtel JM, McGuire EJ. Urethral dilation improves bladder compliance in children with myelomeningocele and high leak point pressures. J Urol 1990; 144:430–433.

24

Urinary diversion

Greg G Bailly and Sender Herschorn

Introduction

The goals of urologic management of neurogenic bladder dysfunction are to achieve and maintain low-pressure urinary storage and voiding, with preservation of the upper urinary tract and achievement of urinary continence. Long-term management has been facilitated by the widespread acceptance of clean self-intermittent catheterization (CIC).[1] The introduction of new medications over the past few years has also contributed to management. The vast majority of patients with neurogenic bladder dysfunction can be managed without resorting to urinary diversion. However, there continues to be patients who are unwilling or unable to perform self-catheterization or to be intermittently catheterized. There are others who despite appropriate management are unable to maintain low-pressure urinary storage and voiding and/or continence. It is these patients who may benefit from lower urinary tract reconstruction and urinary diversion rather than resort to indwelling Foley catheters.

Patients with neurogenic bladder dysfunction are followed regularly with clinical evaluation, laboratory testing with serum creatinine and urine cultures, upper tract imaging (usually ultrasound), and urodynamic studies. The storage and voiding problems are usually addressed with a combination of CIC and various medications. Males with spinal cord injuries are frequently managed with condom drainage with or without CIC. However, outlet-relaxing procedures, such as transurethral sphincterotomy[2] or Urolume stent,[3] are occasionally needed in suprasacral cord injury patients with high detrusor pressures and sphincter dyssynergia. Neurogenic bladders in women may be harder to manage. Urethral CIC may be difficult for wheelchair-bound women and incontinence between CICs may also be more difficult to contain.

The aim of long-term follow-up of patients with neurogenic bladder disease is to prevent any changes that may lead to upper tract compromise. The complications of high intravesical pressures are well described and include upper tract dilatation, reflux, stones, pyelonephritis, and renal failure.[4,5] In addition, the patients may present with clinical symptoms. Changes in overall health can often be the first sign that the bladder may not be functioning satisfactorily. Worsening of incontinence, recurrent urinary tract infections, autonomic dysreflexia, suprapubic or back pain, as well as changes in the neurologic status of some patients, often indicate an alteration in lower urinary tract. These important clues can direct the urologist toward the appropriate investigations.

An outline of management of neurogenic bladder in relation to urinary diversion is shown in Figure 24.1. Urinary diversion, although frequently employed in the past for the treatment of neurogenic bladder dysfunction, is now only required in special circumstances. The commonly accepted indications include hydronephrosis that may be accompanied by progressive renal deterioration secondary to ureteral obstruction from a thick-walled bladder or intractable ureterovesical reflux, recurrent episodes of urosepsis, and persistent storage or emptying failure when CIC is impossible.[6] If, in the opinion of the urologist, the upper tract deterioration and/or storage problem cannot be managed with bladder augmentation surgery alone then urinary diversion may be indicated. Another reason for diversion is when urethral CIC is not feasible.

Unmanageable incontinence, while not life-threatening, may lead to skin breakdown, persistent infection, social isolation, and negative psychological impact on patients. When procedures such as bulking agents, slings, artificial sphincters, and augmentation cystoplasty are unsuccessful or contraindicated, and/or urethral CIC is not possible, urinary diversion may be considered. Often the diversion is as an alternative to an indwelling catheter. Although there have been no randomized prospective long-term trials, patients with indwelling catheters have more morbidity, such as infectious complications, calculi, and radiographic abnormalities, than those managed with CIC.[7,8] Although a long-term Foley catheter may be convenient, safe, and effective for some patients, urinary diversion may be a reasonable option. The various types of diversions will be discussed in this chapter.

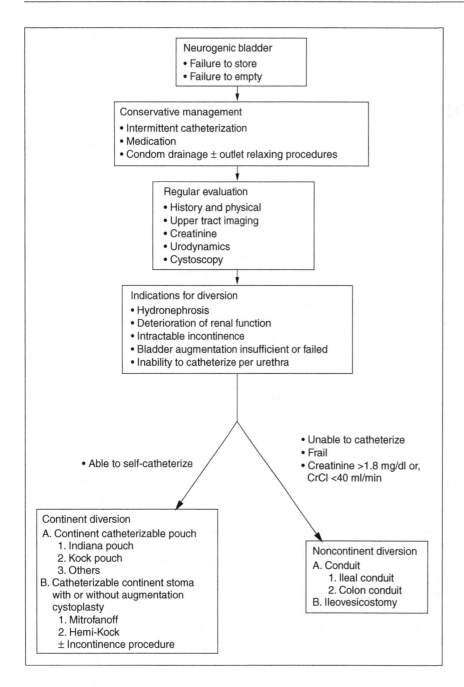

Figure 24.1
Surgical management of patients with neurogenic bladders requiring urinary diversion.

The choice of urinary diversion: patient considerations

The selection of a urinary diversion procedure is largely based on the surgeon's opinion and experience. Several important patient characteristics are considered when choosing an appropriate form of diversion (see Figure 24.1). The patient's ability to self-catheterize must be evaluated as it significantly impacts on whether to construct a noncontinent or continent form of urinary diversion. Patients who cannot perform self-catheterization of an abdominal stoma because of underlying neurologic disease or poor manual dexterity are not well suited for continent diversions. Other medical conditions may also exclude a patient from undergoing a continent diversion. Elderly, debilitated patients with other significant medical co-morbidities are generally not good candidates for continent diversion. In addition to poor outcomes, these patients have higher perioperative risks. Continent diversions often take longer to perform and have increased potential for complications compared with noncontinent diversion, and therefore proper patient selection is paramount to successful outcome.

Renal insufficiency is a relative contraindication to continent forms of diversion.[9,10] Continent diversion allows longer exposure time of urine to the intestinal mucosa, thereby increasing the risk of electrolyte disturbances, particularly in the patient with renal insufficiency. As a general rule, it has been recommended that patients with a preoperative creatinine of greater than 1.8 mg/dl (180 μmol/l) should undergo a noncontinent form of diversion.[10] A patient with borderline renal function should have a creatinine clearance calculated. A minimal creatinine clearance of 40 ml/min should be documented before the patient is deemed an appropriate candidate for a continent diversion.[11] Hepatic function should also be evaluated. Significant hepatic dysfunction increases the risk of developing hyperammonemia if the liver is unable to adequately process the ammonium chloride that may be produced by bacterial growth in retained urine of a pouch.[9]

Once the patient has been assessed it is important that the surgeon work with the patient and family/caregivers, without forcing the patient into one direction or another. The patient's willingness, ability, and motivation to comply with self-care and follow-up are other crucial considerations. Speaking to other patients with various forms of diversion often helps the patient better understand the surgery. The Internet may also provide valuable information on different forms of diversion. The surgeon should inform the patient of all potential risks and benefits of each type of diversion. The surgeon's experience, opinion, and review of the literature are important in protecting the patient from inappropriate or unrealistic expectations. Ultimately the decision is made on an individual basis by the patient and family with physician input.

General principles of surgery

Preoperative preparation

History and physical examination are required to ascertain any risk factors that may affect bowel segment selection. These include previous surgery, regional enteritis, ulcerative colitis, diverticulitis, intraperitoneal malignancy, and prior bowel resection. The patient should be seen preoperatively by the enterostomal therapist to have appropriate marking of the stoma site. The site is selected by patient anatomy and preference. A bag should stay on or the patient (or caregiver) should be able to catheterize comfortably. Usually the site is marked with the patient in the sitting position. The appropriate site will vary depending on the patient's body habitus, spinal column stability, and ability to see and access various abdominal locations. Rather than the traditional right lower quadrant site, other locations such as the left side, umbilicus, or supraumbilical regions may have to be considered. The site should be indicated with ink and then the skin etched with a needle after the patient is anesthetized at the time of surgery.

Bowel preparation

The patient usually receives mechanical bowel preparation prior to surgery, in an attempt to reduce the amount of feces in the colon. An antibiotic bowel preparation may be used to reduce the bacterial count. Bowel preparation has been shown to decrease the rates of wound infection, intraperitoneal abscesses, and anastomotic dehiscence rate.[12,13]

Although the true benefit of mechanical bowel preparation is poorly defined in the literature, most urologic, colon, and rectal surgeons in North America routinely prescribe mechanical bowel preparations.[14,15] The type of preparation varies from center to center, but usually includes Fleet Phospho-soda (sodium phosphate), polyethylene glycol electrolyte (PEG) solution (GoLYTELY or NuLYTELY, Braintree Laboratories, Braintree, Massachusetts), or magnesium citrate. PEG solution requires administration of approximately 4 liters of fluid but is safe in most cases since there is virtually no net absorption of ions or water in the gut.

Oral sodium phosphate, i.e. Fleet Phospho-soda (C.B. Fleet Co., Lynchburg, Virginia), has replaced PEG at many centers, because it appears to be better tolerated by patients.[15] This compound acts as an osmotic cathartic, causing large volumes of water to be translocated into the bowel, which results in diarrhea and bowel cleansing. Two 45 ml doses are usually ingested 4 hours apart on the night before surgery.[16] At least three 8-ounce glasses of water should be consumed after each dose, with as much clear liquid as possible until midnight. When compared with PEG, Phospho-soda has been shown to be better tolerated and equally effective, with similar wound infection rates.[17] Patients appear to prefer Phospho-soda to PEG.[18,19] It is, however, contraindicated in patients with renal insufficiency, symptomatic congestive heart failure, or liver failure with ascites.[14] Most clinical studies have also excluded patients with creatinines greater than 2 mg/dl.[17,18]

Antibiotic coverage

Preoperative antibiotic coverage for elective bowel surgery continues to be controversial. Urologists tend to use prophylactic antibiotics based on information extrapolated from the colorectal surgery literature. However, the literature is not clear on what to give and how to give it, and there are no clear consistent recommendations. In an extensive review of the use of antibiotic and mechanical preparations in urologic diversion surgery, Ferguson and colleagues recommended 1 g of oral-based neomycin and 1 g metronidazole at 5 and 11 p.m. on the night before surgery.[14]

The use of antibiotics administered intravenously within an hour prior to making the skin incision is less controversial.

The Centers for Disease Control and Prevention (CDC) recommends a second-generation cephalosporin, such as cefoxitin or cefotetan, over a first-generation cephalosporin, such as cefazolin, for surgery of the rectum or colon.[20] Additional doses may be required during the surgery based on the half-life of the antibiotic, or if blood loss exceeds 1 liter, and the duration of the surgery. The benefit of continued prophylactic antibiotics during the postoperative period is unproven. The CDC also recommended that prophylactic antibiotics not be continued more than 24 hours.[21]

Surgical principles

Intestinal anastomosis

Since urinary diversion is dependent on reconstructing various segments of bowel, it is important to understand certain basic principles of intestinal surgery. Much of the morbidity and mortality associated with urinary diversion in the immediate postoperative period relates to intestinal complications.[22] The fundamental principles of intestinal anastomoses include adequate mobilization, maintenance of blood supply, apposition of serosa to serosa of the two bowel segments, and creation of a watertight and tensionless anastomotic line. The various methods of performing the enteroenterostomy are well described.[23] Sutures or staples can be used with similar efficacy and complication rates.[23]

Ureterointestinal anastomoses

Many different types of ureterointestinal anastomoses have been used in urinary diversion surgery, but all should follow basic surgical principles. Only as much ureter as necessary should be mobilized to create a tensionless anastomosis. Periadventitial tissue should remain to ensure adequate blood supply. The anastomosis with the intestine should be performed with fine (4-0 or 5-0) delayed absorbable sutures, with the creation of a watertight mucosa-to-mucosa apposition. At our center, we frequently retroperitonealize the anastomoses for further protection.

The issue of antirefluxing ureteric anastomoses is controversial. While some experimental literature indicates a benefit, the results of clinical studies of colonic conduits with antirefluxing anastomoses are equivocal. Deterioration of the upper tracts for ileal and colon conduits has been reported in 10–60% of patients.[23] In one widely quoted historic series, 49% of the upper tracts showed changes after conduit diversion, 16% of which had a blood urea nitrogen increase of 10 mg/dl or more.[24] Deterioration of the upper tracts is usually a consequence of either infection or stones, or less commonly obstruction at the ureteral intestinal anastomosis.[23] In a prospective randomized comparison of ileal and colonic conduits into which one ureter was implanted with and the other without an antireflux technique, renal scarring was more prominent on the refluxing side.[25] However, split renal function tests showed no difference after 10 years.[26] These findings and those of others do not support the use of nonrefluxing ureterointestinal anstomoses for conduits. The final decision often rests with the surgeon's preference. At our center, we use refluxing anastomoses (Bricker or Wallace technique) for ileal conduits (Figures 24.2 and 24.3).

The ureterointestinal anastomoses of continent reservoirs may be refluxing or nonrefluxing.[27] Depending upon which continent reservoir is chosen, the nonrefluxing mechanism can be constructed from intussuscepted bowel, by tunneled implantation of the ureters, or by providing a long proximal loop or other techniques such as the split-nipple or LeDuc mucosal groove.[27]

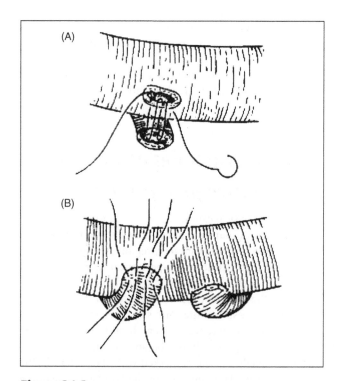

Figure 24.2
Bricker ureterointestinal anastomosis. (A) A full-thickness serosa and mucosal plug is removed from the bowel. Interrupted 5-0 delayed absorbable suture approximates the ureter to the full thickness of the bowel mucosa and serosa. (B) A supportive suture layer can be added from the adventitia of the ureter to the serosa of the bowel. (Reproduced with permission from McDougal.)[23]

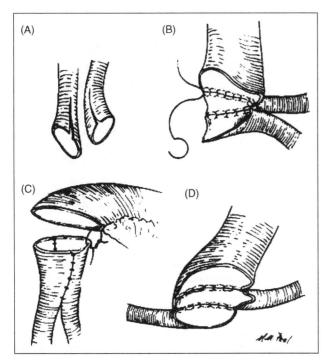

Figure 24.3
Wallace ureterointestinal anastomosis. (A) Both ureters are spatulated and are laid adjacent to each other. (B) The apex of one ureter is sutured to the apex of the other ureter. The medial walls of both ureters are then sutured together with interrupted or running 5-0 delayed absorbable suture. The lateral walls are then sutured to the bowel. (C) A 'Y-type' variant of above. (D) The 'head-to-tail' variant. (Reproduced with permission from McDougal.)[23]

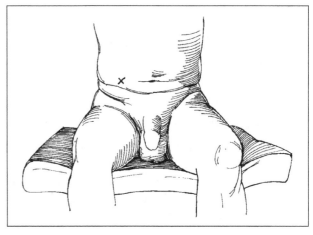

Figure 24.4
The stoma site is selected and marked on the surface of the abdomen where the skin is not rolled into folds while the patient is either sitting or standing. (Reproduced with permission from Hinman.)[27]

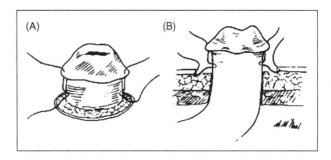

Figure 24.5
Rosebud stoma: 5–6 cm of intestine is brought through the abdominal wall. The open bowel is sutured to the skin with four quadrant sutures of 3-0 delayed absorbable sutures that pass through the skin edge, then catch the adventitia of the bowel well below the level of the skin, and finally go through the mucosal edge, thus everting the stoma. Additional sutures are placed through the skin and bowel edge between the quadrant sutures to close the gap. (Reproduced with permission from McDougal.)[23]

The stoma

The stoma is a very important aspect of the surgery. Much of the success of a stoma can be dependent on appropriate selection of the stomal site, as outlined above. A noncontinent stomal site should accommodate a collection device that does not leak, while maintaining patient comfort when wearing clothes. It should meet these requirements in the standing, sitting, and supine position (Figure 24.4). A commonly used stoma for an incontinent conduit is the nipple, or 'rosebud', described by Brooke in 1954[28] (Figure 24.5). It is usually created as the last step in the conduit construction.

The catheterizing stoma of the continent diversions is often placed in the lower quadrant of the abdomen through the rectus muscle and below the 'bikini line', or at the umbilicus. The umbilicus, or even higher, is the preferred location for someone in a wheelchair, because of easier access.

Diversions
Noncontinent urinary diversion

The first attempt at using isolated segment of bowel for urinary diversion was reported in 1908 by Verhoogen, who described a technique to divert urine into an isolated segment of ileum and ascending colon.[29] Construction of the ileal loop conduit was first reported by Seiffert in 1935.[30] Unfortunately, his procedure lacked effective means to collect and store urine. It was not until Bricker reported his technique that the ileal conduit became an acceptable method of urinary diversion.[31] Noncontinent diversions generally are ileal conduits, although various forms of conduits can be constructed from colon or jejunum. An alternative form of noncontinent diversion to the conduit is an ileovesicostomy.

Ileal conduit

Background. Since 1950, the Bricker ileal conduit has been the standard for noncontinent urinary diversion.[31] Still, today, the ileal conduit remains the most popular form of urinary diversion.[32] It is the most straightforward of the diversionary procedures to construct, with overall fewer potential complications than continent diversions.[32] It is the most appropriate urinary diversion in elderly, debilitated patients and in those who lack the hand–eye coordination or manual dexterity for self-catheterization, or the motivation to care for a continent pouch.

Technique. Little has changed since Bricker described his technique of the ileal conduit in 1950.[32] Blood supply is based on the superior mesenteric artery (SMA). The jejunal and ileal branches of the SMA anastomose to form arcades of vessels, which can be easily transilluminated through the mesentery during the operation for preservation of the blood supply to the conduit.

A lower vertical midline incision is made from the symphysis pubis to the umbilicus or beyond. The ureters are identified and transected approximately 3–4 cm above the bladder. The left ureter is brought under the sigmoid colon through the sigmoid mesentery to the right side, taking care to avoid damage to both the sigmoid and ureteral blood supply. The ileum is inspected to ensure healthy disease-free tissue. About 15–20 cm from the ileocecal valve, a 15–20 cm segment of ileum is selected, a length that will extend from the sacral promontory to the abdominal wall without tension. Two windows are constructed in the mesentery, with care taken to keep the base of the mesentery as wide as possible to prevent ischemia of the segment. The distal window usually measures 10–15 cm, and the proximal window can be much shorter at 3–5 cm. The bowel is transected, and the disconnected ileal segment is placed inferior to the remaining bowel segments. The bowel is reanastomosed using staplers or a standard two-layer closure. The mesenteric trap is closed. The ureteroileal anastomoses are performed either separately, as with the Bricker technique, or the ureters are joined together, as in the Wallace technique, at the proximal end of the loop.[33] The final step is the creation of the stoma (Figure 24.6).

Colon conduit

Background. A colon conduit may be chosen when there are functional or anatomical factors that preclude the use

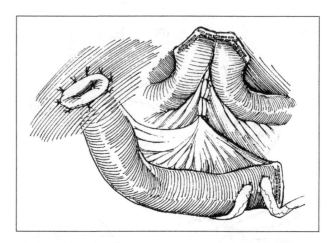

Figure 24.6
The ileal conduit at completion. (Reproduced with permission from Hinman.)[27]

of ileum. It has a larger diameter than ileum and can usually be easily mobilized into any portion of the abdomen or pelvis. The three types of colon conduits are transverse, sigmoid, and ileocecal, each having specific indications with advantages and disadvantages. The transverse colon is used in individuals who have received extensive pelvic irradiation. It is also an excellent segment when an intestinal pyelostomy needs to be performed. The sigmoid conduit is a good choice in patients undergoing a pelvic exenteration who will have a colostomy. An ileocecal conduit has an advantage of providing a long segment of ileum if a distal segment of ureter needs replacement. Because of the large lumen of the colon, stomal stenosis is rare. It is also used in situations in which reflux of urine from the conduit to the upper tracts is thought to be undesirable, as antireflux ureteral anastomoses are relatively easy to perform due to the thick wall. Contraindications to the use of transverse, sigmoid, and ileocecal conduits include the presence of inflammatory large bowel disease and severe chronic diarrhea.[23]

Ileal vesicostomy

The concept of ileal vesicostomy arose from the successful management of pediatric neurogenic bladders by creation of a vesicostomy. It is an alternative to an ileal conduit in some patients. It avoids the complications of ureterointestinal anastomosis, while maintaining the native ureteral antireflux mechanism. The small segment of ileum from the bladder to the abdominal acts to maintain low pressure in the bladder. The ileal segment is often referred to as a 'chimney', the distal end of which is brought up to the abdominal wall and a 'rosebud' stoma fashioned. It is important to use as short a segment of ileum as possible and to avoid a circular anastomosis between the ileum and the bladder. Redundancy of bowel may inhibit urinary flow and lead to electrolyte disturbances, which will be discussed below.[34] Theoretically, this results in a low-pressure reservoir that, if indicated at a later date, can be converted back to normal anatomy.

Technique. With the patient in the supine position, a lower midline incision is usually adequate. A 10–15 cm ileal segment is isolated, depending on what length is required to bridge the gap between the abdominal wall and bladder dome, leaving approximately 20 cm of terminal ileum and the ileocecal valve intact. The bowel anastomosis is performed as described previously. The bladder is mobilized from the pelvic wall by dividing its lateral attachments, and the bladder dome is generously opened transversely. The proximal ileal segment is spatulated approximately 4–6 cm along its antimesenteric border, and anastomosed to the open bladder with 2-0 absorbable sutures. The distal tubularized segment is brought out to the abdominal wall at a predetermined site and a stoma is created, as in the ileal conduit (Figure 24.7). A Foley catheter is left indwelling and exits through the stoma. An ileovesicostomy cystogram is performed 3 weeks postoperatively to ensure adequate healing of the suture line, and if there is no leak, the catheter is removed.[34]

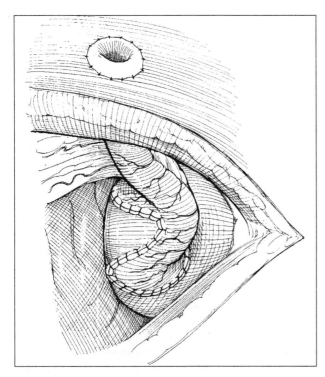

Figure 24.7
The ileovesicostomy. (Reproduced with permission from Hinman.)[27]

Continent urinary diversion

Background

Continent urinary diversion includes any reservoir subserved by a catheterizable efferent mechanism other than the native urethra and bladder neck.[35] Continent urinary diversion is often performed in patients with malignancy who require cystectomy and/or urinary diversion. It may also be used for appropriate patients with neurogenic bladder dysfunction who require diversion and wish to remain continent. In this setting, we generally try to preserve the bladder while adding capacity with an augmentation, thus maintaining the native ureteral antireflux mechanism. When this cannot be achieved due to significant bladder disease, a supravesical continent catheterizable pouch may be a better option. In the next section we will review the continent supravesical reservoirs and the continent bladder stoma.

The continent supravesical reservoir

Continence mechanisms

Although various forms of continent diversions were attempted in the past, it was not until 1982 when Kock et al reported the successful construction of an ileal reservoir that renewed interest in continent diversion was generated.[36] Its use in the neurogenic bladder population requires careful evaluation of physical and mental capabilities to ensure proper patient selection.

Continent catheterizable pouches are more complex to construct than conduits. Perhaps the single most demanding technical aspect of a catheterizable pouch is the creation of the continence mechanism. Four techniques are well described in the literature. The first involves using the appendix or a pseudoappendiceal tube fashioned from ileum or right colon and is sometimes performed for right colon pouches.[10]

The second type of continence mechanism used in right colon pouches is the tapered and/or imbricated terminal ileum and ileocecal valve. It involves imbrication or plication of the ileocecal valve region along with tapering of the more proximal ileum in the fashion of a neourethra.[37–40] This technique has been criticized by some because of the loss of the ileocecal valve and the potential consequence of more frequent bowel movements in some patients.

The third type of continence mechanism is an intussuscepted nipple valve, or more recently, the flap valve. The creation of the nipple valve may be technically demanding, and is associated with the highest complication and reoperation rate.[37] A significant learning curve is required, and thus this technique is not meant for the surgeon who performs the occasional continent pouch. Many modifications have been made to the original Kock pouch description, because of the long-term instability of the nipple valve in some patients. Despite the modifications, nipple valve failure can be observed in 10–15% of cases with the most experienced surgeons.[37] Failure may result from eversion and effacement of the intussusception and ischemic atrophy requiring a new nipple to be constructed. As well, stone formation on eroded or exposed staples can present a problem. Recently, a group from the University of Southern California has developed a new procedure, the T pouch, which uses a simpler and possibly more reliable procedure to create a flap valve, which results in both a continence and antireflux mechanism.[41]

The fourth procedure involves the construction of a hydraulic valve, as in the Benchekroun nipple.[42] This procedure has been largely abandoned because of nipple destabilization and stomal stenosis and will not be discussed.

Types of continent supravesical reservoirs

Indiana pouch

The Indiana pouch was first reported by Rowland and colleagues from the University of Indiana in 1985, and has since become one of the most popular forms of continent urinary diversion.[38] It uses the right colon as a reservoir while using reinforcement of the ileocecal valve for continence and tunneled tenial ureteral implantation for antireflux (Figure 24.8). The remaining ileal limb acts as the 'neourethra', which can be tapered and brought out through the abdominal wall as a stoma (Figure 24.9). Several variations of the Indiana pouch exist, including the Florida (Tampa) pouch[39] and the University of Miami pouch.[40]

Kock pouch (continent ileal reservoir)

Unlike the Indiana pouch, the Kock pouch involves the use of only small bowel to create a low-pressure reservoir.[36] Continence of urine and prevention of reflux to the upper tracts is achieved by constructing 'nipple valves' (Figure 24.10). It has been criticized for being technically difficult and associated with a high complication rate. As such, many urologists have abandoned it. However, the Kock limb (nipple valve) remains an important procedure for constructing a continent catheterizable stoma, such as with the hemi-Kock augmentation cystoplasty.

Other types of pouches that have been reported include the Mainz pouch, the UCLA pouch, the T pouch, and the Penn pouch.[37]

Continent bladder stoma

At our center, we aim to preserve the patient's native bladder if possible, thereby performing an augmentation cystoplasty and incorporating a continent bladder stoma.

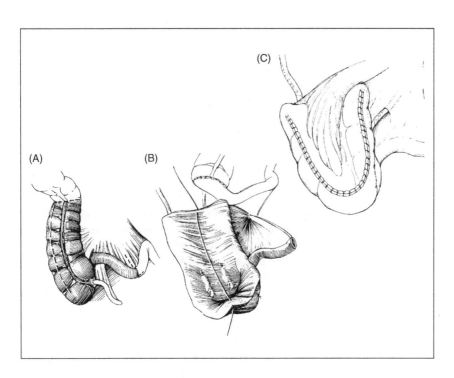

Figure 24.8
Indiana pouch. (A) A 25–30 cm segment of cecum, ascending colon, and hepatic flexure, in addition to an 8–10 cm of terminal ileum, is selected. The ascending colon is split down the antimesenteric border to within 2 cm of the caudal tip. (B) An ileocolostomy is performed using a suture technique or by a stapled method. The ureters are inserted by a submucosal technique. (C) A Malecot catheter is placed through the wall of the lowest part of the complex, in a position to allow direct exit through the abdominal wall. The U-shaped defect is closed by folding the distal portion of the colon into the proximal end and sutured into place with a running 3-0 absorbable suture. A serosal Lembert stitch with occasional lock stitches is added. The ileum is left to form the cutaneous conduit with tapering, as shown in Figure 24.9. (Reproduced with permission from Hinman.)[27]

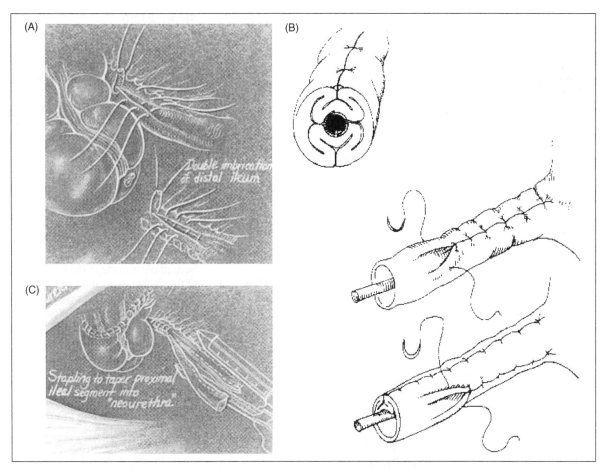

Figure 24.9
Tapering of ileal cutaneous conduit for Indiana pouch. Apposing Lembert sutures are applied on each side of the terminal ileum. Excess ileum can also be tapered by a stapling technique. (Reproduced with permission from Benson and Olsson.)[37]

Preserving the bladder and avoiding the ureterointestinal anstomoses should lead to fewer complications. Two popular methods of achieving a continent catheterizable bladder stoma are the Mitrofanoff procedure and the hemi-Kock (nipple valve) with or without formal augmentation cystoplasty. Urethral continence may be addressed simultaneously if necessary. Depending on the severity, it may involve a pubourethral sling, insertion of an artificial urinary sphincter, or closure of the bladder neck.[43]

The Mitrofanoff principle

In 1980, Mitrofanoff described a procedure in which the isolated appendix was anastomosed to the bladder at one end and the other end brought out to the skin.[44,45] The appendix is mobilized on its mesenteric pedicle and implanted on the bladder dome (Figures 24.11–24.13). The proximal lumen is tunneled under the bladder mucosa as an antireflux mechanism. As the reservoir fills, the rise in intravesical pressure is transmitted through the epithelium and to the implanted conduit, coapting its lumen. This mucosal tunneling technique is key to achieving continence.

The appendix has many advantages over methods for creating a continent catheterizable stoma.[46] The intraluminal pressure can rise nearly threefold that of the reservoir itself.[47] Perhaps the most important aspect of the flap-valve mechanism is the tunnel length to lumen ratio. Urodynamic evaluation has shown that a minimal tunnel length of 2 cm is required to achieve continence.[48] The Mitrofanoff principle can be used in native bladder, enterocystoplasty, or in a continent urinary reservoir. Because it is so reliable in preventing incontinence, it may place the patient at risk for upper tract deterioration or spontaneous rupture of the bladder or reservoir if regular catheterization is not performed. The appendix is particularly well suited for children because it is relatively longer and the abdominal wall is thinner. It also circumvents many of the secondary complications associated with using the ileocecal valve or other bowel segments.

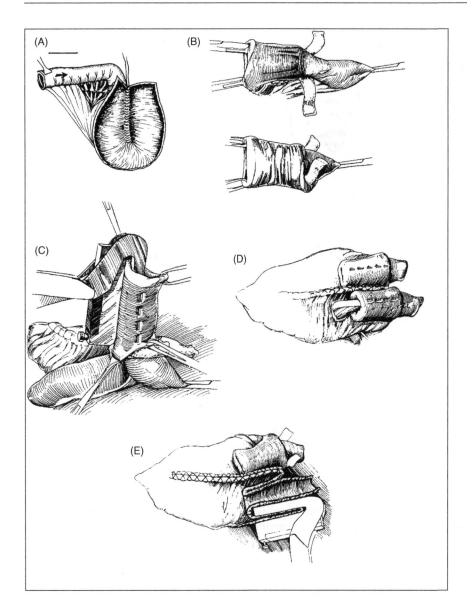

Figure 24.10
Construction of a nipple valve for the Kock pouch. (A) A 15 cm segment of terminal ileum is isolated and opened along its antimesenteric wall. The proximal 10 cm serves as the continent intussusception and the distal 5–10 cm as the patch. The size of the patch varies according to the size of the excised segment. (B) A Babcock clamp is advanced into the terminal ileum, the full thickness of the intussuscipiens is grasped, and it is prolapsed into the pouch. (C) Three rows of 4.8 mm staples are applied to the intussuscepted nipple valve using the TA55 stapler. (D) A small buttonhole is made in the back wall of the ileal plate to allow the anvil of the TA55 stapler to be passed through and advanced into the nipple valve. A fourth row of staples is applied. The figure shows two valve mechanisms. In this instance, there would be only one. (E) The anvil of the stapler can be directed between the two leaves of the intussuscipiens and the fourth row of staples applied in this manner. The figure shows two valve mechanisms. In this instance, there would be only one. (Reproduced with permission: (A) from Ghoneim MA, Kock NG, Lycke G, El-Din AB. An appliance-free, sphincter-controlled bladder substitute. J Urol 1987; 138:1150–1154; (B–E) from Hinman[27] and Benson and Ollson.)[37]

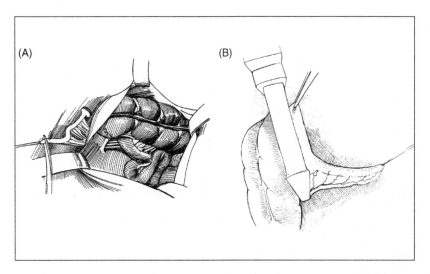

Figure 24.11
Mitrofanoff (appendicovesicostomy). (A) Stay sutures are placed at the base of the appendix, and the wall of the cecum is incised circumferentially to take a small cuff of cecum with the appendix. The appendiceal mesentery is separated a short distance from that of the cecum, preserving all of the appendiceal blood supply. The cecal defect is closed. The appendix is extraperitonealized behind the ileocecal junction. For umbilical placement of the stoma, it is not necessary to extraperitonealize the appendix. (B) For a short appendix or an obese patient, the appendix can be made longer by incorporating some of the cecal wall. (Reproduced with permission from Hinman.)[27]

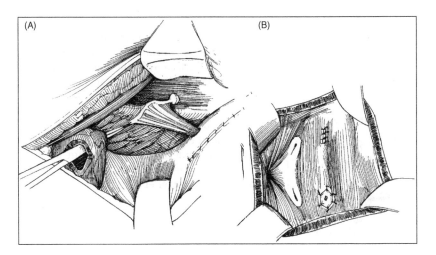

Figure 24.12
Through a cystotomy, a submucosal tunnel is made in the posterolateral wall of the bladder, beginning well above the right ureteral orifice. The appendix tip is implanted. A bladder augmentation is usually done next. (Reproduced with permission from Hinman.)[27]

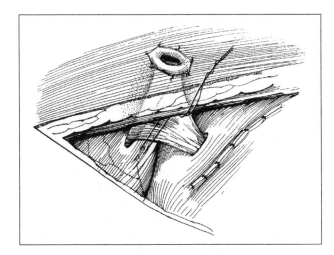

Figure 24.13
The appendiceal base is passed through an opening in the abdominal wall muscles large enough to accommodate a finger. The appendiceal opening is sutured to the skin (sometimes at the umbilicus). The bladder should be hitched to the anterior abdominal wall, and a catheter left in the appendix. (Reproduced with permission from Hinman.)[27]

Hemi-Kock augmentation enterocystoplasty

As an alternative to the Mitrofanoff procedure, patients may undergo a hemi-Kock ileocystoplasty with continent stoma permitting abdominal catheterization into the bladder. At our center, we have performed this procedure on various patients: wheelchair-dependent patients when urethral catheterization is difficult or impossible due to physical disability; patients who are unable to perform intermittent urethral catheterization; or patients who had a urethra that could not be rehabilitated due to trauma or surgery.[49] This procedure can be performed in conjunction with an incontinence procedure, including closure of the bladder neck in select cases.

Through a lower midline incision, the bladder is accessed and, in the case of an augmentation, the bladder is bivalved (clammed) in an anteroposterior direction in the midline from the bladder neck to 1 cm above the trigone. The ileal segment is measured from a point 25–30 cm proximal to the ileocecal valve. The next 15 cm proximal to this segment are for the nipple valve and the efferent limb. Up to another 45 cm is isolated on a mesenteric pedicle if an augmentation is performed. The intussuscepted nipple valve is constructed with three lines of TA55 staples, including one line that attaches the nipple to the segment. If no augmentation is performed, the bowel segment with the nipple is approximated to the bladder incision, and the third TA55 staple line fastens the nipple directly to the bladder wall. The catheterizing limb is brought out through the lower abdominal wall, usually on the right side, although other sites, including the umbilicus, can be used (Figure 24.14).

In a review of 47 patients who had construction of a hemi-Kock nipple valve as a catheterizable bladder stoma, Herschorn reported that 36 were dry or had mild leakage, and 44 (94%) patients considered their surgery to be successful compared with their preoperative management at a mean follow-up of 56 months.[50] Six patients required valve revision and/or stomal hernia surgery within the first 2 years. After the technique was modified by tapering the efferent limb, there was a significant decrease in revision rate. Kreder and colleagues have also reported success with using the hemi-Kock as a catheterizable bladder stoma.[51]

Complications of urinary diversion

The complications of urinary diversion can be categorized as either technical–surgical, metabolic, or neuromechanical.[23] Surgical complications are related to the reconstruction

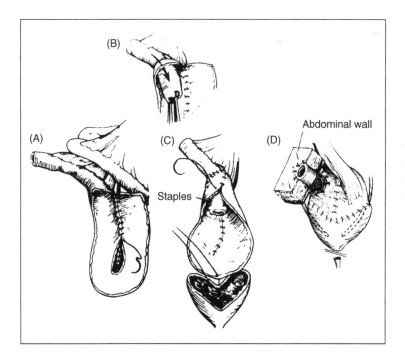

Figure 24.14
Hemi-Kock augmentation cystoplasty. (A) The distal segment of 15 cm for the efferent limb remains tubularized while the 45 cm for the augmentation has been detubularized. (B) Construction of the valve for continence. (C) Anastomosis of the augmentation to the 'clammed' bladder. (D) The efferent limb has been brought through the abdominal wall as a stoma. (A urethral continence procedure or urethral closure may be done for continence.) (Adapted from Kreder et al.)[51]

of the bowel and diversionary unit. Metabolic complications are the result of how the reabsorption of solutes is altered by the contact of urine with the bowel. The neuromechanical aspects involve the configuration of the reconstructed urinary reservoir and conduits and how this impacts on storage of urine.

Surgical complications

The complications associated with intestinal urinary diversion are displayed in Table 24.1. Postoperative surgical complications can also be classified as early or late. Nurmi and co-workers[71] reported on 144 patients with ileal conduits and found that the most common early postoperative complication was wound infection, followed by ureteroileal leakage, intestinal obstruction, intestinal fistulas, and acute pyelonephritis. Long-term complications were related to the delayed sequelae of intestinal surgery: stomal stenosis; ureteroileal stenosis; elongation of the loop; subsequent failure of the loop to propel urine adequately; and deterioration of the upper urinary tract.

The complications that can occur with ureterointestinal anastomosis include leakage, stenosis, reflux in antireflux anastomoses, and pyelonephritis. Urine leakage usually presents within the first 7–10 days postoperatively with an incidence of 3–9%.[72,73] The use of soft ureteral stents has reduced the incidence. Fortunately, most leaks resolve with time and proper drainage, but they have been associated with periureteral fibrosis and scarring, leading to stricture formation.[23] The incidence of ureteric stenosis is approximately 1–14%.[23] Stricture formation can be asymptomatic

and occur at any time in the life of the patient; hence the importance of yearly or biennial upper tract imaging. Strictures can be anywhere along the ureter, as well as at the anastomosis. A common location is where the left ureter crosses over the aorta beneath the inferior mesenteric artery. When a stricture is detected it is usually treated first by endourologic or percutaneous means using balloon dilatation or incision. Although these methods offer less morbidity to the patient, the long-term success rate is lower than open repair (90% vs 50%).[74,75]

Stomal complications are the single most common problem encountered in the postoperative period after diversion.[23] Early problems include bowel necrosis, bleeding, dermatitis, parastomal hernia, prolapse, obstruction, stomal retraction, and stomal stenosis. The incidence of stomal stenosis has been reported in 20–24% of patients with ileal conduits and 10–20% of those with colon conduits.[23] Stomal problems can frequently be improved or prevented with proper stomal care and better-fitting appliances.

Metabolic complications

Electrolyte abnormalities

Electrolyte abnormalities may result from absorption and excretion of water and solutes from the bowel surface. They are dependent on the segment of bowel used, the surface area of the bowel, the amount of time the urine is exposed to the bowel, the concentration of the solutes in the urine, renal function, and pH. Jejunal conduits are rarely performed because of their potential

Table 24.1 *Complications of urinary intestinal diversion*

Complications	Type of diversion	Patients (complications/no.)	Incidence (%)
Bowel obstruction	Ileal conduit	124/1289	10
	Colon conduit	9/230	5
	Gastric conduit	2/21	10
	Continent diversion	2/250	4
Ureteral intestinal obstruction	Ileal conduit	90/1142	8
	Antireflux colon conduit	25/122	20
	Colon conduit	8/92	9
	Continent diversion	16/461	4
Urine leak	Ileal conduit	23/886	3
	Colon conduit	6/130	5
	Continent diversion	104/629	17
	Ileum colon	5/123	4
Stomal stenosis or hernia	Ileal conduit	196/806	24
	Colon conduit	45/227	20
	Continent diversion	28/310	9
Renal calculi	Ileal conduit	70/964	7
	Antireflux colon conduit	5/94	5
Pouch calculi	Continent diversion	42/317	13
Acidosis requiring treatment	Ileal conduit	46/296	16
	Antireflux colon conduit	5/94	5
	Gastric conduit	0/21	0
	Continent diversion		
	Ileum	21/263	8
	Colon or colon-ileum	17/63	27
Pyelonephritis	Ileal conduit	132/1142	12
	Antireflux colon conduit	13/96	13
	Continent diversion	15/296	5
Renal deterioration	Ileal conduit	146/808	18
	Antireflux colon conduit	15/103	15

Source: from McDougal.[23]
[a] Composite from the literature. Follow-up averages 5 years for ileal conduits, 3 years for colon conduits, 2 years for gastric conduits, and 2 years for continent diversions.
[b] Data from references 52–70

metabolic complications. They can cause hyponatremia, hypochloremia, hyperkalemia, and metabolic acidosis, leading to lethargy, nausea, vomiting, dehydration, weakness, and hyperthermia. This syndrome is more profound if the proximal jejunum is used. Ileum and colon diversions may result in similar abnormalities: hyperchloremic metabolic acidosis. Abnormalities may be worse with continent diversions than conduits because of the exposure time of the bowel to urine. However, normal kidneys can usually correct the abnormalities. Clinical symptoms can include easy fatigability, anorexia, weight loss, polydipsia, and lethargy. Regardless of the type of diversion, patients require regular screening of their electrolytes.[23]

Magnesium deficiency, drug intoxication, or abnormalities in ammonia metabolism

These factors are uncommon, but may lead to alteration of the sensorium. Each should be identified and treated accordingly. Drugs more likely to be a problem are those that are absorbed by the gastrointestinal tract and excreted unchanged by the kidneys, e.g. phenytoin.[76] Methotrexate toxicity has been documented in a patient with an ileal conduit.[77] The problems with chemotherapeutic agents, in particular the antimetabolites, are relatively rare, but caution should be given to patients with continent diversions receiving chemotherapy. In this case, it is recommended that a pouch be drained during the time the toxic drugs are being administered.

Osteomalacia

Osteomalacia is loss of mineralized bone while the osteoid component increases. It may occur in patients with urinary diversion secondary to a combination of persistent acidosis, vitamin D resistance, and excessive calcium loss by the kidney.[23] The degree to which each of these factors contributes to the syndrome varies from patient to patient. With this syndrome comes lethargy, joint pain, especially on the weightbearing joints, and proximal myopathy. Serum calcium may be low or normal, and the alkaline phosphatase is usually elevated. Treatment involves correcting the acidosis and providing dietary supplements of calcium and rarely vitamin D. It is especially important to prevent acidosis in patients who are at risk of developing osteoporosis with aging to spare them the possibility of severe bone disease.

Bacteriuria and clinical infection

Bacteriuria and clinical infection are reported in most series of patients with bowel incorporated into the urinary tract, and the theoretical basis is well described.[78] Urine in the bowel may have a higher pH than normal and is less bacteriostatic. Distended bowel may become ischemic, and the disrupted mucosal barrier may allow translocation of bacteria into the systemic circulation. Intestinal mucus may also act as a template for formation of bacterial biofilms and perpetuate the bacteriuria.[79]

Bacteriuria, bacteremia, and sepsis occur with greater frequency when patients have intestinal diversions, especially in those with conduits. About three-quarters of those with conduits have bacteriuria at any time, yet many of them are asymptomatic and do not require treatment for their colonization. The main indication to treat asymptomatic bacteriuria is the presence of cultures dominant for *Proteus* or *Pseudomonas* spp. It has been suggested that these organisms may contribute to upper tract damage.[23]

The majority of patients with catheterized pouches will have chronic bacteriuria. Most urologists do not suggest treating asymptomatic bacteriuria.[80] Patients are usually well protected from pyelonephritis from their nonrefluxing ureterointestinal anastomosis. With a symptomatic pouch infection or pyelonephritis, antibiotic treatment should be administered. True pouch infections may require long courses of antibiotics, and, if frequently recurrent, we occasionally employ regular pouch instillation with antibiotics. A condition known as 'pouchitis' is manifested by pain in the region of the pouch along with increased pouch contractility.[23] The patient may experience sudden explosive

discharge of urine from the continent stoma in this setting. This type of scenario usually responds to longer courses of antibiotics.

Because of the devastating consequences with infection and possibly perforation, these patients and caregivers must be well informed regarding urinary retention. It may occur from simply not catheterizing the stoma or occasionally when the stoma, particularly with the nipple valve, obstructs or does not allow entrance of a catheter. This is considered a true emergency and the patient is instructed to seek attention from experienced medical personnel. It is recommended that various sizes and types of catheters are used, including the coude tip catheter. Sometimes, flexible cystoscopy is necessary. When significant manipulation of the stoma/pouch is required, we recommend leaving a catheter in for a short period due to edema.

Other metabolic complications

There is substantial evidence that urinary intestinal diversion has a negative impact on bone growth and development.[81] These effects are most prominent in children who have diversions performed prior to puberty.

Most *stones* formed in intestinal urinary diversions are composed of calcium, magnesium, and ammonium phosphate. Patients with hyperchloremic metabolic acidosis, pre-existing pyelonephritis, and urinary tract infection with urea-splitting organisms are at the greatest risk of developing stones.[82] A major cause of calculus formation in conduits and pouches is the presence of a foreign body, such as staples or nonabsorbable sutures.

The exact risk of developing *cancer* in a segment of bowel that has been incorporated into the urinary tract is unknown. After bladder augmentation for benign disease, there have been at least 14 cases of malignancy reported in the literature.[83,84] In a series of 2000 patients with a maximum follow-up of 22 years, only 1 case of malignancy was reported.[85]

Neuromechanical complications

Perforation of a cutaneous continent diversion or augmentation cystoplasty with catheterizable stoma occurs infrequently. In the former, the incidence of perforation/rupture is in the range of 1–2%.[86] In a survey of 1700 patients in Scandinavia, 20 episodes of perforation occurred in 18 patients.[87] Rupture may occur from reservoir catheterization, endoscopic examination, a fall, or spontaneously. The signs and symptoms may be vague, especially in patients with neurological disease, who may not sense fullness. This possible complication should be kept in mind when these patients present with pain, and consideration should be given to performing enterocystography or a CT scan. Since the perforation may cause peritonitis, prompt recognition and possible surgical exploration may be necessary.

Quality of life

In addition to maintaining low-pressure urinary storage and protecting the upper tracts, urinary diversion in the patient with a neurogenic bladder aims to improve the patient's quality of life (QoL). Often this translates into providing a reliable state of urinary continence, which positively impacts on the patients' lives. QoL issues in neurogenic bladder patients who have undergone urinary diversion are infrequently described in the literature. Much of what we know is extrapolated from cancer patients, who, in many ways, are a different patient population. Whether one procedure is better than another is very much based on what factors were considered when choosing which type of diversion. Newer or more complicated methods do not always result in a better QoL.[88] Herschorn and Hewitt,[89] in their series of 59 augmentation cystoplasties in neurogenic bladder patients, 35 of whom had a continent bladder stoma, reported the results of a patient questionnaire. Forty-one patients were 'delighted', 12 were 'pleased', and 6 were 'mostly satisfied' with their urinary tract management. This was despite one-third having some degree of incontinence. Most of the patients had been managed with indwelling catheters preoperatively.

Another important issue regarding continent vs noncontinent forms of diversion is the effect on the body image and sexuality of the patient. In a series of 18 neurologically impaired women treated with indwelling catheters, Watanabe and co-workers[90] reported the effect of urinary tract reconstruction on self-esteem and sexual function. On a scale of 0 (worst) to 5 (best), mean scores for self-esteem improved from 1 preoperatively to 4 postoperatively, self-image from 1 to 4, sexual desire from 2 to 4, and ability to cope with disability from 1 to 4, respectively. In 4 of the 15 women who were sexually active preoperatively, the frequency of sexual intercourse doubled from a mean of 3 to 6 times per month, respectively, and all 4 women reported improved sexual satisfaction. All 13 patients with pelvic pain and 5 with symptoms of autonomic dysreflexia noticed significant improvement if not complete resolution of the symptoms.

These reports confirm the positive effect that improvement in urinary tract management has on patients' QoL. It also underscores the need for evaluating patients' QoL in response to treatment and for further studies.

Conclusion

Considerable progress has been made in the surgical management of neurogenic bladder disease. Prior to 1950 the only diversion available was ureterosigmoidostomy, but infections, electrolyte problems, and long-term development of carcinomas discouraged its use. The ileal conduit then became the standard for urinary diversion and has essentially remained so, especially for patients with bladder cancer who need cystectomies. The procedure is standardized and the long-term risks and benefits are well known.

In the last 15 years continent diversions have become established as a reasonable alternative to an ileal conduit. In addition, procedures, such as continent bladder stomas, which address continence and catheterization difficulties with an intact bladder, have emerged as another option. The risks, benefits, and long-term outcomes are becoming more widely known. The availability of these procedures has improved the management and QoL for patients in whom conservative therapy has failed.

References

1. Barkin M, Dolfin D, Herschorn S. The urologic care of the spinal cord injured patient. J Urol 1983; 129:335–339.

2. Madersbacher H, Scott FB. Twelve o'clock sphincterotomy. Urol Int 1975; 30:75–81.

3. Chancellor M, Gajewski J, Ackman CFD, et al. Long-term follow-up of the North American Multicenter Urolume Trial for the treatment of external detrusor-sphincter dyssynergia. J Urol 1999; 161:1545–1550.

4. Rivas D, Karasick S, Chancellor M. Cutaneous ileocystostomy (a bladder chimney) for the treatment of severe neurogenic vesical dysfunction. Paraplegia 1995; 33:530–535.

5. Madersbacher H, et al. Conservative management in the neuropathic patient (Committee 19). In: Abrams P, Khoury S, Wein A, eds. Incontinence. London: Health Publication Ltd, 1999:755–812.

6. Wein AJ. Neuromuscular dysfunction of the lower urinary tract and its management. In: Walsh PC, Wein AJ, Vaughan ED Jr, Retik AB, eds. Campbell's urology, 8th edn. Philadelphia: WB Saunders, 2002:931–1026.

7. Weld KJ, Dmochowski RR. Association of level of injury and bladder behavior in patients with post traumatic spinal cord injury. Urology 2000; 55:490–494.

8. Jamil F, Williamson M, Ahmed YS, et al. Natural fill urodynamics in chronically catheterized patients with spinal cord injury. BJU Int 1999; 83:396–399.

9. Mills RD, Studer UE. Metabolic consequences of continent urinary diversion. J Urol 1999; 161:1057–1066.

10. Benson MC, Olsson CA. Continent urinary diversion. Urol Clin N Am 1999; 26(1):125–147, ix.

11. Kristjansson A, Davidsson T, Mansson W. Metabolic alterations at different levels of renal function following continent urinary diversion through colonic segments. J Urol 1997; 157:2099–2103.

12. Irvin TT, Goligher JC. Aetiology of disruption of intestinal anastomosis. Br J Surg 1973; 60:461.

13. Dion YM, Richards GK, Prentis JJ, Hinchey EJ. The influence of oral versus parenteral preoperative metronidazole on sepsis following colon surgery. Ann Surg 1980; 192:221–226.

14. Ferguson KH, McNeil JJ, Morey AF. Mechanical and antibiotic bowel preparation for urinary diversion surgery. J Urol 2002; 167:2352–2356.

15. Nichols RL, Smith JW, Garcia RY, et al. Current practices of preoperative bowel preparation among North American colorectal surgeons. Clin Infect Dis 1997; 24:609–611.

16. Henderson JM, Barnett JL, Turgeon DK, et al. Single-day, divided-dose oral sodium phosphate laxative versus intestinal lavage as preparation for colonoscopy: efficacy and patient tolerance. Gastrointest Endosc 1995; 42:238–240.

17. Oliveira L, Wexner SD, Daniel N, et al. Mechanical bowel preparation for elective colorectal surgery. A prospective, randomized, surgeon blinded trial comparing sodium phosphate and polyethylene glycol-based oral lavage solutions. Dis Col Rectum 1997; 40:585–587.

18. Thomson A, Naidoo P, Crotty B. Bowel preparation for colonoscopy: a randomized prospective trial comparing sodium phosphate and polyethylene glycol in a predominantly elderly population. J Gastroenterol Hepatol 1996; 11:103–106.

19. Heymann TD, Chopra K, Nunn E, et al. Bowel preparation at home: prospective study of adverse effects in elderly people. BMJ 1996; 313:727–730.

20. Mangram AJ, Horan TC, Pearson ML, et al. Guideline for prevention of surgical site infection, 1999. Centers for Disease Control and Prevention (CDC) Hospital Infection Control Practices Advisory Committee. Am J Infect Control 1999; 27:97–103.

21. Rowe-Jones DC, Peel AL, Kingston RD, et al. Single dose cefotaxime plus metronidazole versus three dose cefuroxime plus metronidazole as prophylaxis against wound infection in colorectal surgery: multicentre prospective randomised study. BMJ 1990; 300:18–22.

22. Mansson W, Colleen S, Stigsson L. Four methods of uretero-intestinal anastomoses in urinary conduit diversion. Scand J Urol Nephrol 1979; 13:191–199.

23. McDougal WS. Use of intestinal segments and urinary diversion. In: Walsh PC, Retik AB, Vaughan ED, et al, eds. Campbell's urology, 8th edn. Philadelphia: WB Saunders, 2002:3745–3788.

24. Schwarz GR, Jeffs RD. Ileal conduit urinary diversion in children: computer analysis of follow-up from 2 to 16 years. J Urol 1975; 114:285–288.

25. Kristjansson A, Wallin L, Månsson W. Renal function up to 16 years after conduit (refluxing or anti-reflux anastomosis) or continent urinary diversion. I. Glomerular filtration rate and patency of uretero-intestinal anastomosis. Br J Urol 1995; 76:539–545.

26. Kristjansson A, Bajc M, Wallin L, et al. Renal function up to 16 years after conduit (refluxing or anti-reflux anastomosis) or continent urinary diversion. II. Renal scarring and location of bacteriuria. Br J Urol 1995; 76:546–550.

27. Hinman F. Atlas of urologic surgery, 2nd edn. Philidelphia: WB Saunders, 1998:682.

28. Brooke BN. Ulcerative colitis and its surgical management, 1st edn. Edinburgh: Churchill Livingstone, 1954:92.

29. Verhoogen J. Neostomie uretero-caecale: formation d'une nouvelle poche vesicale et d'ub nouvel eretre. Assoc Franc Urol 1908; 12:362.

30. Seiffert L. Die Darm-"Siphonblase." Arch Klin Chir 1935; 183:569.

31. Bricker EM. Bladder substitution after pelvic evisceration. Surg Clin N Am 1950; 30:1511.

32. Williams O, Vereb MJ, Libertino JA. Non-continent urinary diversion. Urol Clin N Am 1997; 24(4):735–744.

33. Wallace DM. Uretero-ilestomy. Br J Urol 1970; 42:529–534.

34. Atan A, Konety BR, Nangia A, Chancellor MB. Advantages and risks of ileovesicostomy for the management of neuropathic bladder. Urology 1999; 54:636–640.

35. Kaefer M, Retik AB. The Mitrofanoff principle in continent urinary reconstruction. Urol Clin N Am 1997; 24(4):795–811.

36. Kock NG, Nilson AE, Nilsson LO, et al. Urinary diversion via a continent ileal reservoir: clinical results in 12 patients. J Urol 1982; 128:469.

37. Benson MC, Olsson CA. Cutaneous continent urinary diversion. In: Walsh PC, Retik AB, Vaughan ED, et al, eds. Campbell's urology, 8th edn. Philadelphia: WB Saunders, 2002:3789–3834.

38. Rowland RG, Mitchell ME, Bihrle R. The cecoileal continent urinary reservoir. World J Urol 1985; 3:185–190.

39. Lockhart JL. Remodeled right colon: an alternative urinary reservoir. J Urol 1987; 138:730–734.

40. Bejany DE, Politano VA. Stapled and nonstapled tapered distal ileum for construction of a continent colonic urinary reservoir. J Urol 1988; 140:491–494.

41. Stein JP, Lieskovsky G, Ginsberg DA, et al. The T pouch: an orthotopic ileal neobladder incorporating a serosal lined ileal antireflux technique. J Urol 1998; 159:1836–1842.

42. Benchekroun A. Hydraulic valve for continence and antireflux: a 17 year experience of 210 cases. Scand J Urol Nephrol Suppl 1992; 142:70–72.

43. Leng WW, McGuire EJ. Reconstructive surgery for urinary incontinence. Urol Clin N Am 1999; 26(1):61–80, viii.

44. Mitrofanoff P. Cystostomie continente trans-appendiculaire dans le traitement des vessies neurologiques. Chir Pediatr 1980; 21:297–305.

45. Keating MA, Rink RC, Adams MC. Appendicovesicostomy: a useful adjunct to continent reconstruction of the bladder. J Urol 1993; 149:1091.

46. Hinman F Jr. Functional classification of conduits for continent diversion. J Urol 1990; 144:27.

47. Malone RR, D'Cruz VT, Worth PHL, Woodhouse RJ. Why are continent diversions continent? J Urol 1989; 141:303A.

48. Watson HS, Baur SB, Peters CA, et al. Comparative urodynamics of appendiceal and ureteral Mitrofanoff conduits in children. J Urol 1995; 154:878.

49. Herschorn S, Thijssen AJ, Radomski SB. Experience with the hemi-Kock ileocystoplasty with a continent catheterizable stoma. J Urol 1993; 149:998–1001.

50. Herschorn S. Durability of the hemi-Kock continent bladder stoma. J Urol 2001; 165(5):suppl 88. [Abstract]

51. Kreder K, Anurag KD, Webster GD. The hemi-Kock ileocystoplasty: a versatile procedure in reconstructive urology. J Urol 1992; 147:1248–1251.

52. Adams MC, Mitchell ME, Rink RC. Gastrocystoplasty: an alternative solution to the problem of urological reconstruction in the severely compromised patient. J Urol 1988; 140:1152–1156.

53. Althausen AF, Hagen-Cook K, Hendren WH III. Nonrefluxing colon conduit: experience with 70 cases. J Urol 1978; 120:35–39.

54. Beckley S, Wajsman Z, Pontes JE, Murphy G. Transverse colon conduit: a method of urinary diversion after pelvic irradiation. J Urol 1982; 128:464–468.

55. Boyd SD, Schiff WM, Skinner DG, et al. Prospective study of metabolic abnormalities in patients with continent Kock pouch urinary diversion. Urology 1989; 33:85–88.

56. Castro JE, Ram MD. Electrolyte imbalance following ileal urinary diversion. Br J Urol 1970; 42:29–32.

57. Elder DD, Moisey CU, Rees RWM. A long-term follow-up of the colonic conduit operation in children. Br J Urol 1979; 51:462–465.

58. Flanigan RC, Kursh ED, Persky L. Thirteen year experience with ileal loop diversion in children with myelodysplasia. Am J Surg 1975; 130:535–538.

59. Hagen-Cook K, Althausen AF. Early observations on 31 adults with nonrefluxing colon conduits. J Urol 1979; 121:13–16.

60. Jaffe BM, Bricker EM, Butcher HR Jr. Surgical complications of ileal segment urinary diversion. Ann Surg 1968; 167:367–376.

61. Loening SA, Navarre RJ, Narayana AS, Culp DA. Transverse colon conduit urinary diversion. J Urol 1982; 127:37–39.

62. Malek RS, Burke EC, DeWeerd JH. Ileal conduit urinary diversion in children. J Urol 1971; 105:892–900.

63. Middleton AW Jr, Hendren WH. Ileal conduits in children at the Massachusetts General Hospital from 1955 to 1970. J Urol 1976; 115:591–595.

64. Pitts WR Jr, Muecke EC. A 20-year experience with ileal conduits: the fate of the kidneys. J Urol 1979; 122:154–157.

65. Richie JP. Intestinal loop urinary diversion in children. J Urol 1974; 111:687–689.

66. Schmidt JD, Hawtrey CE, Flocks RH, Culp DA. Complications, results, and problems of ileal conduit diversions. J Urol 1973; 109:210–216.

67. Schwarz GR, Jeffs RD. Ileal conduit urinary diversion in children: computer analysis of follow-up from 2 to 16 years. J Urol 1975; 114:285–288.

68. Shapiro SR, Lebowitz R, Colodny AH. Fate of 90 children with ileal conduit urinary diversions a decade later: analysis of complications, pyelography, renal function, and bacteriology. J Urol 1975; 114:289–295.

69. Smith ED. Follow-up studies on 150 ileal conduits in children. J Pediatr Surg 1972; 7:1–10.

70. Sullivan JW, Grabstald H, Whitmore WF Jr. Complications of ureteroileal conduit with radical cystectomy: review of 336 cases. J Urol 1980; 124:797–801.

71. Nurmi M, Puntala P, Alanen A. Evaluation of 144 cases of ileal conduits in adults. Eur Urol 1988; 15:89–92.

72. Beckley S, Wajsman Z, Pontes JE, Murphy G. Transverse colon conduit: a method of urinary diversion after pelvic irradiation. J Urol 1982; 128:464–468.

73. Loening SA, Navarre RJ, Narayana AS, Culp DA. Transverse colon conduit urinary diversion. J Urol 1982; 127:37–39.

74. Kramolowsky EV, Clayman RV, Weyman PJ. Endourological management of ureteroileal anastomotic strictures: is it effective? J Urol 1987; 137:390–394.

75. Kramolowsky EV, Clayman RV, Weyman PJ. Management of ureterointestinal anastomotic strictures: comparison of open surgical and endourological repair. J Urol 1988; 139:1195–1198.

76. Savarirayan F, Dixey GM. Syncope following ureterosigmoidostomy. J Urol 1969; 101:844–845.

77. Bowyer GW, Davies TW. Methotrexate toxicity associated with an ileal conduit. Br J Urol 1986; 60:592.

78. McDougal WS. Metabolic complications of urinary intestinal diversion. J Urol 1992; 147:1199–1208.

79. Blyth B, Ewalt DH, Duckett JW, et al. Lithogenic properties of enterocystoplasty. J Urol 1992; 148:575–577.

80. Skinner DG, Lieskovsky G, Skinner E, Boyd S. Urinary diversion. Curr Probl Surg 1987; 24:401–471.

81. Kock MO, McDougal WS, Hall MC, et al. Long-term effects of urinary diversion: a comparison of myelomeningocele patients managed by clean, intermittent catheterization and urinary diversion. J Urol 1992; 147:1343–1347.

82. Dretler SP. The pathogenesis of urinary tract calculi occurring after conduit diversion: I. clinical study; II. conduit study; III. prevention. J Urol 1973; 109:204–209.

83. Treiger BFG, Marshall FF. Carcinogenesis and the use of intestinal segments in the urinary tract. Urol Clin N Am 1991; 18:737–742.

84. Carr LK, Herschorn S. Early development of adenocarcinoma in a young woman following augmentation cystoplasty for undiversion. J Urol 1997; 157:2255–2256.

85. Rowland RG, Regan JS. The risk of secondary malignancies in urinary reservoirs. In: Hohenfellner R, Wammack R, eds. Continent urinary diversion. London: Churchill Livingstone, 1992:299–308.

86. Studer UE, Stenzl A, Mansson W, Mills R. Bladder replacement and urinary diversion. Eur Urol 2000; 38(6):1–11.

87. Mansson W, Bakke A, Bergman B, et al. Perforations of continent urinary reservoirs. Scand J Urol Nephrol 1997; 31:529–532.

88. Mansson A, Mansson W. When the bladder is gone: quality of life following different types of urinary diversion. World J Urol 1999; 17:211–218.

89. Herschorn S, Hewitt R. The patient perspective of long-term outcome of augmentation cystoplasty in the management of neurogenic bladders. Urology 1998; 52:672–678.

90. Watanabe T, Rivas DA, Smith R, et al. The effect of urinary tract reconstruction on neurologically impaired women previously treated with an indwelling urethral catheter. J Urol 1996; 156(6):1926–1928.

25

Tissue engineering applications for patients with neurogenic bladder

Anthony Atala

Introduction

Regenerative medicine, a recently defined field, involves the diverse areas of tissue engineering, stem cells, and cloning towards the common goals of developing biological substitutes which would restore and maintain normal tissue and organ function.

Tissue engineering follows the principles of cell transplantation, materials science, and engineering towards the development of biological substitutes which would restore and maintain normal function. Tissue engineering may involve matrices alone, wherein the body's natural ability to regenerate is used to orient or direct new tissue growth, or the use of matrices with cells.

When cells are used for tissue engineering, donor tissue is dissociated into individual cells, which are either implanted directly into the host, or expanded in culture, attached to a support matrix, and reimplanted after expansion. The implanted tissue can be either heterologous, allogeneic, or autologous. Ideally, this approach might allow lost tissue function to be restored or replaced *in toto* and with limited complications.[2] The use of autologous cells would avoid rejection, wherein a biopsy of tissue is obtained from the host, the cells are dissociated and expanded *in vitro*, reattached to a matrix, and implanted into the same host.

One of the initial limitations of applying cell-based tissue engineering techniques to urologic organs had been the previously encountered inherent difficulty of growing genitourinary associated cells in large quantities. In the past, it was believed that urothelial cells had a natural senescence that was hard to overcome. Normal urothelial cells could be grown in the laboratory setting, but with limited expansion. Several protocols were developed over the last two decades which improved urothelial growth and expansion.[3–6] Using these methods of cell culture, it is possible to expand a urothelial strain from a single specimen that initially covers a surface area of 1 cm^2 to one covering

a surface area of 4202 m^2 (the equivalent area of one football field) within 8 weeks.[3]

Biomaterials in genitourinary tissue engineering may function as an artificial extracellular matrix (ECM), and elicit biological and mechanical functions of native ECM found in tissues of the body. The design and selection of the biomaterial is critical in the development of engineered genitourinary tissues. The biomaterial must be capable of controlling the structure and function of the engineered tissue in a predesigned manner by interacting with transplanted cells and/or the host cells. Generally, the ideal biomaterial should be biocompatible, promote cellular interaction and tissue development, and possess proper mechanical and physical properties.

Generally, three classes of biomaterials have been utilized for engineering genitourinary tissues: naturally derived materials, e.g. collagen and alginate; acellular tissue matrices, e.g. bladder submucosa and small intestinal submucosa; and synthetic polymers, e.g. polyglycolic acid (PGA), polylactic acid (PLA), and poly(lactic-co-glycolic acid) (PLGA). These classes of biomaterials have been tested in respect to their biocompatibility with primary human urothelial and bladder muscle cells.[7,8] Naturally derived materials and acellular tissue matrices have the potential advantage of biological recognition. Synthetic polymers can be produced reproducibly on a large scale with controlled properties of their strength, degradation rate, and microstructure.

Tissue engineering of the urethra

Various strategies have been proposed over the years for the regeneration of urethral tissue. Woven meshes of PGA have been used to reconstruct urethras in animals.[9,10] PGA has been also used as a cell transplantation vehicle to engineer tubular urothelium *in vivo*.[11] When using cells for transplantation, it has been shown that cells from an abnormal environment, if genetically stable, are able to be engineered into normal tissues.[12] A homologous free graft of acellular urethral matrix was used in a rabbit model.[13] All tissue components were seen in the grafted matrix after 3 months, with further improvement over time; however, the smooth muscle in the matrix was less than in normal rabbit urethra and was not well oriented.

Acellular collagen matrices obtained from donor bladder submucosa have proven to be suitable grafts for repairing urethral defects both experimentally and clinically at our institution. Rabbit neourethras reconstructed with acellular matrices demonstrated a normal urothelial luminal lining and organized muscle bundles, without any signs of strictures or complications.[14] These results were confirmed clinically in a series of patients with a history of failed hypospadias reconstruction wherein the urethral defects were repaired with human bladder acellular collagen matrices in an onlay fashion, with the size of the created neourethras ranging from 5 to 15 cm (Figure 25.1).[15] The same technique was used to repair urethral strictures on over 40 adult patients.[16] One of the advantages over nongenital tissue grafts used for urethroplasty is that the collagen-based acellular material is 'off the shelf'. This eliminates the necessity of additional surgical procedures for graft harvesting, which may decrease operative time, as well as the potential morbidity due to the harvest procedure.

It has also been noted that although acellular collagen-based grafts may be suitable for partial onlay urethral replacement, they are not effective for the replacement of tubularized segments, as this results in the collapse of the grafts, with subsequent stricture formation.[17] Tubularized urethral repairs require the application of collagen-based grafts seeded with both urothelial and muscle cells.[17] Total urethral replacement is possible with the use of tissue-engineered constructs composed of urothelial and muscle cell seeded matrices.

Tissue engineering of the bladder

Currently, gastrointestinal segments are commonly used as tissues for bladder replacement or repair. However, gastrointestinal tissues are designed to absorb specific solutes, whereas bladder tissue is designed for the excretion of solutes. When gastrointestinal tissue is in contact with the urinary tract, multiple complications may ensue, such as infection, metabolic disturbances, urolithiasis, perforation, increased mucus production, and malignancy.[18] Due to the problems encountered with the use of gastrointestinal segments, numerous investigators have attempted alternative methods, materials, and tissues for bladder replacement or repair.

Seromuscular grafts and de-epithelialized bowel segments, either alone or over a native urothelium, have been attempted.[19–26] The concept of demucosalizing organs is not new to urologists. Over four decades ago, in 1961, Blandy proposed the removal of submucosa from intestinal segments used for augmentation cystoplasty to insure that mucosal regrowth would not occur.[19] Hypothetically, this would avoid the complications associated with using bowel in continuity with the urinary tract.[20,21] Since Blandy's initial report, over 25 years transpired before there was a renewed interest in demucosalizing intestinal segments for urinary reconstruction.[22] Since 1988, several other investigators have pursued this line of research.[23–26] These investigative efforts have emphasized the complexity of both the anatomic and cellular interactions present when combining tissues with different functional parameters. The complexity of these interactions is emphasized by the observation that the use of demucosalized intestinal segments for augmentation cystoplasty is limited by either mucosal regrowth or contraction of the intestinal patch.[23,24] It has been noted that removal of only the mucosa may lead to mucosal regrowth, whereas removal of the mucosa and submucosa may lead to retraction of the intestinal patch.[27,28]

Some researchers have combined the techniques of autoaugmentation and enterocystoplasty. An autoaugmentation is performed and the diverticulum is covered with a demucosalized gastric or intestinal segment. In a series of autoaugmentation[25] enterocystoplasty, patients with a neurogenic bladder had either incorporation of stomach or colon. In both groups of patients the mucosa of the enteric segment was dissected away from the underlying muscle, and the resulting mucosa-free graft was used to cover a newly created bladder diverticulum. A satisfactory increase in bladder capacity and compliance was achieved in most patients. In another series of patients who underwent seromuscular colocystoplasty, the bladder capacity increased an average of 2.4-fold in 14 patients.[26] Ten patients had a postoperative bladder biopsy: 7 patients demonstrated urothelium covering the augmented portion of the bladder, 2 patients had regrowth of colonic mucosa, and 1 patient showed a mixture of colonic mucosa and urothelium. Although colonic mucosal regrowth is seen, there is a subset of patients, that may benefit from these procedures, wherein mucous secretion may be reduced or eliminated.[26]

Bladder grafts, initially used experimentally in 1961, have been used recently by various investigators.[29–32] The allogenic acellular bladder matrix has served as a scaffold for the ingrowth of host bladder wall components. The matrix is prepared by mechanically and/or chemically removing the cellular components.

Allogenic bladder submucosa was utilized as a biomaterial for bladder augmentation in dogs.[31] Biomaterials preloaded with cells prior to their implantation showed better tissue regeneration, compared with biomaterials implanted with no cells in which the tissue regeneration depended on the ingrowth of the surrounding tissue. The bladders showed a significant increase in capacity of 100% when augmented with scaffolds seeded with cells, compared with a capacity of 30% for scaffolds without cells (Figure 25.2).

Small-intestinal submucosa (SIS), derived from pig small intestine, has been used for augmentation cystoplasty in dogs.[33] Preoperative mean bladder capacity was 51 ml compared with a postoperative mean capacity of 55 ml. Histologically, the muscle layer was not fully developed. A large amount of collagen was interspersed between a smaller number of muscle bundles. A computerized assisted image analysis demonstrated a decreased muscle-to-collagen ratio, with a loss of the normal architecture in the SIS regenerated bladders. *In-vitro* contractility studies performed on the SIS regenerated dog bladders showed a decrease in maximal contractile response by 50% from those of normal bladder tissues. Cholinergic and purinergic innervation was present.[34]

In multiple studies using different materials as an acellular graft for cystoplasty, the urothelial layer was able to regenerate normally, but the muscle layer, although present, was not fully developed.[30–33] Engineering tissue using selective cell transplantation may provide a means of creating functional new bladder segments.[11] The success of using cell transplantation strategies for bladder reconstruction depends on the ability to use donor tissue efficiently and to provide the right conditions for long-term survival, differentiation, and growth.

Urothelial and muscle cells can be expanded *in vitro*, seeded onto the polymer scaffold, and allowed to attach and form sheets of cells. The cell–polymer scaffold can then be implanted *in vivo*. A series of *in-vivo* urologic associated cell–polymer experiments were performed in mice, rabbits, and dogs.[3,11,31,35]

To better address the functional parameters of tissue-engineered bladders, an animal model was designed that required a subtotal cystectomy with subsequent replacement with a tissue-engineered organ.[36] Dogs underwent a trigone-sparing cystectomy. The animals were randomly assigned to one of three groups. Animals underwent closure of the trigone without a reconstructive procedure, reconstruction with a cell-free bladder-shaped biodegradable matrix, or reconstruction using a bladder-shaped biodegradable matrix that delivered autologous urothelial and smooth muscle cells. The cell populations had been separately expanded from a previously harvested autologous bladder biopsy. Preoperative and postoperative urodynamic, radiographic, gross, histological, and immunocytochemical analyses were performed serially at 1, 2, 3, 4, 6, and 11 months, postoperatively.[36]

The cystectomy-only controls and polymer-only grafts maintained average capacities of 22% and 46% of preoperative values, respectively. An average bladder capacity of 95% of the original pre-cystectomy volume was achieved in the tissue-engineered bladder replacements. These findings were confirmed radiographically. The subtotal cystectomy reservoirs, which were not reconstructed, and polymer-only reconstructed bladders showed a marked decrease in bladder compliance (10% and 42%, respectively). The compliance of the tissue-engineered bladders showed almost no difference from preoperative values that were measured when the native bladder was present (106%). Histologically, the polymer-only bladders presented a pattern of normal urothelial cells with a thickened fibrotic submucosa and a thin layer of muscle fibers. The retrieved tissue-engineered bladders showed a normal cellular organization, consisting of a trilayer of urothelium, submucosa, and muscle (Figure 25.3). Immunocytochemical analyses for desmin, α-actin, cytokeratin 7, pancytokeratins AE1/AE3, and uroplakin III confirmed the muscle and urothelial phenotype. S-100 staining indicated the presence of neural structures. The results from this study showed that it is possible to tissue engineer bladders which are anatomically and functionally normal.[36] Human bladders have been created using the same techniques.

Clinically, cells used for tissue engineering may be harvested from abnormal bladders. We investigated the contractility of tissue-engineered bladder smooth muscle derived from patients with functionally normal bladders and functionally abnormal neuropathic and exstrophic bladders.[12] The tissue-engineered cells showed similar expression of smooth muscle marker proteins (α-actin and myosin) regardless of their origin. All scaffolds showed similar muscle formation and were α-actin positive. At retrieval, the muscle cell-seeded scaffolds exhibited contractile activity to electrical field stimulation and carbachol. There was no statistical difference between the three different types of muscle cells seeded (normal, neurogenic, and exstrophic). The results of this study were also consistent with prior findings that, in diseased bladders, a large portion of the pathologic effects seen are due to increased fibrosis, whereas the cells retain their genetic stability.

Injectable therapies using tissue engineering techniques

Both urinary incontinence and vesicoureteral reflux are common conditions affecting the genitourinary system, wherein injectable bulking agents can be used for treatment. The goal of several investigators has been to find alternative implant materials that would be safe for human use.[37] Long-term studies were conducted to determine the effect of injectable chondrocytes *in vivo*.[38] It was initially determined that alginate, a liquid solution of gluronic and mannuronic acid, embedded with chondrocytes, could serve as a synthetic substrate for the injectable delivery and maintenance of cartilage architecture *in vivo*. A biopsy of the ear could be easily and quickly performed, followed by chondrocyte processing and endoscopic injection of the autologous chondrocyte suspension for therapy.

Chondrocytes can be readily grown and expanded in culture. Neocartilage formation can be achieved *in vitro* and *in vivo* using chondrocytes cultured on synthetic biodegradable polymers.[38] This system was adapted for the treatment of vesicoureteral reflux in a porcine model.[39] Chondrocytes were harvested from the left auricular surface of surgically created refluxing mini-swine and expanded. The animals underwent endoscopic repair of reflux with the injectable autologous chondrocyte solution on the right side only. Serial cystograms showed no evidence of reflux on the treated side and persistent reflux in the uncorrected control ureter in all animals. The harvested ears had evidence of cartilage regrowth within 1 month of chondrocyte retrieval.

At the time of sacrifice, gross examination of the bladder injection site showed a well-defined rubbery to hard cartilage structure in the suburateral region. Histologic examination of these specimens showed evidence of normal cartilage formation. The polymer gels were progressively replaced by cartilage over time. Aldehyde fuschin-alcian blue staining suggested the presence of chondroitin sulfate.

Using the same line of reasoning as with the chondrocyte technology, the possibility of using autologous muscle cells was also investigated.[40] *In-vivo* experiments were conducted in mini-pigs and reflux was successfully corrected. In addition to its use for the endoscopic treatment of reflux and urinary incontinence, the system of injectable autologous cells may also be applicable for the treatment of other medical conditions, such as rectal incontinence, dysphonia, plastic reconstruction, and wherever an injectable permanent biocompatible material is needed.

Recently, the first human application of cell-based tissue engineering technology for urologic applications has occurred with the injection of chondrocytes for the correction of vesicoureteral reflux in children (Figure 25.4) and for urinary incontinence in adults. The clinical trials are currently ongoing.[37,41–43]

The potential use of injectable, cultured myoblasts for the treatment of stress urinary incontinence has recently been investigated in preliminary experiments.[44] Primary myoblasts obtained from mouse skeletal muscle were transduced *in vitro* to carry the β-galactosidase reporter gene and were then incubated with fluorescent microspheres which would serve as markers for the original cell population. Cells were then directly injected into the proximal urethra and lateral bladder walls of nude mice with a microsyringe in an open surgical procedure. Tissue was harvested up to 35 days post-injection, analyzed histologically, and assayed for β-galactosidase expression. Myoblasts expressing β-galactosidase and containing fluorescent microspheres were found at each of the retrieved time points. In addition, regenerative myofibers expressing β-galactosidase were identified within the bladder wall. By 35 days post-injection, some of the injected cells expressed the contractile filament a-smooth muscle actin, suggesting the possibility of myoblastic differentiation into smooth muscle. The authors reported that a significant portion of the injected myoblast population persisted *in vivo*. The fact that myoblasts can be transfected, survive after injection, and begin the process of myogenic differentiation further supports the feasibility of using cultured cells of muscular origin as an injectable bioimplant.

Gene therapy and tissue engineering

Genetically engineered cells

Cells can be engineered to secrete growth factors for various applications, such as for promoting angiogenesis for tissue regeneration.[45] Angiogenesis, the process of new blood vessel formation, is regulated by different growth factors. These growth factors stimulate endothelial cells, which are already present in the patient's body, to migrate to the implanted area of need, where they proliferate and differentiate into blood vessels.[46] One of the major molecules which promotes and regulates angiogenesis is vascular endothelial growth factor (VEGF).[47] Several methods have been used experimentally to deliver VEGF *in vivo*. The growth factor protein can be directly injected into tissues.[48] However, the rapid clearance of VEGF proteins from the vascular system limits its effect to only minutes. The *VEGF* gene could be delivered to tissues using various techniques; however, the transfection efficiency is low, the onset of action is delayed for up to 48–72 h after the *VEGF* cDNA is incorporated, and the effect is transient, lasting only several days.[48,49]

An approach which has been pursued in our laboratory to increase and stimulate rapid vascularization *in vivo* was to engineer a cell line to secrete high levels of VEGF proteins by gene transfecting the cells with the *VEGF* cDNA. The VEGF-secreting cells were encapsulated in polymeric microspheres. The microspheres allowed nutrients to reach the cells, whereas the VEGF proteins secreted from the cells diffused into the surrounding tissues. The microspheres protected the coated cells from the host immune environment. This novel system of neovascularization was tested *in vitro* and *in vivo* in an animal model. The degree of VEGF secretion and the period of delivery can be regulated by modulating the number of engineered cells encapsulated per microsphere, as well as the number of microspheres injected. A similar strategy has also been pursued for the genetic engineering of antiangiogenic factor secreting cells.[50] These strategies could be useful for antitumor therapy in urology.

Gene therapy for tissue engineered constructs

Based on the feasibility of tissue engineering techniques in which cells seeded on biodegradable polymer scaffolds form tissue when implanted *in vivo*, the possibility was explored of developing a neo-organ system for *in-vivo* gene therapy.[51] In a series of studies conducted in our laboratory, human urothelial cells were harvested, expanded *in vitro*, and seeded on biodegradable polymer scaffolds. The cell–polymer complex was then transfected with *PGL3-luc, pCMV-luc,* and *pCMVß-gal* promoter–reporter gene constructs. The transfected cell–polymer scaffolds were then implanted *in vivo* and the engineered tissues were retrieved at different time points after implantation. Results indicate that successful gene transfer may be achieved using biodegradable polymer scaffolds as a urothelial cell delivery vehicle. The transfected cell–polymer scaffold formed organ-like structures with functional expression of the transfected genes.[51] This technology is applicable throughout the spectrum of diseases which may be manageable with tissue engineering. For example, one can envision the use of effecting *in-vivo* gene delivery through the *ex-vivo* transfection of tissue-engineered cell–polymer scaffolds for the genetic modification of diseased corporal smooth muscle cells harvested from impotent patients. Theoretically, the *in-vitro* genetic modification of corporal smooth muscle cells harvested from an impotent patient, resulting in either a reduction in the expression of the *TGF-1* gene or the overexpression of genes responsible for PGE1 production, could lead to the resumption of erectile functionality once these cells were used to repopulate the diseased corporal bodies.

Stem cells for tissue engineering

Most current strategies for engineering urologic tissues involve harvesting of autologous cells from the host diseased organ. However, in situations where extensive end-stage organ failure is present, a tissue biopsy may not yield enough normal cells for expansion. Under these circumstances, the availability of pluripotent stem cells may be beneficial. Pluripotent embryonic stem cells are known to form teratomas *in vivo*, which are composed of a variety of differentiated cells. However, these cells may be immunocompetent, and may require immunosuppression if used clinically.

The possibility of deriving pluripotent cells from postnatal mesenchymal tissue from the same host, and inducing their differentiation *in vitro* and *in vivo*, was investigated. Pluripotent cells were isolated from human foreskin-derived fibroblasts. Adipogenic, myogenic, and osteoblastic lineages were obtained from these progenitor cells. The cells were grown, expanded, seeded onto biodegradable scaffolds, and implanted *in vivo*, where they formed mature tissue structures. This was the first demonstration that stem cells can be derived from postnatal connective tissue and can be used for engineering tissues *in vivo ex situ.*[52]

Therapeutic cloning for tissue engineering

Recent advances with the cloning of embryos and newborn animals have expanded the possibilities of this technology for tissue engineering and organ transplantation. There are many ethical concerns with cloning in terms of creating humans for the sole purpose of obtaining organs. However, the potential for retrieving cells from early-stage cloned embryos for subsequent regeneration is being proposed as an ethically viable benefit of therapeutic cloning (Figure 25.5). The feasibility of engineering syngeneic tissues *in vivo* using cloned cells was investigated.

Unfertilized donor bovine eggs were retrieved and the nuclear material was removed. Bovine fibroblasts from the skin of a steer were obtained. The nuclear material was removed from the fibroblast and microinjected into the donor egg shell (nuclear transfer). A short burst of energy was delivered, initiating neoembryogenesis. These techniques replicate what was performed to clone the first mammal, Dolly the sheep. However, instead of implanting the embryo into a uterus, the goal would be to harvest stem cells from the embryo, which was created, not from the union of a sperm and an egg, but rather from a skin cell and an egg shell, devoid of any genetic material. To achieve a proof of principle, bypassing the *in-vitro* differentiation, the embryos were placed in the same steer uterus from which the fibroblasts had been obtained. The cloned embryo, with identical genetic material as the steer, was retrieved for tissue harvest. Various cell types were harvested, expanded *in vitro*, and seeded on biodegradable scaffolds. The cell–polymer scaffolds were implanted into the back of the same steer from which the cells were cloned. The implants were retrieved at various time points for analyses. Renal tissue, and cardiac and skeletal muscle were engineered successfully using therapeutic cloning.

These studies demonstrated that cells obtained through nuclear transfer can be successfully harvested, expanded in culture, and transplanted *in vivo* with biodegradable scaffolds where the single suspended cells form and organize into tissue structures, which are the same genetically as the host. These studies were the first demonstration of the use of therapeutic cloning for the regeneration of tissues *in vivo*.[53] One could envision taking one skin cell from a patient, and having the ability to generate most types of tissues for replacement or transplantation, which would be genetically identical and fully biocompatible. Thus, each patient could conceivably have a ready-made supply of their own tissues available on demand.

Conclusion

Tissue engineering efforts are currently being undertaken for every type of tissue and organ within the urinary system. Primary autologous cells, stem cells, and therapeutic cloning are being applied for the creation of tissues and organs. Tissue engineering techniques require expertise in growth factor biology, a cell culture facility designed for human application, and personnel who have mastered the techniques of cell harvest, culture, and expansion. Polymer scaffold design and manufacturing resources are essential for the successful application of this technology.

The first human application of cell-based tissue engineering for urologic applications occurred at our institution with the injection of autologous cells for the correction of vesicoureteral reflux in children. The same technology has been recently expanded to treat adult patients with urinary incontinence. Trials involving urethral tissue replacement using processed collagen matrices are in progress at our center for both hypospadias and stricture repair. Bladder replacement using tissue engineering techniques is being explored. Recent progress suggests that engineered urologic tissues may have a wider clinical applicability in regenerative medicine.

References

1. Murray JE, Merrill JP, Harrison JH. Renal homotransplantation in identical twins. J Am Soc Nephrol 2001; 12(1):201–204.

2. Atala A. Tissue engineering in the genitourinary system. In: Atala A, Mooney D, eds. Tissue engineering. Boston: Birkhauser Press, 1997:149.

3. Cilento BG, Freeman MR, Schneck FX, et al. Phenotypic and cytogenetic characterization of human bladder urothelia expanded in vitro. J Urol 1994;152:655.

4. Scriven SD, Booth C, Thomas DF, et al. Reconstitution of human urothelium from monolayer cultures. J Urol 1997; 158(3 Pt 2): 1147–1152.

5. Liebert M, Wedemeyer G, Abruzzo LV, et al. Stimulated urothelial cells produce cytokines and express an activated cell surface antigenic phenotype. Semin Urol 1991; 9(2):124–130.

6. Puthenveettil JA, Burger MS, Reznikoff CA. Replicative senescence in human uroepithelial cells. Adv Exp Med Biol 1999; 462:83–91.

7. Pariente JL, Kim BS, Atala A. In vitro biocompatibility assessment of naturally-derived and synthetic biomaterials using normal human urothelial cells. J Biomed Mat Res 2001; 55:33–39.

8. Pariente JL, Kim BS, Atala A. In vitro biocompatibility evaluation of naturally derived and synthetic biomaterials using normal human bladder smooth muscle cells. J Urol 2002; 167:1867–1871.

9. Bazeed MA, Thüroff JW, Schmidt RA, Tanagho EA. New treatment for urethral strictures. Urology 1983; 21:53–57.

10. Olsen L, Bowald S, Busch C, et al. Urethral reconstruction with a new synthetic absorbable device. Scand J Urol Nephrol 1992; 26:323–326.

11. Atala A, Vacanti JP, Peters CA, et al. Formation of urothelial structures in vivo from dissociated cells attached to biodegradable polymer scaffolds in vitro. J Urol 1992; 148:658.

12. Lai JY, Yoon CY, Yoo JJ, et al. Phenotypic and functional characterization of in vivo tissue engineered smooth muscle from normal and pathological bladders. J Urol 2002; 168:1853–1858.

13. Sievert KD, Bakircioglu ME, Nunes L, et al. Homologous acellular matrix graft for urethral reconstruction in the rabbit: histological and functional evaluation. J Urol 2000; 163(6):1958–1965.

14. Chen F, Yoo JJ, Atala A. Acellular collagen matrix as a possible "off the shelf" biomaterial for urethral repair. Urology 1999; 54:407–410.

15. Atala A, Guzman L, Retik A. A novel inert collagen matrix for hypospadias repair. J Urol 1999; 162:1148–1151.

16. Kassaby EA, Yoo J, Retik A, Atala A. A novel inert collagen matrix for urethral stricture repair. J Urol 2000;163(supp 4):70.

17. DeFilippo RE, Yoo JY, Chen F, Atala A. Urethral replacement using cell-seeded tubularized collagen matrices. J Urol 2002; 168:1789–1793.

18. McDougal WS. Metabolic complications of urinary intestinal diversion. J Urol 1992; 147:1199.

19. Blandy JP. Neal pouch with transitional epithelium and anal sphincter as a continent urinary reservoir. J Urol 1961; 86:749.

20. Blandy JP. The feasibility of preparing an ideal substitute for the urinary bladder. Ann Roy Coll Surg 1964; 35:287.

21. Harada N, Yano H, Ohkawa T, et al. New surgical treatment of bladder tumors: mucosal denudation of the bladder. Br J Urol 1965; 37:545.

22. Oesch I. Neourothelium in bladder augmentation. An experimental study in rats. Eur Urol 1988; 14:328.

23. Salle J, Fraga C, Lucib A, et al. Seromuscular enterocystoplasty in dogs. J Urol 1990; 144:454.

24. Cheng E, Rento R, Grayhack TJ, et al. Reversed seromuscular flaps in the urinary tract in dogs. J Urol 1994; 152:2252.

25. Dewan PA. Autoaugmentation demucosalized enterocystoplasty. World J Urol 1998; 16:255–261.

26. Gonzalez R, Buson H, Reid C, Reinberg Y. Seromuscular colocystoplasty lined with urothelium (SCLU). Experimental in 16 patients. Urology 1995; 45:124.

27. Atala A. Commentary on the replacement of urologic associated mucosa. J Urol 1995; 156:338.

28. Atala A. Autologous cell transplantation for urologic reconstruction. J Urol 1998; 159:2.

29. Tsuji I, Ishida H, Fujieda J. Experimental cystoplasty using preserved bladder graft. J Urol 1961; 85:42.

30. Probst M, Dahiya R, Carrier S, Tanagho EA. Reproduction of functional smooth muscle tissue and partial bladder replacement. Br J Urol 1997; 79:505–515.

31. Yoo JJ, Meng J, Oberpenning F, Atala A. Bladder augmentation using allogenic bladder submucosa seeded with cells. Urology 1998; 51:221.

32. Sutherland RS, Baskin LS, Hayward SW, Cunha GR. Regeneration of bladder urothelium, smooth muscle, blood vessels, and nerves into an acellular tissue matrix. J Urol 1996; 156:571–577.

33. Kropp BP, Rippy MK, Badylak SF, et al. Small intestinal submucosa: urodynamic and histopathologic evaluation in long term canine bladder augmentations. J Urol 1996; 155:2098–2104.

34. Vaught JD, Kroop BP, Sawyer BD, et al. Detrusor regeneration in the rat using porcine small intestine submucosal grafts: functional innervation and receptor expression. J Urol 1996; 155:374–378.

35. Atala A, Freeman MR, Vacanti JP, et al. Implantation in vivo and retrieval of artificial structures consisting of rabbit and human urothelium and human bladder muscle. J Urol 1993; 150:608.

36. Oberpenning FO, Meng J, Yoo J, Atala A. De novo reconstitution of a functional urinary bladder by tissue engineering. Nat Biotechnol 1999; 17:2.

37. Kershen RT, Atala A. Advances in injectable therapies for the treatment of incontinence and vesicoureteral reflux. Urol Clin 1999; 26:81–94.

38. Atala A, Cima LG, Kim W, et al. Injectable alginate seeded with chondrocytes as a potential treatment for vesicoureteral reflux. J Urol 1993; 150:745.

39. Atala A, Kim W, Paige KT, et al. Endoscopic treatment of vesicoureteral reflux with chondrocyte-alginate suspension. J Urol 1994; 152:641.

40. Cilento BG, Atala A. Treatment of reflux and incontinence with autologous chondrocytes and bladder muscle cells. Dial Pediatr Urol 1995; 18:11.

41. Diamond DA, Caldamone AA. Endoscopic correction of vesicoureteral reflux in children using autologous chondrocytes: preliminary results. J Urol 1999; 162:1185.

42. Caldamone AA, Diamond DA. Long-term results of the endoscopic correction of vesicoureteral reflux in children using autologous chondrocytes. J Urol 2001; 165(6 Pt 2):2224–2227.

43. Bent AE, Tutrone RT, McLennan MT, et al. Treatment of intrinsic sphincter deficiency using autologous ear chondrocytes as a bulking agent. Neurourol Urodyn 2001; 20(2):157–165.

44. Yokoyama T, Chancellor MB, Watanabe T, et al. Primary myoblasts injection into the urethra and bladder as a potential treatment of stress urinary incontinence and impaired detrusor contractility; long term survival without significant cytotoxicity. J Urol 1999; 161:307.

45. Machlouf M, Orsola A, Atala A. Controlled release of therapeutic agents: slow delivery and cell encapsulation. World J Urol 2000; 18:80–83.

46. Polverini PJ. The pathophysiology of angiogenesis. Crit Rev Oral Biol Med 1996; 6:230.

47. Klagsbrun M, D'Amore PA. Regulation of angiogenesis. Ann Rev Physiol 1991; 53:217.

48. Bauters C, Asahara T, Zheng LP, et al. Physiological assessment of augmented vascularity induced by VEGF in ischemic rabbit hindlimb. Am J Physiol 1994; 267:263.

49. Takeshita S, Tsurumi Y, Couffinahl T, et al. Gene transfer of naked DNA encoding for three isoforms of vascular endothelial growth factor stimulates collateral development in vivo. Lab Invest 1996; 75:487.

50. Joki T, Machluf M, Atala A, et al. Continuous release of endostatin from microencapsulated engineered cells for tumor therapy. Nat Biotechnol 2001; 19(1):35–39.

51. Yoo JJ, Atala A. A novel gene delivery system using urothelial tissue engineered neo-organs. J Urol 1997; 158:1066–1070.

52. Bartsch GC, Yoo JJ, De Coppi P, et al. Dermal stem cells for pelvic and bladder reconstruction. J Urol 2002; 167:59a.

53. Lanza RP, Chung HY, Yoo JJ, et al. Generation of histocompatible tissues using nuclear transplantation. Nat Biotechnol 2002;20: 689–696.

26

Restoration of complete bladder function by neurostimulation

Michael Craggs

Introduction

During the past 20 years two key developments using implantable neuroprostheses have had a significant impact on treating and managing patients with a neurogenic bladder. The first of these was the Brindley sacral anterior root stimulator[1] used principally for bladder emptying in (see Chapter 19). The second was the sacral nerve stimulator originally developed by Tanagho and Schmidt for neuromodulating[2,3] a variety of bladder dysfunctions, including the overactive bladder and urinary retention (see Chapter 20). It is timely to consider how these two techniques, among others, may in the future be combined using emerging technologies to restore more complete control of the dysfunctional bladder in people with a suprasacral spinal cord injury (SCI).

Suprasacral lesions to the spinal cord nearly always lead to serious disruption of lower urinary tract function: impairment of voluntary sphincter control and sensation of bladder, fullness, aberrant reflexes of the bladder, and an uncoordinated urinary sphincter[4]. As a consequence, bladder emptying is impaired and the result is reflex incontinence. Reflex incontinence is primarily caused by detrusor hyperreflexia, an aberrant reflex that emerges after a period of spinal shock following SCI (Figure 26.1). It is often associated with dyssynergenic contractions of the striated sphincter muscle of the urethra, preventing efficient emptying of the bladder. Persons with SCI frequently develop large residual volumes and urinary tract infections, and are prone to upper urinary tract damage and subsequent renal failure if managed incorrectly.

Medical treatment is usually by a combination of drugs for suppressing detrusor hyperreflexia and intermittent catheterization for emptying the bladder. However, the antimuscarinic drugs used to treat incontinence often have debilitating side-effects, such as constipation, dry mouth, and visual disturbance.

Emptying the bladder can also be very troublesome, especially in women for whom no reliable collection device exists (other than indwelling catheters and bags or ungainly pads), and intermittent catheterization can often introduce bladder infections. Other more radical approaches such as surgery for augmenting the bladder, sphincterotomies, cutting posterior sacral roots to suppress

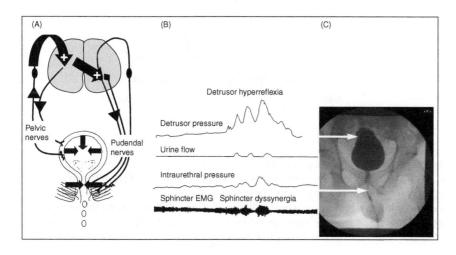

Figure 26.1
The neurogenic bladder in suprasacral spinal cord injury. (A) Aberrant pelvic reflexes causing detrusor hyperreflexia and detrusor-external sphincter dyssynergia. (B) Traces showing the high bladder pressures generated, dyssynergia of the sphincter, associated electromyography (EMG) and urine leakage during videourodynamics. (C) X-ray image shows the bladder and sphincter at the exact time of dyssynergia.

hyperreflexia, or repeated injections of toxins such as Botulinum toxin to paralyse the sphincter and bladder may all have destructive effects which could preclude the use of future developments, including more novel implantable neurostimulating devices.

This chapter briefly reviews some future possibilities for combining existing and emerging science and technologies[5,6] to develop an implantable neuroprosthesis capable of restoring complete control to the bladder and sphincters in SCI. Six areas of development will be addressed:

- sacral anterior root stimulation for emptying the paralysed bladder
- sacral nerve stimulation for suppressing detrusor hyperreflexia
- conditional neuromodulation for automatic control of reflex incontinence
- the sacral posterior and anterior root stimulator implant (SPARSI)
- selective stimulation of sacral roots to prevent detrusor-sphincter dyssynergia
- prospects for complete restoration of bladder control by neuroprosthesis.

Sacral anterior root stimulation for emptying the paralysed bladder

In the 1970s, Brindley and his colleagues developed an implantable device to empty the bladder and control the sphincters[7] (see Chapter 19). The prosthesis uses sacral anterior root stimulation (Finetech–Brindley SARS, Finetech Medical Limited, Welwyn Garden City, UK) to activate bladder motor pathways and produce clinically effective voiding (Figure 26.2). For reflex incontinence and sphincter dyssynergia to be overcome in these patients, the sacral sensory nerve roots from S2 to S4 have to be cut (sacral deafferentation or posterior rhizotomy).

The Finetech–Brindley device has been successfully used in many countries throughout the world.[8] The implant when combined with sacral deafferentation has been shown to be very effective in increasing bladder volume, promoting complete emptying of the bladder, reducing bladder infections, and significantly improving the quality of life for many patients.[9] However, the need for sacral deafferentation (posterior rhizotomy), with the consequent

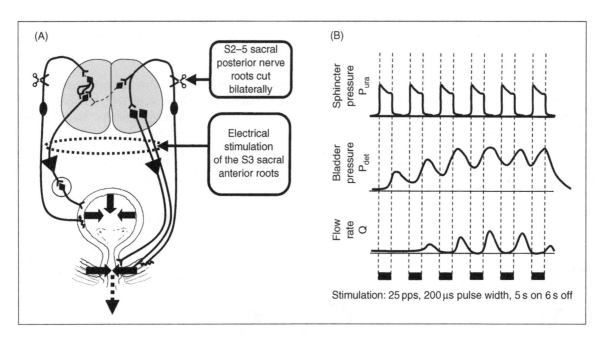

Figure 26.2

Sacral anterior root stimulation (SARS) with sacral deafferention for bladder control. (A) The Finetech–Brindley SARS implantable stimulator uses bilaterally placed intrathecal or extradural electrodes on the S2–S4 sacral roots to activate the preganglionic parasympathetic pathway to produce efficient bladder emptying. A rhizotomy of the corresponding posterior roots (sensory) prevents detrusor hyperreflexia, dyssynergia of the sphincter, and incontinence. (B) Bursts of stimulation activate simultaneously the striated sphincter muscle and detrusor smooth muscle. During the intervals between the bursts the sphincter relaxes rapidly to leave a low urethral resistance whilst the detrusor is still contracting slowly to a higher pressure so as to enable efficient voiding.

loss of reflex erections, reflex ejaculation, bowel problems, and potential pelvic floor weakness can deter many very suitable young male patients from accepting SARS. Furthermore, the hope by some patients of a 'cure' for SCI in the future using neural regeneration and repair techniques is a further obstacle to acceptance. Patients having already suffered accidental damage to their spinal cord are understandably reluctant to then accept deliberate damage. Realistically, a cure for restoring autonomic functions controlling bladder and bowel may take many years to perfect and, meanwhile, management has to try to give the patient the best quality of life. With good medical management of the neurogenic bladder in SCI most patients can now expect a near normal life span and SARS can definitely help many patients, but clearly it would be much more acceptable if it did not involve further destruction of potentially useful reflexes. There may be an alternative solution to sacral deafferentation which involves stimulation of these same afferent pathways rather than cutting them to suppress reflex incontinence.

Sacral root stimulation for suppressing detrusor hyperreflexia

During the 1980s Tanagho and Schmidt developed the use of electrical stimulation of sacral nerves to treat a variety of lower urinary tract problems, including those of the neurogenic bladder[10] (see Chapter 20). Subsequently, a neuroprosthesis was developed (Interstim, Medtronic, Inc., Minneapolis, USA) which comprised an implanted pulse generator attached to a multipole electrode surgically inserted into the S3 sacral foramina for stimulating the

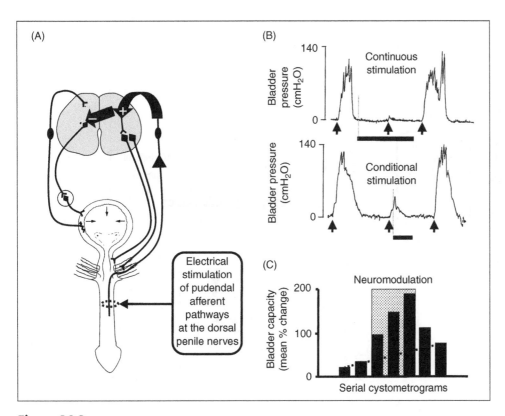

Figure 26.3

Controlling detrusor hyperreflexia by noninvasive neuromodulation through pudendal afferent pathways. (A) By stimulating the dorsal penile (or clitoral) nerves with electrical pulses between 10 and 20 per second and above twice the threshold for the pudendo-anal reflex, it is possible to profoundly suppress detrusor hyperreflexia. (B) The upper trace shows the effect of continuous stimulation of the dorsal penile nerves on the bladder pressure rise associated with a detrusor hyperreflexia contraction provoked at the middle arrow. Control hyperreflexic contractions provoked at the other arrows can be seen before and after stimulation. The lower trace shows the effect of applying neuromodulation conditionally (that is only when detrusor hyperreflexia just appears) in response to provocation at the middle arrow. Again, this response is flanked by control provocations. (C) Repeated cystometrograms with continuous neuromodulation (shaded area), demonstrating significant increases in bladder volume when compared to control fills. Following stimulation the bladder takes some time to restore to its smaller capacity, probably as a result of stretching of the bladder wall during the period of neuromodulation.

mixed sacral nerves.[11] Such stimulation, commonly known as *neuromodulation*, has also been successfully used to increase bladder capacity in patients with an SCI.[12]

Studies using noninvasive multipulse magnetic stimulation over the sacrum to stimulate the mixed extradural sacral roots (S2–4) have demonstrated that the increase in bladder capacity is brought about by suppression of detrusor hyperreflexia in patients with SCI.[13] The mechanism for this 'neuromodulatory' action has yet to be determined in man, but one theory, based on experimental work in animals,[14] suggests that neuromodulation involves inhibitory action by pudendal afferent (sensory) nerve stimulation on pelvic nerve motor pathways to the bladder through spinal cord circuits.[15] Pudendal afferents course through S2–4 posterior (sensory) roots to the spinal cord. Evidence in support of the theory was obtained by electrically stimulating purely pudendal afferent pathways at the level of the dorsal penile[16,17] (or dorsal clitoral) nerves in patients.

Dorsal penile nerve (DPN) stimulation through surface electrodes in patients with SCI produces a profound and repeatable suppression of provoked detrusor hyperreflexia when applied either continuously (pre-emptively) or conditionally (i.e. when bladder pressure just begins to increase)[18,19] (Figure 26.3). Furthermore, in addition to suppressing hyperreflexia, DPN stimulation can produce significant increases in bladder volume, as demonstrated in serial cystometrograms.[20] These effects depend essentially on stimulation, and diminish when stimulation is switched off. Interestingly, intermittent stimulation also appears to produce good results, although the ideal interval between bursts has yet to be determined, balancing the need to suppress every hyperreflexic contraction reliably against preserving the battery life of the stimulator.[21]

In a recent pilot study the same benefit has been shown using a Finetech–Brindley implantable device to stimulate extradural or intradural sacral roots but without

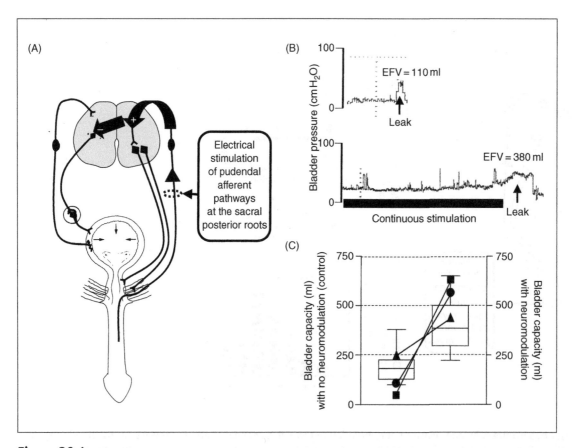

Figure 26.4

Controlling detrusor hyperreflexia and increasing bladder capacity by sacral posterior root stimulation. (A) A Finetech–Brindley implanted stimulator (without deafferentation) is used to apply neuromodulation bilaterally through the S3–S4 sacral roots. (B) Continuous stimulation at about 15 pulses per second (240 μs pulse width) with a current level set to suppress detrusor hyperreflexia significantly increased bladder capacity over control tests (EFV = end-fill volume). (C) The graph shows box and whisker results from a group of 11 patients with SCI tested using continuous neuromodulation through the dorsal penile nerves (DPN) compared with the effect of applying neuromodulation through the posterior roots in 3 patients (solid lines with symbols) from this same group. It can be seen that bladder capacity is markedly increased with stimulation of the roots and compares favorably with the significant group result using DPN stimulation. DPN stimulation may be a good predictor for success with a sacral nerve stimulator.

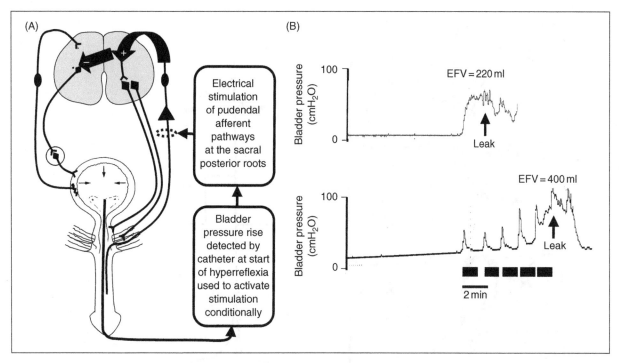

Figure 26.5
Using bladder pressure to automatically control detrusor hyperreflexia with conditional neuromodulation. (A) By measuring bladder pressure with a catheter it is possible to detect exactly when a detrusor hyperreflexic contraction begins and this can be used to activate stimulation of the sacral posterior roots to suppress the contraction automatically. The cystometrograms in this figure were obtained from a patient with an incomplete upper thoracic spinal lesion, but similar results have also been shown in patients with complete lesions. (B) The upper trace shows a cystometrogram without stimulation and a relatively low bladder capacity. The lower trace shows that when a pressure rise is detected, the applied stimulation immediately reduces the pressure, and by automatically repeating this suppression on successive detrusor hyperreflexic contractions a much larger bladder capacity can be achieved. A point is reached at this new maximum capacity when suppression is no longer possible. EFV = end-fill volume.

deafferentation.[22] In a small group of patients with a suprasacral spinal injury, electrodes were placed bilaterally on either the mixed extradural sacral (S2–4) roots or separated anterior and posterior sacral roots (S3) intrathecally. Each patient was assessed preoperatively with DPN stimulation, as described above, to demonstrate the efficacy of neuromodulation. Preliminary results indicated that patients were able to achieve both good suppression of detrusor hyperreflexia and clinically useful increases in bladder volume (Figure 26.4).

Conditional neuromodulation for automatic control of reflex incontinence

In the implant studies described above it was also demonstrated that conditional stimulation, applied only at the onset of hyperreflexic contractions, was at least as good as continuous stimulation at increasing bladder capacity and was sometimes better. Bladder contractions were sensed by measuring intravesical pressure with a standard catheter

and the pudendal afferents stimulated either at the level of the penile dorsal nerve or sacral roots to inhibit bladder contractions (Figure 26.5).[20,22]

A conditional system that detects the onset of unstable bladder contractions and then suppresses them has a number of theoretical advantages. Although continuous neuromodulation is an effective and simple way to increase bladder capacity in spinally injured patients, in many situations it is not ideal. The need for constant current delivery would shorten both battery and electrode life in a completely implanted device, and continuous stimulation of the sacral afferents may have undesirable long-term reflex effects on the anal and urethral sphincters, perhaps exacerbating any residual dyssynergia.

Hence, a device that could stimulate the sacral nerves for neuromodulation only when necessary might have considerable benefits and would have the added advantage that it could provide feedback about bladder fullness to the patient. That is, stimulating pulses associated with the conditional neuromodulation could also be applied to sensate parts of the body to warn of detrusor hyperreflexia at bladder capacity.

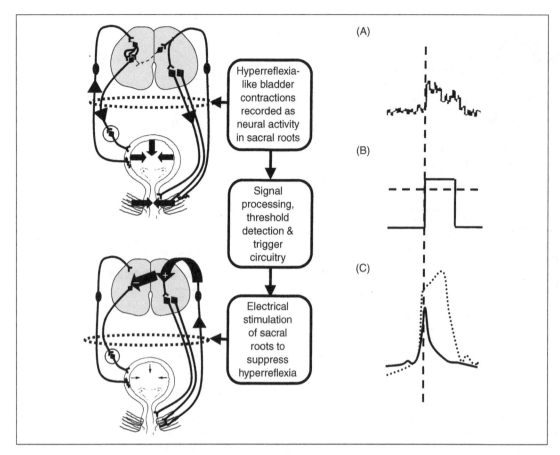

Figure 26.6

Sacral nerve activity as feedback control for conditional neuromodulation. (A) A miniature electrical signal (<0.5 μV) from the sacral nerves associated with a hyperreflexia-like contraction in an experimental animal. (B) Using special signal processing techniques it is possible to detect the changes and then activate stimulation of the sacral posterior roots for conditional neuromodulation. (C) The hyperreflexia-like contraction (dotted line) without neuromodulation is very effectively suppressed (solid line) when stimulation is applied.

What sort of reliable detection system for conditional neuromodulation could be incorporated into an implant? Brindley was the first to suggest that it might be possible to monitor bladder pressure by implant and use the information to control electrical stimulation of the pudendal nerves to inhibit unstable bladder contractions. Subsequently, an implanted applanation tonometer was developed which could be sutured onto the bladder wall to record pressure. However, tests to assess its long-term performance in experimental animals were not very successful, as the device eroded or became dislodged from the bladder.[23] Further obstacles, such as infection and encrustation, preclude the immediate development and implementation of such vesical devices.

Recently it has been shown in experimental animals that it is possible to detect very small electroneurographic signals at fractional microvolt levels, using sophisticated recording techniques, from the afferents in the mixed sacral nerve roots during hyperreflexia-like bladder contractions.[24] The recorded signals could then be used to trigger stimulation of the pudendal or sacral posterior nerves to inhibit conditionally in a feedback loop those same contractions (Figure 26.6).

Some preliminary work in patients with SCI during implantation of sacral anterior root stimulators indicates that detecting bladder contractions from the sacral sensory nerves may also be possible.[25,26] However, although an implanted conditional neuromodulation device may be feasible in people with a spinal cord injury it is likely to be considerably more complex than present devices tried in animals and will have to be very reliable. Implantable microcircuits for detecting minute neural signals in humans which could be used to activate conditional neuromodulation are now being developed for this purpose.[27]

Whether detrusor hyperreflexia is to be controlled by automatic conditional stimulation or simply by continuous neuromodulation the interesting possibility now exists for combining the benefits of bladder emptying with control of reflex incontinence in one implantable sacral root stimulator.

The sacral posterior and anterior root stimulator implant

This new concept is being developed using a single implant (Finetech–Brindley) to combine bladder emptying through sacral anterior root stimulation with posterior sacral root stimulation to prevent reflex incontinence.[28] If successful, the major advantage of SPARSI would be restoration of bladder function without the need for sacral deafferentation.

In a recent study, five patients with a suprasacral spinal injury have been implanted with a standard bilateral extradural Finetech–Brindley device, but without sacral deafferentation, to test the concept of SPARSI. These patients were part of the neuromodulation study described above.[22] A significant finding in this study, reported first in 2001,[29] demonstrated that the benefits of neuromodulation by a SPARSI implant at home were comparable to the effects of oxybutynin in improving functional bladder capacity in the same patient (Figure 26.7). Furthermore, the improvement also compared favorably with the benefits of sacral deafferentation. Another interesting finding, which agrees with other studies of sacral neuromodulation for the overactive bladder (e.g. using the Medtronic sacral nerve stimulator), showed that the effects do not necessarily diminish appreciably with time, but that when stimulation is stopped symptoms such as incontinence return. With SPARSI, bladder capacity always returned to much smaller values in less than 24 h when stimulation was stopped.

Unfortunately in this small group of patients bladder emptying was not always very efficient despite the generation of adequate bladder pressures. The concept of SPARSI using extradural electrodes will only be successful when good bladder emptying (as in the original SARS with posterior rhizotomy) is also achieved. SARS uses post-stimulus voiding to empty the bladder efficiently so that during the intervals between bursts of stimulation, urethral pressure is much lower than bladder pressure, allowing unimpeded urine flow. In SPARSI, where both striated sphincter and bladder reflex pathways are intact, there can be residual increases in urethral pressure as the slow bladder pressure develops in the post-stimulation gap (Figure 26.8). This is reflex detrusor-sphincter dyssynergia, and leads to urinary outflow obstruction, making emptying much less reliable (compare with Figure 26.2).

As Brindley suggested,[9] bladder emptying is improved by posterior rhizotomy, and so implantation of a Finetech–Brindley device for bladder emptying without a rhizotomy in patients with severe detrusor-external sphincter dyssynergia would not currently be advised. Interestingly, Brindley's early patients often did not have a rhizotomy, and most achieved good emptying, but the devices were intrathecal and there was almost certainly posterior root damage in many cases.[30]

The SPARSI concept could achieve its original objective once the problems of bladder emptying are overcome. A number of possible solutions to control detrusor-external sphincter dyssynergia are available – including pharmacotherapy (e.g. Botulinum toxin), stenting, and surgery (sphincterotomy) – but ideally we should find a neurophysiological solution which could be applied through the same stimulating implant.

Selective stimulation of sacral roots to prevent detrusor-sphincter dyssynergia

Sacral anterior roots contain, among other pathways, both the large somatic nerves to the urethral striated sphincter and the small preganglionic parasympathetic nerves to the bladder detrusor smooth muscle. Consequently, during anterior root stimulation, bladder emptying is impaired by coactivation of these two groups of nerve fibers (see Figure 26.2). This is the reason for adopting the post-stimulus voiding technique,[31] which takes advantage of the rapid relaxation of the sphincter and slow contraction of the detrusor to achieve good bladder emptying. This type of voiding is not particularly physiological, but it is efficient. However, in the presence of intact sacral reflexes (i.e. no rhizotomy), the dyssynergia persists in the gap between the bursts of stimulation to prevent efficient emptying, as described above. For this problem to be overcome, tests are now being done using a variety of techniques, including sphincter fatiguing methods and selective nerve blocking ('anode block') of sphincter motor pathways.

The principle of selective electrical stimulation relies on blocking the large nerve fibers to the striated muscles by anodal hyperpolarization to prevent the passage of action potentials down the nerve, while permitting the flow of action potentials along the small motor nerves to the bladder muscle (Figure 26.9). To prevent 'anode-break' excitation when the individual stimulating pulses in the train switch off, they must be switched off slowly.

This method of stimulation was originally shown by Brindley and Craggs to be effective in experimental animals using a specially designed chronically implanted tripolar electrode and triangular-shaped electrical pulses to stimulate the sacral anterior roots selectively.[32] The range of stimulating currents where sphincter motor potentials were blocked while bladder pressure increased was relatively small but effective. However, Brindley and Craggs did not demonstrate bladder emptying in their experiments.

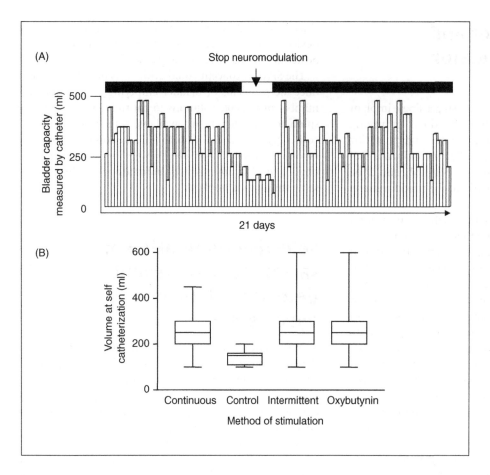

Figure 26.7
Neuromodulation through SPARSI at home. (A) A continuous set of data showing that over a 3-week period neuromodulation through the implant maintained good bladder capacity when compared to a short period during which stimulation was stopped. (B) Continuous stimulation was shown to be comparable to intermittent stimulation given on a 50 s 'on' to 50 s 'off' cycle and both gave bladder volumes statistically greater than no stimulation during a control period. An interesting finding was the near equivalence of benefit with neuromodulation alone or oxybutynin (an anticholinergic drug to block detrusor hyperreflexic contractions) alone.

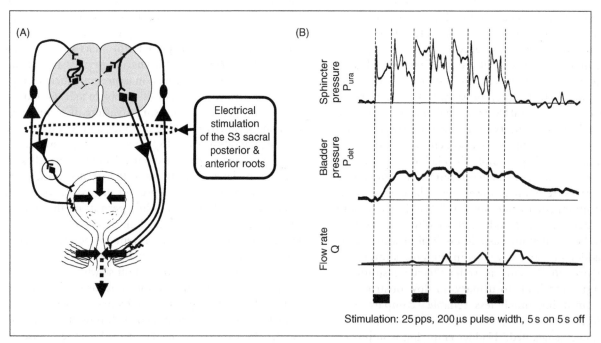

Figure 26.8
Bladder contraction through SPARSI. (A) Stimulation of the mixed sacral roots through extradural electrodes or separated roots through intrathecal electrodes activates both efferent (motor) and afferent (sensory) pathways either directly or reflexly. (B) Good bladder pressures are generated by bursts of stimulation, but voiding is very inefficient in the gaps as a result of reflex contractions of the sphincter, elevating urethral pressure above the bladder pressure (compare with the traces shown in Figure 26.2).

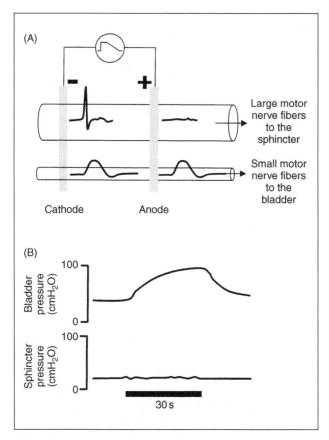

Figure 26.9

Selective blockade of the motor nerves to the sphincter.
(A) Applying triangular or quasitrapezoidal electrical pulses to groups of different diameter nerve fibers in the sacral roots it is possible to find a range of stimulating currents that block the large motor nerves to the striated sphincter at the anode electrode (anode block), while still permitting conduction down the small motor nerves to the bladder detrusor muscle.
(B) Selective anode blockade of the sphincter successfully applied while a good bladder contraction is elicited during stimulation with a train of triangular pulses at 30 pulses per second.

Interestingly, a similar type of tripolar electrode is used in the standard intrathecal Finetech–Brindley SARS implant, so theoretically it should be possible to investigate the possibility of using this technique for actual bladder emptying in patients. However, to prevent reflex effects on all of the motor fibers to the sphincter it may be necessary to apply anode blockade to all of the sacral anterior roots simultaneously.

It has been shown that during implantation of a Finetech–Brindley SARS it is possible to demonstrate intraoperatively that an anode-blocking technique with long rectangular pulses can be used to get selective stimulation in anesthetised patients,[33] but again efficient bladder emptying was not demonstrated. Recently, it has been claimed that physiological micturition (i.e. natural voiding

where the sphincter relaxes during contraction of the bladder to produce a good stream of urine and complete bladder emptying) is possible using a modified Finetech–Brindley intrathecal electrode to activate the bladder in the dog.[34] Unfortunately, this study did not present data to substantiate the claim but did demonstrate a significant lowering of sphincter pressure simultaneous with good bladder pressures during sacral stimulation with quasitrapezoidal pulses.[35]

So, it remains to be seen whether such selective stimulation techniques can produce efficient voiding; the evidence from animal studies is promising[36] but awaits a successful resolution in patients in whom we may wish to preserve all sacral reflexes. When resolved, the concept of SPARSI described above is more likely to become a realistic possibility.

Prospects for complete restoration of bladder control by neuroprosthesis

In this chapter we have considered some old, new, and emerging developments and technologies using sacral root stimulation which together may in the future provide full restoration of bladder control to the neurogenic bladder (Figure 26.10).

In recent times our understanding of the neurophysiology of the lower urinary tract has advanced in ways that may lead to even more sophisticated ways of controlling the neurogenic bladder, bowel, and sexual dysfunction. Of these emerging techniques currently being developed in experimental animal models is the exciting possibility of actually stimulating and recording from the nuclei of origin of the sacral motor pathways in the spinal cord. Intraspinal microstimulation, as it has become known, involves inserting fine wire electrodes into the tracts in these structures.[37–40] Interestingly, as with sacral root stimulation, the problem of controlling the dyssynergia of the urethral sphincter presents as the most difficult problem to be overcome in these experimental studies. Neurophysiological studies have shown that spinal interneurons are very much involved in the segmental coordination of the bladder and sphincters and therefore it may become possible to activate these interneuronal pathways by stimulation to get the synergic control necessary to empty the bladder efficiently.[41] It seems that considerable technical advances will be needed to apply microstimulation, not least the problem of keeping fine microelectrodes in close contact with the appropriate neural substrates while at the same time preventing tethering of the spinal cord, which in itself could cause significant damage.

Whichever future development provides the best and safest solution for controlled neurostimulation it still

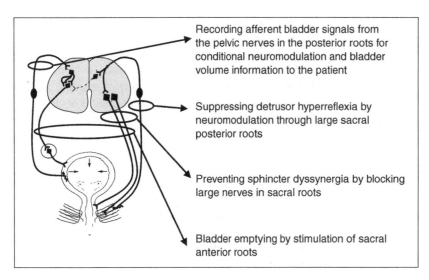

Recording afferent bladder signals from the pelvic nerves in the posterior roots for conditional neuromodulation and bladder volume information to the patient

Suppressing detrusor hyperreflexia by neuromodulation through large sacral posterior roots

Preventing sphincter dyssynergia by blocking large nerves in sacral roots

Bladder emptying by stimulation of sacral anterior roots

Figure 26.10
Possible techniques to overcome problems of the neurogenic bladder in SCI.

remains that for a significant number of patients, with lower motor neuron problems, such as corda equina lesions, the possibilities for restoration of pelvic functions is problematic. For this important group of patients, coordination of the bladder and sphincter is less important than impaired contraction, but problems of incontinence and the inability to void remain impediments to good management and quality of life. Perhaps the new surgical techniques for neural repair and regeneration of the motor pathways may offer some prospect for helping these patients.[42] There may even be a place to assist or combine this neuronal repair with neurostimulation.[43] Although recovery of central afferent pathways is less likely in these repairs, any sacral reflexes that are restored may be more aberrant than in suprasacral injuries and therefore present with new and more difficult challenges to be overcome.

Finally, some of the ideas presented here might be limited by current technology but this is very likely to become realizable in the near future. Such technological advances might include more appropriately designed and stable electrode–nerve interfaces (especially important if the electrodes are to be implanted inside the spinal cord or brain), new implantable integrated electronics capable of processing tiny signals and delivering patterned stimuli, and improved systems for transferring or using power efficiently in implants. A new range of intelligent sensor technology for detecting physiological changes in the body is likely to emerge. The future may also see the increased use of telemetries for computerized control of implants, including the transfer of data to and from these devices to improve function.

Summary

Ultimately, it is hoped that by combining conditional neuromodulation for reflex incontinence with selected neurostimulation for bladder emptying we can completely control the neurogenic bladder without cutting any sacral sensory nerves. The big challenge will probably be to overcome the detrusor-sphincter dyssynergia resulting from the emergence of aberrant reflexes following spinal injury. By preserving all pelvic reflexes, including those for erection, ejaculation, and bowel control, as well as those essential to guard against stress incontinence, we will help to reassure people with a spinal cord injury that this technology will improve their quality of life until the time comes when neural repair becomes a realistic possibility for them.

References

1. Brindley GS, Polkey CE, Rushton DN. Sacral anterior root stimulators for bladder control in paraplegia. Paraplegia 1982; 20:365–381.

2. Schmidt RA. Treatment of the unstable bladder. Urology 1991; 37:28–32.

3. Tanagho EA. Concepts of neuromodulation. Neurourol Urodyn 1993; 12:487–488.

4. Selzman AA, Hampel N. Urologic complications of spinal cord injury. Urol Clin N Am 1993; 20:453–464.

5. Grill WM, Craggs MD, Foreman RD, et al. Emerging clinical applications of electrical stimulation: opportunities for restoration of function. J Rehab Res Dev 2001; 38:641–653.

6. Jezernik S, Craggs M, Grill WM, et al. Electrical stimulation for the treatment of bladder dysfunction: current status and future possibilities. Neurol Res 2002; 24:413–430.

7. Brindley GS. An implant to empty the bladder or close the urethra. J Neurol Neurosurg Psychiatry 1977; 43:1083–1090.

8. van Kerrebroeck PEV. Worldwide experience with the Finetech–Brindley Sacral Anterior Root Stimulator. Neurourol Urodyn 1993; 12:497–503.

9. Brindley GS. The first 500 patients with sacral anterior root stimulator implants: general description. Paraplegia 1994; 32:795–805.

10. Tanagho EA, Schmidt RA. Electrical stimulation in the clinical management of the neurogenic bladder. J Urol 1988; 140:1331–1339.

11. Schmidt RA, Jonas U, Oleson KA, et al. for the Sacral Nerve Stimulation Study Group. Sacral nerve stimulation for the treatment of refractory urinary urge incontinence. J Urol 1999; 162:352–357.

12. Chartier-Kastler EJ, Bosch RJL, Perrigot M, et al. Long-term results of sacral nerve stimulation (S3) for the treatment of neurogenic refractory urge incontinence related to detrusor hyperreflexia. J Urol 2000; 164:1476–1480.

13. Sheriff MKM, Shah PJR, Fowler C, et al. Neuromodulation of detrusor hyperreflexia by functional magnetic stimulation of the sacral roots. Br J Urol 1996; 78:39–46.

14. Lindström S, Fall M, Carlsson CA, Erlandson BE. The neurophysiological basis of bladder inhibition in response to intravaginal electrical stimulation. J Urol 1983; 129:405–410.

15. Craggs MD, McFarlane JP. Neuromodulation of the lower urinary tract. Exp Physiol 1999; 84:149–160.

16. Nakamura M, Sakurai T. Bladder inhibition by penile electrical stimulation. Br J Urol 1984; 56:413–415.

17. Wheeler JS, Walter JS, Zaszczurynski PJ. Bladder inhibition by penile nerve stimulation in spinal cord injury patients. J Urol 1992; 147:100–103.

18. Shah N, Edhem I, Knight SL, Craggs MD. Acute suppression of provoked detrusor hyperreflexia with detrusor sphincter dyssynergia by electrical stimulation of the dorsal penile nerves in patients with a spinal injury. Eur Urol 1998; 33(suppl): 60.

19. Kirkham A, Knight S, Casey A, et al. Conditional neuromodulation of end-fill hyperreflexia to increase bladder capacity in spinally injured patients. Neurourol Urodyn 2000; 19:515–516.

20. Kirkham APS, Shah NC, Knight SL, et al. The acute effects of continuous and conditional neuromodulation on the bladder in spinal cord injury. Spinal Cord 2001; 39:420–428.

21. Zafirakis H, Knight SL, Shah PJR, et al. Intermittent versus continuous electrical stimulation of the dorsal penile nerve on bladder capacity in spinal cord injury. Neurourol Urodyn 2002; 21:400.

22. Kirkham APS, Knight SL, Casey ATM, et al. Neuromodulation of sacral nerve roots 2 to 4 with a Fintech–Brindley sacral posterior and anterior root stimulator. Spinal Cord 2002; 40:272–281.

23. Koldewijn EL, van Kerrebroeck PE, Schaafsma E, et al. Bladder pressure sensors in an animal model. J Urol 1994; 151:1376–1384.

24. Jezernik S, Grill WM, Sinkjaer T. Detection and inhibition of hyperreflexia-like bladder contractions in the cat by sacral nerve root recording and electrical stimulation. Neurourol Urodyn 2001; 20:215–230.

25. Sinkjaer T, Rijkhoff N, Haugland M, et al. Electroneurographic (ENG) signals from intradural S3 dorsal sacral nerve roots in a patient with a suprasacral spinal cord injury. Proc 5th Int Functional Electrical Stimulation Soc Conf, Aalborg, Denmark, 2000:361–364.

26. Grill WM, Creasey GH, Wu K, Takaoka Y. Detection of hyperreflexia-like increases in bladder pressure by recording of sensory nerve activity in human spinal cord injury. Abstract in Proc 5th Int Functional Electrical Stimulation Soc Conf, Aalborg, Denmark, 2000:234.

27. Donaldson N de N, Zhou L, Haugland M, Sinkjaer T. An implantable telemeter for long-term electroneurographic recordings in animals and humans. Proc 5th Int Functional Electrical Stimulation Soc Conf, Aalborg, Denmark, 2000:378–381.

28. Craggs MD, Casey A, Shah PJR, et al. SPARSI: an implant to empty the bladder and control incontinence with posterior rhizotomy in spinal cord injury. Br J Urol Int 2000; 85(suppl 5): 2.

29. Kirkham APS, Knight SL, Casey ATM, et al. Acute and chronic use of a sacral posterior and anterior nerve root stimulator to increase bladder capacity in spinal cord injury. Proc 6th Int Functional Electrical Stimulation Soc Conf, Cleveland, Ohio, USA, 2001:172–174.

30. Brindley GS, Polkey CE, Rushton DN, Cardozo L. Sacral anterior root stimulators for bladder control in paraplegia: the first 50 cases. J Neurol Neurosurg Psychiatry 1986; 49:1104–1114.

31. Jonas U, Tanagho EA. Studies on the feasibility of urinary bladder evacuation by direct spinal cord stimulation. II. Poststimulus voiding: a way to overcome outflow resistance. Invest Urol 1975; 13:151–153.

32. Brindley GS, Craggs MD. A technique of anodally blocking large nerve fibres through chronically implanted electrodes. J Neurol Neurosurg Psychiatry 1980; 43:1083–1090.

33. Rijkhoff NJM, Wijkstra H, van Kerrebroeck PEV, Debruyne FMJ. Selective detrusor activation by electrical sacral root stimulation in spinal cord injury. J Urol 1997; 157:1504–1508.

34. Seif Ch, Braun PM, Bross J, et al. Selective block of urethral sphincter contraction using a modified Brindley electrode in sacral anterior root stimulation of the dog. Neurourol Urodyn 2002; 21:502–510.

35. Fang ZP, Mortimer JT. Selective activation of small motor axons by quasitrapezoidal current pulses. IEEE Trans Biomed Engng 1991; 38:168–174.

36. Grünewald V, Bhadra N, Creasey GH, Mortimer JT. Functional conditions of micturition induced by selective sacral anterior root stimulation. World J Urol 1998; 16:329–336.

37. Carter RR, McCreery DB, Woodford BJ, et al. Micturition control by microstimulation of the sacral spinal cord of the cat: acute studies. IEEE Trans Rehab Engng 1995; 3:206–214.

38. Grill WM, Bhadra N, Wang B. Bladder and urethral pressures evoked by microstimulation of the sacral spinal cord in cats. Brain Res 1999; 836:19–30.

39. Tai C, Booth AM, de Groat WC, Roppolo JR. Colon and anal sphincter contractions evoked by microstimulation of the sacral spinal cord in cats. Brain Res 2001; 889:38–48.

40. Tai C, Booth AM, de Groat WC, Roppolo JR. Penile erection produced by microstimulation of the sacral spinal cord of the cat. IEEE Trans Rehab Engng 1998; 6:374–381.

41. Grill WM. Electrical activation of spinal neural circuits: application to motor system neural prostheses. Neuromodulation 2000; 3:97–106.

42. Carlstedt T. Approaches permitting and enhancing motoneuron regeneration after spinal cord, ventral root, plexus and peripheral nerve injuries. Curr Opin Neurol 2000; 13:683–686.

43. Grill WM, McDonald JW, Peckham PH, et al. At the interface: convergence of neural regeneration and neural prostheses for restoration of function. J Rehab Res Dev 2001; 38:633–639.

27

Neuroprotection and repair after spinal cord injury

W Dalton Dietrich

Introduction

Injury to the spinal cord initiates a cascade of events that ultimately leads to cell death and neurological dysfunction. Various biochemical and molecular pathways are activated after spinal cord injury (SCI) in both the acute and subacute injury setting that may be targeted for therapeutic intervention. Clarification of what dominant injury mechanisms may be attenuated by pharmacological and hypothermic therapies is an active area of investigation. Also, there is much excitement in the area of transplantation and repair therapy in chronic SCI. New strategies are being used to alter the local environment to make it more permissive for axonal regeneration. The replacement of lost cell populations by using transplantation strategies as well as the delivery of genes or proteins to enhance axonal regeneration is another exciting research direction. In this chapter, we review various neuroprotective strategies as well as several transplantation strategies directed toward a cure of paralysis following SCI.

Neuroprotection following spinal cord injury

In acutely injured SCI patients, especially those having incomplete lesions, neuroprotective strategies have the potential of limiting secondary injury mechanisms. Although methylprednisolone (MP) treatment has been reported to benefit a subpopulation of SCI patients,[1] recent publications have questioned the benefits of MP as the standard therapy for acute SCI.[3–5] Thus, new therapies need to be developed and tested. Glutamate, the major endogenous excitatory neurotransmitter in the central nervous system (CNS), has been shown to mediate pathological processes in many injury models, including SCI. With the use of intracerebral microdialysis, sampling

of the extracellular space has shown massive release of glutamate as well as other neurotransmitters during and following SCI.[5]

In recent studies, Wrathall and colleagues[6] have reported that treatment with NBQX, a highly selective antagonist of the non-N-methyl-D-aspartate excitatory amino acid receptor, reduces histopathological and functional deficits following traumatic SCI. Likewise, convincing support for the importance of free radicals and lipid peroxidation in SCI models has been derived from studies reporting that oxygen radical scavengers or the use of inhibitors of lipid peroxidation can limit neuronal damage and improve outcome.[7,8] In a model of traumatic brain injury (TBI), the novel inhibitor of lipid peroxidation, LY341122, was reported to improve histopathological outcome only when the agent was given in the early post-injury period.[9] Thus, when evaluating the potential use of agents that block excitotoxic or free radical-mediated damage, questions regarding the therapeutic window for these strategies must be addressed. Obviously, if the window of opportunity has passed prior to the patient's arrival in the emergency room, these pathomechanisms may not be appropriate targets for therapeutic strategies.

A fundamental question regarding pathophysiology of SCI is the nature of cell death: is it necrosis or apoptosis?[10] Necrosis is characterized by the early compromise of cell membrane integrity, leading to a loss of ionic homeostasis and prominent cell swelling. Apoptosis reflects the activation of intrinsic genetic programs, leading to the endonuclease cleavage of DNA and eventual death of the cell.[11] While the death of neurons induced by ischemia or trauma has been classically considered to be necrosis, growing evidence is suggestive that some cells undergo apoptosis following SCI.[11,12] Indeed, recent experimental and clinical data have suggested that the death of oligodendrocytes following traumatic SCI involves activation of apoptotic pathways.[12,13] This research direction is particularly important because the potential for developing antiapoptotic strategies to target late occurring cell death after SCI is a real possibility.[14-16] For example, the antiapoptotic gene Bcl-2 has been reported to inhibit neuronal death induced by glutamate. The potential use of gene therapy to introduce protective genes into the host to enhance cellular neuroprotective mechanisms or antagonize cytotoxic products associated with apoptosis is an exciting research direction.

An emerging strategy for the treatment of CNS injury is directed toward inflammatory events.[17] Experimental studies have indicated roles of several inflammatory molecules in the pathophysiology, including tumor necrosis factor α (TNFα) and interleukin-β (IL-β), as well as various chemokines.[18,19] In this regard, recent experimental data have demonstrated that the administration of the potent anti-inflammatory cytokine IL-10 improves both histopathological and locomotive function following traumatic SCI in rats.[18] In that study, IL-10 treatment significantly decreased overall contusion volume, preserved the white matter tracts, and improved behavioral recovery as assessed by the Basso, Bresnahan, and Beattie (BBB) open-field test. In terms of therapeutic windows for anti-inflammatory strategies, current investigations are determining how long after SCI IL-10 can be given to promote improved outcome. Interestingly, IL-10 in combination with MP has been reported to reduce tissue injury after SCI.[20] Thus, combination therapy may also be advantageous in specific clinical conditions.

Mild-to-moderate hypothermia has been shown to be neuroprotective in many experimental models of CNS injury.[21,22] Local as well as systemic hypothermia has been used by various laboratories to prevent energy failure, reduce histopathological damage, diminish free radical activity, and elevated levels of glutamate following injury. Recent studies have evaluated the relationship between systemic and epidural temperature after SCI and the effects of moderate systemic hypothermia following traumatic SCI in rats. In one study, post-traumatic hypothermia (32–33°C) initiated 30 min after injury for a 4-hour period significantly protected against locomotive deficits and reduced the area of tissue damage.[23] Experimental findings also indicate that post-traumatic hypothermia following SCI reduces polymorphonuclear leukocyte (PMNL) accumulation.[24] In a recent study, post-traumatic hypothermia significantly reduced myeloperoxidase (MPO) activity (an enzyme for neutrophil infusion) compared with normothermic animals. Thus, a potential mechanism by which hypothermia improves outcome following SCI is by attenuating post-traumatic inflammation. Whether mild systemic or local hypothermia can be used clinically to inhibit the detrimental effects of post-injury hyperthermia and/or protect the spinal cord from secondary injury merits further investigation.

Nitric oxide (NO) has been shown to play an important role in the pathophysiology of SCI.[25,26] Importantly, NO has been reported to be both neurodestructive and neuroprotective, depending on the location and time of release.[27]

In a recent study, the effects of inhibiting inducible NO synthase (iNOS) by aminoguanidine treatment were investigated.[26] Treated rats demonstrated improved hind limb function and decreased histopathological injury compared with nontreated traumatized rats. Immunostaining for iNOS indicated that a significant cellular source of iNOS protein appeared to be invading PMNLs. Thus, in the acute injury state, therapeutic interventions including hypothermia and aminoguanidine may be protective by attenuating the release of NO-induced cytotoxic products from PMNLs. Additional research in the area of neuroprotection is required to clarify what injury mechanisms may be targeted for therapeutic intervention.

Cellular transplantation following spinal cord injury

There is an unprecedented sense of enthusiasm within the scientific community that one day therapeutic strategies will be developed to treat paralysis following SCI. The replacement of lost cell populations by cell transplantation strategies as well as utilizing helper cells to deliver genes or proteins to enhance axonal regeneration is currently being investigated in many laboratories throughout the world.[28] Indeed, several types of intraspinal transplants have effectively treated experimental models of human diseases. The peripheral nervous system provides an appropriate environment for axonal regeneration. David and Aguayo[29] first demonstrated that segments of sciatic nerve could be used as bridges between the medulla and lower cervical or thoracic spinal cord. In that study, evidence was presented that axons from nerve cells in the injured spinal cord and brainstem could elongate for long distances when the glial environment of the CNS was replaced by peripheral nerve. Axonal elongation is thought to be due to the presence of Schwann cells (SCs) that produce neurotrophic factors and synthesize and secrete elements of extracellular matrix, including laminin and cell adhesion molecules. Indeed, the use of guidance channels lined with SCs has been successfully utilized to support axonal regeneration following transection of the adult spinal cord.[30]

Most recently, the axonal growth-promoting properties of adult olfactory ensheathing glia (OEG) and SC-filled guidance channels have been utilized to bridge spinal cord stumps and to enhance regeneration into the host spinal cord.[31] Supraspinal serotinergic axons were reported to cross the transection gap through the bridges and elongate in white and periaqueductal gray. Long-distance regeneration (at least 2.5 cm) of injured ascending propriospinal axons was also observed in the rostral spinal cord. In another study, spinal implantation of OEG was performed in adult rats after rhizotomy to promote axonal regeneration and bladder function.[32] Immediately after rhizotomy,

OEG cells were injected into the vicinity of the sacral parasympathetic nucleus and several roots reattached to the cord with fibrin glue. Importantly, both anatomical regeneration of bladder wall primary afferents as well as recovered bladder function were observed. Taken together, this study and others indicate that EG appear to provide injured spinal axons with factors for long-distance regeneration. Successful regeneration may, therefore, be attained eventually by using a combination of 'helper cell' transplantation strategies following adult CNS injury.

The infusion of various neurotrophins to enhance axonal regeneration following SCI has also been utilized in various experimental models. Grill et al[33] determined the effects of transgenic cellular delivery of neurotrophin-3 (NT-3) on the morphological and functional disturbances following SCI in rats. In that study, experimental subjects received grafts of fibroblasts genetically modified to produce NT-3. Importantly, the local cellular delivery of NT-3 in this model of SCI led to regrowth of corticospinal tracts and improved functional recovery at 1 and 3 months post-injury. In a study of SCs, Tuszynski et al[34] reported robust growth of host neurotrophin-responsive axons after grafting with genetically modified SC, producing high levels of human nerve growth factor (NGF). Thus, the use of genetically engineered cells to locally deliver various neurotrophins represents an important approach to enhancing axonal regeneration.

Neuronal progenitors isolated from the adult CNS may one day be used to replace populations of neurons and oligodendrocytes destroyed following injury. Recently, the consequences of transplanting embryonic stem cells into the injured rat spinal cord on recovery of function has been assessed. McDonald et al[35] transplanted neuro-differentiated mouse embryonic stem cells into the injured spinal cord to determine the fate of these cells as well as to determine whether the transplant procedure led to behavioral recovery. Histological analysis demonstrated that the transplanted cells survived and differentiated into astrocytes, oligodendrocytes, and neurons. Importantly, gait analysis showed improved hind limb function, weight support, and coordination in rats transplanted with stem cells, compared with controls. Ongoing research continues to investigate novel sources of stem cells that one day may be isolated from SCI subjects prior to transplantation procedures.

Although inflammatory processes have been implicated in the pathophysiology of neuronal cell injury following SCI,[18] recent data indicate that activated macrophages may also enhance functional recovery.[36,37] Rapalino et al[37] have reported that bloodborne macrophages stimulated with segments of rat peripheral sciatic nerve and transplanted into the lesion site lead to improved electrophysiological, morphological, and behavioral outcome after SC transection, compared with non-treated animals. Based on these findings, it appears that therapeutic strategies to attenuate inflammatory responses after SCI may have to target early but not later occurring inflammatory processes. Indeed, the inflammatory cascade appears to be extremely complicated, and more experimental work is required to assess what specific inflammatory processes need to be attenuated or promoted after SCI.

Future directions

In terms of both acute neuroprotection and cellular transplantation strategies for the treatment of spinal cord dysfunction, great progress has been made in the last several years. In the area of neuroprotection, future investigations will target combination therapy where multiple strategies may be used to promote more complete protection and recovery of function following SCI. One exciting direction involves the use of mild hypothermia plus pharmacotherapy. Indeed, recent studies in cerebral ischemia found that mild hypothermia plus IL-10 protected the brain better than either therapy alone.[22] Also, following SCI, a synergistic effect of basic fibroblast growth factor (bFGF) and MP on neurological function was reported.[38] In addition, better therapies must be developed to target white matter pathology, which plays an extremely important role in the functional consequences of SCI.

Recent breakthroughs in the cell biology of CNS injury have demonstrated the regenerative capacity of the adult spinal cord to recover function under the right circumstances. Many laboratories throughout the world have reported novel strategies that appear to be successful in converting nonpermissive environments for regeneration into permissive ones. Future studies will continue to investigate combination therapies to target axonal regeneration that may also include neuroprotective strategies to protect cellular transplants and enhance growth. It is conceivable that the use of multiple helper cells in addition to the administration of neuroprotective agents, neurotrophic factors, and antibodies that target inhibitory proteins will all be necessary to one day successfully regenerate the spinal cord. For example, while several recent publications have reported significant degrees of axonal regeneration using peripheral nerve or SC grafts,[39,40] unsuccessful re-entry into the dorsal cord has been a major limitation of this repair procedure.

Recent studies suggest that the formation of an astroglial scar and/or an inhibitory molecular barrier may inhibit fibers from exiting the grafts.[41,42] Thus, strategies including the use of neutralizing antibodies against growth inhibitors or enzyme treatments have been investigated in some regeneration studies.[43–45] In a recent investigation, the effects of degrading chondroitin sulfate proteoglycan with chrondroitinase ABC on sensory and motor projections were studied.[45] Importantly, treatment up-regulated a regeneration-associated protein and promoted regeneration of both ascending sensory and descending corticospinal tract axons. Combination therapies, including bridging strategies, cellular transplantation, growth factor administration, and the blockage of inhibitory factors, may have therapeutic potential for the treatment of human SCI. These reparative strategies, combined with rehabilitative procedures to relearn motor tasks, are critical in the overall cure strategy.[46] As new circuits are formed, remaining as well as new neural pathways must become functional to execute stepping and standing. Thus, the use of robotically based assistive devices may be necessary to promote circuit function and motor recovery as well as improved cardiovascular, pulmonary, and skeletal systems.[46] The correct combination of treatments in both the acute and chronic injury setting continues to be an exciting area of investigation in the field of SCI.

Acknowledgments

I would like to thank The Miami Project faculty and fellows for helpful discussions and Charlaine Rowlette for editorial assistance and manuscript preparation.

References

1. Bracken MB, Shepard M, Holford TR, et al. Administration of methylprednisolone for 24 or 48 hours or tirilazad mesylate for 48 hours in the treatment of acute spinal cord. JAMA 1997; 277:1597–1604.

2. Hulbert RJ. Methylprednisolone for acute spinal cord injury: an inappropriate standard of care. J Neurosurg 2000; 93:1–7.

3. Rabchevsky AG, Fugaccia I, Sullivan PG, et al. Efficacy of methylprednisolone therapy for the injured rat spinal cord. J Neurosci Res 2002; 68:7–18.

4. Short DJ, El Masry WS, Jones PW. High dose methylprednisolone in the management of acute spinal cord injury – a systematic review from a clinical perspective. Spinal Cord 2000; 38:273–286.

5. Painter SC, Wum SW, Faden AI. Alteration in extracellular amino acids after traumatic spinal cord injury. Ann Neurol 1990; 27:96–99.

6. Wrathall JR, Teng YD, Marriott R. Delayed antagonism of AMPA/kainate receptors reduces long-term functional deficits resulting from spinal cord trauma. Exp Neurol 1997; 145:565–573.

7. Behrmann DL, Bresnahan JC, Beattie MS. Modeling of acute spinal cord injury in the rat: neuroprotection and enhanced recovery with methylprednisolone, U-74006F and YM-14673. Exp Neurol 1994; 126:61–75.

8. Liu D, Liu J, Wen J. Elevation of hydrogen peroxide after spinal cord injury detected by using the fenton reaction. Free Rad Biol Med 1999; 27(3/4):478–482.

9. Wada K, Alonso OF, Busto R, et al. Early treatment with a novel inhibitor of lipid peroxidation (LY341122) improves histopathological outcome after moderate fluid percussion brain injury in rats. Neurosurgery 1999; 45:601–608.

10. Keane RW, Kraydieh S, Lotocki G, et al. Apoptotic and anti-apoptotic mechanisms following spinal cord injury. J Neuropathol Exp Neurol 2001; 60:422–429.

11. Kato H, Kanellopoulos GK, Matsuo S, et al. Neuronal apoptosis and necrosis following spinal cord ischemia in the rat. Exp Neurol 1997; 148:464–474.

12. Crowe MJ, Bresnahan JC, Shuman SL, et al. Apoptosis and delayed degeneration after spinal cord injury in rats and monkeys. Nature Med 1997; 3:73–76.

13. Emery E, Aldana M, Bunge M, et al. Apoptosis after traumatic human spinal cord injury. J Neurosurg 1998; 89:911–920.

14. Osawa H, Keane RW, Marcillo AE, et al. Therapeutic strategies targeting caspase inhibition following spinal cord injury in rats. Exp Neurol 2002; 177:306–313.

15. Li M, Ona VO, Chen M, et al. Functional role and therapeutic implications of neuronal caspase-1 -3 in a mouse model of traumatic spinal cord injury. Neuroscience 2000; 99:333–342.

16. Springer JE, Azbil D, Knapp PE. Activation of the caspase-3 apoptosis cascade in traumatic spinal cord injury. Nature Med 1999; 5:943–946.

17. del Zoppo G, Ginis I, Hallenbeck JM, et al. Inflammation and stroke: putative role for cytokines, adhesion molecules and iNOS in brain response to ischemia. Brain Pathol 2000; 10:95–112.

18. Bethea JR, Nagashima H, Acosta MC, et al. Systemically administered interleukin-10 reduces tumor necrosis factor-alpha production and significantly improves functional recovery following traumatic spinal cord injury in rats. J Neurotrauma 1999; 16:851–863.

19. Kinoshita K, Chatzipanteli K, Vitarbo E, et al. Interleukin-1β messenger ribonucleic acid and protein levels after fluid percussion brain injury in rats: the importance of injury severity and brain temperature. Neurosurgery 2002; 51:195–203.

20. Takami T, Oudega M, Bethea JR, et al. Methylprednisolone and interleukin-10 reduce gray matter damage in the contused Fischer rat thoracic spinal cord but do not improve functional outcome. J Neurotrauma 2002; 19(5):653–666.

21. Dietrich WD. Therapeutic hypothermia in experimental models of traumatic brain injury. In: Hayashi N, ed. Brain hypothermia: pathology, pharmacology and treatment of severe brain injury. Tokyo: Springer-Verlag, 2000:39–46.

22. Dietrich WD, Busto R, Bethea JR. Postischemic hypothermia and IL-10 treatment provide long-lasting neuroprotection of CA1 hippocampus following transient global ischemia in rats. Exp Neurol 1999; 158:444–450.

23. Yu CG, Jimenez O, Marcillo AE, et al. Beneficial effects of modest systemic hypothermia on locomotor function and histopathological damage following contusion-induced spinal cord injury in rats. J Neurosurg 2000; 93:85–93.

24. Chatzipanteli K, Yanagawa Y, Marcillo A, et al. Posttraumatic hypothermia reduces polymorphonuclear leukocyte accumulation following spinal cord injury in rats. J Neurotrauma 2000; 17:321–332.

25. Callsen-Cencic P, Hoheisel U, Kask EA, et al. The controversy about spinal neuronal nitric oxide synthase: under which conditions is it up- or down-regulated? Cell Tissue Res 1999; 295:183–194.

26. Chatzipanteli K, Garcia R, Marcillo AE, et al. Temporal and segmental distribution of constitutive and inducible nitric oxide synthases following traumatic spinal cord injury: effect of aminoguanidine treatment. J Neurotrauma 2002; 19:639–651.

27. Sinz EH, Kochanek PM, Dixon CE, et al. Inducible nitric oxide synthase is an endogenous neuroprotectant after traumatic brain injury in rats and mice. J Clin Invest 1999; 104:647–656.

28. Sagen J, Bunge MB, Kleitman N. Transplantation strategies for treatment of spinal cord dysfunction and injury. In: Lanza RP, Langer R, Vacanti JP, eds. Principles of tissue engineering, 2nd edn. New York: Academic Press, 2000:799–820.

29. David S, Aguayo AJ. Axonal elongation into peripheral nervous system "bridges" after central nervous system injury in adult rats. Science 1981; 214:931–933.

30. Xu XM, Guénard V, Kleitman N, Bunge MB. Axonal regeneration into Schwann cell-seeded guidance channels grafted into transected adult rat spinal cord. J Comp Neurol 1995; 351:145–160.

31. Ramón-Cueto A, Plant GW, Avila J, Bunge MB. Long-distance axonal regeneration in the transected adult rat spinal cord is promoted by olfactory ensheathing glia transplants. J Neurosci 1998; 18:3803–3815.

32. Pascual JI, Gudiño-Cabrera G, Insausti R, Nieto-Sampedro M. Spinal implants of olfactory ensheathing cells promote axon regeneration and bladder activity after bilateral lumbosacral dorsal rhizotomy in the adult rat. J Urol 2002; 167:1522–1526.

33. Grill R, Murai K, Blesch A, et al. Cellular delivery of neurotrophin-3 promotes corticospinal axonal growth and partial functional recovery after spinal cord injury. J Neurosci 1997; 17:5560–5575.

34. Tuszynski MH, Weidner N, McCormack M, et al. Grafts of genetically modified Schwann cells to the spinal cord: survival, axon growth and myelination. Cell Trans 1998; 7(2):187–196.

35. McDonald JW, Liu X-Z, Qu Y, et al. Transplanted embryonic stem cells survive, differentiate and promote recovery in injured rat spinal cord. Nature Med 1999; 5:1410–1412.

36. Bethea JR, Dietrich WD. Targeting the host inflammatory response in traumatic spinal cord injury. Curr Opin Neurol 2002; 15:355–360.

37. Rapalino O, Lazarov-Spiegler O, Agranov E, et al. Implantation of stimulated homologous macrophages results in partial recovery of paraplegic rats. Nature Med 1998; 4:814–821.

38. Baffour R, Achanta K, Kaufman J, et al. Synergistic effect of basic fibroblast growth factor and methylprednisolone on neurological function after experimental spinal cord injury. J Neurosurg 1995; 83:105–110.

39. Guest JD, Rao A, Olson L, et al. The ability of human Schwann cell grafts to promote regeneration in the transected nude rat spinal cord. Exp Neurol 1997; 148:502–522.

40. Levi ADO, Dancausse H, Li X, et al. Peripheral nerve grafts promoting central nervous system regeneration after spinal cord injury in the primate. J Neurosurg 2002; (suppl 2) 96:107–205.

41. Snow DM, Lemmon V, Carrino DA, et al. Sulfated proteoglycans in astroglial barriers inhibit neurite outgrowth *in vivo*. Exp Neurol 1990; 109:111–130.

42. Schwab ME, Kapfhammer JP, Bandtlow CE. Inhibitors of neurite growth. Ann Rev Neurosci 1993; 16:565–595.

43. Oudega M, Rosano C, Sadi D, et al. Neutralizing antibodies against neurite growth inhibitor NI-35-250 do not promote regeneration of sensory axons in the adult rat spinal cord. Neuroscience 2000; 100(4):873–883.

44. Bregman BS, Kunkel-Bagden E, Schnell L, et al. Recovery from spinal cord injury mediated by antibodies to neurite growth inhibitors. Nature 1995; 378:498–501.

45. Bradbury EJ, Moon LD, Popat RJ, et al. Chondroitinase ABC promotes functional recovery after spinal cord injury. Nature 2002; 416:636–640.

46. Edgerton VR, deLeon RD, Harkema SJ, et al. Topical review. Retaining the injured spinal cord. J Physiol 2001; 533:15–22.

Part IV

Synthesis of treatment

Treatment alternatives for different types of neurogenic bladder dysfunction in adults

Erik Schick and Jacques Corcos

Introduction

Vesicourethral dysfunction secondary to degenerative processes, traumas, or neoplasias of the central or peripheral nervous system will most certainly have a deleterious effect on the patient's quality of life.

For centuries, the prognosis of these pathologies on patient survival was bad. We know from the Edwin Smith papyrus that as far back as 1600 BC the ancient Egyptians were aware of the relationship between the nervous system and urinary bladder function.[1] They considered spinal cord trauma as a 'disease not to treat'.[2]

Statistics on spinal cord trauma are available since World War I. The mortality rate was extremely high in those days – more than 90% – mainly due to urinary complications such as urosepsis and renal insufficiency. Dramatic improvements in prognosis came during World War II when Sir Ludwig Guttmann, in England, established specialized units to take care of these patients, and introduced the method of intermittent catheterization.[3] During the 1970s the use of urodynamics became more widespread, allowing a better understanding of the physiology and pathophysiology of the lower urinary tract. Translation of these new notions has significantly improved the prognosis of these patients.

The main goals in treating patients with neurogenic bladder dysfunction are threefold:

1. to preserve upper urinary tract integrity
2. to insure adequate continence
3. to minimize stone formation and urinary infection.

All these therapeutic goals aim to improve the patient's quality of life and prolong life expectancy.

In the ideal situation, these objectives should be attainable without the necessity of having to rely on a foreign body (i.e. a catheter) permanently installed in the urinary tract.

Therapeutic classification of vesicourethral dysfunction

Several classifications of vesicourethral dysfunction have been proposed in the literature. The latest, and probably the most original, is developed elsewhere in this book by A Matthiasson (see Chapter 12). Based mainly on Krane and Siroky's work, we have elaborated a simple and practical classification that is derived from observations obtained from urodynamic studies, and which focuses on therapeutic goals.[4]

The bladder, as a reservoir, can exhibit only three types of dysfunction:

1. hypo- or areflexia
2. hyperreflexia (including those with decreased contractility)
3. small capacity bladder with or without decreased compliance.

The urethra, the outlet, can be obstructive owing to an anatomical cause (e.g. stenosis, or benign prostatic hyperplasia), functional alterations (e.g. vesicosphincteric dyssynergia), or it can be hypotonic (e.g. incontinence). In clinical practice, most often, both structures function abnormally to varying degrees (Table 28.1).

Urodynamics investigation is the cornerstone of any treatment strategy in neurogenic bladder dysfunction. It allows us to separately evaluate the reservoir function and outlet function, as well as the coordination of these structures during micturition. A well-conducted urodynamics study should answer at least the following questions:

- During the filling phase, is the bladder hyper-, hypo-, or areflexic?
- What is the bladder wall compliance?
- At what bladder volume does the first desire to void appear?
- What is the post-void residual volume and the cystometric capacity?

Table 28.1 *Urodynamic classification of neurogenic bladder dysfunction*

Bladder function	Urethral function
Normal	Hypotonic
Normal	Hypertonic
Hyperreflexic[a]	Normal
Hyperreflexic[a]	Hypotonic
Hyperreflexic[a]	Hypertonic
Hypo- or areflexic	Normal
Hypo- or areflexic	Hypotonic
Hypo- or areflexic	Hypertonic

[a] With or without decreased compliance; with or without impaired contractility.

- Does the bladder represent a high-pressure or a low-pressure system?
- During micturition, is there any kind of infravesical obstruction?
- What is the detrusor contractility, and what is its power?
- As far as the urethra is concerned, what is its 'tonicity' (hypo- or hypertonic) at rest?
- How is increased abdominal pressure transmitted to the urethra in females?
- Is micturition synergic or dyssynergic?

In any kind of neurological pathology associated with vesicourethral dysfunction, even complex situations can be logically analyzed by urodynamics evaluation, which estimates the component of the lower urinary tract that is dysfunctional and to what extent. This allows us to elaborate a logical therapeutic plan that is adapted or personalized to each patient's condition.

Altered reservoir function

As mentioned above, neurological pathology can modify bladder function with three possible end results.

The hypo- or areflexic bladder

In this situation, the bladder cannot empty itself, or can do so only partially, leaving a high post-void residual volume behind. Complete bladder emptying can be promoted by the following techniques.

Clean intermittent catheterization

Whenever the clinical situation permits, clean intermittent catheterization is one of the major approaches taken to ensure adequate bladder emptying. The credit goes to Lapides, who demonstrated that self-catheterization does not need to be sterile and is safe and harmless if the catheter is simply clean.[5–7] His observations, which revolutionized the management of patient bladder evacuation problems, are based on the premise that one of the mechanisms the bladder has to resist bacterial colonization is its periodic and complete emptying.

Transurethral electrical stimulation of the detrusor

Katona et al,[8] who stimulated the bladder wall with a monopolar electrode placed in the bladder *per urethram*, proposed direct stimulation of the detrusor muscle itself. Continuous 60–100 mA current stimulates the mechanoreceptors of the bladder, provoking reflex detrusor contraction.[9] The sacral reflex arc must be intact and the patient must feel the desire to void during the sessions to successfully apply this technique. Daily stimulation sessions of 60–90 min for up to 80 days are necessary. This approach differs significantly from neurostimulation of the sacral roots, since the aim here is to rehabilitate the bladder to regain voluntary control of micturition. The 75% success rate claimed by the original investigators has been confirmed by others[10–13] (see Chapter 21).

Myoplasty of the detrusor

To decrease a large, decompensated bladder, Klarskov et al[14] suggested a partial cystectomy. It has been postulated that this will not only decrease bladder volume but also might increase the contractile efficiency of the detrusor. Hanna,[15] on the other hand, proposed 'remodeling' of the bladder, whereby a part of the bladder wall, stripped of its mucosa, covers the remaining bladder wall, much like a double-breast closure of the abdominal cavity. This would double the thickness of the detrusor, increasing its overall contractility. He operated on 11 patients (9 adults and 2 children): 10 of them have been improved.

Bladder wall strengthening by striated muscle flap

More recently, the group of Tanagho[16] demonstrated in the dog that use of the skeletal muscle, which can be stimulated, may serve to facilitate bladder emptying. Stenzl et al[17] proposed detrusor myoplasty in humans, which consists of transposing a part of the latissimus dorsi muscle around the bladder in such a way that 75% of the bladder wall will be covered by this striated muscle. Of the 11 patients operated on, all were able to void volitionally, and 8 of them no longer required catheterization throughout the follow-up period of 12–46 months.

Pharmacological therapy

Because motor innervation of the detrusor is mainly cholinergic, it seems logical to use this type of medication to enhance bladder emptying. Despite the theoretical advantages of this approach, very little success has been achieved in clinical practice. Awad et al[18] pointed out the importance of the agent's route of administration. They succeeded in obtaining spontaneous voiding and decreasing post-void residual by injecting the medication subcutaneously. Comparable results were not obtained with oral administration. However, it should be noted that side-effects increased with prolonged subcutaneous treatment.

Decreasing urethral resistance

Obviously, decreasing or eliminating urethral resistance should improve bladder emptying. This will be discussed in more detail below.

Summary

The hypo- or areflexic bladder is best managed, whenever possible, by clean intermittent catheterization. Electrostimulation becomes an increasingly valuable alternative, but is still expensive. Direct electrical stimulation of the bladder wall should be attempted when the sacral reflex arc

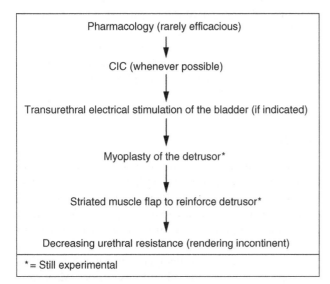

Pharmacology (rarely efficacious)

↓

CIC (whenever possible)

↓

Transurethral electrical stimulation of the bladder (if indicated)

↓

Myoplasty of the detrusor*

↓

Striated muscle flap to reinforce detrusor*

↓

Decreasing urethral resistance (rendering incontinent)

* = Still experimental

Figure 28.1
Algorithm for the treatment of hypo- or areflexic bladder. CIC, clean intermittent catheterization.

is preserved. The time-consuming nature of this approach and the relatively limited indications might prevent its widespread use, in spite of the favorable results reported in the literature. Striated muscle flap is still in its experimental phase. Long-term results in a substantial number of patients are not yet available.

Pharmacological manipulation in this group of patients has limited success and, at the present, has no real indication (Figure 28.1).

The hyperreflexic bladder

The physiopathological consequences of bladder hyperreflexia are threefold:

1. urinary incontinence can be provoked when the amplitude of bladder contractions exceeds urethral closure pressure
2. a low-pressure system can become a high-pressure system if the uninhibited contractions are frequent, with an amplitude over 40 cmH$_2$O, and/or bladder compliance decreases as a result of progressive bladder wall fibrosis
3. vesicoureteral reflux can develop as a result of hyperreflexia.

Hyperreflexia can be controlled by pharmacological and/or surgical means.

Pharmacological manipulation

Oral administration. In the last decade, a large number of pharmacological substances have been developed to control bladder hyperreflexia. All of these substances have antimuscarinic properties, interfering with M$_3$ type receptors. Their overall efficacy in neurogenic hyperreflexia is about 50%.[19] No published randomized clinical trials have been performed on the newly developed anticholinergics – Ditropan XL (oxybutynin), tolterodine, Darifenacine, etc. – in the neurogenic bladder patient population. However, 15–30 mg daily doses of Ditropan XL have been found to be very effective in the hyperreflexic bladder in clinical practice.[20,21]

Transcutaneous administration. James et al[22] in a pilot study used nitroglycerin dermal patches to control bladder instability. They observed a reduction in diurnal and nocturnal frequency as well as a decrease in incontinence episodes per 24 hours. More recently, Davila et al[23] reported the results of a multicenter trial with transcutaneous oxybutynin. Compared with oral administration, the transdermal route had equal efficacy and a significantly improved side-effect profile in adults with urge urinary incontinence. This subject is examined in more detail in Chapter 16.

Intravesical treatment. Bladder hyperreflexia involves an intact sacral reflex arc. Intravesically administered substances can act on the efferent or on the afferent branches of this reflex arc.

Anticholinergics block the efferent part of the reflex. Brendler et al[24] used 5 mg of oxybutynin chloride in 20–30 ml of water in 10 incontinent patients. All of them became continent. Madersbacher et al[25] studied oxybutynin in 13 hyperreflexic bladder patients: in 10 of them who presented incontinence between clean intermittent catheterizations, 9 became continent. Even if the oxybutynin serum level was higher after intravesical administration than orally, the side-effects of anticholinergics were totally absent in the intravesical group. In patients with enterocystoplasty, the side-effects were identical to the oral group. This observation led Massad et al[26] to conclude that a hepatic metabolite of oxybutynin is probably responsible for the side-effects. In a recent study of 12 patients with hyperreflexic bladder, Di Stasi et al[27] found that oral oxybutynin had no effect. When administered intravesically, passive diffusion of oxybutynin significantly reduced urinary leakage, but with electromotive diffusion it caused significantly greater post-void residual urine volume and fewer episodes of urinary leakage, together with measurable changes in urodynamic parameters: decreased duration and amplitude of uninhibited contractions as well as increased bladder wall compliance.

Multisite botulinum A toxin injection in the bladder (up to a total of 300 units) has been proposed to control hyperreflexia. Schurch et al[28] reported their experience recently in 31 spinal cord injury (SCI) patients. Bladder capacity and mean reflex volume increased significantly, mean maximum voiding pressure decreased, and post-void residual volume rose. The duration of bladder paresis was at least 9 months, when repeated injections were required.

Among substances interfering with the afferent branch of the reflex arc, one should mention capsaicin, resiniferatoxin and Marcain (bupivacaine). Capsaicin and resiniferatoxin, both vanilloids, block neurotransmission via small demyelinized C fibers, which come into function only after spinal disruption when myelinized Aδ fibers cannot transmit information to the central nervous system. In idiopathic detrusor instability and in suprapontine pathology, where the C-fiber-mediated reflex does not emerge, these substances seem not to be effective.[29] A controlled trial by de Sèze et al[30] showed that capsaicin was significantly more effective than placebo for continence, frequency, urgency, and patient satisfaction. In a meta-analysis by this same group,[31] 84% of patients (97 out of 115) with detrusor hyperreflexia presented some improvement in their symptoms when treated with intravesical capsaicin. Worldwide experience suggests that 60–100% of patients might respond favourably to this kind of therapy by decreasing or eliminating incontinence episodes between clean intermittent catheterizations for 1–9 months without systemic toxicity.[21]

At 1000-fold more potent than capsicin, resiniferatoxin is mainly interesting for the reduced local reaction that it provokes in the bladder.[32] Resiniferatoxin trials were recently summarized by De Ridder and Baert.[33] The results on vanilloids are updated in Chapter 15.

Local anesthetics block axonal conduction in unmyelinated nerve fibers. The clinical response is of very short duration, and no protocol has been proposed using this approach to control detrusor hyperreflexia. An extensive review on the intravesical administration of drugs in patients with bladder hyperreflexia has been published by Ekström.[34]

Intrathecal administration. According to the experience of Steers et al,[35] intrathecal infusion of baclofen, a γ-aminobutric acid (GABA) agonist, proved to be successful in patients with severe spasticity and hyperreflexia. In all of them, hyperreflexia disappeared, bladder capacity increased by 72%, and bladder compliance improved in 16%. Kums et al[36] made similar observations in 9 quadriplegics. In the last decade, however, no report on this approach to treat detrusor hyperreflexia has been found in the literature.

Neurostimulation

Neurostimulation is the term used when electrical stimulation is applied directly to a nerve fiber to achieve a desired function (sphincter contraction or detrusor relaxation). Neuromodulation is the term used when electrical stimulation is applied to indirectly modify sensory and/or motor functions of the lower urinary tract.

Neurostimulation is applied mainly in patients with complete SCI and preserved detrusor function. (It excludes patients with areflexic bladder.) Introduced by Tanagho[37] and Brindley,[38] this technique is most often associated with bilateral sacral posterior rhizotomy to reduce hyperreflexia and autonomic dysreflexia. The success rate is high for bladder function, but less for rectal function.[39–41]

Surgery

Two main surgical procedures have been proposed in the literature to decrease detrusor hyperreflexia and/or to manage low-compliant bladders: partial detrusorectomy (autoaugmentation) and enterocystoplasty. The ultimate goal with each procedure is to increase reservoir capacity and reduce the amplitude of detrusor contractions.

Enterocystoplasty is contemplated in patients with bladder capacity less than 300 ml under anesthesia. Most commonly, a detubularized segment of the distal ileum is used for this purpose, but a detubularized colic segment or part of the gastric wall can also be used.

Excellent long-term results were reported in about 75% of patients, with improvement in another 20%. The most frequent complications were stone formation in the reservoir (20%) and reoperation (15%) to reaugment the bladder.[42]

The main advantages of autoaugmentation over enterocystoplasty are its lower morbidity (the peritoneal cavity is not opened, the gastrointestinal tract is not violated) and, in case of failure, further intestinal substitution is not precluded. We reserve partial detrusorectomy for patients with bladder capacity over 300 ml under general anesthesia. Detrusor myomectomy and enterocystoplasty offer comparable success or improvement.[43]

Summary

The first step in the management of the hyperreflexic bladder should be a pharmacological one. The oral route of administration is used most frequently. Among transdermal anticholinergic patches, oxybutynin is the only one which underwent clinical trials. It showed equal efficacy and a better side-effect profile than the traditional oral route. Intravesical capsaicin will probably be replaced by the better-tolerated resiniferatoxin, but clinical trails have been recently suspended by the sponsoring pharmaceutical companies.[30] Botulinum A toxin injections in the detrusor are promising, but must be repeated, probably on an annual basis or so. No long-term results exist. Intrathecal baclofen is not indicated at present for the treatment of hyperreflexic bladder, but one should remember that if a baclofen infusion pump is installed for other reasons (e.g. uncontrollable skeletal muscle spasticity), the patient might have some benefit from the urological point of view as well. Neurostimulation constitutes the less-invasive surgical alternative. The still very expensive nature of this treatment modality limits its widespread use. More invasive surgical procedures include bladder autoaugmentation or enterocystoplasty, with equally good long-term results and an acceptable complication rate (Figure 28.2).

Altered outlet function

Infravesical obstruction

From the functional point of view, distinction should be made between occlusion and obstruction. Occlusion is a static phenomenon, as it can be observed: e.g., during a cystoscopic examination. Viewing the lateral lobes of the prostate from the verumontanum, one is looking at a static image. It is impossible to extrapolate from this observation how the proximal urethra will relax in response to detrusor contraction and to what degree urethral funneling will allow the normal passage of urine. In contrast, obstruction

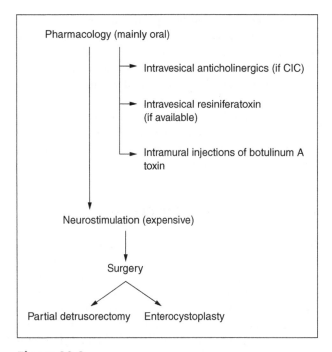

Figure 28.2
Algorithm for the treatment of hyperreflexic bladder. CIC, clean intermittent catheterization.

is a dynamic phenomenon which, in hydrodynamics, means high pressure associated with decreased flow. This can only be objectively demonstrated by urodynamics. Infravesical urethral obstruction can be anatomical (e.g. urethral stenosis) or functional (e.g. vesicosphincteric dyssynergia). We will concentrate on functional obstructions.

The pharmacological approach

From the theoretical point of view, alpha-blocking agents and those that might relax the striated sphincter (together with the pelvic floor) should decrease urethral resistance during micturition. This approach can be beneficial in the neurologically intact patient, but their use in the neurological patient is not very effective. It should be noted, however, that no randomized, double-blind study has demonstrated the role of these substances in the neurological bladder.

Dykstra and Sidi[44] injected botulinum A toxin locally in the striated sphincter once a week for 3 consecutive weeks in 5 patients with proven vesicourethral dyssynergia. Electromyographic (EMG) activity in the striated sphincter has been abolished after injections, while maximum urethral closure pressure, voiding pressure, and post-void residual all decreased. Follow-up of these patients was not provided.

Fowler et al[45] also injected botulinum A toxin in the external sphincter of 6 non-neurological women who exhibited chronic urinary retention. None of the women improved, a failure that might be explained by the fact that these patients were neurologically normal.

Phelan et al[46] recently reported on the efficacy of botulinum toxin injection in the urethral sphincter of men and women with acontractile bladder. All but 1 of the 21 patients treated voided without catheterization, post-void residual decreased by 71%, and voiding pressure by 38%. Transient incontinence was sometimes observed.[47]

In the previously quoted study by Steers et al,[35] intrathecal infusion of baclofen not only abolished bladder hyperreflexia in all patients but also eliminated vesicosphincteric dyssynergia in 40% of them.

Reversible surgical procedures

Intraurethral stents. Growing experience suggests that intraurethral stents are effective in eliminating vesicosphincteric dyssynergia. According to the North American experience, 13% of the prosthesis were withdrawn during the 24-month observation period.[48] The result was 11% in a European study, with a global complication rate of 38%.[49] An excellent in-depth review of the subject, including sphincterotomy, and comparison between the two treatment modalities, have been presented recently by Rivas and Chancellor.[50]

Transurethral balloon dilatation. Chancellor et al[51] proposed hydraulic dilatation of the striated urethral sphincter. Their study, of 17 male patients with vesicourethral dyssynergia, demonstrated interesting results 1 year later: micturition pressure decreased significantly (83 ± 35 cmH$_2$O vs 37 ± 15 cmH$_2$O), as well as post-void residual (163 ± 162 vs 68 ± 59 cmH$_2$O). One year postoperatively, 82% of the patients voided adequately. Even autonomic dysreflexia, when present, was improved. No long-term follow-up was provided.

Overdistention of the female urethra. Overdistention should be very generous to rupture the helicoidal fibers of the urethra. If the bladder neck is competent, stress incontinence should not result from this approach.[52] Transurethral resection of the bladder neck in females should be avoided, as stress incontinence will most likely be its consequence.

Credé's maneuver. This maneuver is more efficacious, especially in females, when the pelvic floor muscles are paralyzed. The increased abdominal pressure is dissipated in part by the flaccid pelvic floor, and lesser pressure will be exerted simultaneously on the proximal urethra. Bladder evacuation, however, is never complete with this technique.

Irreversible surgical procedures

Transurethral bladder neck/prostate incision/resection. If the patient is able to void during urodynamic testing, distinction can be made between constrictive and compressive obstruction.[53] If the obstruction is constrictive in nature and there is no anatomical stenosis at the level of the anterior urethral, we prefer transurethral incision of the bladder neck, as described a number of years ago by Turner-Warwick.[54] Our incision, however, is not limited strictly to the bladder neck, but goes down to the level of the verumontanum, including the lateral lobes of the prostate as well. We observed less restenosis after incision than after resection of the bladder neck, which is contrary to the experience of others.[52]

Sphincterotomy. In the absence of videourodynamics, it is not always easy to decide when to perform sphincterotomy alone and when to combine it with bladder neck incision. Gardner et al[55] combined cystography and static urethral pressure measurements: their algorithm is illustrated on Figure 28.3. In our experience, X-ray studies are recommended, but not absolutely mandatory. When pressure–flow assessment demonstrates obstruction and maximum urethral closure pressure (MUCP) is high, transurethral surgery can include sphincterotomy as well. If MUCP is low, sphincterotomy is probably not useful.

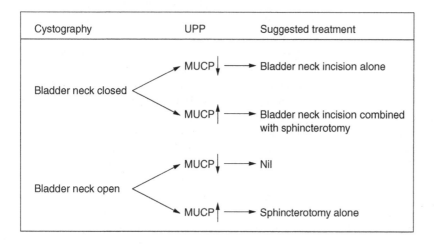

Figure 28.3
Algorithm to decrease urethral resistance. UPP, static urethral pressure profile; MUCP, maximum urethral closure pressure. (Reproduced with permission from Gardner et al.)[55]

Summary

Increased urethral resistance can be weakened by pharmacological means, which, in the form of oral medication, is less efficacious than in the non-neurologic patient. However, it should be the first-line treatment. In case of failure, transurethral injection of botulinum A toxin can be offered. Clinical experience with this form of treatment is limited, and the toxin is not readily available worldwide. Intraurethral stents are effective, but not exempt from causing morbidity and their removal after a prolonged time period can be quite challenging. Balloon dilatation has never gained wide acceptance, despite the fact that it is easy to perform, relatively inexpensive, produces limited complications, and gives good results. Unfortunately, no long-term results are available with this form of therapy. Overdilation of the female urethra should not result in stress urinary incontinence. Sphincterotomy with or without bladder/prostate incision/resection, although the most invasive alternative, remains the gold standard in the management of the obstructive male urethra (Figure 28.4).

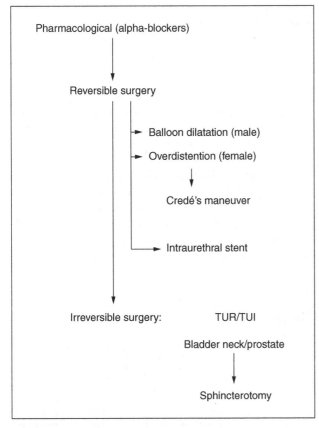

Figure 28.4
Algorithm for the treatment of functional bladder outlet obstruction. TUR, transurethral resection; TUI, transurethral incision.

The hypotonic outlet – incontinence

Urinary incontinence can result from an alteration in reservoir function (hyperreflexia, decreased compliance, small capacity) or a sphincteric failure at the level of the urethra. How to obviate alterations in reservoir function has been discussed previously. In the following sections we will summarize the possibilities of increasing urethral resistance. It should be pointed out that the prerequisite to augmented resistance is a low-pressure bladder reservoir.

Urethropexy

When intrinsic sphincter deficiency and abdominourethral pressure transmission failure are demonstrated in patients with neurogenic bladder, urethropexy can be performed. A detailed description of the multiple techniques proposed in the literature to achieve this is beyond the scope of our chapter. At the moment, Burch urethropexy[56] is the gold standard, as modified by Tanagho.[57] After having been used mainly for the failure of previous urethropexy, and the treatment of stress urinary incontinence without bladder neck hypermobility, sling operations became more popular during the last decade, and indications have been enlarged. However, no randomized study has yet been published to compare retropubic open urethropexy with sling operations. Different sling materials have been used, such as autologous fascia, cadaveric fascia, and a variety of artificial materials. Among the commercially available materials, the tension-free vaginal tape (TVT) technique has gained much popularity, and has the potential to replace the traditional retropubic approach.[58] The precise indications for TVT use are not yet clearly defined in the literature.

Periurethral injections

Berg was the first to report on periurethral injection of Teflon paste in the submucosa of the vesical neck to increase urethral resistance.[59] Because microparticles of this paste have been recovered from the lymphatic ganglia, liver, spleen, brain, and kidney, alternative substances have been proposed.[60] Collagen has been the most widely used substance,[61] followed by autologous fat tissue[62] and silicone microspheres (Genisphere).[63] Pineda and Hadley recently published an extensive review on the subject.[64] The overall success rate in the reported series in females is between 54% and 83% for collagen and 43% and 86% for fat. In men, the overall success rate is between 36% and 100% for collagen. No series were found with fat injection in males. This treatment modality has not been studied in detail in the neurogenic population. Only a few reports reflect the experience in patients with neurogenic bladder dysfunction.[65]

Neurostimulation

Neurostimulation has been summarized previously.

Artificial urinary sphincter

Artificial urinary sphincter remains the gold standard, especially in males, for the treatment of urinary incontinence secondary to sphincter weakness. Fulford et al[66] reported on 68 patients, all of them followed for more than 10 years: 75% of them had satisfactory continence, but only 13% still retained their original device. This suggests that the lifetime of the artificial sphincter is around 10–15 years, which has been confirmed recently by Spiess et al,[67] who studied 30 meningomyelocele children in whom an artificial sphincter was implanted at the bladder neck or the bulbar urethra. Survival analysis of the sphincter device revealed a sharp drop after 100 months, with only 8.3% of the sphincters still functioning beyond this point.

Urethra replacement

When the urethra is judged nonsalvageable from the functional point of view, it can be replaced by a muscular tube obtained from the detrusor. Two main surgical techniques have been described. The Young–Dees–Leadbetter technique creates a muscular tube from the trigone. This necessitates reimplantation of both ureters in an extratrigonal site. Long-term results showed perfect continence in 57% of adults and 70% of children.[68] Tanagho[69] proposed creation of the tube from the anterior bladder wall. This leaves the ureterovesical junction undisturbed. Good to excellent results were obtained in 71.5% of the 56 patients operated on.

Supraurethral derivation

When the clinical situation is such that neither the Young–Dees–Leadbetter operation nor the Tanagho technique is feasible, supraurethral derivation might become necessary. This creates an abdominal stoma which can be continent or incontinent. It frequently implies, especially in females, the simultaneous closure of the bladder neck.

Summary

Failure of the sphincter mechanism in males is best treated by the implantation of an artificial sphincter, which might even be the first line of treatment. Pharmacological substances are rarely effective enough in ensuring continence, and periurethral injections do not resist time. In females suburethral

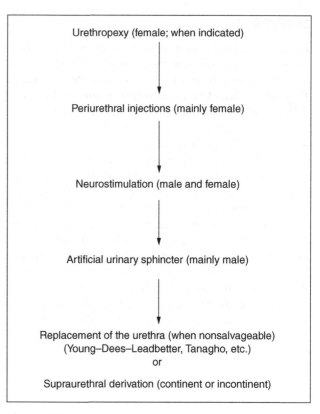

Figure 28.5
Algorithm for the hypotonic outlet: incontinence.

slings are an interesting option, especially if the patient is on a clean intermittent catheterization regimen. In this case, the sling might even be overstretched to some extent to allow continence, bladder emptying being secured by catheterization. When complete replacement of a nonsalvageable urethra is indicated, both posterior (trigonal) and anterior bladder wall tubes give almost the same good results. It should be kept in mind, however, that these are complex surgical procedures with some degree of associated morbidity. Supraurethral derivation (continent or incontinent) should be considered as a last resort treatment (Figure 28.5).

References

1. Küss R, Grégoire W. Histoire illustrée de l'urologie de l'Antiquité à nos jours. Paris (France): R. Dacosta, 1988.

2. Gutierrez PA, Young RR, Vulpe M. Spinal cord injury – an overview. Urol Cl N Am 1993; 20:373–382. [Quote]

3. Guttman L, Frankel H. The value of intermittent catheterization in the early management of traumatic paraplegia and tetraplegia. Paraplegia 1966; 4:63–84.

4. Schick E. Synthèse thérapeurique: traitement des grands types de vessies neurogènes. In: Corcos J, Schick E, eds. Les vessies neurogènes de l'adulte. Paris (France): Masson et Cie, 1996:203–226.

5. Lapides J, Diokno AC, Silber SJ, Lowe BS. Clean, intermittent self-catheterization in the treatment of urinary tract disease. J Urol 1972; 107:458–461.

6. Lapides J, Diokno AC, Lowe BS, Kalish MD. Follow-up on unsterile, intermittent self catheterization. J Urol 1974; 111:184–187.

7. Diokno AC, Sonda P, Hollander JB, Lapides J. Fate of patients started on clean intermittent self-catheterization therapy 10 years ago. J Urol 1983; 129:1120–1122.

8. Katona F, Berényi M. Intravesical transurethral electrotherapy in meningomyelocele patients. Acta Paediatr Acad Sci Hung 1975; 16:363–374.

9. Ebner A, Jiang C, Lindström S. Intravesical electrical stimulation – an experimental analysis of the mechanism of action. J Urol 1992; 148:920–924.

10. Madersbacher H, Hetzel H, Gottinger F, Ebner A. Rehabilitation of micturition in adults with incomplete spinal cord lesions by intravesical electrotherapy. Neurourol Urodyn 1987; 6:230–232. [Abstract]

11. Kaplan WE, Richards I. Intravesical transurethral electrotherapy for the neurogenic bladder. J Urol 1986; 136:243–246.

12. Decter RM, Snyder P, Rosvanis TK. Transurethral electrical bladder stimulation: initial results. J Urol 1992; 148:651–653.

13. Lyne CJ, Bellinger MF. Early experience with transurethral electrical bladder stimulation. J Urol 1993; 150:697–699.

14. Klarskov P, Holm-Bentzen M, Larsen S, et al. Partial cystectomy for the myogenous decompensated bladder with excessive residual urine. Urodynamics, histology and 2–13 years follow-up. Scand J Urol Nephrol 1988; 22:251–256.

15. Hanna MK. New concept in bladder remodeling. Urology 1982; 19:6–12.

16. von Heyden B, Anthony JP, Kaula M, et al. The latissimus dorsi muscle for detrusor assistance: functional recovery after nerve division and repair. J Urol 1994; 151:1081–1087.

17. Stenzl A, Strasser H, Klima G, et al. Reconstruction of the lower urinary tract using autologous muscle transfer and cell seeding: current status and future perspectives. World J Urol 2000; 18:44–50.

18. Awad SA, McGinnis RH, Downie JW. The effectiveness of bethanechol chloride in lower motor neuron lesions: the importance of mode of administration. Neurourol Urodyn 1984; 3:173–178.

19. Barrett DM, Wein AJ, Parulkar BG. Surgery for neuropathic bladder. AUA Update Series 1990; 9:298–303.

20. Appell RA. Treatment of overactive bladder with once-daily extended release tolterodine or oxybutynin: the antimuscarinic clinical effectiveness trial (ACET). Curr Urol Rep 2002; 3:343–344.

21. Elliott DS, Barrett DM. Surgical and medical management of the neurogenic bladder. AUA Update Series 2002; 21:138–143.

22. James MJ, Iacovon JW. The use of GNT patches in detrusor instability: a pilot study. Neurourol Urodyn 1993; 12:399–400. [Abstract]

23. Davila GW, Daugherty CA, Sanders SW. Transdermal Oxybutynin Study Group. A short-term, multicenter, randomized double-blind dose titration study of the efficacy and anticholinergic side effects of transdermal compared to immediate release oxybutynin treatment of patients with urge urinary incontinence. J Urol 2001; 166:140–145.

24. Brandler CB, Radebaugh LC, Mohler JL. Topical oxybutynin chloride for relaxation of dysfunctional bladders. J Urol 1989; 141:1350–1352.

25. Madersbacher H, Jilg G. Control of detrusor hyperreflexia by the intravesical installation of oxybutynin chloride. Paraplegia 1991; 29:84–90.

26. Massad CA, Kogan BA, Trigo-Rocha FE. Pharmacokinetics of intravesical and oral oxybutynin chloride. J Urol 1992: 595–597.

27. Di Stasi SM, Giannantoni A, Navarra P, et al. Intravesical oxybutynin: mode of action assessed by passive diffusion and electromotive administration with pharmacokinetics of oxybutynin and N-desethyl-oxybutynin. J Urol 2001; 166:2232–2236.

28. Schurch B, Stöhrer M, Kramer G, et al. Botulinum-A toxin for treating detrusor hyperreflexia in spinal cord-injured parients: a new alternative to anticholinergic drugs? Preliminary results. J Urol 2000; 164:692–697.

29. Fowler CJ. Bladder afferents and their role in overactive bladder. Urology 2002; 59(suppl 5A):37–42.

30. de Sèze M, Wiart L, Joseph PA, et al. Capsaicin and neurogenic detrusor hyperreflexia: a double-blind placebo-controlled study in 20 patients with spinal cord lesions. Neurourol Urodyn 1998; 17:513–523.

31. de Sèze M, Wiart L, Ferrière JM, et al. Intravesical installation of capsaicin in urology: a review of the literature. Eur Urol 1999; 36:267–277.

32. Maggi CA, Patacchini R, Tramontana M, et al. Similarities and differences in the action of resiniferatoxin and capsaicin on central and peripheral endings of primary sensory neurons. Neuroscience 1990; 37:531–539.

33. De Ridder D, Baert L. Vanilloids and the overactive bladder. BJU Int 2000; 86:172–180.

34. Ekström B. Intravesical instillation of drugs in patients with detrusor hyperactivity. Scand J Urol Nephrol 1992; 149(suppl):1–67.

35. Steers WD, Meythaller JM, Haworth C, et al. Effects of acute bolus and chronic continuous intrathecal Baclofen on genito-urinary dysfunction due to spinal cord pathology. J Urol 1992; 148:1849–1855.

36. Kums JJM, Delhaas EM. Intrathecal Baclofen infusion in patients with spasticity and neurogenic bladder disease. Preliminary results. World J Urol 1991; 9:99–104.

37. Tanagho EA, Schmidt RA. Electrical stimulation in the clinical management of the neurogenic bladder. J Urol 1988; 140:1331–1339.

38. Brindley GS, Pulkey CE, Rushton DN, Cardozo L. Sacral anterior root stimulators for bladder control in paraplegia: the first 50 cases. J Neurol Neurosurg Psychiatry 1986; 49:1104–1114.

39. Chartier-Katler EJ, Denys P, Chancellor MB, et al. Urodynamic monitoring during percutaneous sacral nerve neurostimulation in patients with neurogenic detrusor hyperreflexia. Neurourol Urodyn 2001; 20:61–71.

40. Van Kerrebroeck PE, Koldewijn EL, Debruyne FM. Worldwide experience with the Finetech-Brindley sacral anterior root stimulator. Neurourol Urodyn 1993; 12:497–503.

41. Van Kerrebrock PE. Neurostimulation. In: Corcos J, Schick E, eds. The urinary sphincter. New York: Marcel Dekker, 2001:553–563.

42. Flood HD, Malhotra SJ, O'Connell HE, et al. Long-term results and complications using augmentation cystoplasty in reconstructive urology. Neurourol Urodyn 1995; 14:297–309.

43. Leng WW, Blalock HJ, Frederiksson WH, et al. Enterocystoplasty or myomectomy? Comparison of indications and outcomes for bladder augmentation. J Urol 1999; 161:758–763.

44. Dykstra DD, Sidi AA. Treatment of detrusor-sphincter dyssynergia with Botulinum A toxin: a double-blind study. Arch Phys Med Rehab 1990: 71:24–26.

45. Fowler CJ, Betts CD, Christmas TJ, et al. Botulinum toxin in the treatment of chronic urinary retention in women. Br J Urol 1992; 70:387–389.

46. Phelan MW, Franks M, Somogyi GT, et al. Botulinum toxin urethral sphincter injection to restore bladder emptying in men and women with voiding dysfunction. J Urol 2001; 164:1107–1110.

47. Boyd RN, Britton TC, Robinson RO, Borzyskowski M. Transient urinary incontinence after Botulinum A toxin. Lancet 1996; 348(9025):481–482. [Letter]

48. Oesterling JE, Kaplan SA, Epstein HB, et al., and The North American Urolume Study Group. The North American experience with the Urolume endoprosthesis as a treatment for benign prostatic hyperplasia. Long term results. Urology 1994; 44:353–362.

49. Guazzone G, Montorsi F, Coulange Ch, et al. A modified prostatic wallstent for healthy patients with symptomatic benign prostatic hyperplasia: a European multicenter experience. Urology 1994; 44:364–370.

50. Rivas DA, Chancellor MB. Sphincterotomy and sphincter stent prosthesis placement. In: Corcos J, Schick E, eds. The urinary sphincter. New York: Marcel Dekker, 2001:565–582.

51. Chancellor MB, Karasick S, Strup S, et al. Transurethral balloon dilation of the external urinary sphincter: effectiveness in spinal cord-injured men with detrusor-sphincter dyssynergia. Radiology 1993; 187:557–560.

52. Parsons KF. Difficulty with voiding or acute urinary retention having previously voided satisfactorily. In: Parsons KF, Fitzpatrick JM, eds. Practical urology in spinal cord injury. London: Springer-Verlag, 1991:27–42.

53. Schäfer W. Principles and clinical application of advanced urodynamic analysis of voiding function. Urol Cl N Am 1990; 17:553–566.

54. Turner-Warwick R. Clinical problems associated with urodynamic abnormalities with spacial reference to the value of synchronous cinepressure-flow cystography and the clinical importance of detrusor function studies. In: Lutzeyer W, Melchior H, eds. Urodynamics – upper and lower urinary tract. Berlin: Springer-Verlag, 1970:237–263.

55. Gardner BP, Parsons KF, Machin DG, et al. The urological management of spinal cord damaged patients: a clinical algorithm. Paraplegia 1986; 24:138–147.

56. Burch JC. Cooper's ligament urethrovesical suspension for stress incontinence. Nine year's experience – results, complications, technique. Am J Obstet Gynecol 1968; 100:764–774.

57. Tanagho EA. Colpocystourethropexy: the way we do it. J Urol 1976; 116:751–753.

58. Ulmsten U, Falconer C, Johnson P, et al. A multicenter study of tension-free vaginal tape (TVT) for surgical treatment of stress urinary incontinence. Int Urogynec J Pelvic Floor Dysfunc 1998; 9:210–213.

59. Berg S. Polytef augmentation urethroplasty. Arch Surg 1973; 107:379–381.

60. Malizia AA, Reiman HM, Myers RP, et al. Migration and granulomatous reaction after periurethral injection of polytef (Teflon). JAMA 1984; 251:3277–3281.

61. Corcos J, Fournier C. Periurethral collagen injection for the treatment of female stress urinary incontinence: 4-year follow-up results. Urology 1999; 54:815–818.

62. Santarosa RP, Blaivas JG. Periurethral injection of autologous fat for the treatment of sphincteric incontinence. J Urol 1994; 151:607–611.

63. Barrett DM, Ghoniem G, Bruskewitz R, et al. The Genisphere: a new percutaneously placed anti-incontinence device. J Urol 1990; 141:224A. [Abstract # 141]

64. Pineda EB, Hadley HR. Urethral injection treatment for stress urinary incontinence. In: Corcos J, Schick E, eds. The urinary sphincter. New York: Marcel Dekker, 2001:497–515.

65. Kassouf W, Capolechio J, Bernardinucci G, Corcos J. Collagen injection for treatment of urinary incontinence in children. J Urol 2001; 165:1666–1668.

66. Fulford SC, Sutton C, Bales G, et al. The fate of the 'modern' artificial urinary sphincter with a follow-up of more than 15 years. Br J Urol 1997; 79:713–716.

67. Spiess PE, Capolicchio JP, Kiruluta G, Salle JP, Berardinucci G, Corcos J. Is an artificial sphincter the best choice for incontinent boys with spina bifida? Review of our long term experience with the AS-800 artificial sphincter. Can J Urol 2002; 9:1486:91.

68. Leadbetter GW Jr. Surgical reconstruction for complete urinary incontinence: a 10 to 22 year follow-up. J Urol 1985; 113:205–206.

69. Tanagho EA. Bladder neck reconstruction for total urinary incontinence: 10 years of experience. J Urol 1981; 125:321–326.

29

Treatment alternatives for different types of neurogenic bladder dysfunction in children

Roman Jednak and Joao Luiz Pippi Salle

Introduction

Congenitally acquired lesions of spinal cord development collectively referred to as neurospinal dysraphisms are the most common cause of neurogenic bladder dysfunction in children. Abnormal bladder innervation is found in the overwhelming majority of patients with myelodysplasia, and, consequently, impaired drainage of the lower and upper urinary tract, if not managed appropriately, can be a significant cause of morbidity.

Management goals include establishing satisfactory bladder emptying, maintaining safe bladder storage pressures to prevent upper urinary tract deterioration, avoiding urinary tract infections, and, in the long term, achieving urinary continence. Fortunately, significant advances in the treatment of children with myelodysplasia have resulted in an impressive decrease in the incidence of upper urinary tract deterioration and marked improvements in the achievement of urinary continence. Naturally, this has translated into decreased morbidity and notable improvements in the quality of life for affected children.

Renal damage, nevertheless, remains a real risk and patients require careful evaluation and follow-up. It should also be emphasized that in the myelodysplastic child, the neurologic lesion and bladder dynamics can change with time. Regular urodynamic testing should be performed both in order to identify worsening parameters before upper urinary tract deterioration occurs and to appropriately select management strategies when trying to establish urinary continence.

Here we outline some of the medical and surgical alternatives available when managing the child with neurogenic bladder. The reported outcomes of various surgical techniques in the pediatric population are reviewed.

Management of the bladder

Anticholinergic medications and clean intermittent catheterization

Bladder management is tailored according to the results of urodynamic evaluation.[1–4] Management goals are the maintenance of a compliant low-pressure reservoir that can be regularly emptied in order to both protect the upper urinary tract from deterioration and achieve urinary continence.

Not all children require early clean intermittent catheterization and/or anticholinergic medications.[2,5] Children who empty the bladder effectively in association with synergic or incompetent sphincter function can be observed closely. Clean intermittent catheterization should be started in those patients with a flaccid bladder that empties poorly.[6–8] Latex catheters should be avoided in order to minimize the risk of developing a latex allergy.[9–12] Antibiotic prophylaxis need not be routinely administered in all children but should be considered in those with documented vesicoureteral reflux.[13–15]

Catheterization is ideally performed at intervals of every 3–4 hours. Clean intermittent catheterization used in combination with an anticholinergic medication is indicated in patients with a poorly compliant or hyperreflexic bladder or in those with detrusor-sphincter dyssynergia.[16–24] Detrusor contraction is primarily mediated by the action of acetylcholine.[25,26]

Anticholinergic agents effectively increase the bladder capacity achieved prior to the onset of an uninhibited contraction, decrease the magnitude of uninhibited contractions, and produce an increase in total bladder capacity. Oxybutynin is the most commonly used anticholinergic and in children can be introduced 2–3 times

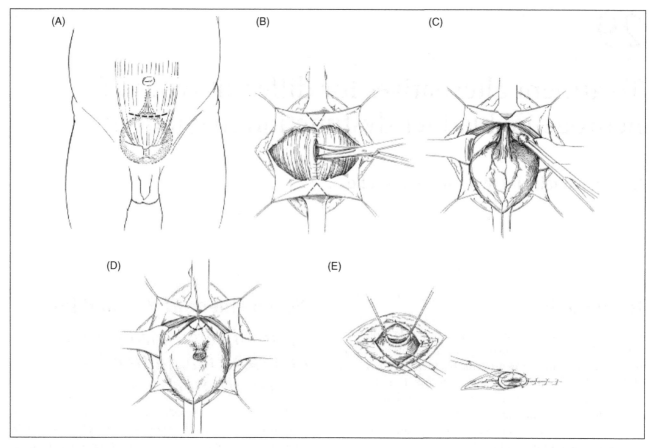

Figure 29.1
Cutaneous vesicostomy. (A) Transverse incision made midway between the umbilicus and symphysis pubis. (B) Modified Pfannenstiel approach. Fascial flaps are raised and the rectus muscles separated in the midline. (C) Urachal remnant, dome, and posterior bladder gradually accessed by progressively retracting the bladder inferiorly and sweeping away the peritoneum. (D) Site for cystostomy selected behind the ligated urachus. (E) Detrusor circumferentially anastomosed to the fascia below the cystostomy. The musosa is matured to the skin with interrupted sutures. (From Keating MA: Incontinent urinary diversion. In Marshall FF (ed): Textbook of Operative Urology. Philadelphia, WB Saunders, 1996, with permission Dr FF Marshall.)

per day at a dose of 0.1–0.2 mg/kg. The medication can be safely used, even in the neonatal period. The most common anticholinergic side-effects encountered in children are dry mouth, constipation, flushing of the skin, blurred vision, and hyperactivity.[27] A newer extended-release formulation that can be administered once daily and may produce fewer adverse effects is also available. Alternatively, intravesical instillation can also be performed. It should be remembered, however, that intravesical instillation is also associated with a similar spectrum of side-effects.[27–33]

Cutaneous vesicostomy

Occasionally, despite maximal efforts, clean intermittent catheterization and anticholinergics are unsuccessful in managing high-risk bladders, controlling reflux, avoiding infections, or preventing upper urinary tract deterioration. In addition, clean intermittent catheterization may not be reliably instituted because of social or anatomic factors. In these cases, cutaneous vesicostomy is a useful and reliable form of temporary urinary diversion in neonates and infants.[34–36] The procedure involves creating a communication between the bladder and the skin of the lower abdominal wall, which allows for free and unobstructed drainage of urine (Figure 29.1).[37] Complications include prolapse, stomal stenosis, stomal eversion, stones, and peristomal dermatitis.[38,39] Anterior bladder wall stomas can allow for posterior bladder wall prolapse. The incidence of prolapse can therefore best be minimized by using a posterior portion of the bladder wall cephalad to the urachus for the vesicostomy.

Bladder augmentation

The objective of bladder augmentation is to create a low-pressure storage reservoir of sufficient capacity to preserve upper urinary tract function and maintain or establish urinary continence when maximal medical therapy is unsuccessful. Advances in surgical techniques have enabled the attainment of these goals with a high degree of reliability, and the experience with bladder enlargement has been extended to a variety of materials and techniques.[40] Most commonly, intestinal segments are selected for bladder augmentation.[41] More recent developments have focused on techniques attempting to preserve the bladder urothelium and thereby avoiding the introduction of intestinal mucosa into the urinary tract.[42–45] Irrespective of the technique used, bladder emptying is usually impaired to some degree and, consequently, most children require clean intermittent catheterization postoperatively. All patients should additionally be made aware of the risk of bladder perforation, a potentially life-threatening complication that may occur following any form of bladder augmentation.[46]

Techniques which do not preserve the urothelium

Ileo- and colocystoplasty. Bladder augmentation using ileum or colon has proven to be a reliable means of increasing bladder capacity and reducing bladder pressures.[47–52] The incorporation of these intestinal segments into the urinary tract, however, is associated with a number of long-term complications.[41] Because of the young patient population typically being treated, this long-term exposure to these complications is of significant concern. Complications most commonly observed include mucus production, bacterial colonization, electrolyte imbalances, metabolic acidosis, somatic growth retardation, and vitamin B_{12} deficiency.[53–57] Other concerns are the risk of calculus formation and the development of malignancy (Table 29.1).[58–66]

Gastrocystoplasty. Stomach first gained popularity as an alternative to colon or ileum in children with chronic renal failure and azotemia as a direct result of its natural acid-secreting ability, which does not worsen the metabolic acidosis.[67,68] The technique is also useful when bowel resection is not an option, as is the case with short-bowel syndrome. Mucus production is less problematic and the acidic urine may also reduce bacterial colonization and the incidence of urinary tract infections. Specific complications include intermittent hematuria, metabolic alkalosis, and the hematuria–dysuria syndrome, which is characterized by bladder or urethral pain and hematuria in

Table 29.1 *Long-term complications associated with ileo- and colocystoplasty*

	Ileum	Colon
Medical		
Hyperchloremic metabolic acidosis	+	+
Vitamin B_{12} deficiency	+	−
Bile salt malabsorption	+	−
Somatic growth retardation	+	−
Osteomalacia/rickets	+	+
Alterations in drug metabolism	+	+
Mucus production	+	+
Bacterial colonization	+	+
Malignancy	+	+
Surgical		
Calculus formation	+	+
Bladder perforation	+	+
Bowel obstruction	+	+

Table 29.2 *Complications associated with gastrocystoplasty*

Hyperchloremic metabolic alkalosis
Hypergastrinemia
Hematuria–dysuria syndrome
Peptic ulcer disease
Dumping syndrome

the absence of infection (Table 29.2).[69,70] Children with incontinence or renal insufficiency/oliguria tend to experience more problems with the hematuria–dysuria syndrome. Since the hematuria–dysuria syndrome does not always respond well to histamine antagonists, this may pose a significant problem in children with normal bladder and urethral sensation.

Techniques which preserve the urothelium

Ureterocystoplasty. The dilated ureter serving a non-functioning kidney can occasionally be used for bladder augmentation (Figure 29.2).[71,72] Success with ureterocystoplasty has been excellent and, since the urothelium is preserved, acid–base disturbances and mucus production are not a problem.[73] In addition, the procedure can be performed using an exclusively extraperitoneal approach.[74] Since the procedure requires a severely dilated ureter and

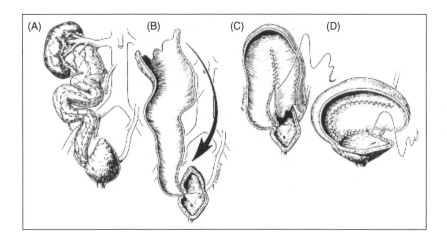

Figure 29.2
Operative stages of ureteral bladder augmentation. (A) Normal blood supply to ureter. (B) Ureteral detubularization following mobilization. (C) Reconfiguration of ureter into U-shaped patch. (D) Anastomosing ureteral patch to native bivalved bladder. (From Churchill BM, et al. Ureteral bladder augmentation. J Urol 1993; 150:716–720.)

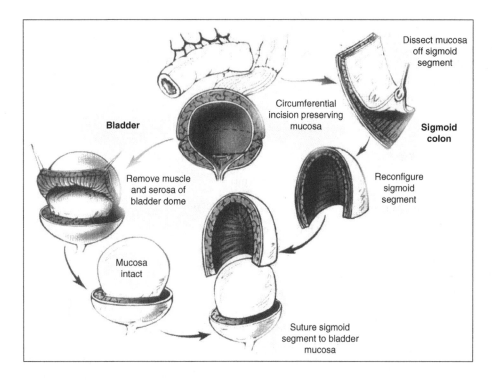

Figure 29.3
Operative technique of seromuscular colocystoplasty lined with urothelium. (Reprinted with modification from Urology 44, Buson et al, Seromuscular colocystoplasty lined with urothelium: experimental study, pp. 743–748, Copyright 1994, with permission from Elsevier Science.)

nonfunctioning kidney, however, its usefulness is limited to specific clinical situations.

Autoaugmentation. Excision or incision of the diseased detrusor with preservation of the urothelium creates a urothelium diverticulum that serves to augment the bladder.[75,76] The benefits of preserving the urothelium are maintained but the reported urodynamic outcomes have varied. Some reports have described only slight improvements in bladder capacity, whereas others have noted improvements in capacity with persistently high bladder pressures.[77–79] One series has reported lower success rates in patients with neurogenic bladder dysfunction.[80]

Seromuscular enterocystoplasty. The complications associated with enterocystoplasty are attributable to the

presence of intestinal mucosa within the urinary tract.[41,53–57] Seromuscular enterocystoplasty makes use of demucosalized segments of ileum, colon, or stomach to augment the bladder and thereby avoid the potential disadvantages of urine contact with intestinal mucosa.[43–45] The procedure can be performed with or without preservation of the urothelium. When the urothelium is preserved the detrusor is excised, leaving a urothelial diverticulum over which the seromuscular patch is then placed (Figure 29.3).[81–86] When no attempt is made to preserve the urothelium, a standard clam enterocystoplasty technique is used and the seromuscular patch is used to augment the bladder using the standard enterocystoplasty technique.[87–89]

The importance of postoperative bladder distention has consistently been stressed as essential to achieving an optimal result in all reports describing the technique.[83,86–88,90] This can be achieved by one of two methods. When the urothelium is preserved and the seromuscular patch is positioned over the exposed urothelial bubble, a Foley catheter can be left to straight drainage and positioned 20–30 cm above the level of the symphysis pubis for a period of 4–5 days.[81–83,86,90] A competent bladder outlet is important to optimize bladder distention in this case, and a concomitant bladder outlet procedure is recommended in patients with poor outlet resistance. In addition, since urothelial integrity is critical to minimizing postoperative leaks, performing concomitant procedures that violate the urothelium should be avoided.[83,86,90]

An alternative method makes use of an intravesical silicone mold that maintains the seromuscular patch in a distended state for a period of 10–14 days.[87,88] This technique can be used both when the urothelium is and is not preserved. Short-term results to date have been encouraging, with postoperative urodynamic parameters and continence rates paralleling those of standard augmentation techniques. Mucus production and electrolyte abnormalities do not appear to be a problem.

Management of the bladder outlet

Medications to increase outlet resistance

Adrenergic nerves innervate the muscular fibers of the bladder base. Alpha agonists (ephedrine, pseudoephedrine) produce an increase in bladder outlet resistance and on occasion may improve urine storage.[91–93] The results with these agents, however, are often less than satisfactory, but improvements in continence can occasionally be obtained in children with mild degrees of wetting due to sphincteric incompetence. In addition, side-effects, including hypertension, anxiety, headaches, and insomnia, may be problematic, so that the use of these agents in managing the incompetent bladder outlet remains limited.

Periurethral injection of bulking agents

Bulking agents such as collagen, Teflon, and, more recently, dextranomer/hyaluronic acid copolymer can be injected submucosally at the bladder neck to facilitate mucosal coaptation and achieve continence.[93–103] Continence rates are difficult to interpret since variable criteria have been reported to define success. In addition, some authors have failed to show a durable response with long-term follow-up.[101] When

defined as a dry interval of 4 hours, continence rates are in the range of 5–63%. Success is often dependent on more than one injection, and as a result cost may become an important issue. Predictors of response to the injection of bulking agents are inconsistent but at least one group has noted improved outcomes in patients with detrusor areflexia and low-pressure bladders.[100] Attempts at defining urodynamic characteristics that may serve as predictors of long-term success have been unsuccessful.[104] Importantly, collagen injection has not been found to interfere with bladder neck surgery if this is subsequently required.

Bladder neck suspension and fascial sling procedures

The use of bladder neck suspension techniques for the treatment of the pediatric neurogenic bladder has not gained widespread use. Reported continence rates achieved in girls in association with bladder augmentation have been at least 80%, with the longest period of follow-up being 30 months.

Fascial slings improve outlet resistance by compression and elevation of the urethra. Reported continence rates have varied from 40 to 100% over a follow-up period of at most 4.5 years.[109–118] The majority of patients have been girls. Attempts at improving outlet resistance have led to a number of modifications, including concomitant bladder neck tapering or circumferentially wrapping the bladder neck with rectus fascia, a rectus myofascial flap, or a strip of anterior bladder wall.[119–125] Bladder augmentation is often necessary to improve continence rates and intermittent catheterization is frequently required. Success using the procedure in boys has been reported in several series.[110,113,115–119,121,122,124,125]

Urethral lengthening procedures

The Kropp and Pippi Salle procedures create a fixed increase in bladder outlet resistance by using a portion of the anterior bladder wall to construct a one-way valve. The Kropp procedure consists of performing urethral lengthening with a tubularized segment of anterior bladder wall, which is reimplanted in the posterior intertrigonal area, creating a one-way valve mechanism similar to the antireflux mechanism procedures used for correction of vesicoureteral reflux (Figure 29.4).[126] Increases in intravesical pressures are transmitted to the submucosal urethral tube, thereby increasing closure pressure and preventing incontinence.

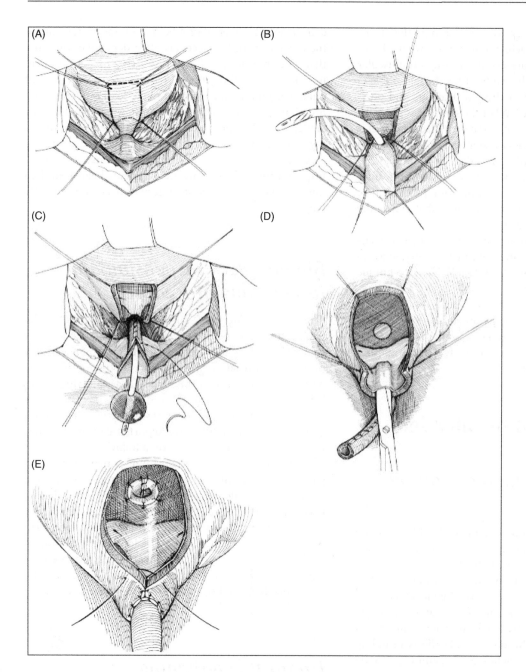

Figure 29.4
(A) An anterior bladder wall flap (5 to 7 cm x 2.5 cm wide) is outlined. (B) The junction of the trigone and the bladder neck is identified from within and the mucosa of the bladder neck separated from the urethra. (C) The anterior bladder flap is tubularized with a one-layer suture (interrupted suture in the last 2 cm). (D) A posterior trigonal tunnel (6 x 3 cm wide) is created beginning at the bladder neck and carried upward beyond the ureteral orifices. (E) The tubularized flap is reimplanted in the posterior submucosal tunnel and the anterior bladder wall is sutured over the bladder neck at the base of the neourethra. (Reprinted from Pippi Salle JL: Urethral lengthening for urinary incontinence. In Gearhart, Mouriquand, Rink (eds): Pediatric Urology, Copyright 2001, with permission from Elsevier Science.)

The procedure is technically demanding and, consequently, revisions have been proposed to facilitate creation of the submucosal tube. Mollard and colleagues described resection of the muscular layer of the distal 50% of the tube to make it more pliable and facilitate submucosal tunneling.[127] Snodgrass made use of a longitudinal bladder incision starting from the bladder neck and extending up between the ureteral orifices into which the detrusor tube was laid. Lateral mucosal flaps are then secured to either side of the tube.[128] The Pippi Salle procedure consists of fashioning an anterior bladder wall flap, which is then sutured to the posterior bladder wall in an onlay fashion. The neourethra is then covered with bladder wall and lateral mucosal flaps to fashion a submucosal tunnel (Figure 29.5).[129–131]

Both these techniques commit the patient to intermittent catheterization, which at times may be difficult.[126,128,130,132–134] Overall, more catheterization difficulties seem to be encountered with the Kropp procedure. As a result, thought should be given to performing a concomitant continent catheterizable channel to facilitate intermittent catheterization postoperatively.[135] Because bladder wall is sacrificed to lengthen the urethra, the postoperative development of low bladder capacity and poor compliance is a risk and, consequently, concomitant bladder augmentation is often required with both techniques.[128,130–133,135–137]

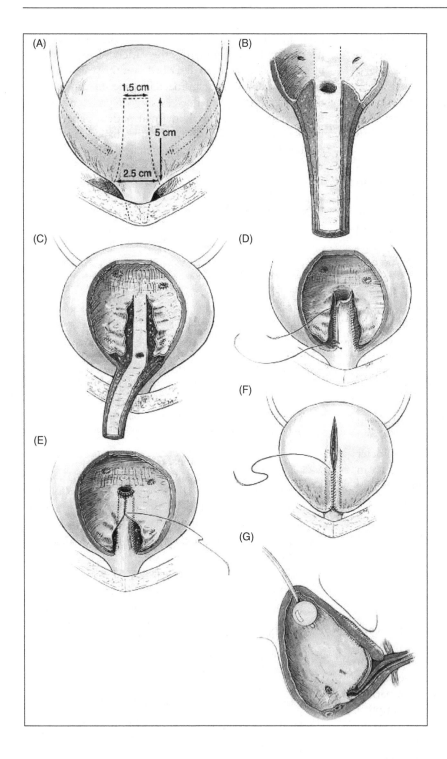

Figure 29.5
(A) Anterior bladder wall flap with a wide base to improve vascular supply. (B) The flap mucosal edges are excised from the muscle to achieve a narrow rectangular mucosal strip with a rich blood supply. This allows a non-overlapping two-layer anastomosis. (C) Parallel incisions are made in the posterior trigonal mucosa. If reimplantation is necessary, both ureters are disconnected and reimplanted superiorly in a cross-trigonal fashion. (D) The anterior flap is dropped onto the incised posterior mucosa and sutured in two layers (mucosa–mucosal and muscle–muscular) to the posterior wall in an onlay fashion. (E) The posterior mucosa lateral to either side of the trigonal incision is mobilized from the detrusor and used to cover the neourethra. (F) The anterior bladder wall is closed in front of the intravesical urethra in a tension-free manner. Tension over the neourethra can cause impairment of the flap vascular supply. (G) Schematic lateral view of the neourethra demonstrating its intravesical position and the flap-valve mechanism when the bladder fills. (From Pippi Salle JL, et al. Modifications of and extended applications for the Pippi Salle procedure. World J Urol 1998; 16: 279–284, Spinger-Verlag publishers, with permission.)

As a result of the potential risk for upper tract deterioration should bladder storage characteristics worsen, careful radiologic and urodynamic follow-up is essential.

Reported continence rates are in the range of 77–91% for the Kropp[126–128,132,133] procedure, whereas those rates for the Pippi Salle[128,130–133,135–137] procedure are in the range of 64–94%. Outcome with the Pippi Salle procedure tends to be more favorable in girls.[136–138]

The artificial urinary sphincter

The artificial urinary sphincter was first introduced in 1974 and has since undergone a number of improvements in design. Continence is achieved by compression of the bladder neck or urethra by an inflatable cuff that can be intermittently deflated to allow for catheterization or voiding. The preferred site of placement in children is around the bladder neck. Patients that empty their bladder without the need for catheterization prior to surgery may continue to do so following sphincter placement[142–150] but, if necessary, intermittent catheterization can be instituted safely.[151,152] It is essential that bladder capacity and compliance be evaluated prior to placing an artificial sphincter, but admittedly this may be difficult in the presence of an incompetent bladder neck.

Some centers have found that preoperative urodynamics may not accurately predict which patient will go on to require bladder augmentation[154] but, nevertheless, failure to recognize a clearly noncompliant bladder preoperatively may put the upper urinary tracts at an unnecessary and significant risk when outlet resistance is increased. In cases where bladder augmentation is required, this can be performed concomitantly without increasing the risk of complications.[155,156]

Despite having favorable preoperative bladder dynamics some patients may develop deterioration in bladder compliance and, therefore, postoperative urodynamic studies and careful radiological and urodynamic follow-up are essential.[143,145–149,157,158] The most common complications include mechanical failure, erosion, and infection. Both erosion and infection result in permanent failure. Revision of the device has been high in most published series, but more recent reports have noted a considerable improvement in the revision rate. Given that the artificial sphincter is a mechanical device with a finite life span, however, it can be expected that most patients will at some time require surgery for revision. Overall, continence rates from 61% to over 95% have been reported in those children having a functional artificial urinary sphincter still in place.[143,144,146–149,159–161]

Conclusions

The treatment of neurogenic bladder dysfunction in children has been a major driving force behind a myriad of innovative surgical solutions: unfortunately, we must accept that none of these are perfect. It also needs to be kept in mind that the successful management of any given patient is defined by a multitude of variables and is not simply a good surgical outcome. Management goals are consistent from patient to patient, but the management strategies are not simply defined by urodynamic studies and urinary tract imaging. Often, the patient's physical limitations as well as their emotional and social needs play a critical role in determining a rational therapeutic strategy.

Before any surgical reconstruction is entertained, available medical management options should be exhausted. Bladder augmentation remains a reliable and highly successful means of dealing with the small capacity, poorly compliant, or hyperreflexic bladder. Far more controversy surrounds the management of the incompetent bladder

neck and the inherent difficulty of dealing with bladder neck incompetence underlies the variety of reconstructive techniques that has been described over the years. The most favorable management approach in a specific clinical situation is therefore often defined by surgeon preference against the background of clearly defined patient expectations. Urodynamic studies performed with a balloon catheter to occlude the bladder neck may facilitate the process.

References

1. McGuire EJ, Woodside JR, Borden TA, Weiss RM. Prognostic value of urodynamic testing in myelodysplastic patients. J Urol 1981; 126:205–209.

2. Bauer SB, Hallett M, Khoshbin S, et al. Predictive value of urodynamic evaluation in newborns with myelodysplasia. JAMA 1984; 252:650–652.

3. Sidi AA, Peng W, Gonzalez R. The value of urodynamic testing in the management of newborns with myelodysplasia: a prospective study. J Urol 1986; 135:90–93.

4. Wang SC, McGuire EJ, Bloom DA. A bladder pressure management system for myelodysplasia – clinical outcome. J Urol 1988; 140:1499–1502.

5. Fernandes ET, Reinberg Y, Vernier R, Gonzalez R. Neurogenic bladder dysfunction in children: review of pathophysiology and current management. J Pediatr 1994; 124:1–7.

6. Lapides J, Diokno AC, Silber S, Lowe BS. Clean, intermittent self-catheterization in the treatment of urinary tract disease. J Urol 1972; 107:458–461.

7. Lapides J, Diokno AC, Lowe BS, Kalish M. Followup on unsterile, intermittent self-catheterization. J Urol 1974; 111:184–187.

8. Lapides J, Diokno AC, Gould FR, Lowe BS. Further observations on self-catheterization. J Urol 1976; 116:169–171.

9. Slater JE, Mostello LA, Shaer C. Rubber-specific IgE in children with spina bifida. J Urol 1991; 146:578–579.

10. Ellsworth PI, Merguerian PA, Klein RB, Rozycki AA. Evaluation and risk factors of latex allergy in spina bifida patients: is it preventable? J Urol 1993; 150:691–693.

11. Pasquariello CA, Lowe DA, Schwartz RE. Intraoperative anaphylaxis to latex. Pediatrics 1993; 91:983–986.

12. Nguyen DH, Burns MW, Shapiro GG, et al. Intraoperative cardiovascular collapse secondary to latex allergy. J Urol 1991; 146:571–574.

13. Kass EJ, Koff SA, Diokno AC, Lapides J. The significance of bacilluria in children on long-term intermittent catheterization. J Urol 1981; 126:223–225.

14. Ottolini MC, Shaer CM, Rushton HG, et al. Relationship of asymptomatic bacteriuria and renal scarring in children with neuropathic bladders who are practicing clean intermittent catheterization. J Pediatr 1995; 127:368–372.

15. Schlager TA, Anderson S, Trudell J, Hendley JO. Nitrofurantoin prophylaxis for bacteriuria and urinary tract infection in children with neurogenic bladder on intermittent catheterization. J Pediatr 1998; 132:704–708.

16. Diokno AC, Kass E, Lapides J. New approach to myelodysplasia. J Urol 1976; 116:771–772.

17. Crooks KK, Enrile BG, Wise HA. The results of clean intermittent catheterization on the abnormal upper urinary tracts of children with myelomeningocele. Ohio State Med J 1981; 77:377–379.

18. Perez-Marrero R, Dimmock W, Churchill BM, Hardy BE. Clean intermittent catheterization in myelomeningocele children less than 3 years old. J Urol 1982; 128:779–781.

19. Geraniotis E, Koff SA, Enrile B. The prophylactic use of clean intermittent catheterization in the treatment of infants and young children with myelomeningocele and neurogenic bladder dysfunction. J Urol 1988; 139:85–86.

20. Joseph DB, Bauer SB, Colodny AH, et al. Clean, intermittent catheterization of infants with neurogenic bladder. Pediatrics 1989; 84:78–82.

21. Klose AG, Sackett CK, Mesrobian H-GJ. Management of children with myelodysplasia: urological alternatives. J Urol 1990; 144:1446–1449.

22. Baskin LS, Kogan BA, Benard F. Treatment of infants with neurogenic bladder dysfunction using anticholinergic drugs and intermittent catheterisation. Br J Urol 1990; 66:532–534.

23. Kasabian NG, Bauer SB, Dyro FM, et al. The prophylactic value of clean intermittent catheterization and anticholinergic medication in newborns and infants with myelomeningocele at risk of developing urinary tract deterioration. Am J Dis Child 1992; 146:840–843.

24. Edelstein RA, Bauer SB, Kelly MD, et al. The long-term urological response of neonates with myelodysplasia treated proactively with intermittent catheterization and anticholinergic therapy. J Urol 1995; 154:1500–1504.

25. de Groat WC, Yoshimura N. Pharmacology of the lower urinary tract. Ann Rev Pharmacol Toxicol 2001; 41:691–721.

26. Yamanishi T, Chapple CR, Chess-Williams R. Which muscarinic receptor is important in the bladder? World J Urol 2001; 19:299–306.

27. Andersson KE, Chapple CR. Oxybutynin and the overactive bladder. World J Urol 2001; 19:319–323.

28. Greenfield SP, Fera M. The use of intravesical oxybutynin chloride in children with neurogenic bladder. J Urol 1991; 146:532–534.

29. Kasabian NG, Vlachiotis JD, Lais A, et al. The use of intravesical oxybutynin chloride in patients with detrusor hypertonicity and detrusor hyperreflexia. J Urol 1994; 151:944–945.

30. Kaplinsky R, Greenfield S, Wan J, Fera M. Expanded followup of intravesical oxybutynin chloride use in children with neurogenic bladder. J Urol 1996; 156:753–756.

31. Painter KA, Vates TS, Bukowski TP, et al. Long-term intravesical oxybutynin chloride therapy in children with myelodysplasia. J Urol 1996; 156:1459–1462.

32. Palmer LS, Zebold K, Firlit CF, Kaplan WE. Complications of intravesical oxybutynin chloride therapy in the pediatric myelomeningocele population. J Urol 1997; 157:638–640.

33. Ferrara P, D'Aleo CM, Tarquini E, et al. Side-effects of oral or intravesical oxybutynin chloride in children with spina bifida. BJU Int 2001; 87:674–677.

34. Cohen JS, Harbach LB, Kaplan GW. Cutaneous vesicostomy for temporary urinary diversion in infants with neurogenic bladder dysfunction. J Urol 1978; 119:120–121.

35. Mandell J, Bauer SB, Colodny AH, Retik AB. Cutaneous vesicostomy in infancy. J Urol 1981; 126:92–93.

36. Snyder HM III, Kalichman MA, Charney E, Duckett JW. Vesicostomy for neurogenic bladder with spina bifida: followup. J Urol 1983; 130:724–726.

37. Duckett JW Jr. Cutaneous vesicostomy in childhood: the Blocksom technique. Urol Clin N Am 1974; 1:485–495.

38. Hurwitz RS, Ehrlich RM. Complications of cutaneous vesicostomy. Urol Clin N Am 1974; 10:503–508.

39. Duckett JW, Ziylan O. Uses and abuses of vesicostomy. AUA Update Series 1995; 14:130–135.

40. Duel BP, Gonzalez R, Barthold JS. Alternative techniques for augmentation cystoplasty. J Urol 1999; 159:998–1005.

41. Gough DCS. Enterocystoplasty. BJU Int 2001; 88:739–743.

42. Ureterocystolasty: the latest developments. BJU Int 2001; 88:744–751.

43. Jednak R, Schmike CM, Ludwikowski B, González R. Seromuscular colocystoplasty. BJU Int 2001; 88:752–756.

44. Close CE. Autoaugmentation gastrocystoplasty. BJU Int 2001; 88:757–761.

45. Lima SVC, Araújo LAP, Vilar FO, et al. Experience with demucosalized ileum for bladder augmentation. BJU Int 2001; 88:762–764.

46. Shekarriz B, Upadhyay J, Demirbilek S, et al. Surgical complications of bladder augmentation: comparison between various enterocystoplasties in 133 patients. Urology 2000; 55:123–128.

47. Hendren WH, Hendren RB. Bladder augmentation: experience with 129 children and young adults. J Urol 1990; 144:445–453.

48. Mitchell ME, Kulb TB, Backes DJ. Intestinocystoplasty in combination with clean intermittent catheterization in the management of vesical dysfunction. J Urol 1986; 136:288–291.

49. Decter RM, Bauer SB, Mandell J, et al. Small bowel augmentation in children with neurogenic bladder: an initial report of urodynamic findings. J Urol 1987; 138:1014–1016.

50. Mitchell ME, Piser JA. Intestinocystoplasty and total bladder replacement in children and young adults: followup in 129 cases. J Urol 1987; 138:579–584.

51. Krishna A, Gough DCS, Fishwick J, Bruce J. Ileocystoplasty in children: assessing safety and success. Eur Urol 1995; 27:62–66.

52. Wang K, Yamataka A, Morioka A, et al. Complications after sigmoidocolocystoplasty: review of 100 cases at one institution. J Pediatr Surg 1999; 34:1672–1677.

53. McDougal WS. Metabolic complications of urinary intestinal diversion. J Urol 1992; 147:1199–1208.

54. Stampfer DS, McDougal WS, McGovern FJ. Metabolic and nutritional complications. Urol Clin N Am 1997; 24:715–722.

55. Nurse DE, Mundy AR. Metabolic complications of cystoplasty. Br J Urol 1989; 63:165–170.

56. Wagstaff KE, Woodhouse CRJ, Duffy PG, Ransley PG. Delayed linear growth in children with enterocystoplasties. Br J Urol 1992; 69:314–317.

57. Mundy AR, Nurse DE. Calcium balance, growth and skeletal mineralisation in patients with cystoplasties. Br J Urol 1992; 69:257–259.

58. Blyth B, Ewalt DH, Duckett JW, Snyder HM. Lithogenic properties of enterocystoplasty. J Urol 1992; 148:575–577.

59. Palmer LS, Franco I, Kogan SJ, et al. Urolithiasis in children following augmentation cystoplasty. J Urol 1993; 150:726–729.

60. Nurse DE, McInerney PD, Thomas PJ, Mundy AR. Stones in enterocystoplasties. Br J Urol 1996; 77:684–687.

61. Khoury AE, Salomon M, Doche R, et al. Stone formation following augmentation cystoplasty: the role of intestinal mucus. J Urol 1997; 158:1133–1137.

62. Kronner KM, Casale AJ, Cain MP, et al. Bladder calculi in the pediatric augmented bladder. J Urol 1998; 160:1096–1098.

63. Mathoera RB, Kok DJ, Nijman RJM. Bladder calculi in augmentation cystoplasty in children. Urology 2000; 56:482–487.

64. Filmer RB, Spencer JR. Malignancies in bladder augmentations and intestinal conduits. J Urol 1990; 143:671–678.

65. Trieger BFG, Marshall FF. Carcinogenesis and the use of intestinal segments in the urinary tract. Urol Clin N Am 1991; 18:737–742.

66. Malone MJ, Izes JK, Hurley LJ. Carcinogenesis. The fate of intestinal segments used in urinary reconstruction. Urol Clin N Am 1997; 24:723–728.

67. Adams MC, Mitchell ME, Rink RC. Gastrocystoplasty: an alternative solution to the problem of urological reconstruction in the severely compromised patient. J Urol 1988; 140:1152–1156.

68. Sheldon CA, Gilbert A, Wacksman J, Lewis AG. Gastrocystoplasty: technical and metabolic characteristics of the most versatile childhood bladder augmentation modality. J Pediatr Surg 1995; 30:283–287.

69. Nguyen DH, Bain MA, Salmonson KL, et al. The syndrome of dysuria and hematuria in pediatric urinary reconstruction with stomach. J Urol 1993; 150:707–709.

70. Kinahan TJ, Khoury AE, McLorie GA, Churchill BM. Omeprazole in post-gastrocystoplasty metabolic alkalosis and aciduria. J Urol 1992; 147:435–437.

71. Bellinger MF. Ureterocystoplasty: a unique method for vesical augmentation in children. J Urol 1993; 149:811–813.

72. Churchill BM, Aliabadi H, Landau EH, et al. Ureteral bladder augmentation. J Urol 1993; 150:716–720.

73. Landau EH, Jayanthi VR, Khoury AE, et al. Bladder augmentation: ureterocystoplasty versus ileocystoplasty. J Urol 1994; 152:716–719.

74. Dewan PA, Nicholls EA, Goh DW. Ureterocystoplasty: an extraperitoneal urothelial bladder augmentation technique. Eur Urol 1994; 26:85–89.

75. Cartwright PC, Snow BW. Bladder autoaugmentation: partial detrusor excision to augment the bladder without use of bowel. J Urol 1989; 142:1050–1053.

76. Cartwright PC, Snow BW. Bladder autoaugmentation: early clinical experience. J Urol 1989; 142:505–508.

77. Reid C, Moorehead JD, Hadley HR. Experience with detrusorectomy procedures. J Urol 1990; 143:331A.

78. Stothers L, Johnson H, Arnold W, et al. Bladder autoaugmentation by vesicomyotomy in the pediatric neurogenic bladder. Urology 1994; 44:110–113.

79. Skobejko-Wlodarska L, Strulak K, Nachulewicz P, Szymkiewicz C. Bladder autoaugmentation in myelodysplastic children. Br J Urol 1998; 81(Suppl 3):114–116.

80. Swami KS, Feneley RCL, Hammonds JC, Abrams P. Detrusor myectomy for detrusor overactivity: a minimum 1-year follow-up. Br J Urol 1998; 81:68–72.

81. Dewan PA, Stefanek W. Autoaugmentation colocystoplasty. Pediatr Surg Int 1994; 9:526–528.

82. Dewan PA, Stefanek W. Autoaugmentation gastrocystoplasty: early clinical results. Br J Urol 1994; 74:460–464.

83. González R, Buson H, Churphena R, Reinberg Y. Seromuscular colocystoplasty lined with urothelium: experience with 16 patients. Urology 1995; 45:124–129.

84. Nguyen DH, Mitchell ME, Horowitz M, et al. Demucosalized augmentation gastrocystoplasty with bladder autoaugmentation in pediatric patients. J Urol 1996; 156:206–209.

85. Dayanç M, Kilciler M, Tan Ö, et al. A new approach to bladder augmentation in children: seromuscular enterocystoplasty. Br J Urol 1999; 84:103–107.

86. Jednak R, Schimke CM, Barroso U Jr, et al. Further experience with seromuscular colocystoplasty lined with urothelium. J Urol 2000; 164:2045–2049.

87. Lima SVC, Araújo LAP, Vilar FO, et al. Nonsecretory sigmoid cystoplasty: experimental and clinical results. J Urol 1995; 153:1651–1654.

88. Lima SVC, Araújo LAP, Montoro M, et al. The use of demucosalized bowel to augment small contracted bladders. Br J Urol 1998; 82:436–439.

89. de Badiola F, Ruiz E, Puigdevall J, et al. Sigmoid cystoplasty with argon beam without mucosa. J Urol 2001; 165:2253–2255.

90. Vates TS, Smith C, Gonzalez R. Importance of early bladder distension for the success of the seromuscular colocystoplasty lined with urothelium. Pediatrics 1997; 100:564.

91. Diokno AC, Taub M. Ephedrine in treatment of urinary incontinence. Urology 1975; 5:624–625.

92. Raezer DM, Benson GS, Wein AJ, Duckett JW Jr. The functional approach to the management of the pediatric neuropathic bladder: a clinical study. J Urol 1977; 117:649–654.

93. Decter RM. Pharmacologic management of the neurogenic bladder. Probl Urol 1994; 8:373–388.

93. Vorstman B, Lockhart JL, Kaufman MR, Politano V. Polytetrafluoroethylene injection for urinary incontinence in children. J Urol 1985; 133:248–250.

94. Wan J, McGuire EJ, Bloom DA, Ritchey ML. The treatment of urinary incontinence in children using glutaraldehyde cross-linked collagen. J Urol 1992; 148:127–130.

95. Capozza N, Caione P, De Gennaro M, et al. Endoscopic treatment of vesico-ureteric reflux and urinary incontinence: technical problems in the paediatric patient. Br J Urol 1995; 75:538–542.

96. Leonard MP, Decter A, Mix LW, et al. Treatment of urinary incontinence in children by endoscopically directed bladder neck injection of collagen. J Urol 1996; 156:637–641.

97. Bomalaski MD, Bloom DA, McGuire EJ, Panzl A. Glutaraldehyde cross-linked collagen in the treatment of urinary incontinence in children. J Urol 1996; 155:699–702.

98. Pérez LM, Smith EA, Parrott TS, et al. Submucosal bladder neck injection of bovine dermal collagen for stress urinary incontinence in the pediatric population. J Urol, part 2, 1996; 156:633–363.

99. Sundaram CP, Reinberg Y, Aliabadi HA. Failure to obtain durable results with collagen implantation in children with urinary incontinence. J Urol 1997; 157:2306–2307.

100. Silveri M, Capitanucci ML, Mosiello G, et al. Endoscopic treatment for urinary incontinence in children with a congenital neuropathic bladder. Br J Urol 1998; 82:694–697.

101. Kassouf W, Capolicchio G, Berardinucci G, Corcos J. Collagen injection for treatment of urinary incontinence in children. J Urol 2001; 165:1666–1668.

102. Caione P, Capozza N. Endoscopic treatment of urinary incontinence in pediatric patients: 2-year experience with dextranomer/hyaluronic acid copolymer. J Urol, part 2, 2002; 168:1868–1871.

103. Lottmann HB, Margaryan M, Bernuy M, et al. The effect of endoscopic injections of dextranomer based implants on continence and bladder capacity: a prospective study of 31 patients. J Urol 2002; 168:1863–1867.

104. Kim YH, Kattan MW, Boone TB. Correlation of urodynamic results and urethral coaptation with success after transurethral collagen injection. Urology 1997; 50:941–948.

105. Woodside JR, Borden TA. Suprapubic endoscopic vesical neck suspension for the management of urinary incontinence in myelodysplastic girls. J Urol 1986; 135:97–99.

106. Raz S, Ehrlich RM, Zeidman EJ, et al. Surgical treatment of the incontinent female patient with myelomeningocele. J Urol 1988; 139:524–527.

107. Gearhart JP, Jeffs RD. Suprapubic bladder neck suspension for the management of urinary incontinence in the myelodysplastic girl. J Urol 1988; 140:1296–1298.

108. Freedman ER, Singh G, Donnell SC, et al. Combined bladder neck suspension and augmentation cystoplasty for neuropathic incontinence in female patients. Br J Urol 1994; 73:621–624.

109. McGuire EJ, Wang C-C, Usitalo H, Savastano J. Modified pubovaginal sling in girls with myelodysplasia. J Urol 1986; 135:94–96.

110. Raz S, McGuire EJ, Ehrlich RM, et al. Fascial sling to correct male neurogenic sphincter incompetence: the McGuire/Raz approach. J Urol 1988; 139:528–531.

111. Bauer SB, Peters CA, Colodny AH, et al. The use of rectus fascia to manage urinary incontinence. J Urol 1989; 142:516–519.

112. Elder JS. Periurethral and puboprostatic sling repair for incontinence in patients with myelodysplasia. J Urol 1990; 144:434–437.

113. Decter RM. Use of the fascial sling for neurogenic incontinence: lessons learned. J Urol 1993; 150:683–686.

114. Gormley EA, Bloom DA, McGuire EJ, Ritchey ML. Pubovaginal slings for the management of urinary incontinence in female adolescents. J Urol 1994; 152:822–825.

115. Kakizaki H, Shibata T, Shinno Y, et al. Fascial sling for the management of urinary incontinence due to spincteric incompetence. J Urol 1995; 153:648–649.

116. Pérez LM, Smith EA, Broecker BH, et al. Outcome of sling cystourethropexy in the pediatric population: a critical review. J Urol 1996; 156:642–646.

117. Dik P, van Gool JG, De Jong TPVM. Urinary continence and erectile function after bladder neck sling suspension in male patients with spinal dysraphism. BJU Int 1999; 83:971–975.

118. Austin PF, Westney OL, Leng WW, et al. Advantages of rectus fascial slings for urinary incontinence in children with neuropathic bladders. J Urol, part 2, 2001; 165:2369–2372.

119. Herschorn S, Radomski SB. Fascial slings and bladder neck tapering in the treatment of male neurogenic incontinence. J Urol 1992; 147:1073–1075.

120. Ghoniem GM. Bladder neck wrap: a modified fascial sling in treatment of incontinence in myelomeningocele patients. Eur Urol 1994; 25:340–342.

121. Walker RD, Flack CE, Hawkins-Lee B, et al. Rectus fascial wrap: early results of a modification of the rectus fascial sling. J Urol 1995; 154:771–774.

122. Kurzrock EA, Lowe P, Hardy BE. Bladder wall pedicle wraparound sling for neurogenic urinary incontinence in children. J Urol 1996; 155:305–308.

123. Barthold JS, Rodriguez E, Freedman AL, et al. Results of the rectus fascial sling and wrap procedures for the treatment of neurogenic sphincteric incontinence. J Urol 1999; 161:272–274.

124. Walker RD, Erhard M, Starling J. Long-term evaluation of rectus fascial wrap in patients with spina bifida. J Urol 2000; 164:485–486.

125. Mingin GC, Youngren K, Stock JA, Hanna MK. The rectus myofascial wrap in the management of urethral sphincter incompetence. BJU Int 2002; 90:550–553.

126. Kropp KA, Angwafo FF. Urethral lengthening and reimplantation for neurogenic incontinence in children. J Urol 1986; 135:533–536.

127. Mollard P, Mouriquand P, Joubert P. Urethral lengthening for neurogenic urinary incontinence (Kropp's procedure): results of 16 cases. J Urol 1990; 143:95–97.

128. Snodgrass W. A simplified Kropp procedure for incontinence. J Urol 158:1049–1052.

129. Pippi Salle JL, de Fraga JCS, Amarante A, et al. Urethral lengthening with anterior bladder wall flap for urinary incontinence: a new approach. J Urol 1994; 152:803–806.

130. Pippi Salle JL, McLorie GA, Bagli DJ, Khoury AE. Urethral lengthening with anterior bladder wall flap (Pippi Salle procedure): modifications and extended indications of the technique. J Urol 1997; 158:585–590.

131. Pippi Salle JL, McLorie GA, Bagli DJ, Khoury AE. Modifications of and extended indications for the Pippi Salle procedure. World J Urol 1999; 16:279–284.

132. Belman AB, Kaplan GW. Experience with the Kropp anti-incontinence procedure. J Urol 1989; 141:1160–1162.

133. Nill TG, Peller PA, Kropp KA. Management of urinary incontinence by bladder tube urethral lengthening and submucosal reimplantation. J Urol 1990; 144:559–563.

134. Waters PR, Chehade NC, Kropp KA. Urethral lengthening and reimplantation: incidence and management of catheterization problems. J Urol 1997; 158:1053–1056.

135. Koyle MA. The Kropp bladder neck reconstruction and its variations in the incontinent patient with neurogenic bladder. Pediatrics 1996; 98:602.

136. Mouriquand PD, Sheard R, Phillips N, et al. The Kropp-onlay procedure (Pippi Salle procedure): a simplification of the technique of urethral lengthening. Preliminary results in eight patients. Br J Urol 1995; 75:656–662.

137. Hayes MC, Bulusu A, Terry T, et al. The Pippi Salle urethral lengthening procedure; experience and outcome from three United Kingdom centres. BJU Int 1999; 84:701–705.

138. Rink RC, Adams MC, Keating MA. The flip-flap technique to lengthen the urethra (Salle procedure) for treatment of neurogenic urinary incontinence. J Urol 1994; 152:799–802.

139. Scott FB, Bradley WE, Timm GW. Treatment of urinary incontinence by an implantable prosthetic urinary sphincter. J Urol 1974; 112:75–80.

140. Furlow WL, Barrett DM. The artificial urinary sphincter: experience with the AS 800 pump-control assembly for single-stage primary deactivation and activation – a preliminary report. Mayo Clin Proc 1985; 60:255–258.

141. Light JK, Reynolds JC. Impact of the new cuff design on reliability of the AS800 artificial urinary sphincter. J Urol 1992; 147:609–611.

141. Leo ME, Barrett DM. Success of the narrow-backed cuff design of the AMS800 artificial urinary sphincter: analysis of 144 patients. J Urol 1993; 150:1412–1414.

142. Mitchell ME, Rink RC. Experience with the artificial urinary sphincter in children and young adults. J Pediatr Surg 1983; 18:700–706.

143. Gonzalez R, Koleilat N, Austin C, Sidi AA. The artificial sphincter AS800 in congenital urinary incontinence. J Urol 1989; 142:512–515.

144. Bosco PJ, Bauer SB, Colodny AH, et al. The long-term results of artificial sphincters in children. J Urol 1991; 146:396–399.

145. Belloli G, Caampobasso P, Mercurella A. Neuropathic urinary incontinence in pediatric patients: management with artificial sphincter. J Pediatr Surg 1992; 27:1461–1464.

146. González R, Merino FG, Vaughn M. Long-term results of the artificial urinary sphincter in male patients with neurogenic bladder. J Urol 1995; 154:769–770.

147. Levesque PE, Bauer SB, Atala A, et al. Ten-year experience with the artificial urinary sphincter in children. J Urol 1996; 156:625–628.

148. Kryger JV, Barthold JS, Fleming P, González R. The outcome of artificial urinary sphincter placement after a mean 15-year follow-up in a paediatric population. BJU Int 1999; 83: 1026–1031.

149. Hafez AT, McLorie G, Bägli D, Khoury A. A single-centre long-term outcome analysis of artificial urinary sphincter placement in children. BJU Int 2002; 89:82–85.

150. Toh K, Diokno AC. Management of intrinsic sphincter deficiency in adolescent females with normal bladder emptying function. J Urol 2002; 168:1150–1153.

151. Diokno AC, Sonda LP. Compatibility of genitourinary prostheses and intermittent self-catheterization. J Urol 1981; 125:659–660.

152. Barrett DM, Furlow WL. Incontinence, intermittent self-catheterization and the artificial genitourinary sphincter. J Urol 1984; 132:268–269.

153. de Badiola FIP, Castro-Diaz D, Hart-Austin C, Gonzalez R. Influence of preoperative bladder capacity and compliance on the outcome of artificial sphincter implantation in patients with neurogenic sphincter incompetence. J Urol 1992; 148:1493–1495.

154. Kronner KM, Rink RC, Simmons G, et al. Artificial urinary sphincter in the treatment of urinary incontinence: preoperative urodynamics do not predict the need for future bladder augmentation. J Urol 1998; 160:1093–1095.

155. Strawbridge LR, Kramer SA, Castillo OA, Barrett DM. Augmentation cystoplasty and the artificial genitourinary sphincter. J Urol 1989; 142:297–301.

156. Gonzalez R, Nguyen DH, Koleilat N, Sidi AA. Compatibility of enterocystoplasty and the artificial urinary sphincter. J Urol 1989; 142:502–504.

157. Bauer SB, Reda EF, Colodny AH, Retik AB. Detrusor instability: a delayed complication in association with the artificial sphincter. J Urol 1986; 135:1212–1215.

158. Murray KHA, Nurse DE, Mundy AR. Detrusor behavior following implantation of the Brantley Scott artificial urinary sphincter for neuropathic incontinence. Br J Urol 1988; 61:122–128.

159. Simeoni J, Guys JM, Mollard P, et al. Artificial urinary sphincter implantation for neurogenic bladder: a multi-institutional study in 107 children. Br J Urol 1996; 78:287–293.

160. Castera R, Podesta ML, Ruarte A, et al. 10-year experience with artificial urinary sphincter in children and adolescents. J Urol 2001; 165:2373–2376.

161. Spies PE, Capolicchio JP, Kiruluta G, et al. Is an artificial sphincter the best choice for incontinent boys with spina bifida? Review of our long term experience with the AS-800 artificial sphincter. Can J Urol 2002; 9:1486–1491.

30

The vesicourethral balance

Erik Schick and Jacques Corcos

Introduction

In Chapter 28, we summarized the different treatment modalities that can be considered to correct bladder dysfunction or urethral dysfunction, independently of each other. In clinical practice, however, most patients present simultaneous alterations of reservoir and outlet functions.

The ultimate goal in neurogenic bladder management is the preservation of normal kidney function. The most important factor to achieve is to maintain the lower urinary tract at a low pressure. Ensuring regular bladder emptying, decreasing outlet resistance in patients who void spontaneously, preventing infection by eliminating foreign bodies from the urethra and/or the bladder, and treating infection when it becomes symptomatic are some of the modalities used to attain this goal. Additionally, maintaining or restoring continence will significantly increase the patient's quality of life. To avoid or minimize potential complications, these objectives have to be constantly kept in mind when dealing with the problem of neurogenic bladder dysfunction.

Vesicourethral balance and balanced bladder are by no means synonymous. The balanced bladder concept emerged after World War II and was part of the bladder rehabilitation process. It implied reflex bladder voiding and a post-void residual urine volume of less than 100 ml. Clinicians felt safe in trying to achieve this goal. Later experience proved that the approach was not necessarily safe, because it could not prevent infection, sepsis, loss of renal function, etc. The flaw with this empirical therapy is that elevated bladder filling and emptying pressures can occur, causing silent renal damage despite low post-void residual urine volume.[1]

The concept of vesicourethral balance helps us to understand the pathophysiological consequences of vesicourethral dysfunction. It indicates how to modify reservoir function, outlet function, or both in order to restore normal vesicourethral function to a safe, normal, low-pressure zone. Urodynamics are essential in this respect, because

they allow bladder and urethral function to be evaluated independently along with the interaction between them.

Normal vesicourethral balance

The vesicourethral unit can be compared to a balance where the bladder represents one arm, and the urethra with its sphincteric mechanism the other arm of the balance. Figure 30.1 illustrates this concept.

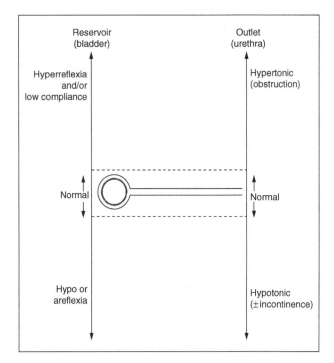

Figure 30.1

Normal vesicourethral balance. Bladder filling and micturition under normal pressure conditions, within the 'security zone' of <40 cmH$_2$0.

During the filling phase of the voiding cycle, the bladder is accommodating a progressively increasing volume. Because of normal bladder wall compliance, pressure inside the bladder remains constant, about 15–20 cmH$_2$O, and never exceeds 40 cmH$_2$O. The system is in a low-pressure state, and the upper urinary tract is safe.[2,3] During the voiding phase, the detrusor contracts, the urethral sphincteric mechanism relaxes, and there is normal vesicourethral synergia.

Under pathological conditions, this relatively delicate balance can easily be disturbed. Bladder function can be normal or altered by some pathological process in several ways. It may become hypo- or areflexic, or hyperreflexic, with or without impaired contractility, with or without decreased compliance. Urethral function can be normal, hypotonic (incontinence), or hypertonic (obstruction). The different combinations of these vesicourethral alterations can lead to eight different clinical situations, as illustrated in Table 30.1.

The aim of any therapeutic intervention is to ensure the restoration of normal balance in the security zone – security from the point of view of the preservation of renal function.

Alterations in vesicourethral balance

Normal bladder contractility and compliance

The hypotonic outlet

This is characteristic of the stress incontinent patient. By simply improving outlet function, normal vesicourethral conditions in normal pressure ranges can be restored (Figure 30.2).

The obstructive outlet

Early benign prostatic obstruction is a good example of this situation. The treatment strategy should not be to increase bladder contractility, but rather to decrease urethral resistance (Figure 30.3). Often, however, infravesical obstruction induces bladder instability. In this eventuality, vesicourethral balance could be considered to be acceptable,

Table 30.1 *Summary of vesico–urethral balance*

Figure number	Bladder activity	Bladder compliance	Outlet	Clinical example	Treatment
60.2	Normal	Normal	Low	SUI	↑ outlet
60.3	Normal	Normal	High	Early BPH	↓ outlet
60.4	OAB	Normal or Low	High	Symptomatic BPH	↑ outlet ↓ OAB
60.5	OAB	Normal	Normal	Primary OAB	↓ OAB
60.6	OAB	Normal or Low	Low	Mixed urinary incontinence	↑ outlet ↓ OAB
60.7	Hypo – or areflexia	High	Normal	'Primary' hypotonic bladder; diabetes	CIC (±↓ outlet?)
60.8	Hypo – or areflexia	High	Low	Cauda equina syndrome	CIC (±↑ outlet?)
60.9	Hypo – or areflexia	Normal or High	High	Late BPH with decompensated bladder	CIC (±↓ outlet?)

BPH = Benign Prostatic Hypertrophy
CIC = Clean Intermittent Catheterization
OAB = Overactive Bladder
SUI = Stress Urany Incontinence

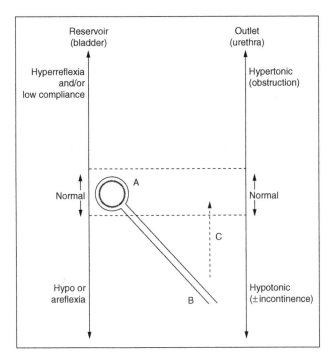

Figure 30.2
The bladder is normal (A), but the urethra hypotonic (B), a condition favorable for incontinence. By increasing urethral tonicity (C), continence is re-established. Overcorrecting may induce urinary retention, as in Figure 30.3.

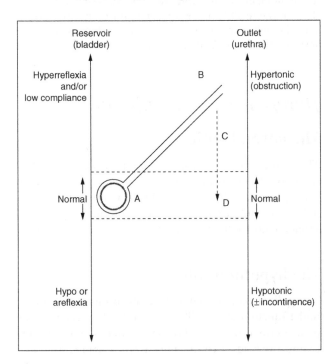

Figure 30.3
The bladder is normal (A), and the urethra obstructive (B), as in benign prostatic hyperplasia or distal urethral stenosis. Correction of outlet conditions (C) allows the re-establishment of micturition under normal pressure conditions (D).

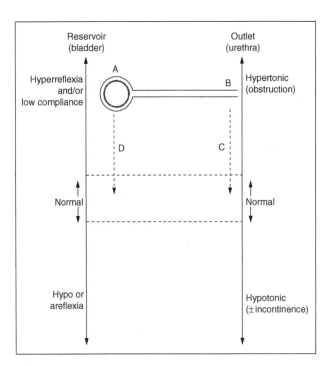

Figure 30.4
The bladder is hyperreflexic and/or low compliant (A), associated with overactive or obstructed outlet (B). The patient is probably continent, but the upper tract is in real danger of decompensation. Therapeutic measures should be directed toward the urethra (C) and the bladder (D) simultaneously to establish normal balance in the security zone.

but this balance is established in the high-pressure zone, compromising renal function in the long term. By eliminating obstruction and controlling hyperreflexia, the system will return to normal equilibrium in the security zone (Figures 30.3 and 30.4).

Bladder hyperreflexia and/or low-compliant bladder

The normotonic outlet

When the bladder is hyperreflexic and/or low compliant, but the urethra still has normal closure pressure, the patient will probably be incontinent. The solution to this problem is not to increase urethral closure pressure, because – although the patient will become continent – the system will be transformed to a high-pressure one, jeopardizing the integrity of the upper urinary tract. Treatment should be directed to controlling hyperreflexia or to improving bladder wall compliance. Thus, the system will be balanced in the security zone (Figure 30.5).

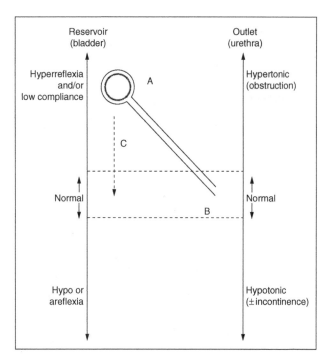

Figure 30.5
The bladder is hyperreflexic and/or low compliant (A) with a normal outlet (B), predisposing to incontinence. Treatment should correct the hyperreflexia (C) without interfering with urethral function (D). Continence should be re-established.

The hypotonic outlet

This clinical situation is relatively rare. With decreased outlet resistance, the patient will almost certainly be incontinent, but because of this hypotonicity a high-pressure system is unlikely to develop. Correcting urethral function alone might put the upper urinary tract in a precarious situation, as in the preceding example. Together with the improvement of urethral hypotonicity, one should also control bladder hyperreflexia and/or compliance (Figure 30.6).

The hypertonic outlet

It is estimated that more then 50% of males with outlet obstruction will develop bladder overactivity.[4,5] Elimination of obstruction will normalize urethral function, but might expose the patient to incontinence. In a non-neurological context, bladder overactivity will subside spontaneously within 1 year after the removal of the obstruction in a significant proportion of patients.[6] In the neurological patient, however, therapeutic measures should be taken to control hyperreflexia, in conjunction with the correction of outlet function (Figure 30.4).

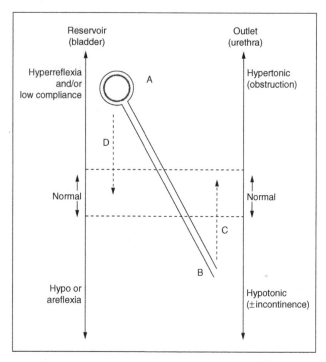

Figure 30.6
The bladder is hyperreflexic and/or low compliant (A), associated with a hypotonic outlet (B). The patient will almost certainly be incontinent. Increasing urethral resistance (C) will probably not be sufficient; conditions similar to those in Figure 30.5 will be created. Detrusor hyperreflexia should also be controlled (D) in order to reach normal vesicourethral equilibrium.

Hypo- or areflexic bladder

The normal outlet

This is the case of the patient who underwent prostatectomy for chronic urinary retention, but who is unable to void spontaneously. Increasing bladder contractility without other modification of outlet conditions should allow spontaneous voiding (Figure 30.7).

The hypotonic outlet

The patient may or may not be incontinent. Improving outlet function alone will almost certainly precipitate the patient into urinary retention. Every effort should be made to improve bladder contractility as well (Figure 30.8).

The obstructive outlet

In this case, the patient will be in chronic urinary retention. Decreasing outlet resistance by eliminating the obstructive factor will not necessarily permit normal voiding without

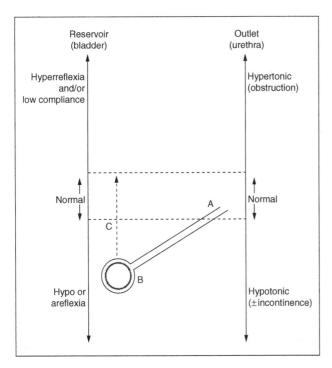

Figure 30.7
The outlet is normal (A), and the bladder is hypo- or areflexic (B). Spontaneous voiding might be possible but with significant post-void residual volume. Treatment should reinforce detrusor contractility (C) without interfering with outlet conditions (A).

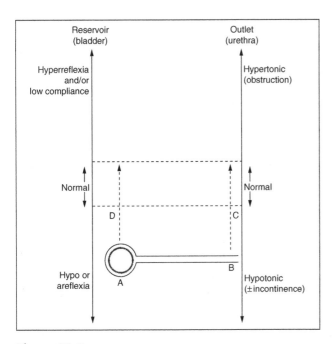

Figure 30.8
Hypo- or areflexic bladder (A) with a hypotonic outlet (B). If the patient is continent, one might adopt a watchful waiting policy, because the system is a low-pressure one. In case of incontinence, the outlet (C) and bladder (D) should be reinforced together. If only the outlet is corrected, the patient might not void spontaneously.

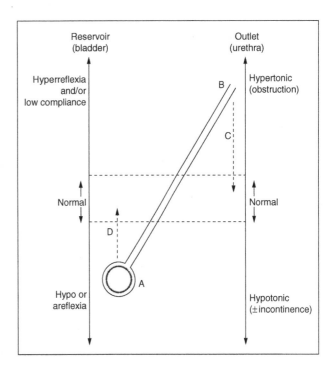

Figure 30.9
Hypo- or areflexic bladder (A) combined with an obstructed outlet (B). No spontaneous voiding is expected. Urethral resistance must be decreased (C) and bladder contractility increased (D) to ensure normal vesicourethral balance.

significant post-void residual volume. Attempts should also be made to improve bladder contractility simultaneously (Figure 30.9).

Conclusion

Normal vesicourethral balance signifies a low-pressure system with normal contractility and compliance, together with no outlet obstruction, and normal urethral tone. Urodynamics allow us to determine which elements are responsible for vesicourethral dysfunction or the disruption of vesicourethral balance. Urodynamics help to identify the element(s) responsible for this dysfunction. Treatment is directed towards restoring vesicourethral balance in the normal pressure ranges.

References

1. Chancellor MB, Blaivas GJ. Spinal cord injury. In: Chancellor MB, Blaivas JG, eds. Practical neurourology: genitourinary complications in neurologic diseases. Boston: Butterworth-Heinemann, 1995: 99–118.

2. McGuire EJ, Cespedes RD, O'Connell HE. Leak point pressures. Urol Clin N Am 1996; 23:253–262.

3. Stöhrer M, Goepel M, Kondo A, et al. The standardization of terminology in neurogenic lower urinary tract dysfunction with suggestions for diagnostic procedures. Neurourol Urodyn 1999; 18: 139–158.

4. Abrams PH, Griffiths DJ. The assessment of prostatic obstruction from urodynamic measurements and from residual urine. Br J Urol 1979; 51:129–134.

5. Dorflinger T, Frimodt-Møller PC, Bruskewitz RC, et al. The significance of uninhibited detrusor contractions in prostatism. J Urol 1985; 133:819–821.

6. Frimodt-Møller PC, Jensen KM, Iversen P, et al. Analysis of presenting symptoms in prostatism. J Urol 1984; 132:272–276.

Part V

Complications

31

Complications related to neurogenic bladder dysfunction – I: infection, lithiasis and neoplasia

Andrew Z Buczynski

Infection

Definition

The term urinary tract infection (UTI) is defined by urine culture showing more than 100,000 bacterial colonies in 1 ml of urine. This criterion has been widely adopted to define this condition. Its usefulness, however, depends on the method of urine collection and the clinical situation.[1] The presence of bacteria in the urine is termed bacteriuria but it does not necessarily mean UTI. Bacteriuria, and even UTI, can be clinically asymptomatic. Proper assessment of UTI is more difficult in patients with neurogenic bladder dysfunction (NBD) compared to the neurologically normal patient. UTI can be acute or chronic, relapsing or recurrent. The term relapse implies infection with the same bacteria, while recurrent infection implies infection with a different strain of bacteria.[2] UTI is the most common cause of fever in spinal cord injury (SCI) patients.[3]

Pyuria alone is not diagnostic of infection, because it may occur from the irritative effect of the catheter, especially if pyuria is at a low level of less than or equal to 30 white blood cells per high power field.[4] Any detectable bacteria from indwelling or suprapubic catheter aspitrates should be considered significant.[5] In patients on clean intermittent catheterization (CIC) 10^2 colonies/ml should be considered significant, while in catheter-free males, a clean voided specimen of 10^4 colonies/ml is significant for infection.[6]

Urine specimen collection for culture and antibiogram

In both sexes, external urethral meatus must be exposed, and cleansed by antiseptic solution. The first 50 ml is passed without collection. Afterwards, approximately 50 ml (= mid-stream) should be collected in a sterile container. Urine should be cultured as soon as possible. If this is impossible, it should be kept refrigerated and cultured within 24 h of refrigeration. It has been shown, that no clinically significant changes in cultures or colony counts occurred between fresh and refrigerated urine samples for up to 24 h.[7] Proper urine collection is best accomplished under the supervision of professional staff in hospital, outpatient clinic or laboratory.

For obtaining urine specimen from patients with NBD, one can use external stimulation (usually suprapubic percussion). If this is impossible, urine should be obtained by a single catheterization. Collection of urine for culture from the drainage bag is not a reliable technique.

Microorganisms involved

The most frequently cultured bacteria from urine specimens, particularly in female patients, is *Escherichia coli*.[1,2] This kind of bacteria is cultured from most patients with uncomplicated cystitis, pyelonephritis or from asymptomatic spinal injured patients. Other, quite often cultured microorganisms are *Klebsiella*, *Pseudomonas*, *Enterobacter*, *Providencia*, *Serratia* and *Proteus*. These are most likely hospital-acquired.[1,8] Especially harmful are the bacteria producing urease, an enzyme causing significant alkalization of urine, which promotes the precipitation of struvite stones (ammonio-magnesium triphosphates and calcium phosphates) in the upper and lower urinary tract.[9] If such a bacteria is cultured, appropriate antibiotics should be administered to prevent further complications. Other, rarely cultured organisms, especially if multiple strains are present, usually indicate contamination rather than true infection. However, patients on catheter drainage for a prolonged period of time (over 1 month) often have polymicrobial flora.

Risk factors

The main risk factors for UTI associated with SCI are impaired voiding, overdistension of the bladder, elevated intravesical pressure, vesicoureteral reflux, urinary tract obstruction, instrumentation and increased incidence of stone formation.[6]

Whenever possible, CIC is the preferred method of adequate bladder drainage. It has been demonstrated, that CIC decreases intravesical pressure and reduces the incidence of bladder stone formation.[10] In general, patients on CIC have significantly lower rates of complications compared to those with indwelling urethral catheterization.[11]

Lower genitourinary tract complications

Urethritis

Since indwelling catheter almost always causes urethritis in patients with NBD, the best is to remove the catheter if in place and start with intermittent catheterization as soon as possible. Occasionally, the blockade of the periurethral glands by the catheter with secondary infection is responsible for the development of periurethral abscess.[2,12] In the acute stage, when Buck's fascia is penetrated, necrosis of the subcutaneous tissue and fascia can represent a life-threatening condition. Immediate suprapubic cystostomy is mandatory, together with wide debridement of all nonviable tissues. Agressive intravenous antibiotherapy should be instituted.

In a less acute, or more chronic stage, the infected gland can evolve in three different directions. It can drain spontaneously to the penile skin and heal without sequel. More often, however, it will drain inside the urethral lumen. The drained cavity will create a urethral diverticulum that needs surgical treatment, because urine trapped in the diverticulum will cause permanent infection and lead eventually to a recurrence of the periurethral abscess (Figure 31.1). Finally, when the abscess drains simultaneously at both sides, via the skin and via the urethral lumen, it results in a urethrocutaneous fistula, which can only be treated surgically. Periurethral abscesses develop mostly in patient with long-term indwelling catheters. However, if proper catheter care is provided, periurethral abscess develops rarely.

Epididymitis and epididymo-orchitis

Epididymitis and epididymo-orchitis are catheter-related complications of UTI. Infection gains the epididymis via the vas deferens in a retrograde fashion.[1,12] Symptoms are usually unilateral. As neurologically impaired patients often do not have sensation of pain, the only clinical sign of

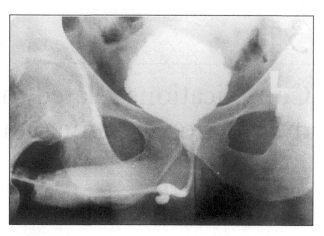

Figure 31.1
Urethral diverticulum, a consequence of a periurethral abscess in a tetraplegic patient.

epididymitis is swelling and flare. Significant enlargement of testicle may develop, which becomes hard and sometimes the scrotal skin reddish. Treatment consists of specific antibiotics based on culture results. Antibiotic therapy is usually successful. In rare instances, when treatment is initiated too late, inadequate or the patient is not treated at all, infection may gain the testicle and cause orchitis with eventually the formation of a testicular abscess. In this circumstance, drainage of the abscess and antibiotherapy gives a chance for spontaneous healing but the affected testicle loses its function.[12,13] Orchidectomy sometimes becomes necessary.

Bacterial infection of the prostate

It is generally admitted, that most often bacteria gains the prostate by infected urine refluxing into the prostatic ducts. Hematogenous and lymphatic spread, however, should also be considered. *Escherichia coli* is the most frequent bacteria.[2] Bacterial prostatitis in NBD is generally chronic and asymptomatic, and chronic bacterial prostatitis is the most common cause of relapsing UTI.[1,2] Only during episodes of acute cystitis, urinalysis will show pyuria and bacteriuria. In other cases, segmented lower tract urine cultures, as suggested by Meares and Stamey[14] should be used in an attempt to localize the infection in the prostate. Unfortunately most antibiotics diffuse poorly into prostatic tissue. Trimethoprim[15] and Ofloxacin[16] are among the recommended antibiotics because they penetrate best into the chronically infected prostatic tissue.

Cystitis

Infection of the lower urinary tract is the most common complication of neurogenic bladder. Almost all patients with NBD will, sooner or later, be in contact with catheters. Indwelling or suprapubic catheter in the acute stage of spinal injury, CIC, all represent risk factors for infection. If sterile catheterization is strictly observed, the risk of introducing infection into the lower urinary tract is theoretically low.[12] Practically, however, all patients with NBD will have UTI from time to time.

Another favorable factor for the development of cystitis is residual urine. Complete bladder emptying is one of the most important defense mechanisms against UTI.[1,12] When residual urine volumes are high, large numbers of bacteria remain in the urine having perfect conditions for growing. The ability to expel bacteria is complete when voiding is complete. This concept is important when considering the association between urinary infection and neurogenic disorders of lower urinary tract.[17]

Urinalysis reveals pyuria in almost all instances of bacterial infection. Recurrent infections, through cicatrization of the bladder wall, gradually reduces bladder capacity and wall compliance, similarly to indwelling catheter, and may result in a small fibrotic bladder.[6]

In some instances, acute bladder infection may cause bleeding, which needs a combination of antibiotherapy with bladder drainage and periodic irrigations to prevent catheter blockade by blood clots. In our experience, bladder irrigation with neomycine solution (5 gm in 500 ml of water) using three-way Foley catheter is very useful in combination with systemic antibiotherapy.

Due to partial or complete loss of sensation in patients with neuropathic bladders, the only signs of cystitis may be increased frequency of micturition, intensification of spasticity and changes in urinalysis.[13] Chronic cystitis in these patients, even with significant changes in urinalysis, are often clinically asymptomatic. Fever is generally absent, although low-grade temperature elevations are not uncommon.[2,13]

Asymptomatic UTI should not be treated.[12,18] Unnecessary or prolonged use of antibiotics will only increase the likelihood of selecting out more resistant microorganisms. Treatment of septic complications under these circumstances may then become very challenging.

Upper urinary tract complications

Prolonged or recurrent infection in the lower urinary tract is one of the factors, that might interfere with antireflux mechanism causing reflux of infected urine to the kidney.[12] This situation may lead to stone formation in the kidney and to the development of progressive failure of the affected kidney. Although infected vesicoureteral reflux significantly increases the risk of pyelonephritis, many patients with pyelonephritis do not have demonstrable reflux.[1] Similarly, not all patients with reflux will have

clinical evidence of pyelonephritis. Acute pyelonephritis, which is most commonly caused by aerobic gram-negative bacteria, reaches the kidney from the lower urinary tract.

Functional infravesical obstruction, such as detrusor-external sphincter dyssynergia (DESD), common in NBD, contributes to the development of pyelonephritis through stasis of urine. Additionally, high intravesical pressure, also common in these patients, creates risk of reflux[12] of an already infected urine.

As the sensation of pain is often absent in neurological patients, the main clinical symptom of acute pyelonephritis is fever up to 40°C. Urinalysis shows pyuria, bacteriuria and microscopic hematuria. Hemogram reveals significant leukocytosis. Intravenous pyelography (IVP) could show some degree of renal enlargement and decreased nephrogram.

Treatment of noncomplicated pyelonephritis consists of specific antibiotherapy according to the results of urine culture and sensitivity studies. An important aspect of the problem however, is the recognition and elimination of complicating factors such as functional infravesical obstruction, infected stones or high intravesical pressures. Ultrasonography may provide similar information than IVP concerning presence of obstruction, stones or abscess.

Catheter care

Catheters should be used only when absolutely necessary. CIC create much less risk of UTI than does indwelling catheter[12,18] so, whenever possible, the former method is recommended. If indwelling catheter must be applied, instillation of suprapubic puncture drainage should be considered. Suprapubic catheters, even if they do not eliminate complications associated with a foreign body in the urinary tract, significantly reduce the incidence of urethral and prostato-epididymal infections. Insertion of the catheter should be performed under aseptic conditions. Closed drainage by gravity should be maintained, with the collecting bag lower than the level of the pubic symphysis. Additionally, the bag should have a valve for prevention of reflux of urine into the bladder when the bag is accidentally raised above the level of the bladder. Until the catheter is in place, antimicrobial treatment of asymptomatic, catheter-associated, bacteriuria is not recommended.[1,19]

Lithiasis

The occurrence of stones within the urinary tract is a problem as old as mankind. Many methods of dealing with stones have been developed in the past, but none have had as much of an impact as had the development of endourology and extracorporeal shock wave lithotripsy (ESWL). Those two innovations significantly reduced the necessity for open surgery in the treatment of lithiasis.

The stone disease affects male patients 3 times as commonly than females, and whites 4–5 times more commonly then blacks.[9] The development of stones in the urinary tract is a complex, incompletely understood, multifactorial process. In patients with NBD, the stone formation is relatively well recognized. The main factors responsible for stone formation in these patients are chronic or recurrent infections, especially those caused by urease-forming organisms, infravesical obstruction producing stasis, hypercalciuria related to immobilization (especially in young men),[9,12] and high specific gravity of urine, especially for kidney stones.[20] This last point was challenged by others,[21] suggesting that total fluid intake does not determine stone occurrence, but rather the fluid type (juice) which influences stone formation. Struvite stones form only when urine pH is significantly increased (>7.24).[22] Organisms that produce the enzyme urease, split urea into ammonium which, in turn, causes significant alkalinization of urine. Proteus species are the most common urea-splitting organisms and are identified in most patients with struvite stones.[8,9,13] Other organisms may produce urease also, including *Klebsiella*, *Pseudomonas*, *Providencia* and *Staphylococcus*. According to several authors 10–20% of SCI patients have struvite calculi.[5,23,24]

Renal calculi

Patients with NBD develop almost exclusively struvite stones.[9,13] Important minerals involved in struvite stone formation include calcium, magnesium, ammonium and phosphates. A protein matrix, such as fragments of papillae or urinary epithelium, is common and constitutes the nidus of the stone. In a large series of 1669 SCI patients, the overall incidence of renal calculi was estimated to be about 3.5%.[25] Risk factors included indwelling catheters (49%), bladder stones (52%) and vesicoureteral reflux (28%). The recurrence rate was 69%. Chen et al[26] compared two large cohort of patients: 8314 patients between 1986 and 1999, vs 5850 patients between 1973 and 1982. They estimated that within 10 years after injury, 7% of patients will develop their first kidney stone. This trend has not changed over the past 25 years. Interestingly, they could not demonstrate any significant differential effect on kidney stone formation in relation to the type of urinary drainage used, including indwelling catheter, intermittent catheterization or condom catheter.[26,27] Once a kidney stone developed, there is a 34% chance of a second stone developing episode within the next five years.[28] Male patients with complete spinal cord lesion represent an increased risk for kidney stone formation.[29] Regular position changing of paralysed patients, high fluid intake,[20] early mobilization, proper treatment of urinary infection and prevention of subsequent reinfection are important factors in the prophylaxis of renal calculi. Struvite stones may grow to fill the entire renal pelvis and

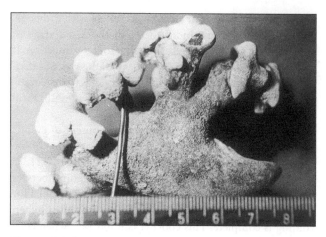

Figure 31.2
Staghorn calculus removed from the kidney of a paraplegic man 10 years after his accident.

collecting system creating staghorn calculi (Figure 31.2). It is interesting to note that staghorn calculi, even those which fill the collecting system completely of kidney, rarely cause complete obstruction of urine outflow. Sometimes, however, they can be responsible for silent hydronephrosis or even pyonephrosis which is not perceived by the patient, because a number of them lost pain sensation due to the neurological lesion. Nonspecific symptoms, such as feeling unwell, abdominal discomfort, increased spasms and autonomic dysreflexia can alert the well-informed physician.[30]

Kidney calculi are diagnosed by ultrasonography and plain X-ray of the abdomen. Struvite stones are more or less radioopaque, depending on their content in calcium but usually they are quite well visualized. An IVP will confirm the presence of calculi and show the degree of obstruction, if any. Successful treatment of renal stones depends on complete elimination of the calculus, eradication of infection and removing the obstruction causing stasis of urine. Selection of the best method of treatment should be individualized and adapted to every given patient. In paraplegic and quadriplegic patients typical ESWL alone is not recommended because of the difficulty in eliminating crushed stone fragments.[31,32] The recommended technique for treatment of renal stones in patients with NBD is percutaneous nephrolithotripsy (PCNL), in some selected cases in combination with ESWL. Stowe et al[33] reported in 9 out of 52 SCI patients (17.3%) who developed autonomic dysreflexia after ESWL. If ESWL is considered in a quadriplegic patient, this can be performed without the added risk of general or regional anesthesia. In a small series of 5 patients undergoing 10 ESWL treatments, no incidence of complete clinical syndrome of autonomic dysreflexia occurred. These patients, however, should be monitored closely by an anesthetiologist, because significant hypertension developed intraoperatively in 2 patients.[34] Effective prophylaxis can be obtained with 10–20 mg of nifedipine sublingually, 15–20 min before the procedure.[35] Intraoperative monitoring remains mandatory. Exacerbation of post-traumatic syringomyelia following ESWL has also been reported,[36] presumably caused by the shock waves reverberating the fluid within the intramedullary cavity producing further damage to the spinal cord. ESWL usually needs to be repeated for complete elimination of calculi from the kidney. In rare cases, patients will require open surgery. Nephrectomy should be performed when the affected kidney is practically non-functional, or in case of pyonephrosis.

In the prevention of struvite calculi it is essential to eliminate the infection with urea-splitting organisms. When chronic infection cannot be eradicated, urease inhibitors may be used to decrease pH of urine and ammonia level. Methenaminhippurat should be recommended in a dose of 1 gm twice a day for the prevention of recurrent infection and struvite calculosis in patients with NBD.[37]

Ureteral calculi

Most ureteral stones originate in the kidney. Only stones caused by ureteral obstruction like stricture or tumor may be formed or develop in the ureter. Small stones will pass down the ureter and will block the ureterovesical junction. These can be evacuated endoscopically using ureterorenoscope (URS). Sometimes fragmentation by ultrasonic or laser lithotripsy becomes necessary. Contrary to the neurologically healthy people, patients with NBD, because of immobilization, have less chance to spontaneously expel ureteral calculi. If ureteric stone is big enough and remains blocked in the middle third of the ureter, open surgical intervention could be considered.

Bladder stones

Infection of lower urinary tract by urea splitting, mainly nosocomial microorganisms, indwelling catheter and residual urine are the main reasons for bladder stone formation.

From 1973 to 1996 Chen et al[38] observed a decline in the incidence for an initial bladder stone (from 29% down to 8%). During the first year following the SCI, bladder stone risk increased with decreasing age, and was greater for whites. During the subsequent years, neurologically complete lesions, males, persons with indwelling catheter or on intermittent catheterization, also had a higher risk. At least in quadriplegics, suprapubic catheter drainage carried a statistically higher risk for bladder stone formation than did CIC.[27] Often bladder stone starts from the small pieces of thin struvite calculus formed around the balloon of a Foley catheter and left behind after the removal of the catheter. Those calculi may grow but they will retain the typical egg-shell or bowl shape (Figure 31.3). These calculi are usually multiple and are common in patients who have had indwelling

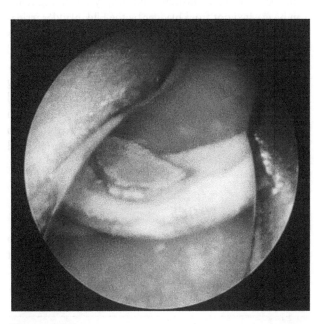

Figure 31.3
Typical bowl shaped struvite bladder calculi in a paraplegic patient.

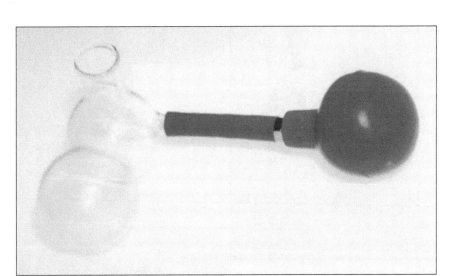

Figure 31.4
The Ellik bladder irrigator. The evacuated stone or tissue fragments are trapped in the bottom of the second glass recipient.

catheters for a long period of time. In other instances, debris, sloughs, pus cells and bacterial bodies are the nidus for struvite stone formation.[39] Bladder stones may cause severe irritative symptoms, hematuria and perpetuate infection. Unless bladder stones are removed, eradication of infection is impossible and antibiotics are not efficacious. Park and Linsenmeyer[40] suggested that weekly catheter changes might dramatically reduce catheter incrustation rates.

It should be mentioned that small struvite stones with low calcium content can easily be missed on X-ray and are often incidentally discovered during cystoscopy.

The treatment of bladder stones is easy, because of easy access, endoscopical and surgical, to the bladder. Additionally, struvite stones are not hard and easily fragmented. After fragmentation by mechanical forceps, ultrasonic, laser or electrohydraulic lithotripsy, small fragments can be washed out from bladder by the Ellik bladder irrigator (Figure 31.4). Vespasiani et al[41] reported excellent results with the endoscopic ballistic Swiss Lithoclast lithotripsy. All patients were stone free at 6 months postoperatively. They noticed, however, 5 intraoperative complications, including crisis of autonomic dysreflexia in 3 patients. Open surgical intervention for bladder stones is indicated only when bladder capacity is very small or the size of the stone is so big, that endoscopical litholapaxy would be too late and extremely difficult.

Urethral stones

Calculi lodged in the urethra are rare and mainly due to obstruction, sometimes from an unexpected cause,[42] but can also develop in preexisting urethral diverticulum. Figure 31.5A illustrates a stone which was growing slowly

inside the urethral diverticulum and became a "staghorn calculus" growing into both sides of the urethral lumen without creating clinically significant outflow obstruction.

Treatment of urethral stones is surgical (Figure 31.5B). If the reason for stone formation is stricture, endoscopic urethrotomy and subsequently lithotripsy is probably the best solution. In case of a stone inside a diverticulum, open surgery is necessary.

Neoplasm

It is generally accepted that the incidence and mortality of bladder cancer are heightened in SCI patients compared to the neurologically normal population.[43] The risk was estimated to be 16–28 times higher, especially for squamous cell carcinoma of the bladder in this group of patients.[44,45]

Bejany et al[46] found an incidence of 2.3% of bladder tumor in their SCI unit. Of these 9 (81%) had squamous cell carcinoma, 1 transitional cell carcinoma and 1 a mixed type (transitional and squamous cell) carcinoma. All of them had chronic bacteriuria, 44% had gross or microscopic hematuria, and 5 had stone disease. At 3 years follow-up, only 55% were free of disease. They did not find urine cytology helpful in the diagnosis of these patients. As 55% of them had had urethral recurrence, they suggested that urethrectomy should also be performed together with radical cystectomy.

Stonehill et al[47] evaluated the role of urinary cytology in this group of patients, especially because endoscopy is often nonspecific, difficult to interpret and sometimes even may be normal. They studied patients with indwelling

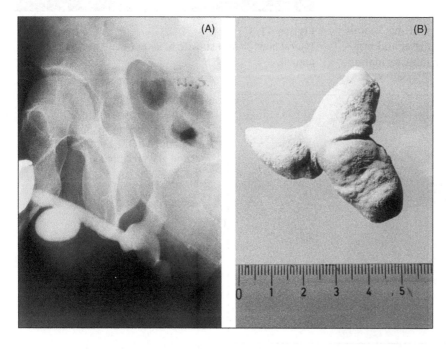

Figure 31.5
(A) X-ray of the urethra showing two diverticuli. The proximal one contains a stone. (B) Stone removed surgically.

catheter for more than 5 years. Positive cytology had a sensitivity of 71% and a specificity of 97% when evaluating patients with suspicious finding. Based on these observations the authors recommended yearly cytology in all high risk SCI patients, followed by biopsy, if any abnormal finding was noted on cystoscopy. Indwelling catheter and history of bladder stones were statistically significant risk factors.[48]

Locke et al[49] found an 8% incidence of squamous cell carcinoma in 25 SCI patients catheterized for a minimum of 10 years. Two patients had positive cytology, and both of them had hematuria as well.

Esrig et al[50] discovered in 37 patients with long-term indwelling catheter drainage (mean: 18.6 years), transitional cell carcinoma (grade 2 to 3) in 2 patients.

Bickel et al[51] pointed out that with appropriate management of these patients the survival is not different from the ambulatory, neurologically normal, population.

Pannek[52] reported, recently, the results of a mail survey sent to all SCI centers in Germany, Switzerland and Austria treating SCI patients between 1995 and 1999. Only 64.6% of the centers responded. The charts of 43,564 patients were reviewed, which represent the largest cohort published so far. Fourty-eight of them (0.11%) developed bladder cancer. This is somewhat lower than that reported by West et al[53] in a cohort of 33,656 patients, where they found a bladder cancer incidence of 0.39%. In the Pannek-survey, 81% of the tumors were urothelial and 19% squamous cell carcinomas. The majority of tumors were muscle-infiltrating at the initial diagnosis. Of these 48 patients only 18.9% had indwelling catheter (suprapubic or transurethral), with a mean duration of 8.5 $\pm$ 11.2 years. Intermittent catheterization was used by 32.4% of them. As pointed out by the author, this decline in incidence might be secondary at least in part to the avoidance of indwelling catheters, which have to be regarded as an important risk factor for bladder cancer.

The follow-up of patients with indwelling catheter is controversial. Some advocate for screening cystoscopy,[54] arguing that this will detect malignant lesions in an earlier stage. Others[55] believe that cystoscopy does not fulfill the accepted criteria for screening for primary bladder cancer in SCI patients.

This review of the literature suggests that SCI patients with long-standing indwelling catheterization (certainly after 10 years, perhaps even after 5 years post-trauma) should undergo yearly (or every second year?) cystoscopy, combined with urine cytology. If cytology is doubtful or positive, cold cup biopsy should be done randomly if no suspicious lesion is found endoscopically. History of bladder stone and chronic UTI should be considered as significant risk factors for the development of bladder cancer in SCI patients. New onset of gross hematuria should be investigated in the same way as in the neurologically normal population.

References

1. Levine FS, Staskin DR. Genitourinary infection. In: Siroky MB, Krane RJ, eds. Manual of urology, 1st edn. Boston: Little, Brown and Company, 1990:205–224.

2. Ward TT, Jones SR. Genitourinary tract infections. In: Reese RE, Betts RF, eds. A logical approach to infectious diseases, 3rd edn. Boston: Little, Brown and Company, 1991:357–389.

3. Beraldo PS, Neves EG, Alves CM, Khan P, Cirilo AC, Alencar MR. Pyrexia in hospitalized spinal cord injured patients. Paraplegia 1993; 31:186–191.

4. Menon EB, Tan ES. Pyuria: index of infection in patients with spinal cord injuries. Br J Urol 1992; 69:144–146.

5. Cardenas DD, Hooton TM. Urinary tract infection in persons with spinal cord injury. Arch Phys Med Rehabil 1995; 76:272–280.

6. National Institute on Disability and Rehabilitation Research Consensus Statement: the prevention and management of urinary tract infections among people with spinal cord injury. SCI Nurs 1993; 10:49–61.

7. Horton JA 3rd, Kirshblum SC, Lisenmeyer TA, Johnston M, Rustagi A. Does refrigeration of urine alter culture results in hospitalized patients with neurogenic bladder? J Spinal Cord Med 1998; 21:342–347.

8. Menon EB, Tan ES. Urinary tract infection in acute spinal cord injury. Singapore Med J 1992; 33:359–361.

9. Babayan RK. Urinary Calculi and Endourology. In: Siroky MB, Krane RJ, eds. Manual of urology, 1st edn. Boston: Little, Brown and Company, 1990:123–131.

10. Stover SL, Lloyd LK, Waites KB, Jackson AB. Urinary tract infection in spinal cord injury. Arch Phys Med Rehabil 1989; 70:47–54.

11. Weld KJ, Dmochowski RR. Effect of bladder management on urological complications in spinal cord injured patients. J Urol 2000; 163:768–772.

12. Buczynski AZ. Principles for urological management of SCI patients. Ortopedia Traumatologia Rehabilitacja 2000; 2:57–60.

13. Buczynski AZ. Urological complications in paraplegic and quadriplegic patients. New Medicine 1999; 89:13–15.

14. Meares EM Jr, Stamey TA. Bacteriologic localization patterns in bacterial prostatitis and urethritis. Invest Urol 1968; 5:492–518.

15. Stamey TA, Meares EM Jr. Chronic bacterial prostatitis and the diffusion of drugs into prostatic fluid. J Urol 1970; 103:187–194.

16. Bjerklund Johansen TE, Gruneberg RN, Guilbert J, Hofstetter A, Lobel B, Naber KG, Palon Redorta J, van Cangh PJ. The role of antibiotics in the treatment of chronic prostatitis: a concensus statement. Eur Urol 1998; 34:457–466.

17. Kunin CM. Detection, prevention and management of urinary tract infections. Philadelphia: Lea & Febiger 1987:

18. Stover SL, Lloyd LK, Waites KB, Jackson AB. Neurogenic urinary tract infection. Neurol Clin 1991; 9:741–755.

19. Warren JW, Tenney JH, Hoopes JM, Muncie HL, Anthony WC. A prospective microbiologic study of bacteriuria in patients with indwelling urethral catheters. J Infect Dis 1982; 146:719–723.

20. Chen Y, Roseman JM, Funkhouser E, DeVivo MJ. Urine specific gravity and water hardness in relation to urolithiasis in persons with spinal cord injury. Spinal Cord 2001; 39:571–576.

21. Chen Y, Roseman JM, DeVivo MJ, Funkhouser E. Does fluid amount and choice influence urinary stone formation in persons with spinal cord injury? Arch Phys Med Rehabil 2002; 83:1002–1089.

22. Nomura S, Ishido T, Teranishi J, Makiyama K. Long-term analysis of suprapubic cystostomy drainage in patients with neurogenic bladder. Urol Int 2000; 65:185–189.

23. Buczynski AZ. Urolithiasis as complication of traumatic lesions of spinal cord. Pol Med Week 1980; 4:129–131.

24. Takasaki E, Suzuki T, Honda M, Imai T, Maeda S, Hosoya Y. Chemical Compositions of 300 lower urinary tract calculi and associated disorders in the urinary tract. Urol Int 1995; 54:89–94.

25. Donnellan SM, Bolton DM. The impact of contemporary bladder management technics on struvite calculi associated with spinal cord injury. BJU Int 1999; 84:280–285.

26. Chen Y, DeVivo MJ, Roseman JM. Current trend and risk factors for kidney stones in persons with spinal cord injury: a longitudinal study. Spinal Cord 2000; 38:346–353.

27. Mitsui T, Minami K, Furuno T, Morita H, Koyanagi T. Is suprapubic cystostomy an optimal urinary management in high quadriplegics? A comparative study of suprapubic cystostomy and clean intermittent catheterisation. Eur Urol 2000; 38:434–438.

28. Chen Y, DeVivo MJ, Stover SL, Lloyd LK. Recurrent kidney stone: a 25-year follow-up study in persons with spinal cord injury. Urology 2002; 60:228–232.

29. DeVivo MJ, Fine PR, Cutter GR, Maetz HM. The risk of renal calculi in spinal cord injury patients. J Urol 1984; 131:857–860.

30. Vaidyanathan S, Singh G, Soni BM, Hughes P, Watt JM, Dundas S, Sett P, Parsons KF. Silent hydronephrosis/pyonephrosis due to upper urinary tract calculi in spinal cord injury patients. Spinal Cord 2000; 38:331–338.

31. Robert M, Bennani A, Ohanna F, Guiter J, Averous M, Grasset D. The management of upper urinary tract calculi by piezoelectric extracorporeal shock wave lithotripsy in spinal cord injury patients. Paraplegia 1995; 33:132–135.

32. Niedrach WL, Davis RS, Tonetti FW, Cockett AT. Extracorporeal shock-wave lithotripsy in patients with spinal cord dysfunction. Urology 1991; 38:152–156.

33. Stowe DF, Bernstein JS, Madsen KE, McDonald DJ, Ebert TJ. Autonomic hyperreflexia in spinal cord injured patients during extracorporeal shock wave lithotripsy. Anesth Analg 1989; 68:788–791.

34. Spirnak JP, Bodner D, Udayashankar S, Resnick MI. Extracorporeal shock wave lithotripsy in traumatic quadriplegic patients: can it be safely performed without anasthesia? J Urol 1988; 139:18–19.

35. Sugiyama T, Fugelso P, Avon M. Extracorporeal shock wave lithotripsy in neurologically impaired patients. Semin Urol 1992; 10:109–11.

36. Di Lorenzo N, Maleci A, Williams BM. Severe exacerbation of post-traumatic syringomyelia after lithotripsy: case report. Paraplegia 1994; 32:694–696.

37. Banovac K, Wade N, Gonzales F, Walsh B, Rhamy RK. Decreased incidence of urinary tract infections in patients with spinal cord injury: effect of methenamine. J Am Paraplegic Soc 1991; 14:52–54.

38. Chen Y, DeVivo MJ, Lloyd LK. Bladder stone incidence in persons with spinal cord injury: determinants and trends, 1973–1996. Urology 2001; 58:665–670.

39. Boyarsky S. Labay P, Hanick P, Abramson AS, Boyarsky R. Care of the patient with neurogenic bladder, 1st edn. Boston: Little, Brown and Company, 1979.

40. Park YI, Linsenmeyer TA. A method to minimize indwelling catheter calcification and bladder stones in individuals with spinal cord injury. J Spinal Cord Med 2001 Summer; 24:105–108.

41. Vespasiani G, Pesce F, Finazzi Agro E, Virgili G, Giannantoni A, Micali S, Micali F. Endoscopic ballistic lithotripsy in the treatment of bladder calculi in patients with neurogenic voiding dysfunction. Endourol 1996; 10:551–554.

42. Vaidyanathan S, Singh G, Sett P, Soni BM. Complication of penile sheath drainage in a spinal cord injury patient: calculus impacting in the urethra proximal to the rim of a condom. Spinal Cord 2001; 39:240–241.

43. Groah SL, Weitzenkamp DA, Lammertse DP, Whiteneck GG, Lezotte DC, Hamman RF. Excess risk of bladder cancer in spinal cord injury: evidence for an association between indwelling catheter use and bladder cancer. Arch Phys Med Rehabil 2002; 83:346–351.

44. El-Masri WS, Fellows G. Bladder cancer after spinal cord injury. Paraplegia 1981; 19:265–270.

45. van Velzen D, Kirshnan KR, Parsons KF, Soni BM, Frazer MH, Howard CV, Vaidyanathan S. Comparative pathology of dome and trigone of urinary bladder mucosa in paraplegics and tetraplegics. Paraplegia 1995; 33:565–572.

46. Bejany DE, Lockhart IL, Rhamy RK. Malignant vesical tumors following SCI. J Urol 1987; 138:1390–1392.

47. Stonehill WH, Goldman HB, Dmochowski RR. The use of urine cytology for diagnosing bladder cancer in spinal cord injured patients. J Urol 1997; 157:2112–2114.

48. Stonehill WH, Dmochowski RR, Patterson AL, Cox CE. Risk factors for bladder tumors in spinal cord injury patients. J Urol 1996; 155:1248–1250.

49. Locke JR, Hill DE, Walzer Y. Incidence of squamous cell carcinoma in patients with long term catheter drainage. J Urol 1985; 133:1034–1035.

50. Esrig D, McEvoy K, Bennett CJ. Bladder cancer in the spinal cord-injured patient with long-term catheterisation: a causal relationship? Semin Urol 1992; 10:102–108.

51. Bickel A, Culkin DJ, Wheeler JS Jr. Bladder cancer in spinal cord injury patients. J Urol 1991; 146:1240–1242.

52. Pannek J. Transitional cell carcinoma in patients with spinal cord injury: a high risk malignancy? Urology 2002; 59:240–244.

53. West DA, Cummings JM, Longo WE, Virgo KS, Johnson FE, Parra RO. Role of chronic catheterisation in the development of bladder cancer in patients with spinal cord injury. Urology 1999; 53:292–297.

54. Navon JD, Soliman H, Khonsari F, Ahlering T. Screening cystoscopy and survival of SCI patients with squamous cell carcinoma of the bladder. J Urol 1997; 157:2109–2111.

55. Yang CC, Clowers DE. Screening cystoscopy in chronically catheterised SCI patients. Spinal Cord 1999; 37:204–207.

32

Complications related to neurogenic bladder dysfunction – II: reflux and renal insufficiency

Imre Romics, Antal Hamvas, and Attila Majoros

Introduction

After World War I, 80% of the spinal cord injury (SCI) patients died from urological complications,[1] mostly from urinary infection, which was untreatable at that time in the absence of antibiotics, and from secondary upper urinary tract damage. Urodynamics being unknown, the accepted approach was the 'balanced bladder' method, i.e. if voiding took place with no or minimal residual urine, the patient's condition was considered satisfactory. With no information on intravesical pressures during storage and voiding, there was no way to prevent upper urinary tract damage resulting from lower tract dysfunction.[2]

Today, widespread use of antibiotics, urodynamic evaluation, clean intermittent self-catheterization (CIC), and up-to-date management of urolithiasis have led to considerable improvements in life expectancy and, indeed, in the quality of life of SCI patients.

Nevertheless, urinary infections are still considered the most frequent complication in SCI patients. In a follow-up study of paraplegics from World War II, renal disease was the most common cause of death in the first 20 years post-injury, accounting for 40% of all deaths.[3]

Pathophysiology of upper urinary tract damage caused by neurogenic bladder dysfunction

Abnormally high intravesical storage and/or voiding pressure may predispose to vesicoureteral reflux (VUR), urinary retention, and urinary infection, leading ultimately to renal insufficiency. The most frequent urological abnormality associated with vesicoureteral reflux appears to be uninhibited bladder contraction. Koff et al found uninhibited detrusor contractions during the storage phase in the majority of neurologically normal children with recurrent urinary infections; nearly 50% of them had VUR, and 30% had an abnormal ureteric orifice but without VUR. Their findings were confirmed by the fact that after reducing intravesical pressure with anticholinergic medication, 58% of urinary infections were cured without the use of antibiotics.[4]

Urinary infection in itself will increase intravesical pressure, reduce compliance, and weaken the uretero-vesical junction, thus predisposing to reflux. The incidence of VUR in SCI patients varies between 17 and 25%,[5,6] and can be found in 20% of neonates with meningomyelocele.[7] Soygur et al examined a group of children with reflux and without neurological symptoms, noting unilateral reflux in 40.3% and bilateral reflux in 59.7%. Urodynamic evaluation revealed asymptomatic voiding dysfunction in 28% of the unilateral and in 72% of the bilateral reflux cases. This significant difference seems to indicate that bilateral reflux is caused by some (perhaps silent) voiding dysfunction, whereas unilateral reflux may be attributed in patients with intact bladder function to primary damage of the vesicoureteral junction.[8] Apart from high intravesical pressure, VUR may also be related directly to urinary infection and high-pressure bladder function. Retention, high intrapyelic pressure, and proliferation of mostly urease-producing microorganisms may lead to the formation of renal calculi, to hydronephrosis, pyonephrosis, and renal insufficiency. Intrapyelic pressure rises may cause pyelocaliceal reflux and reduce postglomerular blood flow, resulting in ischemic damage.[9]

Gerridzen et al examined 140 SCI patients with voiding dysfunction and found detrusor hyperreflexia in 100 and areflexia in 40, with kidney damage in 16 and 7 patients, respectively. The 7 patients in the areflexic group with kidney damage showed significantly higher storage pressures (58 cmH$_2$O on average) than the rest of the same group (24 cmH$_2$O on average). In the hyperreflexic group, the 16 patients with kidney damage also showed significantly higher detrusor pressure values (115 cmH$_2$O on average) than the 84 patients with no renal impairment (72 cmH$_2$O on average). However, the pathologically high bladder pressures in this group were taken during the voiding phase.[10] High-pressure hyperreflexia was combined with detrusor-sphincter dyssynergia (DSD) in 55% of cases. In 4 of 23 patients, there was only radiographic evidence of kidney damage, 7 developed VUR, and 9 had hydronephrosis. Kidney damage from VUR was found in less than 1% of the cases.[10,11]

Patients with neurogenic bladder dysfunction secondary to suprasacral lesions (injuries above the sacral micturition center) usually develop detrusor hyperreflexia with or without DSD. High-pressure values are measured both during the storage and the voiding phase, more than 40 and 90 cmH$_2$O, respectively. This may be the consequence of protracted, intensive, uninhibited contractions, reduced bladder compliance, or functional (DSD) or organic (benign prostatic hyperplasia) urinary obstruction.[12–14] Therefore, the chances of upper tract damage are higher than in the case of lower motoneuron lesions (level of injury within or below the sacral micturition center). In this latter circumstance, the detrusor will be hypo- or areflexic so that even with reduced bladder compliance, pathologically high pressure values will only appear during the storage phase. Among patients voiding spontaneously via reflex contractions and exhibiting normal pressure values, both in the storage and voiding phases, there are still a few who will show some degree of reflux or urinary retention.

Linsenmeyer et al found 4 cases of VUR and 9 cases of upper tract dilatation in 84 patients voiding via reflex contraction. The only significant difference between the two groups was in the duration of the reflexly induced contractions.[15]

However, it does happen that an intially areflexic bladder decreases compliance and changes into a hyperreflexic state, which may lead to upper tract damage. This is suggested by the results of Jamil et al, who performed natural-fill urodynamics in 30 patients with indwelling catheters. Intravesical pressure rises of >40 cmH$_2$O were found in 11 and renal scarring in 9 patients, 6 of them from the high-pressure group.[16]

On the other hand, 'silent' voiding dysfunctions with no lower tract symptoms may also result in upper tract complications.[17,18]

Tables 32.1–32.3 summarize the risk factors that are associated with kidney damage.

Table 32.1 *Risk factors associated with kidney damage*

General risk factors:
   Newborns
   Old age
   Immobilization
   Diabetes mellitus
   Immunosuppression
   Polymorbidity

Neurological risk factors:
   Quadriplegia > paraplegia
   Complete lesion > incomplete lesion

Table 32.2 *Urological abnormalities representing risk for kidney damage*

Urinary tract infection

Bladder outlet obstruction (BPH, stricture, etc.)

Urinary lithiasis

Bladder diverticulum

VUR with secondary reflux nephropathy

Foreign body in the urinary tract (catheter, urethral stent, etc.)

BPH, benign prostatic hypertrophy; VUR, vesicoureteral reflux.

Table 32.3 *Urodynamic abnormalities representing risk factors for kidney damage*

Decreased bladder compliance (>10 ml/cmH$_2$O)

LPP or storage pressure >40 cmH$_2$O

Reduced bladder capacity

Sustained high-pressure detrusor contraction

Voiding pressure >90 cmH$_2$O

DESD or detrusor-bladder neck dyssynergia

High post-void residual (>30% of bladder capacity)

LPP, leak point pressure; DESD, detrusor-external sphincter dyssynergia.

Etiology of neurogenic bladder dysfunction leading to reflux and renal failure

Spinal cord injury

Spinal cord injury due to an accident, disc prolapse, acute myelitis, operation of thoracic aorta aneurysms, etc., occurs in the United States approximately 12,000 times a year. Half of these victims end up quadriplegic, and the rest paraplegic, 53% with complete and 47% with incomplete lesions, half of the total number in the upper thoracal section above the 12th thoracic level, and 75% are male.[19] As a consequence, most SCI patients have a hyperreflexic bladder. Reports suggest a 7–32% incidence of renal lithiasis in SCI patients. Bors and colleagues found an 8.2% incidence of renal lithiasis.[20] Hall et al[21] examined 898 SCI patients after an average of 27 years, detecting renal calculi in 14.8%, in association with VUR in 37.7%, and without reflux in 10%. Of those with renal calculi, 56.6% were on indwelling catheters. This contrasts with the 700 patients with no renal calculi, where only 28% were on indwelling catheters. They also found 261 patients with bladder stones, 17.7% of them combined with renal stones. There was no correlation with the prevalence of VUR. A review of this large population suggested three conclusions:

1. the incidence of renal calculi is significantly higher in patients with renal reflux
2. bladder stones and simultaneous reflux will not significantly increase the number of renal calculi
3. indwelling catheters significantly raise the incidence of renal and bladder stones.

The incidence of reflux among SCI patients varies from 5% to 23%.[10,11,20,21] Killorin et al reported upper tract damage in 7% of their SCI patients with areflexic bladder; 32% had hyperreflexic bladder, and there was no upper tract damage in those with normal detrusor function.[22]

Neural tube defects

Neural tube defects (spina bifida occulta, meningocele, meningomyelocele) are the most frequent reasons for bladder dysfunction in infancy. In the majority of the patients, the lumbar section (at the conus medullaris) is involved, resulting in an areflexic bladder and often an open bladder neck. Hydronephrosis was found in less than 10%, VUR in 16%, and bladder diverticuli in 23.5% of these newborns. Based on data in a pediatric myelodysplastic population, in 1981, McGuire et al described the correlation between storage pressure and chances of upper tract damage. He identified the so-called leak point pressure (LPP) at which urine will leak at the urethral meatus, and showed the risk of upper tract damage to be high with LPP >40 cmH$_2$O, but significantly lower with LPP <40 cmH$_2$O. In the low-LPP group, he observed no VUR and only two intravesicular diverticuli, in contrast to 68% VUR and 81% retention in the high-LPP (>40 cmH$_2$O) group.[12]

Iatrogenic damage

Iatrogenic damage is associated with various perioperative complications, the most frequent of which are upper motoneuron lesions due to operations on aneurysms of the thoracic aorta or areflexic bladders resulting from peripheral neural lesions due to radical surgery of the pelvis. Both types of damage may lead to upper tract injury or deteriorated function.

Diagnosis of upper tract damage

Laboratory tests

Serum creatinine, urea nitrogen, serum bicarbonate, blood pH, urine pH, urine gravity and osmolarity, proteinuria, and cylindruria are good indicators of renal function.

Videourodynamic examination

Storage and voiding pressure, maximum bladder capacity, bladder compliance, bladder neck condition, bladder configuration, detrusor-external sphincter or detrusor-bladder neck dyssynergia, passive and/or active VUR are well-documented with this test. It is essential for neurogenic bladders to be initially evaluated by videourodynamics and to repeat the test at least on an annual basis (Madersbacher, pers comm), because bladder dysfunction may change later on. In myelodysplasia, for instance, areflexic bladder dysfunction is likely to change with time to hyperreflexia.[23] In other cases (e.g. control of bladder compliance in meningomyelocele), conventional urodynamics without video control may be all that is needed for follow-up.

Ultrasonography

This is the simplest and least-invasive way to gather information on vesicoureteral dilatation, nephrolithiasis, renal parenchyma thickness, and residual urine. Urine transport abnormalities, both functional (or nonobstructive type, e.g. VUR, brimming bladder, overhydrated condition, acute pyelonephritis) and organic (or obstructive type, e.g. stones, strictures), are easily detected using furosemide (frusemide).

The Doppler technique can define the arterial resistance index. Increased arterial resistance index values are present even before actual dilatation of the collecting system has appeared. Values of 0.7 or more are indications of obstruction. The color Doppler technique demonstrates reflux with no X-ray exposure: a transducer directed toward the ureteral orifices will image retrograde flow in the ureter as a colored jet. Virgili et al sonographed 115 SCI patients and found upper tract anomalies (vesicorenal dilatation, chronic pyelonephritis) in 21.7% of them.[24] Calenoff et al compared ultrasonography with conventional intravenous urograms in 54 SCI patients and observed that all abnormalities seen on intravenous urograms (retention in 36% and VUR in 56% of cases) can also be detected by ultrasonography. They suggested the use of ultrasonography for follow-up rather than intravenous urography.[25] Ozer et al used ultrasonography in a prospective study to screen SCI patients with no urological symptoms and reported that upper tract abnormalities which needed therapeutic intervention were only detected in symptomatic patients. Therefore, they did not recommend ultrasonography for large-scale preventive early diagnosis in asymptomatic patients.[26] Bih et al compared ultrasonographic results before and after micturition and noted that upper tract ultrasonography performed on a full bladder was more likely to show urine transport abnormalities.[27]

Intravenous urography

Intravenous urography is considered to be the gold standard for the detection of upper tract abnormalities due to neurogenic bladder dysfunction. Even if it involves X-ray exposure and possible allergic reactions to the contrast material (very rare, though, today with tri-iodides), the fact remains that this is the most reliable source of information on the morphology and, to some extent, also on the function of the upper urinary tract. In cases of renal damage, it will provide the following information: focal or diffuse atrophy of the parenchyma; dilated, bulky calices; and decreased excretion of the contrast material. In cases of VUR, 30% of the urograms were negative, 5% showed ureteral dilatation, 25% renal scars and calyceal dilatation, 10% cortical atrophy, and 30% a nonfunctioning kidney.[14] Rutuu et al performed 206 intravenous urograms on 119 patients with neurogenic bladder dysfunction and detected 42% upper tract abnormalities, mostly delayed renal emptying. Among patients with pathological urograms, 40% had at least one acute urinary infection episode within the last year, whereas among those with no pathological signs in their urograms, the incidence was only 8%.[28] Rao et al compared secretory urography and ultrasonography in a prospective study of 202 asymptomatic SCI patients to assess their respective effectiveness in diagnosing upper tract damage. Hydronephrosis was detected by urography in 100% of cases vs 86% by ultrasonography; for renal stones, the detection ratios were 87 and 78%, and for signs of chronic pyelonephritis, 100 and 25%, respectively. However, the discrepancy decreased if ultrasonography was combined with plain X-rays of the abdomen.[29]

Cystography and voiding cystourethrography

Cystography at bladder capacity will show low-pressure or passive reflux, in contrast to the Valsalva maneuver, made during micturition effort, which will provide information on high-pressure or active reflux. The same results are, however, available also by videourodynamic testing, which gives exact intravesical pressure values for storage and voiding while imaging the bladder filled with contrast material, and will reveal VUR, if any. The same applies to intravenous urography (provided that all contrast material has been discharged from the kidneys). Stover et al studied the influence of retrograde cystography on excretory urograms when the former was performed immediately before the latter. They showed that iatrogenic dilatation, indistinguishable from true pathological dilatation of the upper tract, occurred in patients with upper motor neuron lesions when intravenous urography was conducted immediately after cystography. They suggested a time delay between the two examinations to avoid this artifact.[30]

Renal scintigraphy

The renal isotope technetium 99m glucoheptonate defines renal function quantitatively and also helps to differentiate obstructive from nonobstructive types of uropathy. Scintigraphy, a dynamic imaging technique, is highly sensitive in depicting minute renal lesions, but is less specific for any given renal pathology. Fabrizio et al used it with good effect in acute septic conditions of SCI patients to identify a urologic cause of the sepsis. Scintigrams localized the renal damage every time when fever was due to a urological condition.[31]

Cystoscopy

Cystoscopy plays an important role in differentiating functional from organic lower tract obstructions in patients with upper tract abnormalities. For this group of patients, it is advisable to use a flexible cystoscope, considering the frequent occurrence of sphincter spasticity.

Therapy

The principal aim of neurogenic bladder dysfunction treatment is the maintenance of renal function. This requires successful and complete rehabilitation of the lower urinary tract, which means a complete and concerted neuro-urological intervention. The maintenance or creation of a low-pressure reservoir with no residual urine, the control of urinary infection, and the avoidance of an indwelling catheter are all measures that will promote the main goal, which is upper tract protection. Together with the adequate control of continence, they will ensure quality of life improvement as well. Whenever possible, a program of CIC should be implemented, but this demands some manual dexterity from the patient. After a well-designed rehabilitation program, even quadriplegics may be able to use CIC, if not via the urethra, then at least via a continent abdominal stoma. Therapeutic measures may be divided into acute intervention, to avoid some imminent complication, or elective treatment, fitting into the long-term management program.

Treatment of acute conditions

Lower urinary tract drainage

In the acute phase of SCI and cerebrovascular injuries, the so-called spinal or cerebral shock that will develop is characterized by an areflexic bladder. At this stage, the main goal is to avoid overflow incontinence. The condition will improve within 2–12 weeks, but in the meantime, until CIC (operated by the patient or nursing caregiver) can be implemented, continuous bladder drainage must be assured.[23] If no contraindication exists, a suprapubic cystostomy should be done with ultrasonographic guidance. A thin 8–10F catheter is recommended. If suprapubic catheterization is not possible, an indwelling urethral catheter should be introduced for the shortest possible duration. Silicone tubes are recommended, size 14–16F for females and 12–14F for males.[32]

Upper urinary tract drainage

If after successful lower tract drainage, upper tract dilatation still exists (bladder wall fibrosis, stricture, stone), causing renal dysfunction, then percutaneous nephrostomy must be done.

Hemodialysis

If the upper tract passage is free but renal failure persists or progresses, acute dialysis may be necessary.

Antibiotic treatment

Urinary tract infections combined with urosepsis require an antimicrobial treatment.[13]

Nephrectomy

Nephrectomy may become necessary if a septic condition (acute pyelonephritis, renal abscess, etc.) is maintained in spite of adequate drainage and appropriate antibiotics.

Conservative treatments

Spontaneous micturition

Spontaneous micturition is advisable after reflex contraction of the detrusor in response to the Credé maneuver or to various trigger mechanisms, only if intravesical pressure values are below 40 cmH$_2$O during the storage phase and less than 90 cmH$_2$O during the voiding phase, if residual urine is less than 30% of cystometric bladder capacity, and if bladder capacity is more than 200 ml. Lower tract obstruction, DSD, VUR, and reduced bladder compliance constitute contraindications for this approach. Reflex micturition usually means incontinence, and, therefore, the use of absorbent pads or, for males, urinary condoms, is indicated. However, 70% of patients using condom catheters are reported to suffer from chronic urinary infection. Skin problems are often due to allergic reactions to latex.[13,32]

Urine drainage

Drainage may be indicated in any form of bladder dysfunction: in the case of detrusor hyperreflexia, to maintain low bladder pressure (kidney protection) and continence; in the case of DSD, to eliminate the obstruction; in the case of areflexia, to eliminate any residual urine; in the case of decreased compliance, to reduce bladder pressure.

Intermittent catheterization. This technique was introduced in the 1940s by Sir Ludwig Guttman[33] to clear the bladder in SCI patients during the spinal shock phase. In 1972, Lapides et al suggested CIC for patients with neurogenic bladders. Follow-up in 66 patients showed no upper tract alteration.[34] In contrast, Perkas reported VUR and hydronephrosis in CIC patients.[23] Among 85 SCI patients using CIC, Naninga et al found 28 incidents of upper tract damage, detrusor hyperreflexia, and DSD in subjects presumed to have areflexic bladders.[35] This study emphasizes once again the importance of regular urodynamic follow-up in such patients. Three patients had sphincterotomy, 15 needed more frequent catheterization, and 10 failed to cooperate and so had to be placed on indwelling catheter drainage.[35] Mollard et al, from Paris, reported on 50 CIC cases. They found that girls and young boys accepted CIC better than did adolescent males.[36] Brem et al studied renal dysfunction and structural abnormalities in 28 children with meningocele on CIC. They reported VUR in 9 cases, renal dysfunction in 14%, and bacteriuria in 38%. They concluded that complications occurred in those patients who had small, noncompliant, trabeculated bladders.[37]

CIC has its own complications. Urinary infection is the most frequent, but urethral damage, stricture, and autonomous dysreflexia have also been noted. Kuhn et al reported a 5-year follow-up of 22 patients on CIC, with sterile urine in 23%, *Escherichia coli* infection in 36.5%, and other pathogenic bacteria (*Pseudomonas, Proteus, Klebsiella*) in another 36% of patients. They found urethral stricture in 1 patient, and autonomous dysreflexia in another. There was no upper tract damage. None of the patients was on anticholinergics, alpha-blockers, or on any continuous antibiotic prophylaxis.[38]

Cass observed that 87.5% of CIC patients with hypo- or areflexic bladders had a stable upper urinary tract with sterile urine in 90%, diminished VUR in 7%, and complete dryness between catheterizations in 34–39%. He reported, however, some complications, such as VUR, renal dysfunction, chronic pyelonephritis, and renal stones.[23] McGuire and Savastano compared patients on CIC for 2–12 years with those on indwelling catheters, finding significantly less acute urinary infections, bladder stones, and episodes of autonomic dysreflexia in the CIC group.[39] According to Madersbacher's experience, 20% of CIC patients had urethral complications, 40% had intermittent and 30% chronic urinary infections, whereas 30% had permanently sterile urine (Madersbacher, pers comm.).

For intermittent catheterization, we may use PVC catheters with a lubricant that contains some anesthetics, or with a hydrophilic coating, size 12–14F for males and 14–16F for females. The control of fluid intake is important: no more than 2000 ml per day. In the case of a normally compliant bladder, catheterization should be repeated 4–6 times a day. However, the catheter should be passed before the amount of urine in the bladder reaches 500 ml. In the case of decreased bladder compliance, urodynamic studies will indicate at what volume the bladder pressure reaches the critical level of 40 cmH_2O. The frequency of catheterization should be adjusted, so that this critical intravesical pressure is not reached. It should also be kept in mind that the more frequent the catheterizations, the less frequent is the incidence of urinary infections, and vice versa. Antibiotic prophylaxis is not unanimously recommended: there are some physicians who would only give antibiotics in the case of acute urinary infections, whereas others advocate prophylactic administration of small doses of varied antibiotic types.[32]

Indwelling bladder catheters. They are the worst solution and should only be used as a last resort. If possible, it should be a suprapubic diversion to eliminate urethral complications, particularly in males. In females, simultaneous surgical closure of the bladder neck is often required to ensure continence. Regular daily care of the catheter, together with changing it every 4 or 6 weeks (silicone catheters), is necessary. Although it seems to be a contradiction, several authors confirmed the occurrence of high bladder pressures, even in the chronically catheterized, a consequence of decreasing compliance. Jamil et al found storage pressures of more than 40 cmH_2O in 11, and renal damage in 9 of 30 patients on indwelling catheters, renal damage presenting merely in the high-pressure group.[16]

Chao et al compared the upper tract situation of 41 patients on CIC and 32 on indwelling catheters, noting a statistically higher number of renal damage and radiological alterations in the second group.[40] The most frequent complications were ever-present urinary infection, urethral damage and strictures, urethro-cutaneous fistulae, epididymitis, and bladder stones. In a retrospective study of a large SCI population, Hall et al found a 56.6% renal stone and 62.5% bladder stone incidence in patients on indwelling catheters.[21] They recommended prophylactic administration of small doses of varied antibiotic types.

Temporary urethral stents. They are an alternative to indwelling catheters. The Nissenkorn polyurethane or the Urolume endourethral Wallstent prosthesis may be placed at the level of the external sphincter under local anesthesia. Within 6 months after placement, there was no evidence of upper tract damage. Migration and secondary bladder neck obstruction were noted in 27% of patients. After a certain period of time the temporary stents were removed, and a final solution implemented. This is a less-invasive and, to some extent, a reversible solution than sphincterectomy.[41,42]

In summary, whenever possible, the best method of managing the neurogenic bladder is CIC, which will provide regular emptying of a low-pressure bladder and often ensure continence as well. At the same time, it will protect the upper tract. It may be combined, if necessary, with medication (overactive bladder), sphincterotomy (DSD), artificial sphincter implantation (reduced sphincter function), or bladder augmentation cystoplasty (reduced capacity, restricted compliance that fails to respond to other conservative treatments). Indwelling urethral catheters mean permanent urinary infection and several complications; they do not necessarily entail a low-pressure reservoir and often lead to renal damage. They should only be used as a last resort; urethral stents may serve as a temporary solution (see also Chapter 23).

Dietetic treatment

Avoidance of alcohol and spices and also urine acidification may help to prevent urinary infections; a low-protein diet may be indicated in renal dysfunction.

Medication

Hyperreflexia. In detrusor hyperreflexia medication is targeted to eliminate, or at least to decrease, reflex contractions, to normalize high-pressure bladder dysfunction, and to improve the effectiveness of intermittent catheterization. Oral anticholinergics, spasmolytics, and mixed-action products (oxybutynin, propiverine, trospium chloride, tolterodine) are meant to increase bladder capacity and to reduce detrusor contractility, but since they have considerable side-effects (dry mouth, troubled vision, arrhythmia), they are not readily tolerated by many patients. Oxybutynin is the standard medication in the United States, but 61% of the patients do not tolerate it orally, while it is ineffective in 48% (see also Chapter 14). Intravesical oxybutynin solution is more easily tolerated, has less side-effects, and the same efficacy on the detrusor.[9,32,43] Intravesically administered capsaicin and resiniferatoxin provide permanent receptor blockade for 2–7 months, increasing bladder compliance and intravesical pressure while protecting kidney function with no systemic side-effects (except for autonomic dysreflexia, which may occur sometimes)[32] (see also Chapter 15).

Areflexia. In areflexia, we may try cholinergic agents (bethanecol), but there is not much to expect from them, partly because of poor intestinal absorption and partly because they act simultaneously on the bladder, bladder neck, and urethra, so that they do not decrease outlet resistance.[9,32]

Intravesical electrostimulation

This method was developed by Katona in 1959 to ameliorate bladder emptying by strengthening the detrusor reflex and simultaneously improving bladder sensation and compliance.[44] Cheng et al enhanced bladder compliance in children with meningocele; upper tract conditions improved, and augmentation cystoplasty became unnecessary (see also Chapter 21).[9]

Elective surgery

Surgical treatments cause irreversible changes. Therefore, they should only be used if other conservative treatments will not achieve a low-pressure reservoir, effective protection of the upper urinary tract, and/or continence.

Denervation techniques

Surgical or chemical interference with the nerve fibers of the pelvic plexus will increase bladder capacity, reduce reflex incontinence, and improve compliance. Injective techniques imply locally injected anesthesic agents or phenol (the latter being irreversible). The early results with phenol are generally very good, but after a year or so, the symptoms will relapse in about 80% of patients. Also, many complications (fistulae, complete areflexia) have been reported; therefore, this technique has been virtually abandoned.[9]

Bladder transection through the entire thickness of the detrusor above the trigone will also increase bladder capacity. Early cure rates are reported to be 74%, but after 5 years the success rate goes down to 65%.[11] Intradural posterior root rhizotomy combined with the implantation of an extradural anterior root stimulator is the most frequently used method.[45,46] Rhizotomy will suppress bladder spasticity, normally low-pressure storage will be achieved, and voiding can be programmed through the anterior root nerve stimulator.

Brindley et al reported on the first 50 implantations in 1986: 60% of patients were continent. Deafferentation was not yet done routinely in every case at that time.[45] Sauerwein tried this method in 45 patients from 1986 to 1989: 95% were cured from hyperreflexia, 91% became continent, and 84% were spontaneous voiders. Postoperatively, 6 patients showed low-pressure reflux, which was corrected by antireflux surgery. No renal damage was noted.[47] Schurch et al reported that implantation of a Brindley stimulator cured reflex incontinence, while increasing bladder compliance and reducing post-void residual urine volume from an average of 340 ml to 140 ml: VUR disappeared in 3 and was improved in 2 patients.[48] Egon et al implanted the stimulator in 93 patients, 82 of whom became continent and 83 became spontaneous voiders. Before surgery, 3 had had VUR, which disappeared after the intervention (see also Chapter 20).[49]

Bladder augmentation techniques

Augmentation techniques should only be used when bladder compliance is reduced because of organic causes.

Autoaugmentation. This technique is a means of partial myectomy, i.e. the detrusor muscle is excised from the upper half of the bladder, which will then dilate, forming a diverticulum. Follow-up results after 5 years show a success rate of 65%. This surgery is easier to perform than conventional intestinal augmentation, and no postoperative carcinoma is to be feared, but there is a high risk of intraoperative mucosal tear. The bladder takes a long time, almost 1 year, to expand sufficiently, so that in the meantime 45% of patients have to be put on intermittent catheterization. As a result of a lower intravesical pressure decrease than that found in intestinal augmentation, the risk of renal damage is somewhat higher.[50,51]

Enterocystoplasty. This technique is indicated in patients with small bladder capacity, reduced compliance, and renal damage, or incontinence between catheterizations, should the condition be refractory to medication. Augmentation can be done either with the small or the large intestine. The patient may develop metabolic acidosis and runs the risk of intestinal carcinoma due to urine contact with the bowel mucosa. The intestine to be used must first be detubularized. In ileum augmentation, the reported success rate is 52–80%, but 20% of patients need to be put on intermittent catheterization due to increased residual urine volume.[23,50] Flood et al evaluated the results of 122 augmentation cystoplasties performed during an 8-year period on patients with reduced bladder compliance (77%), or refractory detrusor hyperreflexia/instability (23%). The clinical diagnosis in over 50% of cases was neuropathic bladder dysfunction (28% SCI, 23% myelodysplasia). They performed detubularized ileal augmentation in 67% of the patients, detubularized ileocecocystoplasty in 30%, and detubularized sigmoid in 3%. Seventy-five percent of patients were cured, and 20% improved. The reported complications included bladder stones in 21%, incontinence in 13%, and pyelonephritis in 11% of these patients. The re-operation rate was 16%.[52] Renal insufficiency is a relative contraindication for this type of surgery.

Supravesical diversion

Supravesical stomas are made if urethral catheterization is not viable, augmentation cystoplasty fails, or if there is an infiltrating bladder tumor. Incontinent stomas (ileal or colonic conduit) mean less comfort than continent stomas. Brem et al created ileal conduits in 14 children with meningomyelocele, and found ureteral reflux in all patients after the intervention, with renal dysfunction in 28% and bacteriuria in 70%.[37] Continent stomas (Mitrofanoff, Koch pouch, Mainz I, II pouch) induce fewer upper tract complications. The most important complications are stomal stenosis, catheterization difficulty, stone formation in the pouch, and incontinence (i.e. incompetence of the continent stoma).

Antireflux surgery

Reflux in neurogenic bladder dysfunction is mostly the result of high intravesical pressures, large residual urine volumes, poor bladder capacity, restricted compliance, or serious urinary infections. Antireflux surgery by itself will not be the unique solution in the majority of cases, as it does not decrease bladder pressure or improve compliance and capacity. Therefore, this type of surgery is mostly done in combination with some other surgical intervention.

The less-invasive endoscopic method to correct VUR consists of submucosal Teflon or collagen injection at the ureteral orifice. The choice of the material used makes no difference as far as the results are concerned. Silveri et al[17] administered endoscopic injections in 15 children with meningomyelocele and performed open surgery in 2. Follow-up results showed renal failure in 8 cases. Casals et al[53] pointed out that the endoscopic method is fast, simple, and repeatable.

The success rate of open surgery is 80–95%. The Lich–Gregoir method consists of elongating of the intramural portion of the distal ureter by burying a 3–4 cm segment between the bladder mucosa and the detrusor muscle via an entirely extravesical route. A success rate of more than 98% has been claimed by Heimbach et al.[54] The Politano–Leadbetter antireflux procedure, which consists of elongating of the submucosal portion of the refluxing ureter, is probably used most widely. The Cohen method is mainly undertaken to correct bilateral reflux, with the ureters crossing each other on the midline through a submucous tunnel. Burbidge[55] compared the results of the two latter techniques and found an equal success rate (97–98%) for both types of repairs.

Sphincterotomy

This type of intervention is only indicated in males with high-pressure storage due to a DSD causing upper tract deterioration. The intervention reduces LPP theoretically to zero. The resulting incontinence may be managed by a condom catheter. Sphincterotomy is performed particularly when CIC is not possible (e.g. in quadriplegics). Upper tract abnormalities and VUR respond favorably to sphincterotomy in 70–90% of cases.[56] The 12 o'clock incision suggested by Madersbacher involves less complications than conventional 3 or 9 o'clock incisions (lower risk of bleeding and postoperative erectile dysfunction).[57]

Nephrectomy

Nonfunctioning kidneys with pyelonephritis or hydronephrosis – especially if they cause hypertension – should eventually be removed.

References

1. Graham SD. Present urological treatment of spinal cord injury patients. J Urol 1981; 126:1–4.

2. Bors E. Neurogenic bladder. Urol Surg 1957; 7:177–250.

3. Donelly J, Hackler RH, Bunts RC. Present urologic status of the World War II paraplegic: 25-year follow-up. Comparison with status of the 20-year Korean war paraplegic and 5-year Vietnam paraplegic. J Urol 1972; 108:558–562.

4. Koff SA, Lapides J, Piazza DH. Association of urinary tract infection and reflux with uninhibited bladder contractions and voluntary sphincteric obstruction. J Urol 1979; 122:373–376.

5. Cosbie-Ross J. Vesico-ureteric reflux in the neurogenic bladder. Br J Surg 1965; 52:164–167.

6. Thomas DG, Lucas MG. The urinary tract following spinal cord injury. In: Chisholm GD, Fair WR, eds. Scientific foundations of urology. Chicago: Year Book Medical, 1990:289–299.

7. Light K, Blerk JP. Causes of renal deterioration in patients with meningomyelocele. Br J Urol 1977;49:257–260.

8. Soygur T, Arikan N, Yesilli C, Gogus O. Relationship among voiding dysfunction and vesicoureteral reflux and renal scars. Urology 1999; 54:905–908.

9. Madersbacher H. Neurogene Harninkontinenz. In: Höfner K, Jonas U, eds. Praxisratgeber Harninkontinez. Bremen: UNI-MED Verlag AG, International Medical Publishers 2000:221–230.

10. Gerridzen RJ, Thijssen AM, Dehoux E. Risk factors for upper tract deterioration in chronic spinal cord injury patients. J Urol 1992; 147:416–418.

11. Mundy AR. Vesicouretheric reflux in adults. In:Whitfield HN, Hendy WF, Kirby RS, Duchet JW, eds. Textbook of genitourinary surgery. Oxford: Blackwell Science, 1998:440–447.

12. McGuire EJ, Woodside JR, Borden TA, Weiss RM. Prognostic value of urodynamic testing in myelodysplastic patients. J Urol 1981; 126:205–209.

13. Society of German Urologists. Guideline for urological treatment of spinal cord injured patients, 1998.

14. Heidler H. Neurogene Blasenfunktionsstörungen. In: Altwein J, Rübben H, eds. Urologie. Ferdinand Enke Verlag Stuttgart, Heinz Neubert GmbH Druckerei Bayreuth, 1993:379–394.

15. Linsenmeyer TA, Bagaria SP, Gendron B. The impact of urodynamic parameters on the upper tracts of spinal cord injured men who void reflexly. J Spin Cord Med 1998; 21:15–20.

16. Jamil F, Williamson M, Ahmed YS, Harrison SC. Natural fill urodynamics in chronically catheterized patients with spinal cord injury. BJU Int 1999; 83:396–399.

17. Silveri M, Capitanucci ML, Capozza N, et al. Occult spinal dysraphism: neurogenic voiding dysfunction and long term urologic follow-up. Pediatr Surg Int 1997; 12:148–150.

18. Vaidyanathan S, Singh G, Soni BM, et al. Silent hydronephrosis/pyonephrosis due to upper urinary tract calculi in spinal cord injury patients. Spinal Cord 2000; 38:661–668.

19. DeVivo MJ, Rutt RD, Black KJ, et al. Trends in spinal cord injury demographics and treatment outcomes between 1973 and 1986. Arch Phys Med Rehab 1992; 73:424–430.

20. Comarr AE, Kawaichi GK, Bors E. Renal calculosis of patients with traumatic cord lesions. J Urol 1962, 87:647.

21. Hall MK, Hackler RH, Zampieri TA, Zampieri JB. Renal calculi in spinal cord-injured patient: association with reflux, bladder stones, and Foley catheter drainage. Urology 1989; 34:126–128.

22. Killorin W, Gray M, Bennet JK, Green BG. The value of urodynamics and bladder management in predicting upper urinary tract complications in male spinal cord injury patients. Paraplegia 1992; 30:437–441.

23. Sukin SW, Boone TB. Diagnosis and treatment of spinal cord injuries and myeloneuropathy. In: Rodney AA, ed. Voiding dysfunction. Totowa: Humana Press, 2000:115–139.

24. Virgili G, Finazzi AE, Giannantoni A, et al. Ultrasonography of the upper urinary tract in patients with spinal cord injury. Arch Ital Urol Androl 2000; 72:225–227.

25. Calenoff L, Neimen HL, Kaplan PE, et al. Urosonography in spinal cord injury patients. J Urol 1982; 128:1234–1237.

26. Ozer MN, Shannon SR. Renal sonography in asymptomatic persons with spinal cord injury: a cost-effectiveness analysis. Arch Phys Med Rehab 1991; 72:35–37.

27. Bih LI, Tsai SJ, Tung LC. Sonographic diagnosis of hydronephrosis in patients with spinal cord injury: influence of bladder fullness. Arch Phys Med Rehab 1998; 79:1557–1559.

28. Ruutu M, Kivisaari A, Lehtonen T. Upper urinary tract changes in patients with spinal cord injury. Clin Radiol 1984; 35:491–494.

29. Rao KG, Hackler RH, Woodlief RM, et al. Real-time renal sonography in spinal cord injury patients: prospective comparison with excretory urography. J Urol 1986; 135:72–77.

30. Stover SL, Witten DM, Kuhlemeier KV, et al. Iatrogenic dilatation of the upper urinary tract during radiographic evaluation of patients with spinal cord injury. J Urol 1986; 135:78–82.

31. Fabrizio MD, Chancellor MB, Rivas DA, et al. The role of renal scintigraphy in the evaluation of spinal cord injury with presumed urosepsis. J Urol 1996; 156:1730–1734.

32. Madersbacher H. Konservative Therapie der neurogenen Blasendysfunktion. Urologe 1999; 38:24–29.

33. Guttman L, Frankel H. The value of intermittent catheterization in the early management of traumatic paraplegia and tetraplegia. Paraplegia 1966; 4:63.

34. Lapides J, Diokono A, Silber S, Lowe B. Clean intermittent self-catheterisation in the treatment of urinary tract disease. J Urol 1972; 107:458–461.

35. Nanninga JB, Wu Y, Hamilton B. Long-term intermittent catheterization in the spinal cord injury patient. J Urol 1982; 128:760–763.

36. Mollard P, Meunier P, Berard C, Henriet M. Treatment of urinary incontinence of neurologic origin in children and adolescents. J Urol (Paris) 1984; 90:227–236.

37. Brem AS, Martin D, Callaghan J, Maynard J. Long term renal risk factors in children with meningomyelocele. J Pediatr 1987; 110:51–55.

38. Kuhn W, Rist M, Zaech GA. Intermittent urethral self catheterisation: long term results (bacteriological evolution, continence, acceptance, complications). Paraplegia 1991; 29:222–232.

39. McGuire EJ, Savastano J. Comparative urological outcome in women with spinal cord injury. J Urol 1986; 135:730–731.

40. Chao R, Clowers D, Mayo ME. Fate of upper urinary tracts in patients with indwelling catheters after spinal cord injury. Urology 1993; 42:259–262.

41. Chartier-Kastler EJ, Thomas L, Bussel B, et al. Feasibility of a temporary urethral stent through the striated sphincter in patients in the early phase (6 months) of spinal cord injury. Eur Urol 2001; 39:326–331.

42. Rivas DA, Chancellor M. Sphincterotomy and sphincter stent prosthesis placement. In: Corcos J, Schick E, eds. The urinary sphincter. New York: Marcel Dekker, 2001:565–583.

43. Szollar SM, Lee SM. Intravesical oxybutynin for spinal cord injury patients. Spinal Cord 1996; 34:284–287.

44. Katona F. Stages of vegetative afferentation in reorganisation of bladder control during electrotherapy. Urol Int 1975; 30:192–203.

45. Brindley GS, Polkey CE, Rushton DN, Cardozo L. Sacral anterior root stimulators for bladder control in paraplegia. The first 50 cases. J Neurol Neurosurg Psychiatry 1986; 49:1104–1114.

46. Tanagho EA, Schmidt RA, Orvis BR. Neural stimulation for the control of voiding dysfunction: a preliminary report on 22 patients with serious neuropathic voiding disorders. J Urol 1989; 142:340–345.

47. Sauerwein D. Die operativen Behandlung der spastischen Blasenlahmung bei Querschnittlahmung. Urologe A 1990; 19:196–203.

48. Schurch B, Rodic B, Jeanmonod D. Posterior sacral rhizotomy and intradural anterior sacral root stimulation for treatment of the spastic bladder in spinal cord injured patients. J Urol 1997; 157:610–614.

49. Egon G, Barat M, Colombel P, et al. Implantation of anterior sacral root stimulators combined with posterior sacral rhizotomy in spinal injury patients. World J Urol 1998; 16:342–349.

50. Müller SC. Chirurgische Therapie. In: Höfner K, Jonas U, eds. Praxisratgeber Harninkontinez. Bremen: UNI-MED Verlag AG, 2000: 144–177.

51. Christmas TJ, Kirby RS. Principles of management of the neurogenic bladder. In: Whitfield HN, Hendy WF, Kirby RS, Duchet JW, eds. Textbook of genitourinary surgery. Oxford: Blackwell Science, 1998: 918–926.

52. Flood HD, Malhotra SJ, O'Connel HE, et al. Long-term results and complications using augmentation cystoplasty in reconstructive urology. Neurourol Urodyn 1995; 14:297–309.

53. Casals J, Rivero A, Rivero J. Endoscopic treatment of vesico-ureteral reflux in the neurogenic bladder. Arch Esp Urol 1997; 50:381–387.

54. Heimbach D, Bruhl P, Mallmann R. Lich–Gregoir antireflux procedure; indications and results with 283 vesicoureteral units. Scand J Urol Nephrol 1995; 29:311–316.

55. Burbidge KA. Ureteral reimplantation: a comparison of results with the cross trigonal and Politano–Leadbetter techniques in 120 patients. J Urol 1991; 146:1352–1353.

56. Ruutu ML, Lehtonen TA. Bladder outlet surgery in men with spinal cord injury. Scand J Urol Nephrol 1985; 19:241–246.

57. Madersbacher H. The twelve o'clock sphincterotomy: technique, indications, results. Paraplegia 1976; 13:261–267.

Index

Page numbers in italics indicate *figures* and *tables*. LUT refers to lower urinary tract.

abdominal leak point pressure (ALPP) 62–3
Abrams–Klevmark classification of voiding
    diaries 15–16
abscesses, periurethral 318
alginate 262
alpha-adrenergic blockers
    DESD therapy 141–2
    reduction of neurologic sweating 140
anal reflex 5
anandamide *149*, 150
anastomoses
    intestinal 244
    ureterointestinal 244–5
angiogenesis 262
anode block technique 273, 275
antibacterial prophylaxis
    bowel surgery 243–4
    urinary tract infection 130
anticholinergic drugs
    drugs 138–40
    intravesical administration 157, 290
    oral administration 289
    use in children 297–8
    see also specific drugs
antimuscarinic drugs *see* anticholinergic drugs
antireflux surgery 331
apoptosis following SCI 279
appendicovesicostomy (Mitrofanoff procedure)
    249, *250*, *251*
areflexic bladder
    balance with urethra 312–13
    management 288–9, 331
        see also specific methods
artificial urinary sphincters
    advantages/disadvantages *212*
    AMS 800 218
    background 215
    in children 303–4
    complications 220, *221–2*, 223
    cost 215
    design evolution 218
    device lifetime 294
    indications and patient selection 218–19
    results 220, *221–2*
    surgical technique 219–20
autoaugmentation 331–2
    in children 300
    compared with other methods 204, 291
    demucosalized enterocystoplasty 260
    indication 202
    procedure 202–3
    results 203–4

autonomic dysreflexia (AD)
    management
        acute 105, 167–8
        anesthesia 168, 169
        pregnancy and labor 168–9
        prophylaxis 105, 168
        summarized *106*
    prevention 167, 169
autonomic nervous system tests 97–8
axon regeneration following SCI 280–1

baclofen 142, 143, 290
bacteria
    artificial sphincter infection 220
    prostate infection 318
    urease-producing 320
    in urine specimens 317
    see also urinary tract infections (UTI)
bacteriuria, after urinary diversion 254
balanced bladder 309, 325
    see also vesicourethral balance
Bcl-2 280
behavioral techniques, adjustments to daily life 125
benign prostatic hypertrophy (BPH) 121, 310
benzodiazepines 142–3
beta-adrenergic agonists 143
biofeedback 52, 126
biomaterials for tissue engineering 259
bladder
    areflexic *see* areflexic bladder
    augmentation 204, 290–1, 299–301, 332
    balanced 309, 325
    cancer 39, *40*, 322–3
    compliance *see* compliance
    development *see* development of bladder function
    expression maneuvers 127
    filling 171
    foreign bodies 39, *40*
    hyperreflexic *see* detrusor hyperreflexia
    mucosa *37*
    normal capacity in children 54, *55*, 74–5
    open neck 43–5
    pressures in children 54–5
    stones 39, 321
    tissue engineering 260–1
    tumors 39, *40*, 322–3
    voiding reflexes in infants 68
    wall
        abnormalities 37
        electrical stimulation 177–8
        trabeculations 37–8
    see also micturition; vesicourethral balance

bladder cooling test 72, 76
bladder emptying improvement techniques 288–9
  see also specific techniques
bladder leak point pressure (BLPP) 61–2, 72
bladder muscle cell injections 262
bladder neck closure
  disadvantages 229
  indications 229
  results and complications 231
  surgical technique
    transabdominal approach 229–30
    transvaginal approach 230–1
bladder neck reconstruction
  background 223
  indications and patient selection 225–6, 229
  procedures
    Kropp 224–5, 226, *227*, 301–3
    Pippi Salle 225, 226, *228*, 229, 302–3
    Young–Dees–Leadbetter 223–4, 226, *228*
  results and complications 226–9
bladder neck slings 301
  advantages/disadvantages *212*
  and bladder augmentation 213
  complications 215
  indications 213
  patient selection 213
  results 215, *216–17*
  surgical techniques 213–15
bladder neck wraps 215
bladder relaxant drugs 137–40
bladder-specific K$^+$ channel openers 144
α-blockers *see* alpha-adrenergic blockers
Bors ice water test (bladder cooling test) 72, 76
botulinum-A toxin
  administration 200
  clinical experience with 155–6, 200, 291–2
  cost 157
  formulations 155, 200
  indication 200
  mode of action 155, 200
  results 200–2, 290
bowel preparation for surgery 243
Bricker ileal conduit 245–6
Bricker ureterointestinal anastomosis *244*
bulbocavernosus reflex (BCR) 5, 93–5, 99
bulking agents, urethral
  background 207–8
  collagen 208
  complications 212
  contraindications 210
  delivery methods 209
  indications 210
  mechanism of action 208–9
  patient selection 210
  postoperative care 209
  results 210–12
  skin test 209
bupivacaine 290
Burch urethropexy 293

calculi *see* lithiasis
capsaicin
  intravesical use
    clinical experience 150–2, 290
    procedure 155
    rationale 150
    safety 152

molecular structure *149*
captopril 168
catheters
  condom 132
  for cystometry in children 71
  indwelling 330
  transurethral and suprapubic 71, 132
  see also clean intermittent catheterization (CIC)/
    self-catheterization (CISC)
cauda equina syndrome 98–9
cell transplantation strategies, SCI therapy 280–1, 281–2
cell-based tissue engineering 259
  bladder 261
  bladder muscle cell injections 262
  chondrocyte injections 262
  genetically engineered cells 262–3
  urethra 259–60
  using stem cells 263
children
  bladder management
    anticholinergic drugs 297–8
    bladder augmentation 299–301
    clean intermittent catheterization 297
    cutaneous vesicostomy 298
  bladder outlet management
    artificial urinary sphincter 303–4
    bulking agents *see* bulking agents, urethral
    drugs to increase resistance 301
    fascial slings 301
    urethral lengthening 301–3
  management goals 297
  normal voiding values 18
  open bladder neck in 44
  pad tests in 30, 71
  patient factors in management 304
  sedation of 70
  see also development of bladder function; urodynamics in
    children
chlorpromazine 105, *106*
chondrocyte injections 262
clam cystoplasty 204, 300
classification of LUT disorders 111–22
  according to nervous system involvement 114
  basis in structure and function 111
  bladder outlet obstruction 117–18
  consequences of disorders 121–2
  current system, need for revision 111
  female incontinence groups 118–19
  harmonic/disharmonic disruptions of micturition 116–17
  interdependence of disorder, consequences and
    comorbidity 114–15
  LUT overactivity 119–20
  micturition cycle 112–13
  neurogenic bladder in spina bifida children 77–8
  patterns of recognition 115–16, *121*
  simplified LUT model 116, *120*
  simplified structure and function-based 120–1
  therapeutic 287–8
  time-related changes 117
  Wein functional classification system 57
clean intermittent catheterization (CIC)/self-catheterization
  (CISC)
  adjunctive therapy 129
  background 288, 329–30
  catheter introduction 128
  catheters and lubricants 127, 330
  frequency 129

infants/children 297
reasons for discontinuation 129
results of studies *128*
reuse of catheters 128–9
sterile technique (SIC) 127–8
urethral trauma 131
urinary tract infections 129–31, 330
other complications 131, 330
clinical evaluation
history *see* history
physical examination 5, 58
see also specific conditions
clinical neurophysiological tests *see* electrophysiological
evaluation
CNEMG *see* concentric needle electromyography (CNEMG)
collagen urethral injections *see* bulking agents, urethral
colocystoplasty, in children 299
colon conduits 246
comorbidity 115
compliance
in children 54, 76–7
defined 60
high intravesical pressure 60–1
impaired 60
normal 60, 76
computed tomography (CT) 47
computer analysis of voiding diary data 17
concentric needle electromyography (CNEMG)
assessment of interference patterns 92
assessment of motor unit potentials (MUPs) 88–92
insertion activity 88
procedure 88
spontaneous denervation activity 88
vs. single fiber electromyography 92
condom catheters 132
conservative treatment of neurogenic bladder 125
see also specific treatments
continent ileal reservoir (Kock pouch) 248, *250*
conus medullaris
electrical stimulation 178
electrophysiological assessment of lesions 98–9
cranberry juice 130
Credé maneuver 127, 292
cremasteric reflex 5
cutaneous vesicostomy 298
cystitis 318–19
cystitis glandularis/follicularis 37
cystography 328
cystometry
in children, FAQs 71–3
compliance assessment 60–1
involuntary detrusor contractions 59–60, *61*
natural fill 73–4
urinary storage assessment 61–3
videocystometry 73
cystoscopes 35
cystourethrography 45
cystourethroscopy *see* endoscopy
cytology/cytoscopy screening 323

dantrolene 143
deafferentation 204
demucosalized intestine for urinary reconstruction 260
DESD *see* detrusor external sphincter dyssynergia (DESD)
N-desethyloxybutinin 161
detrusor areflexia (DA) *see* areflexic bladder
detrusor contractility in children 54–5, 75–6

detrusor external sphincter dyssynergia (DESD)
defined 231
drug therapy 140–3
surgical treatment
balloon dilation 235
indications and patient selection 232
see also sphincteric stenting techniques; sphincterotomy
therapies summarized *141*
urodynamics *62*, *64*
detrusor hyperreflexia
balance with urethra 311–12
drug therapy 137–40, 289–90, 331
neurostimulation treatment 269–71, 290
pathophysiological consequences 289
penile electrical stimulation 175
surgical treatment 199, 290–1
treatment summarized 291
see also specific treatments
detrusor myectomy *see* autoaugmentation
detrusor overactivity *see* detrusor hyperreflexia
detrusor sphincter dyscoordination in infants 68
development of bladder function
bladder capacity 68
bladder control 69
detrusor-sphincter dyscoordination 68
voiding reflex 68
diagnosis, practical guide 105–7
see also specific diagnostic modalities
diet 331
distal urethral electrical conductance (DUEC) test 30
drug intoxication after urinary diversion 253–4
drug therapy
intravesical
advantages 149
anticholinergic drugs 157, 290
botulinum-A toxin *see* botulinum-A toxin
vanilloids *see* vanilloids: intravesical use
systemic/intrathecal
detrusor hyperreflexia/low-compliant detrusor 137–40,
289–90, 331
facilitation of bladder emptying 140
neurogenic sphincter deficiency 140
sphincter dyssynergia 140–3, 291–2
research areas 143–4
transdermal oxybutynin administration 161–6
see also specific drugs

elderly patients, pad test 32–3
electrical stimulation
aims 189
intravesical *see* intravesical electrical stimulation (IVES)
modalities summarized 189
peripheral *see* peripheral electrical stimulation
see also neuromodulation
electrical stimulation, for bladder emptying 177–85
costs 183
detrusor-sphincter dyssynergia 184–5
disadvantages 268–9
methods
equipment 179, *180*, 268
preoperative investigation 179–80
surgery 179, 184
postoperative management 180
patient selection 183–4
principles 177
results 180–1
autonomic dysreflexia 182

electrical stimulation, for bladder emptying (*Continued*)
bowel function 183
continence 181
CSF leakage 182–3
implant infection 183
implant reliability 183
micturition 181
nerve damage 182
pain 182
penile erection 183
upper tract 182
urinary tract infection 181
urodynamics 181–2
role of posterior rhizotomy 185
sites of stimulation 177–8
see also neurostimulation, developments
electrolyte abnormalities after urinary diversion 252–3
electromotive drug administration (EMDA) 157
electromyography *see* electrophysiological evaluation:
electromyography
electrophysiological evaluation 83–100
autonomic nervous system 97
corpus cavernosum electromyography 98
sympathetic skin response 97–8
classification of tests 86, 87
electromyography 64
concentric needle 88–92
coupled with uroflowmetry 53–4
kinesiological 87–8
role in children 71, 72
single fiber 92
general considerations 83–4
patient groups
tests of clinical value 98–9
tests of research interest 99–100
physiological principles 86–7
pudendal somatosensory evoked potentials 93, 95
sacral motor system
assessment of central motor pathways 96
cauda equina stimulation 96
motor nerve conduction studies 95–6
sacral reflexes 93–5
sacral sensory system
cerebral somatosensory evoked potentials 97
dorsal penile nerve electroneurography 96–7
dorsal sacral root electroneurography 96–7
Ellik bladder irrigator *322*
endoscopy 35–41, 106–7
bladder stones 39
equipment 35
foreign bodies 39, *40*
limitations 35
structural bladder anomalies 37–8
technique 36
tumors 39, *40*
ureteral orifices 38–9
urethral stent evaluation 37
urethral strictures 36
enterocystoplasty *see* bladder: augmentation
epididymitis 318
epididymo-orchitis 318
erosion, complicating artificial sphincter use 220
Escherichia coli 317, 318
Euphorbia resinifera 149
extracorporeal shock wave lithotripsy (ESWL) 320–1

families of SCI patients 8
fascial slings *see* bladder neck slings
females
autonomic dysreflexia in pregnancy 168–9
electrophysiological evaluation of urinary
retention 99
incontinence groups 118–19
normal voiding values 18–19
open bladder neck in 44
Finetech–Brindley device 268, 270–1, 273, 275
flavoxate 140
follow-up
neurogenic bladder patients, summarized *107*
renal function 106
free radicals 279
frequency–volume charts *see* voiding diaries

gastrocystoplasty 299
gene therapy
diabetic neurogenic bladder 144
neuroprotective 280
vascular endothelial growth factor delivery 262–3
genomics 144
glutamate, release following SCI 279
glyceryl trinitrate 167–8

hemi-Kock augmentation cystoplasty 251, *252*
hemodialysis 329
history
bowel function 4
LUT symptoms
current symptoms 4
duration 3–4
previous history 4
neurologic disease 3, 58, 85
in preparation for urodynamic testing 58
sexual 4–5
human nerve growth factor 281
hydronephrosis 47
hyperreflexic bladder *see* detrusor hyperreflexia
hyporeflexic bladder
balance with urethra 312–13
management 288–9
see also specific methods
hypothermia, neuroprotective effects 280, 281

ileal conduits 245–6
ileal vesicostomy 246–7
ileocystoplasty, in children 299
imaging techniques 43–8
CNS assessment 45
LUT 45–7
suggesting neurogenic etiology
lumbrosacral spine X-rays 43
open bladder neck and proximal urethra at rest 43–4
upper urinary tract 47–8
imipramine 140
in-and-out catheterization 46
incontinence *see* urinary incontinence
Indiana pouch 248, *249*
indwelling bladder catheters 330
infections *see* urinary tract infections (UTI)
inflammatory response to SCI 281
interleukin-10 (IL-10) 280, 281
intermittent catheterization (IC) *see* clean intermittent
catheterization (CIC)/self-catheterization (CISC)

International Continence Society classification of voiding diaries 16
intestinal anastomoses 244
intra-abdominal pressure measurement 72–3
intraspinal microstimulation 275
intraspinal transplants 280
intrathecal baclofen pump 143, 290
intravenous urography (IVU) 328
intravesical electrical stimulation (IVES) 193–6
    background 193–4, 331
    cost-effectiveness 195, 196
    efficacy 195
    feedback training 194
    further research 196
    mechanism of action 193
    prerequisites for success 195
    recommendations 196
    results 194–5
    safety 195
    technique 194
involuntary detrusor contractions (IDCs) 59–60, *61*

kidney
    bacterial infection 319
    risk factors for damage 326
    stones 320
kinesiological electromyography 87–8
Kock pouch 248, *250*
Kropp bladder neck reconstruction 224–5, 226, *227*, 301–3

leak point pressure measurement 61–3, 72
Lich–Gregoir antireflux procedure 332
lipid peroxidation 279
lithiasis
    after urinary diversion 254
    background 319–20
    bladder stones 39, 321
    renal stones 320
    in SCI patients 327
    ureteral stones 321
    urethral stones 322
lubricants 127
lumbosacral spine X-rays 43
LY341122 279

magnetic resonance imaging (MRI)
    spinal 45
    upper urinary tract 47–8
males, normal voiding values 19
Marcain 290
matrices in tissue engineering 259
    bladder repair 260–1
    urethral repair 260
mechanical bowel preparation 243
Memokath urethral stent 231, 232, 233, 235
mental status assessment 5
methotrexate toxicity 253
methylprednisolone 279
micturition
    cycle 112–13
    harmonic and disharmonic disruptions 116
    neuronal pathways *150*
    spontaneous 329
    see also voiding diaries
midazolam 70

Mitrofanoff procedure 249, *250, 251*
motor innervation of the LUT 85–6
multiple sclerosis (MS) 138
multiple system atrophy (MSA) 98
muscles
    motor reflexes 5
    striated 171
myelodysplasia 44, 327
myelomeningocele (MMC) *46*
myoblast injections 262

NBQX 279
necrosis 279
neoplasms, bladder 39, *40*, 322–3
nephrectomy 329, 332
neural tube defects (NTDs) 327
neurogenic detrusor overactivity (involuntary contractions) 59–60, *61*
neuroimaging 45
    see also specific imaging modalities
neurologic assessment 5
neuromodulation
    conditional system 271–2
    mode of action 190
    noninvasive *269*, 270
    permanent electrode implantation 190
    success rate 191
    trial stimulation 190
    using Finetech–Brindley device 270–1
    see also neurostimulation, developments;
neurophysiological tests *see* electrophysiological evaluation
neuroprotection following SCI 279–80, 281
neurostimulation, developments
    background 267–8, 290
    conditional neuromodulation 271–2
    prospects 275–6
    selective sacral root stimulation 273, 275
    SPARSI 273, *274*
    techniques summarized *276*
    see also electrical stimulation, for bladder emptying; neuromodulation
neurotrophin-3 (NT-3) 281
nifedipine 105, *106*, 167
nitric oxide (NO) 280
nocturnal polyuria, voiding diary 22, *23, 24*
nuclear transfer 263

olfactory ensheathing glia (OEG) 280–1
osteomalacia, after urinary diversion 254
overactivity, LUT 119–20
overflow incontinence 4
oxybutynin
    controlled release 138
    intravesical use 157, 161, 290, 331
    mechanism of action 161
    transdermal administration
        background 161–2
        clinical efficacy 163–4
        convenience 165
        dose escalation and dry mouth 164–5
        matrix-type delivery system 162
        pharmacokinetic advantage over oral delivery 162–3, 165–6
        and quality of life 165, *166*
        side-effect profile 164

pad test 29–33
  continence/incontinence discrimination 29, *30*
  patient populations
    adults 31–2
    children 30–1, 71
    elderly 32–3
  qualitative 30
  quantitative 30
Parkinson's disease (PD) 98
partial detrusor myectomy *see* autoaugmentation
pelvic examination 5
pelvic innervation 85–6
pelvic muscle exercises 125
penile clamps 132
percutaneous nephrolithotripsy (PCNL) 320
peripheral electrical stimulation 171–5
  clinical techniques
    acute maximal stimulation 174
    long-term 173–4
  continence reflex activation
    re-education effect 173, 174
    stimulation parameters 172–3
    utilization of natural reflexes 172
  indications 174–5
  problem of randomized controlled trials 174
  see also electrical stimulation, for bladder emptying;
    intravesical electrical stimulation (IVES)
periurethral abscesses 318
pharmacogenomics 144
pharmacological treatment *see* drug therapy
phenoxybenzamine 167
phentolamine 105, *106*, 141
physical examination 5, 58
physiotherapy
  bladder expression 127
  detrusor hypoactivity 126
  detrusor overactivity 125–6
  triggered reflex voiding 126–7
Pippi Salle bladder neck reconstruction 225, 226,
  228, 229, 302–3
Politano–Leadbetter antireflux procedure 332
polyglycolic acid (PGA) 259
polyuria, voiding diary 22, *23*, 24
positron emission tomography (PET) 45
post-void residual urine (PVR)
  in infants 55, 68
  measurement 46–7, 52, 71
potty-training 69
pouchitis 254
prazosin 105, *106*
pregnancy, autonomic dysreflexia 168–9
progressive supranuclear palsy (PSP) 98
propantheline 138
propiverine 139
prostate, bacterial infection of 318
pudendal nerve lesions 99
pudendal nerve terminal motor latency (PNTML)
  measurement 95–6
pudendal somatosensory evoked potentials (SEPs) *93*, 95
pyelonephritis 319
pyuria 317

quality of life after urinary diversion 255
quality of life in SCI 7–13
  family influences 8
  measurement 8–9

  need for specific questionnaire 9, 12–13
  questionnaire development/validation 9–10
  Qualiveen questionnaire findings 10–12
  Swedish study 7–8

reflex incontinence 267
reflex volume 199
renal damage, risk factors *326*
renal infection 319
renal scintigraphy 328
renal stones 320
renal surveillance 106
renography 47
residual urine *see* post-void residual urine
resiniferatoxin (RTX)
  intravesical use
    clinical experience 152, *153*, *154*, 290
    procedure 154–5
    safety 152
  molecular structure *149*
rosebud stoma *245*

S2-S4 deafferentation 204
sacral agenesis 43
sacral anterior root stimulation (SARS) *see* electrical
  stimulation, for bladder emptying
sacral motor system neurophysiology *see* electrophysiological
  evaluation: sacral motor system
sacral plexus lesions, electrophysiological assessment 99
sacral posterior and anterior root stimulator implant (SPARSI)
  273, *274*
sacral reflex arc *83*, 86
sacral reflex testing 93–5
sacral sensory system neurophysiology *see* electrophysiological
  evaluation: sacral sensory system
St Mark's electrodes 96
Salle bladder neck reconstruction 225, 226, *228*, 229, 302–3
Schwann cells 280
SCI *see* spinal cord injury (SCI)
scintigraphy, renal 328
sedation of children 70
sensory innervation of the LUT 86
seromuscular enterocystoplasty, in children 300–1
sexual function, effect of urinary tract reconstruction 255
sexual history 4–5
Short-Form 36-item questionnaire (SF-36) 8
Shy–Drager syndrome 44
sildenafil 168
single fiber electromyography (SFEMG) 92
single-photon emission computed tomography
  (SPECT) 45
small intestinal submucosa, in bladder
  augmentation 261
SPARSI (sacral posterior and anterior root
  stimulator implant) 273, *274*
sphincteric stenting techniques 231–2
  complications 235, *236*, 237
  indications and patient selection 232
  results 235, *236*
  surgical procedures 233, 235
sphincterotomy 231, 292
  complications 233, *234*
  indications and patient selection 232, 332
  results 233, *234*, 332
  surgical procedures 232–3
sphincters, artificial *see* artificial urinary sphincters

spinal cord injury (SCI)
  autonomic dysreflexia *see* autonomic dysreflexia (AD)
  causes 7
  causes of death 7
  cell death pathways 279–80
  cell transplantation strategies 280–1, 281–2
  electrophysiological assessment 98–9
  incidence of renal stones 327
  neuroprotective strategies 279–80, 281
  patient quality of life 7
    see also quality of life in SCI
  reflux and renal failure 326–7
  renal surveillance 106
  spinal shock and the bladder 329
spinal shock 329
staghorn calculi 320, 322
stem cells
  in tissue engineering 263
  transplantation in SCI 281
stents *see* urethral stents
stomas
  complications 252
  site selection 243, *245*
  see also urinary diversion
stones *see* lithiasis
stress urinary incontinence
  classification 44, 118–19
  electrical stimulation treatment 174–5
  evaluation 4
  management 310, *311*
  see also bulking agents, urethral
striated muscles 171
strictures
  ureterointestinal anastomosis complication 252
  urethral 36
struvite stones 320–1
Subjective Quality of Life Profile (SQLP) 9
suprapubic catheterization 132
surgery
  antireflux 332
  autoaugmentation *see* autoaugmentation
  bladder augmentation 204, 290–1, 299–301, 332
  bladder denervation 331
  bladder neck closure 229–31
  bladder neck reconstruction *see* bladder neck reconstruction
  bladder neck slings *see* bladder neck slings
  bowel preparation for 243
  clam cystoplasty 204
  for DESD 231–7
  for detrusor hyperreflexia 199, 290–1
    see also specific techniques
  electrical stimulation 179, 184, 190
  incompetent bladder outlet 207–31
  intestinal anastomoses 244
  nephrectomy 329, 332
  S2–S4 deafferentation 204
  sphincteric stenting *see* sphincteric stenting techniques
  sphincterotomy *see* sphincterotomy
  transurethral balloon dilation 235, 292
  ureterointestinal anastomoses 244–5, 252
  urethral lengthening procedures 301–3
  urethral obstruction 292–3
  urethral replacement 294
  urethral stents *see* urethral stents

urethropexy 293
urinary diversion *see* urinary diversion
  see also artificial urinary sphincters; *specific conditions*

tachykinin antagonists 144
Teflon injections 207
terazosin 142, 168
tethered cord syndrome 45
tissue engineering 144, 259–64
  background 259
  biomaterials 259
  bladder 260–1
  cell culture 259
  gene therapy delivery 263
  genetically engineered cells 262–3
  injectable therapies 261–2
  therapeutic cloning for 263–4
  urethra 259–60
  using stem cells 263
tolterodine 138–9
transcutaneous electrical nerve stimulation (TENS) 126
transdermal drug delivery systems 162, 289
  see also oxybutynin: transdermal administration
transurethral balloon dilation 235, 292
transurethral bladder stimulation 126, 288
transurethral catheterization 132
tricyclic antidepressants 140
triggered reflex voiding 126–7
trospium 139–40
TRPV1 (vanilloid) receptor 149–50
tumors
  bladder 39, *40*, 322–3
  urethral 39, *40*

Ultraflex urethral stent 231, 233
ultrasonography
  bladder 58
  PVR measurement 46–7
  renal 58, 106
  upper urinary tract 47, 327–8
upper urinary tract damage
  diagnosis
    cystography 328
    cystoscopy 328
    intravenous urography 328
    laboratory tests 327
    renal scintigraphy 328
    ultrasonography 47, 327–8
    videourodynamics 327
  etiology 326–7
  pathophysiology 325–6
  risk factors for kidney damage, summarized *326*
urapidil 140
urease 317, 320
ureteral stones 321
ureteroceles *39*
ureterocystoplasty, in children 299–300
ureterointestinal anastomoses 244–5, 252
urethra
  obstruction vs. occlusion 106, 291
  replacement 294
  tissue engineering 259–60
  treatment of obstructions 291–3
  treatment to increase resistance 293–4, 301–4
  see also vesicourethral balance

urethral stents 231–2, 292, 330
   see also sphincteric stenting techniques
urethral stones 322
urethral tumors 39, *40*
urethritis 318
urethrocystoscopy *see* endoscopy
urethropexy 293
urge incontinence 4, 45
Urilos system 30
urinary bladder *see* bladder
urinary diaries 16
urinary diversion 241–55
   choice of procedure 242–3
   complications *253*
      metabolic 252–4
      neuromechanical 254–5
      surgical 252
   continent, background 247
   continent bladder stoma 248–9
      hemi-Kock augmentation cystoplasty 251, *252*
      Mitrofanoff procedure 249, *250*, 251
   continent supravesical reservoirs
      continence mechanisms 247–8
      Indiana pouch 248, *249*
      Kock pouch 248, *250*
   indications 241, *242*
   noncontinent
      colon conduits 246
      ileal conduits 245–6
      ileal vesicostomy 246–7
   patients who may benefit 241
   preoperative preparation 243
      antibiotic coverage 243–4
      bowel preparation 243
   quality of life 255
   surgical management of patients *242*
   surgical principles
      intestinal anastomoses 244
      stoma 243, 245
      ureterointestinal anastomoses 244–5
urinary incontinence
   definitions 29
   overflow 4
   reflex 267
   stress *see* stress urinary incontinence
   urge 4, 45
urinary retention in women, electrophysiological
   evaluation 99
urinary sphincters, artificial *see* artificial urinary sphincters
urinary tract infections (UTI)
   after urinary diversion 254
   artificial sphincter 220
   asymptomatic 319
   bacteria involved 317
   catheter care 319
   clean intermittent catheterization 129–31, 330
   defined 317
   lower tract complications 318–19
   risk factors 318
   upper tract complications 319
   urine collection for culture 317
urodynamics
   evaluation components 59
      cystometry 59–63
      electromyography 64
      leak point pressures 61–3, 72
      videourodynamics *see* videourodynamics

      voiding pressure–flow studies 63–4
   goals of testing 59
   noninvasive studies 58
   patient assessment before testing 58
   questions to be answered 287–8
urodynamics in children 51–5, 67–80
   age and 70
   care of the child 51, 69–70
   clinical history 51
   common patterns in neurogenic bladder 78–80
   cystometry
      FAQs 71–3
      natural fill 73–4
      videocystometry 73
   historical perspective 67
   indications for 54, 69
   normal variables 54, *55*
      bladder capacity 54, *55*, 74–5
      bladder compliance 54, 76–7
      bladder evacuation 55, 77
      detrusor contractility 54–5, 75–6
      LUT sensation 77
      voiding pressures 54–5, 75–6
   pad test 71
   pelvic electromyography 71
   post-void residual urine 71
   sedation 70
   sphincter contractility 76
   uroflowmetry 70–1
      advantages/disadvantages *51*
      electromyography-coupled 53–4
      indications for 51–2
      interpretation 52–3
      normal parameters *52*
      residual volume determination 52
uroflowmetry 58
   see also urodynamics in children: uroflowmetry
Urolome prosthesis 231, 232, 233, 235

Valsava leak point pressure 62–3
Valsava maneuver 127
vanilloid receptor 1 (VR1) 149–50
vanilloids
   intravesical use
      patient factors 152, 154
      procedures 154–5
      rationale 150
      safety 152
   mechanism of action 290
   molecular structures *149*
vascular endothelial growth factor (VEGF) 262
vesicoureteral reflux
   assessment 58, *63*, 64
   pathophysiology in SCI patients 325–6
   see also antireflux surgery; upper urinary tract
      damage
vesicourethral balance
   altered
      clinical situations 310–13
      summarized *310*
   normal 309–10
videocystometry 73
videourodynamics 46, 64, 73, 327
voiding diaries 15–27
   classification
      Abrams–Klevmark 15–16
      International Continence Society 16

completion by the patient 20
computer data analysis 17
duration 19–20
frequency–volume charts as diagnostic
  tools 20–1
interpretation
  effect of neuromodulation 24, 26, *27*
  nocturnal polyuria 22, *23, 24*
  normal 21–2
  polyuria 22, *23, 24*
  sensory urgency 22, 24, *25*
normal values 17–18
  children 18

females 18–19
  males 19
rationale for use 16–17
reliability 20
voiding reflexes in infants 68

Wallace ureterointestinal anastomosis *245*
women *see* females

X-rays, lumbrosacral spine 43

Young–Dees–Leadbetter bladder neck
  reconstruction 223–4, 226, *228*

9780367393434

T - #0037 - 311024 - C0 - 276/219/20 - PB - 9780367393434 - Gloss Lamination